D0140366

CONTEMPORARY WOMEN'S HEALTH
Issues for Today and the Future

FIFTH EDITION

Cheryl A. Kolander, HSD
Department of Health and Sport Science
University of Louisville

Danny Ramsey Ballard, EdD, FAAHE
Department of Health and Kinesiology
Texas A&M University

Cynthia K. Chandler, EdD, LPC, LMFT
Department of Counseling and Higher Education
University of North Texas

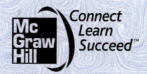

Connect
Learn
Succeed™

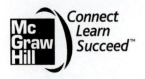

The McGraw-Hill Companies

CONTEMPORARY WOMEN'S HEALTH: ISSUES FOR TODAY AND THE FUTURE, FIFTH EDITION

Published by McGraw-Hill, a business unit of The McGraw-Hill Companies, Inc., 1221 Avenue of the Americas, New York, NY 10020. Copyright © 2014 by The McGraw-Hill Companies, Inc. All rights reserved. Previous editions © 2009, 2006, and 2003. Printed in the United States of America. No part of this publication may be reproduced or distributed in any form or by any means, or stored in a database or retrieval system, without the prior written consent of The McGraw-Hill Companies, Inc., including, but not limited to, in any network or other electronic storage or transmission, or broadcast for distance learning.

This book is printed on acid-free paper.

4 5 6 7 8 9 0 LKV 21 20

ISBN: 978–0–07–8028540
MHID: 0–07–802854X

Senior Vice President, Products & Markets: *Kurt L. Strand*
Vice President, General Manager, Products & Markets: *Michael Ryan*
Vice President, Content Production & Technology Services: *Kimberly Meriwether David*
Executive Director of Development: *Lisa Pinto*
Managing Director: *Gina Boedeker*
Senior Brand Manager: *Bill Minick*
Development Editor: *Sara Jaeger*
Marketing Specialist: *Alexandra Schultz*
Director, Content Production: *Terri Scheisl*
Senior Project Manager: *Joyce Watters*
Buyer: *Susan K. Culbertson*
Media Project Manager: *Sridevi Palani*
Cover Designer: *Studio Montage, St. Louis, MO.*
Cover Images: *© Jose Luis Pelaez Inc./Blend Images LLC (top left); © Terry Vine/Blend Images LLC (top right); © Daniel Koebe/Corbis (bottom left); Pixtal/AGE Fotostock (bottom right)*
Typeface: *9/12 Stone Serif*
Compositor: *S4Carlisle Publishing Services*
Printer: *LSC Communications*

Credits: A credits section for this book begins on page 459 and is considered an extension of the copyright page.

Library of Congress Cataloging-in-Publication Data

Kolander, Cheryl A.
Contemporary women's health/Cheryl A. Kolander. — Fifth edition.
    pages cm
    Includes bibliographical references and index.

    ISBN-13: 978–0–07–802854–0—ISBN-10: 0–07–802854–X   1. Women—Health
and hygiene. I. Title.

RA778.K7245 2014
613'.04244—dc23   2012036860

www.mhhe.com

Dedication

◇ *With gratitude and love to my parents and family for the joy and happiness they bring to my life; to my friends for the fun, adventure, and camaraderie we share; and to the students, whose intellectual curiosity and creativity remind me daily that life as a professor is the best job in the world.* —CAK

◇ *To the fabulous women, both family and friends, who have inspired, guided, loved, listened, supported and brought joy, laughter and meaning to my life! Each of you has made life more meaningful and fulfilling. Thank you with all my heart— I appreciate and love you dearly: Fay, Ruby, Marcelle, Rita, AnnaBelle, Suzanne, Betty, Barbara, Josey, Kristy, Cheryl, Carolyn, Katy, Sue, Jan, Sherry, DeAun, Jill, Beverly, Janene, Kathy, Pat, Nita, Ruth, Aleen, Altha, Judy, Shirley, Carol, Tedi, Frances, Lillian, Priscilla, Diane, Ellen, Linda, Ebbie, Monica, Mary Jane, Katherine, and Christine. . . . and to my wonderful former students!* —DRB

◇ *To my loving and supportive family, my mother and father Billie and Orbie Chandler; my sisters Betty Bush and Bonnie Thomas and brother-in-law Sam Thomas; my brother Charlie Chandler and sister-in-law Vicki Chandler; my nieces Rachel Thomas Little (and husband Tommy), Terra Chandler, and Niki Chandler; and my nephews, Lonnie Bush (and wife Heather), Brandon Bush (and wife Shasta), and Rowdy Bush (and wife Jessica); and Jason Thomas.* —CKC

Brief Contents

Contents

Part Two

MENTAL AND EMOTIONAL WELLNESS 87

Part Three
SEXUAL AND RELATIONAL WELLNESS   154

Part Four

CONTEMPORARY LIFESTYLE AND SOCIAL ISSUES 268

Part Five

COMMUNICABLE AND CHRONIC CONDITIONS   363

CHAPTER FOURTEEN • Preventing and Controlling Infectious Diseases   364

CHAPTER FIFTEEN • Preventing and Controlling Chronic Health Conditions   391

List of Boxes

Health Tips

Her Story

Journal Activity

Viewpoint

Women Making a Difference

Preface

The landscape of women's health has changed dramatically since the first edition of this textbook, nearly 15 years ago. We now have specialized clinics focusing exclusively on women's health and hospitals with entire units dedicated to women. A plethora of goods and services are designed specifically for women's health, and books, journals, and professional conferences are devoted solely to women's health issues. At the time of this writing, the Affordable Health Care Act has been enacted and upheld by the U.S. Supreme Court. Obama Care, as some may call it, has significant positive implications for women's health. For instance, for the first time in the history of the United States, all women and children will be covered by some level of health care. Well-women care, including contraception, domestic violence screening, and breast feeding equipment, will be covered. At the same time, we are experiencing persistent efforts to dismantle *Roe v Wade* and women's reproductive rights, while the number of unintended pregnancies continues to rise. This textbook, in its fifth edition, has been written for women, by women, who have devoted much of their academic careers in the endeavor to promote and enhance the health of all women. Being wise consumers of health care and health care products and advocates for women's reproductive rights is essential for women of all ages. *Contemporary Women's Health* attempts to review and synthesize women's health information and research findings in a manner that appeals to women and the men who want a better understanding of women's health issues.

APPROACH

In the fifth edition of *Contemporary Women's Health* we continue to emphasize health promotion and the impact of multicultural and diversity issues on women's health. Although we focus on "women-only" topics, we believe that both women and men can benefit from discussions of women's issues in the context of societal concerns, and our experiences in diverse classrooms have supported this belief. In the fifth edition we keep the applied approach of the previous editions, with a format that encourages students to examine their health-related preconceptions, attitudes, and behaviors and to explore new ways of thinking critically about the health issues that impact their lives. We believe the classroom can and should be a dynamic environment for empowering and strengthening women's positive health behavior, and our text is designed to support that goal.

Contemporary Women's Health may be used by instructors and students in health education, general education, medical education, and women's studies courses that emphasize a holistic approach to health. The text is written from a woman-centered perspective and is appropriate for both nontraditional and traditional students. The personal pronouns used throughout the text assume a female reader; we have found that men as well as women understand and appreciate this convention.

ORGANIZATION

Contemporary Women's Health is organized into five distinct parts. Part One, "Foundations of Women's Health," emphasizes the scope of women's health issues and introduces students to wellness and prevention concepts, as well as methods for facilitating life-long changes in health behaviors. Chapters devoted to making wise consumer choices are also included in this section. Part Two, "Mental and Emotional Wellness," focuses on strategies for enhancing emotional well-being and managing stress. Part Three, "Relational and Sexual Wellness," addresses building and maintaining healthy relationships, violence against women, and gynecological health and designing a reproductive life plan. Part Four, "Contemporary Lifestyle and Social Issues," offers comprehensive information about nutrition, exercise, and the deleterious effects of tobacco, alcohol, and other drugs. Part Five, "Communicable and Chronic Conditions," includes information about sexually transmitted infections, communicable diseases, cardiovascular health, cancer and other chronic diseases.

FEATURES AND UPDATES

The fifth edition of *Contemporary Women's Health* retains a variety of boxed features that support the text's approach and extend its coverage.

- *Assess Yourself* boxes provide interactive exercises and inventories to help students determine their own level of wellness and need for behavior change. Assessments include an inventory for improving your chances for accurate test results, a stress checklist, and a quiz to determine what you know about the foods you eat, among many others.
- *FYI* boxes succinctly highlight key information. They cover such topics as the inequities in wages between women and men, types of eating disorders, tips for reading food labels, yoga, and more.
- *Health Tips* boxes provide practical, helpful recommendations intended to enhance each student's personal health journey. These boxes cover a broad range of topics, such as questions to ask when taking prescription medicines, calculating fat intake, and tips for successful smoking cessation.
- *Her Story* boxes are based on real-life women confronting such challenges as postpartum depression, negative self-image, and alcoholism. In some instances, the names of the women whose lives are being discussed have been changed to protect their identity, but in other cases real names are used. Each box concludes with follow-up questions that allow students to apply the chapter content to the situation being discussed.
- *Journal Activity* boxes provide opportunities for students to record their thoughts and feelings about their health as well as the social issues affecting the health of all women. These boxes present questions for students to consider, such as "How do you handle stress?" and "Do you know someone in an abusive relationship?" They also give students tips on activities like managing time and browsing the Internet for AIDS research.
- *Viewpoint* boxes highlight controversial issues and ask students to reflect on and form their own opinions about those issues. Topics addressed by these boxes include state laws that discriminate against homosexuality, women's health versus giant pharmaceutical companies, and surrogate grandmothers.
- *Women Making a Difference* boxes feature real-life women who have faced and overcome challenges in their lives and have assumed leadership roles. Included in these boxes are such women as Maggie Kuhn.

The fifth edition has been thoroughly updated with the most current health information and statistical data available. Key content updates and additions to each chapter are listed below.

CHAPTER 1: INTRODUCING WOMEN'S HEALTH
- Updated all statistics and research related to introductory material on women's health including gender discrimination and sexual harassment
- Added more life stories of women from diverse backgrounds
- Updated reference list
- Updated list of web sites and addresses

CHAPTER 2: BECOMING A WISE CONSUMER
- Updated all statistics and research on becoming a wise consumer including information on the new health care program initiated by President Obama
- Updated reference list
- Updated list of web sites and addresses

CHAPTER 3: DEVELOPING A HEALTHY LIFESTYLE
- Updated all statistics regarding life span and causes of death of women of the world
- Updated reference list
- Updated list of web sites and addresses

CHAPTER 4: MENTAL AND EMOTIONAL WELLNESS
- Updated all statistics and research regarding emotional health including prevalence rates and the most prescribed medications for emotional disorders
- Updated statistics on suicide rates of women by ethnic origin
- Updated reference list
- Updated list of web sites and addresses

CHAPTER 5: MANAGING THE STRESS OF LIFE
- Updated all statistics and research on stress and health including prevalence rates for stress/anxiety disorders and most prescribed medications
- Updated reference list
- Updated list of web sites and addresses

CHAPTER 6: SEXUAL AND RELATIONAL WELLNESS
- Updated all statistics and research on healthy relationships
- Updated reference list
- Updated list of web sites and addresses

CHAPTER 7: PREVENTING ABUSE AGAINST WOMEN
- Changed the order of chapters in Part Three (Sexual and Relational Wellness) for better and more meaningful content flow.
- Updated all statistics related to intimate partner violence, sexual assault, murder and child abuse

- Rewrote the Cycle of Violence for better clarity and extension of thoughts and actions for both the victim and the perpetrator.
- Reduced the number of boxes throughout the chapter
- Added section regarding the economic impact of Intimate Partner Violence
- Updated reference list
- Updated list of web sites and addresses

CHAPTER 8: EXPLORING WOMEN'S SEXUALITY

- Updated ACS guidelines for breast cancer screening
- Updated ACS guidelines for cervical cancer screening
- Updated data on hysterectomies
- Revised viewpoint on hormone replacement therapy
- Revised discussion of natural or alternative therapies
- New section on biological bases of human sexuality
- New section on psychosocial bases of human sexuality
- New section on female sexual response
- Updated section on sexual dysfunction
- Updated all references, web sites, and contact information

CHAPTER 9: DESIGNING YOUR REPRODUCTIVE PLAN

- Updated statistics on teen pregnancy
- Revised viewpoint on sexuality education
- Updated table on birth control methods and costs
- Updated information on emergency contraception
- Updated figures on current contraceptives
- Updated information on births to unmarried women
- Updated information on unplanned pregnancies
- Updated information on cesarean deliveries
- Updated information on multiple births
- Updated all references, web sites, and contact information

CHAPTER 10: EATING WELL

- Replaced the Food Guide Pyramid with MyPlate
- Replaced all Dietary Guidelines 2005 information with Dietary Guidelines for Americans 2010
- Increased focus on obesity prevention
- Revised *FYI* on reducing the overall calorie intake and increasing physical activity
- New *FYI* on changes in food availability since 1970
- New section on foods and food products to reduce
- New section on foods and nutrients to increase
- New *FYI* on dietary guidelines for Americans 2010

- Revised dietary guideline recommendations for pregnancy
- Revised organic food information
- Revised food safety information
- Updated all references, web sites, and contact information

CHAPTER 11: KEEPING FIT

- Added a new *Access Yourself: Could You Be a Compulsive Exerciser?*
- Added information on women and obesity
- Added *FYI: How Much Exercise Do Adults Need?*
- Updated information on *Principles of Conditioning*
- Updated Table 11.3, *Fitness Assessments*
- Updated section on *Managing Weight Through Exercise*
- Updated information on *Exercising During the Later Years*
- Updated reference list
- Updated list of web sites and addresses

CHAPTER 12: USING ALCOHOL RESPONSIBLY

- Eliminated information on *Alcohol: The Beverage*
- Reduced number of tables to enhance flow of narrative
- Updated information on *College-Age Women and Alcohol*
- Added section on *Alcohol and Ethnicity*
- Updated *FYI: Annual Alcohol-Related Consequences for College Students*
- Updated and rewrote section on *Alcohol and Pregnancy*
- Updated statistics related to women and alcohol use/abuse
- Updated web sites and addresses
- Updated reference list

CHAPTER 13: MAKING WISE DECISIONS ABOUT TOBACCO, CAFFEINE AND DRUGS

- Updated all statistics related to tobacco, caffeine, and drugs
- Updated reference list
- Updated web sites and addresses
- Updated information section *Substances in Tobacco*
- Included information on harm to pets exposed to tobacco smoke
- Added table on new information regarding *Nicotine Replacement Products*
- Added new introduction and information regarding *Caffeine*
- Added information about energy drinks to Table 13.2 *Comparision of Caffeine in Common Products*

CHAPTER 14: PREVENTING AND CONTROLLING
INFECTIOUS DISEASES

- Updated data on chlamydia
- Updated data on gonorrhea
- Updated data on syphilis
- Updated information on HPV vaccine
- Updated data on HPV infections
- Updated figure on HIV/AIDS diagnoses by race/ethnicity
- Updated epidemiology for hepatitis A, B and C
- Updated epidemiology on tuberculosis
- Updated data on Lyme disease
- Updated all references, web sites, and contact information

CHAPTER 15: PREVENTING AND CONTROLLING
CHRONIC HEALTH CONDITIONS

- Updated all statistics related to chronic diseases
- New guidelines from American Heart Association for age-standardized prevalence of heart disease
- Updated atrial fibrillation information
- Updated endocarditis information
- Updated high blood pressure information
- Revised table on healthy levels of cholesterol
- Updated information on stroke
- Revised warning symptoms of stroke
- Revised table on bone mineral density
- Updated all references, web sites, and contact information

CHAPTER 16: REDUCING YOUR RISK OF CANCER

- Updated Table 16.1: *Leading Sites of New Cancer Cases and Death in Women* with the most current statistics
- Update information on hormone replacement therapy (HRT) and cancer
- Rearranged sections of chapter for better content flow
- Updated information regarding types of cancers and treatment of cancer
- Update on colon cancer screening requirements
- Updated information on types of *Complementary and Alternative Treatment in Cancer Management*
- Updated reference list
- Updated web sites and addresses

PEDAGOGY AND LEARNING AIDS

To maximize its usefulness to students and instructors, *Contemporary Women's Health* provides these learning aids in every chapter:

- *Chapter Objectives* provide students with a succinct overview of the material in the chapter and may be used as a self-check prior to quizzes and exams.

- *Chapter Summaries* reinforce chapter content.
- *Review Questions* help students apply the concepts learned in the chapter and may be used by students to study for exams.
- *Resources* sections list a variety of information sources related to chapter content, including national organizations and hotlines, Web sites, books and articles, and videotapes and audiotapes.
- *References* list the research citations included in the chapter, giving students the opportunity to access key supporting information.

SUPPLEMENTS

The fifth edition of *Contemporary Women's Health* features an Instructor's Web site (www.mhhe.com/ kolander5e) that offers a variety of resources, including an Instructor's Manual and PowerPoint lecture slides. Additional information is available from your McGraw-Hill sales representative.

The fifth edition of *Contemporary Women's* Health is available as an eTextbook at www.CourseSmart.com. CourseSmart is a new way to find and buy eTextbooks. At CourseSmart you can save up to 50% off the cost of a print textbook, reduce your impact on the environment, and gain access to powerful web tools for learning. CourseSmart has the largest selection of eTextbooks available anywhere, offering thousands of the most commonly adopted textbooks from a wide variety of higher education publishers. CourseSmart eTextbooks are available in one standard online reader with full text search, notes and highlighting, and email tools for sharing notes between classmates. For further details contact your sales representative or go to www.coursesmart.com.

ACKNOWLEDGMENTS

We would like to thank the reviewers of all five editions for their excellent comments and suggestions. Our text has benefited significantly from their input.

M. Basti
Cuesta Community College

Linda Bernhard
The Ohio State University

Rebecca Brey
Ball State University

Ni Bueno
Cerritos College

Linda C. Campanelli
American University

Vivian Chavez
San Francisco State University

Joanne Chopak-Foss
Georgia Southern University

Maggie Chrismon
The University of North Carolina at Greensboro

Susanne Christopher
Portland Community College

Susan Craddock
University of Minnesota

Sandra K. Cross
University of North Carolina at Pembroke

Rebecca Crow
The University of Texas at Arlington

Becky Damazo
California State University, Chico

Jennifer Dearden
Morehead State University

Andrea DeMaria
University of Texas Medical Branch at Galveston

Rosalie DiBrezzo
University of Arkansas

Karen Elliott
Oregon State University

Gloria C. Essoka
Hunter College

Eileen R. Fowles
Illinois Wesleyan University

Emogene Fox
University of Central Arkansas

June M. Goemer
St. Cloud State University

Shelley Hamill
Winthrop University

Tammy C. James
West Chester University

Donna G. Knauth
Georgetown University

Becky K. Koch
The Ohio State University

Raeann Koerner
Ventura College

Richard C. Krejci
Columbia College (Columbia, SC)

Melissa Raschel Larsen
Chemeketa Community College

Susan Cross Lipnickey
Miami University (Oxford, OH)

Susan Ann Lyman
University of Louisiana at Lafayette

Margie Maddox
University of Scranton

Deborah A. Miller
College of Charleston

Sue Moore
University of Central Oklahoma

M. Christine Nagy
Western Kentucky University

Willena Pearson
Indiana University-Bloomington

Margaret V. Pepe
Kent State University

Vibeke Rutzon Peterson
Drake University

Laurie Pilotto
Formerly of Hawkins County Health Department

Michelle Salisbury
Vanderbilt University

Ellen D. Schulken
University of Maryland

Felicia Taylor
University of Central Arkansas

Lori Turner
University of Arkansas

Barbara A. Tyree
Valparaiso University

Deborah VanBuren
Dutchess Community College

Jean Worfolk
Fitchburg State College

Diane Kholos Wysocki
University of Nebraska at Kearney

Jenny K. Yi
University of Houston

We appreciate the care and attention to detail provided by the knowledgeable and experienced editorial, marketing, and production teams at McGraw-Hill. Special thanks to Wendy Langerud for her unwavering encouragement, supportive responses to numerous e-mails, kind reminders, and expertise as this edition was being completed. We have also had the pleasure of working with some incredible women in the past editions, and for that we are greatly thankful to McGraw-Hill.

Special appreciation to the women who provided more in-depth support during the previous edition: Kristina Dunham for her research support, Barb Mercer and Carol O'Neal for their expertise in nutrition, Cynthia Saffell for her expertise in chronic disease control, and Donna Julian for her health expertise.

We want to recognize the many women and students who touched our lives with their personal stories. Thank you for sharing your stories and providing further insight, encouragement, and support. Your personal stories and insightful comments have enriched our lives and the lives of others, and we hope that the content of this text-book reflects that information sharing. We know that the contributions of women and students have and will continue to make a difference in the lives of others.

About the Author

Cheryl A. Kolander

Cheryl Kolander is the associate dean for Academic Affairs in the College of Education and Human Development, University of Louisville. She is a professor in the Department of Health and Sport Sciences and previously served as a program director for health education. She received her baccalaureate degree from Luther College, Decorah, Iowa, and her master's and doctoral degrees from Indiana University, Bloomington. She is an advocate for social justice and equity, and has a particular interest in advancing health equity for women. Her primary research focus is prevention science, with an emphasis on women's health, school health education, and accreditation. She directs the Center for Health Promotion and Prevention Science Research, a center for collaborative studies and advocacy related to prevention science. She is a member of the performance team for U of L collegiate athletics, serves on the advisory board for Get Healthy Now, and chairs the curriculum committee for Fit4Me, an after-school program for at-risk girls.

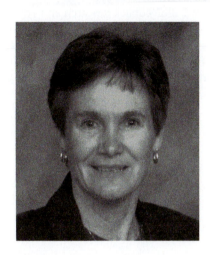

Danny Ramsey Ballard

Danny Ramsey Ballard is Professor Emerita in the Department of Health and Kinesiology at Texas A&M University, where she was former Associate Department Head and Chair of the Health Education Division and the holder of the Ponder Endowed Chair. Dr. Ballard taught graduate and undergraduate courses on women's health as well as a multitude of other health-related courses. In addition to co-authorship of *Contemporary Women's Health: Issues for Today and the Future,* she also was co-author of an elementary textbook series entitled *Health.* She has published multiple research papers, technical papers, book chapters, and other professional materials; and has made more than 230 national, regional, and state presentations. She has been the co-principal investigator and consultant of over $1.7 million in funded projects. Dr. Ballard is past president of the American Alliance for Health, Physical Education, Recreation and Dance (AAHPERD) and Southern District AAHPERD. She is a Fellow in the American Association for Health Education (AAHE) and American School Health Association. She was named Outstanding Health Educator of the Year at the national, district, and state levels for AAHE. She received the Honor Award for the AAHPERD national professional association and the Emma Gibbons Legacy Award from the Texas A&M Department of Health and Kinesiology.

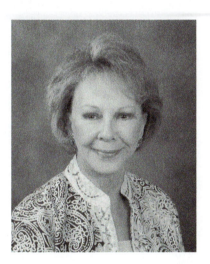

Cynthia K. Chandler

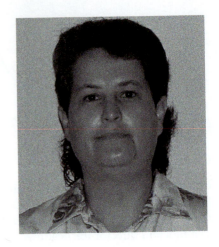

Cynthia K. Chandler, a professor of counseling at the University of North Texas, received her doctoral degree in educational psychology from Texas Tech University in 1986 and has served on the graduate faculty at UNT since 1989. Every year, Dr. Chandler teaches counseling graduate courses, organizes and leads a variety of institutes and workshops, and supervises an abundance of counseling interns. She is the founder and director of the UNT Biofeedback Research and Training Laboratory and the UNT Center for Animal Assisted Therapy. Dr. Chandler is a Licensed Professional Counselor, a Licensed Marriage and Family Therapist, a nationally certified Biofeedback Therapist, and an Animal Assisted Therapist. The coauthor of four books and numerous journal articles, she has given professional presentations in the United States, Korea, Austria, Greece, Hong Kong, and Canada.

FOUNDATIONS OF WOMEN'S HEALTH

Part One

Chapter One

Introducing Women's Health

CHAPTER OBJECTIVES

When you complete this chapter, you will be able to do the following:

◇ Discuss the relevance of having a text dedicated to women's health concerns

◇ Describe three common types of health action

◇ Explain the significance of cultural and international diversity and women's health

◇ Cite important events in the history of the women's social movement and in the history of women's health

◇ Identify sexual discrimination in diverse settings and situations

WHY FOCUS ON WOMEN'S HEALTH?

Why do we need a text on women's health? An obvious reason is that women and men are different. In addition, many general health texts tend to relay information from studies based primarily on the male standard. A text geared specifically to women's health concerns will help to ensure that women's health issues are fairly represented.

By dedicating an entire text to women's health, we have an opportunity to provide a comprehensive presentation of the vast number of issues and concerns that affect women. Many health texts focus only on physiological conditions, whereas this text incorporates the mental, emotional, and spiritual health dimensions as well.

A text dedicated to women's health sends a message to the public that women are important. Too often, issues regarding the welfare of women are completely ignored, and when they are given consideration, it is often as an afterthought. Through long and difficult struggles women have made some progress toward being given equal consideration by the larger society, yet significant discrimination toward women still exists.

A text dedicated to women's health is not meant to subjugate the importance of men's health concerns. It is meant to serve as a forum through which a presentation of issues regarding women's health can be understood and viewed as important and significant in and of themselves. Many aspects of women's health are different from those of men and need to be given ample consideration. Through a text specific to women's issues, information regarding women's status can be shared, examined, and addressed.

Education is the keystone to progress. Education about women is the door through which women can be empowered. The performance of research studies regarding women must be emphasized. Information about the status of women must be made public, and the public must pressure politicians to make women's issues a priority. The health of the world, a country, a city, or a community rests on the health and well-being of its women and children as well as its men.

EMPHASIS ON HEALTH PROMOTION

Why is the concept of **health promotion** so important to the women's health field? The concept of health promotion is not limited to the idea that health is a condition we lose from time to time and try to gain back. Rather, health promotion includes the idea that health is something to be nurtured and by doing so we can prevent the onset of much illness and disease. Three common types of health action are proactive care, health care maintenance, and reactive care. **Proactive care** involves designing and living a lifestyle that reduces the risks of illness and also improves one's current health status. **Health care maintenance** is the continuation of what one is doing to maintain one's current health status. **Reactive care** is the treatment of any illness, disorder, or disease that may develop. The greatest emphasis in health promotion is placed on proactive care.

Proactive health care serves to reduce health care costs by preventing the onset of many illnesses, disorders, and diseases, thereby avoiding the great expense involved in their treatment. Proactive health care is a holistic lifestyle model as opposed to a medical model. The traditional medical model is primarily reactive and attends to the individual's needs after an unhealthy condition has developed. Holistic health care considers the interaction of the mind, body, and spirit: One area cannot be affected without the other areas also being affected. Understanding this interactive process is vital in providing proactive care to yourself and to others. Holistic health care incorporates all that we know about health and utilizes this information to keep the body, mind, and spirit healthy. A proactive, holistic focus empowers women to have a strong voice in their own health care.

WOMEN'S HEALTH IN A GLOBAL SOCIETY

Our text is based primarily on studies of women in the United States of America; however, women around the globe share many of the same concerns. All over the world women are living in poverty, experiencing discrimination and violence, having limited access to birth control information and materials, lacking accessible child care services, developing diseases and disorders specific to women, suffering with low selfesteem and distorted body image, and facing serious gynecological health concerns.

Women in many countries experience significant suppression of their civil rights. They may have no right to vote, to dress as they please, or to divorce. Even the slightest hint of premarital sex or adultery can lead to their death by a family member; this is referred to as "honor killing." Some women and girls as young as 10 years old are sold by their parents into pornography or to be used as sex slaves. According to the World Health Organization (WHO), more than 130 million girls worldwide are at risk of being subjected to genital mutilation, which can cause lifelong pain and medical problems. Women worldwide are dying of HIV/AIDS and cannot afford proper medical treatment. Women in countries at war are gang-raped by troops occupying their territory or are forced into prostitution or pornography to survive.

(See *FYI*: "Rape as a Weapon of War"; *Viewpoint*: "Sex Trafficking in the United States"; *Viewpoint*: "Honor Killing; and *Viewpoint*: Outlawing Female Genital Mutilation").

FYI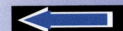

Rape as a Weapon of War

Amnesty International reported in 2004 that women's bodies have become part of the terrain of conflict—rape and sexual abuse are not just a by-products of war but are used as a deliberate military strategy.[1] Amnesty International cited as examples at the time of the report the ongoing conflicts in Colombia, Iraq, Sudan, Chechnya, Nepal, and Afghanistan. The use of rape as a weapon of war has many examples and goes back very far—for example, the systematic rape of women in Bosnia in the 1990s, the estimated 200,000 women raped by state-backed Pakistani troops during the battle for Bangladeshi independence in 1971, and the rapes by the Japanese of hundreds of thousands of women from 1928 to the end of World War II when women from China, Korea, Taiwan, the Philippines, Malaysia, and East Timor were severely coerced into military sexual slavery. "Rape is often used in ethnic conflicts as a way for attackers to perpetuate their social control and redraw ethnic boundaries. Women are seen as the reproducers and caregivers of the community. Therefore if one group wants to control another they often do it by impregnating women of the other community because they see it as a way of destroying the opposing community. And whether a woman is raped at gunpoint or trafficked into sexual slavery by an occupying force, the sexual abuse will shape not just her own but her community's future for years to come. Survivors face emotional torment, psychological damage, physical injuries, disease, social ostracism and many other consequences that can devastate their lives," reports Amnesty International.

On June 20, 2008, the United Nations Security Council unanimously approved a resolution classifying rape as a weapon of war.[2] While the vote was hailed by human rights groups as historic, do you think this action will significantly impact the use of rape as a weapon of war? If so, in what ways do you think it will have a significant impact? If not, why do you think it will not have a significant impact?

Viewpoint

Sex Trafficking in the United States[3]

The U.S. State Department estimates that between 600,000 and 800,000 people are trafficked for forced labor and sex worldwide each year—and that 80 percent are women and girls. Most trafficked females are exploited in commercial sex outlets. The U.S. State Department estimates that between 14,500 and 17,500 human trafficking victims are brought into the United States each year. Some advocacy groups claim this estimate is too low and place the number much higher; for instance the Coalition Against Trafficking Women places the estimate of victims brought into the United States annually at 50,000. The United States is among the top three destination countries for sex traffickers, along with Japan and Australia. It is difficult to enforce laws against sex traffickers because it is easy to cross borders and victims are kept locked up as slaves. Sex traffickers who get caught are rarely convicted. Would-be witnesses, the victims themselves, are afraid to testify because those who have testified have experienced violence and intimidation. Sex trafficking is a growing problem, with relatively little attention being paid to it. What type of social and legal action would make sex trafficking a higher priority for law enforcement officials and assist these officials in obtaining more convictions? How can communities make victims safer and help them to escape their slavery? What special health services will victims need to help their recovery from the psychological and physical trauma of slavery? A web source for combating human trafficking is www.humantrafficking.org.

Many issues are specific to the time, place, and culture in which women live. Countries may have differing policies and attitudes toward women. In addition, religious or family traditions of certain countries place a special emphasis on certain images and roles women are expected to fulfill. The level of economic and technological development, the threat of international terrorism, or the state of war versus peace in a country may also influence the status of women and their health. It is our special obligation to pay attention to world events regarding the health and well-being of women and of all persons in the world community.

Two important concepts to consider when studying issues and events that impact women's health are sexism and misogyny. **Sexism** is an attitude of bias or an act of discrimination against a person because of his or her gender that usually involves economic exploitation or social domination. The most common practice of sexism is by men toward women. One example of sexism

Viewpoint

Honor Killing

The United Nations Population Fund estimates that 5000 women are killed each year for dishonoring their families, though many think this is an underestimate. Victims of honor killings are largely teenage daughters or young women. "Families that kill for honor will threaten girls and women if they refuse to cover their hair or faces, or their bodies or act as a family's domestic servant; wear makeup or Western clothing; choose friends from another religion; refuse an arranged marriage; seek a divorce from a violent husband; marry against their parents' wishes; or behave in ways that are considered too independent, which might mean anything from driving a car to spending time or living away from home or family."[4] Honor killings are most prevalent in Middle East countries. However, Middle East immigrants to Western countries also perform honor killings. Such was the case for teenage sisters Amina (age 18) and Sarah Said (age 17), who were shot dead in Irving, Texas, in January 2008 by their Egyptian-born father, who said he was upset with his daughters for having Western boyfriends and living "Western ways." The girls, who were high school students in Lewisville, Texas, had fled their home after their father threatened them. In another case, three members of an immigrant Afghan family were found guilty of first-degree murder in January 2012 in what was thought to be Canada's first "honor killing" trial—in 2009, Mohammad Shafia (age 58), and his wife, Tooba Mohammad Yahya (age 42), along with son Hamed (age 21), drowned their three daughters (Zainab, Sahar, and Geeti, ages 19, 17, and 13) and Shafia's first wife, Rona Amir Mohammad (age 52), for "living a westernized lifestyle." The family had been living in Canada since 2007. Prior to this Canadian verdict in 2012, "honor killings" in the United States and Canada were categorized as "domestic violence;" but since the verdict, consideration is being given to recognizing this type of family violence as unique and classified as "honor killings." While domestic violence against women is committed by men all over the world, honor killing is committed mostly by men from Middle East cultures that are strongly patriarchal and consider women as the property of men. The governments and press of these cultures often look the other way or condone such acts of violence against women for the sake of family honor. For instance, in 2003 the Jordanian Parliament voted down a provision designed to stiffen penalties for honor killings; as a sad consequence of this, early in 2007, a Jordanian man who murdered his sister because he thought she had a lover was given a 3-month sentence, which was suspended for time served, allowing him to walk free. And in December of 2007, the *Yemen Times* published an article insisting that violence against women is necessary for the stability of the family and the society.[5] In your opinion, are honor killings simply a form of domestic violence, or are they more a cultural tradition?

Viewpoint

Outlawing Female Genital Mutilation (FGM) [6,7]

FGM in infants and young girls, also known as female circumcision and female genital cutting, is common in parts of Africa and, to a lesser extent, Asia and the Middle East. It is considered a religious ritual, rite of passage, a hygienic measure, a means for controlling sexuality and sexual promiscuity, and a prerequisite for marriage. FGM is problematic in that it can cause lifelong pain and health problems for women, and it greatly reduces the pleasure that normally can be obtained from genital stimulation. Immigrants have brought the practice of FGM to the United States. A law making FGM illegal in the United States was introduced by Congresswoman Patricia Schroeder and passed as part of President Clinton's 1996 immigration legislation. As of 2007, 17 U.S. states have passed similar statues. In November, 2006, an Ethiopian immigrant received a 10-year prison sentence for cutting off the clitoris of his 2-year-old daughter. This was hailed as the first conviction for FGM in the U.S. FGM is outlawed in other countries including: Australia (six states), Burkina Faso, Canada, Central African Republic, Djibouti, Ghana, New Zealand, Nigeria (3 states), Norway, Senegal, Sweden, Tanzania, Togo, and the United Kingdom. Since FGM is a cultural and religious practice, is it right to outlaw it? Given that FGM practice is outlawed in the United States, is it problematic that the first conviction for FGM practice occurred 11 years after the legislation to outlaw it passed? Why do you think so little attention has been paid to FGM practice in the United States even though it is illegal?

commonly practiced today is paying a woman less than a man for the same job. Another example is the practice of a financial lending institution, such as a bank, giving fewer loans to women because they are viewed as less capable than men of repaying the debt.

Misogyny is a hatred of women. An example of misogyny would be how the women of Afghanistan were treated in the two decades prior to the Taliban being overthrown in 2001. Women were required to wear burkas in public. These floor-length, dark veils cover every inch of a woman's body and have only a small mesh-covered opening for a woman's face. Women under Taliban rule were not allowed to get an education, hold a job, go anywhere in public alone, or wear makeup. To break the Taliban's rules meant a public flogging with sticks, death by stoning, or a rifle shot to the head. A 1999 report by Physicians for Human Rights revealed shocking statistics regarding Afghan women: 97 percent had major depression, 42 percent suffered from

posttraumatic stress disorder, and 21 percent had suicidal thoughts. In 2009, 8 years after the removal of the government rule of the radical Taliban in Afghanistan, schools had been built and women and girls were once again allowed to work and pursue an education. But members of the Taliban continued to attempt to terrorize them into staying home. Shamsia Husseini and her sister were walking to school when a man pulled alongside them on a motorcycle and posed the question, "Are you going to school?" Then he pulled Shamsia's burqa off of her head and sprayed her face with burning acid. The incident left her partially blinded and badly scarred, but Shamsia continues to go to school despite the terrorist attack to keep her from an education[8] (see *Women Making a Difference*: Rana Husseini and *Her Story:* Fawzia Koofi).

Sexist and misogynistic attitudes are held by people throughout the world, including the United States, but the impact of these attitudes and the practices they inspire are more obvious in some cultures than in others. In one effort to battle oppression, *Newsweek* and *The Daily Beast* sponsored in March 2011 in New York City the 3-day, second annual Women in the World summit, which was brought together by U.S. Secretary of State Hillary Clinton, Egyptian bloggers, Facebook's Sheryl Sandberg, and dozens of inspiring activists from around the globe. Hillary Clinton told Middle Eastern women they "deserve a voice and a vote." An Egyptian blogger urged young Middle Eastern women to harness the Internet to battle an oppressive regime. Women survivors of violence and oppression shared emotional stories from Cambodia and Congo. Human rights activists debated France's controversial veil-wearing ban (which was designed to protect young women from being forced by their families to wear a face-covering veil). Women leaders offered creative solutions to problems facing women in developing and developed countries. Goldman Sachs' Dina Habib Powell and Iraqi-American activist Zainab Salbi explained how equipping women with basic business skills and providing them with small lines of credit transforms entire communities; "Once women in developing nations have an income, they send their daughters to school. And a modest 1 percentage point increase in female education boost GDP growth by 0.2 on average," Powell said.[9]

THE WOMEN'S HEALTH MOVEMENT IN THE UNITED STATES

The branch of medicine that specializes in female health is **gynecology.** This term is derived from the Greek *gyneco* (or *gyne*), meaning "woman," and from the suffix *ology*, meaning "the study of."[13] Gynecology deals with all female reproductive health issues. Obstetrics

Women Making a Difference

Rana Husseini, Fighting Against Honor Killing in Jordan

Rana Husseini is a journalist, feminist, and human rights defender who broke the silence and exposed the shame of Jordan when she unveiled the common but unspoken crime of honor killings there. "Imagine what it means in Jordan, where women who are raped are considered to have compromised their families' honor. Fathers, brothers, and sons see it as their duty to avenge the offense, not by pursuing the perpetrators but by murdering the victims; their own daughters, sisters, mothers." Honor killings accounted for one-third of the murders of women in Jordan in 1999. Husseini wrote a series of reports on the killings and launched a campaign to stop them. Husseini is the author of the book *Murder in the Name of Honor*, published in 2011. This is one of the few books available on the topic. Husseini described various reasons for honor killing including pregnancy outside of marriage. "If a woman becomes pregnant out of wedlock, she will turn herself into the police, and they'll put her in prison to 'protect her life.' Anywhere else in the world you would put the person who is threatening someone's life in prison, but in my country and elsewhere in the Arab world it is the opposite."[10, 11] Husseini has won numerous awards for her activism and journalism. Many people in her country of Jordan consider Husseini a traitor because she told the truth about honor killing. She has put her own life at risk by speaking the truth about this terrible practice. What type of courage do you think it takes for Husseini to face such ridicule and keep on fighting for the cause in which she believes?

Her Story

Fawzia Koofi, Leading Afghan Women into a Better Future

In 2012, Fawzia Koofi published her memoir, *The Favored Daughter: One Woman's Fight to Lead Afghanistan into the Future*, describing the hardship of being a woman in Afghanistan. Fawzia Koofi's name is being floated around in political circles as possibly the first female president of Afghanistan. She plans to announce her intent to run for the presidential office in the near future. Koofi's mother made sure she went to school even when the city streets were civil war zones in the early 1990s. Koofi had plans to become a medical doctor. But when the Taliban regime took over the government, she was prevented from going to school entirely. "I could've been a medical doctor now," imagining what her life would have been without the Taliban. "I could see in front of my eyes, that Afghanistan's talent and capacity—55 percent of the society which is women are deprived of all this progress. And that was a disaster for the country's future."[12] Taliban groups still hold much influence in Afghanistan politics and have threatened the life of Koofi. With the leadership of courageous women such as Fawzia Koofi, women are reclaiming their public voice and having a say in the direction of their country's future. Why do you think governmental regimes oppress the rights of women even though these actions greatly damage their country's welfare and economy?

is a branch of medicine concerned with the treatment of women during pregnancy, labor, childbirth, and the time after childbirth. Obstetrics is often combined with gynecology as a medical specialty.

The care of women during childbirth was originally in the hands of women called midwives, and for centuries these women were the overseers during the process of birthing. In ancient Greece and Rome midwives received some formal training, but the medical arts declined during medieval times. The skills a midwife possessed then were gained only from experience and were passed down via oral storytelling from generation to generation.

In sixteenth-century Europe physicians grew interested in the field of childbirth and began to practice

this form of medicine.[14] As physicians began to formalize the training and licensing of medical practitioners, midwives also began to formalize their training and licensing practice. Professional schools of midwifery were established in Europe at this time. However, midwifery did not become recognized as an important branch of medicine until the practice of obstetrics was formally established in the 1800s.

The physician largely responsible for gaining acceptance of gynecology as a medical and surgical specialty was an American, James Marion Sims (1813–1883).[15] Until then there had been opposition to it on moral grounds from midwives, the clergy, and the medical profession. Sims, a surgeon of international repute, introduced new operations and instruments (including a vaginal speculum) and in 1855 founded Woman's Hospital in New York City. He also wrote an important work, *Clinical Notes on Uterine Surgery,* in 1866. Surgical gynecology was very dangerous prior to the 1800s, but anesthesia (introduced by William Morton in 1846 at the Massachusetts General Hospital in Boston) and

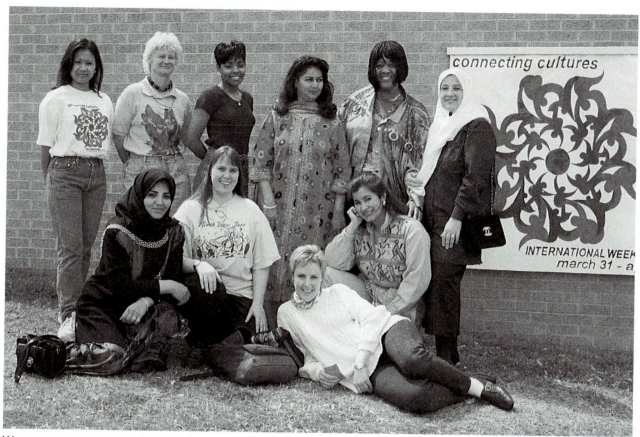

Women represent many different cultures.

antiseptic use (introduced by Joseph Lister in 1865 in London) paved the way for many advances.

The first woman to receive a medical degree in the United States was Elizabeth Blackwell (1821–1910), an American physician who was born in London.[16] The degree was granted in 1849 by Geneva Medical College, now known as Hobart College. With her sister Emily Blackwell (1826–1910), who was also a doctor, and Marie Zackrzewska, she founded the New York Infirmary for Women and Children in 1857, which was expanded in 1868 to include a Women's College for the training of doctors, the first of its kind. In 1869 Elizabeth Blackwell settled in England, and in 1875 she became a professor of gynecology at the London School of Medicine for Women, which she had helped to establish. She wrote *Pioneer Work in Opening the Medical Profession to Women* in 1895 and many other books and papers on health and education.

One of the best-known early American nurses was Dorothea Dix (1802–1887), who was dedicated to reforming the institutions that cared for the mentally ill.[17] This work led her to be appointed superintendent of nurses for the Union Army during the Civil War. The first U.S. schools for the training of nurses were established in 1873, and Linda Richards (1841–1930) was the first recipient of a nursing diploma. Richards dedicated

her life to the creation of training schools for nurses. She spent some time learning from Florence Nightingale in England, and she was the first president of the American Society of Superintendents of Training Schools.[18]

The first nurse to earn a PhD in the United States was Louise McManus (1896–1993).[19] She was central to establishing schools of nursing in colleges and universities, which provided the fundamental basis for a nursing science to evolve. She was a committed patient advocate and developed a "Patient's Bill of Rights," which was adopted by the Joint Commission in Accreditation of Hospitals.

The hospice movement, nursing care for the terminally ill, was brought to the United States from Europe by Florence Wald (1916–2008).[20] She received her nursing degree from Yale University in 1941 and later taught nursing at Yale and served as the dean of Yale's prestigious School of Nursing.

The American leader in the birth control movement was Margaret (Higgins) Sanger (1883–1966).[21] As a public health nurse, she dealt with many health and welfare issues that affect the family, such as poverty and an abundance of children for each family. She studied in London with Havelock Ellis, an English psychologist and physician whose landmark work, titled *Studies in the Psychology of Sex* (seven volumes, 1897–1928), was initially banned on charges of obscenity. Sanger returned to the United States to campaign for the legalization of birth control and practice. She was indicted in 1915 for sending birth control information through the mail and was arrested in 1916 for conducting a birth control clinic in Brooklyn. Her tireless efforts succeeded, however, and a clinic opened in 1923 in New York City and functioned until the 1970s. She organized the first American (in 1921) and international (in 1925) birth control conferences and formed (in 1923) the National Committee on Federal Legislation for Birth Control. She was president of this committee until its dissolution in 1937, once birth control under medical direction had been legalized in most states. Sanger visited many countries in Europe, Africa, and Asia, lecturing and helping to establish clinics.

The first U.S. effort to establish midwifery as a profession was undertaken by Mary Breckinridge (1881–1965).[22] A trained nurse and midwife, she established the Frontier Nursing Service (originally named the Kentucky Committee for Mothers and Babies) in 1925 at Wendover, Kentucky. Until the 1930s an American woman was more likely to die in childbirth than from any other disorder except tuberculosis. Breckinridge chose rural Kentucky as the site for her organization because she believed rural women ran a higher risk of complications and death than urban women. Breckinridge was able to organize existing midwives, recruit new ones, formalize their training, and coordinate their efforts to serve more than 1000 families in 700-plus square miles of Kentucky. Designed around a central hospital and one physician with many nursing outposts, the nurses traveled on horseback to reach the most remote areas.

Over time more hospitals were built in smaller towns and transportation improved, making it easier for expectant mothers to travel to a physician for obstetric care. However, there was a resurgent interest in midwifery in the 1970s as a response to rising health care costs and an interest in natural childbirth. Today, contemporary midwives attend births in hospitals, birthing centers, and private homes.

Women had very little voice in the arena of women's health until the end of the 1960s. Women's advocacy groups had formed during the civil rights movement, and in 1969 a group of women angry about the way the medical establishment viewed women and their bodies gathered at a workshop in Boston and spent the summer studying the health care system and giving courses on women's health.[23] This group came to be known as the Boston Women's Health Collective, and they authored the landmark work *Our Bodies, Ourselves*. Little information on women's health issues was available at that time, and this book encouraged many women to explore health issues. This was followed by *The New Our Bodies, Ourselves* in 1984 and 1996; *Our Bodies, Ourselves: A New Edition for a New Era* in 2005; and *Ourselves, Growing Older*, which was published in 1987 and again in 1994. These works empowered women by giving them the information they needed to make informed choices about their own bodies. Additional publications by this group include *Our Bodies, Ourselves: Menopause* (2006) and *Our Bodies, Ourselves: Pregnancy and Birth* (2008).

The efforts of the Boston Women's Health Collective resulted in a national women's health movement in the 1970s. In March 1971, 800 women gathered in New York City for the first women's health conference in the United States.[24] Here, women challenged the traditional treatment of women by the medical profession, including radical mastectomies and the high incidence of cesarean deliveries and hysterectomies. The work of the women at this conference contributed to the agenda of the National Women's Health Network, founded in 1975, and advanced considerably the treatment of women's health.

THE WOMEN'S SOCIAL MOVEMENT

The social stigmas attached to being a woman have significant influence on a woman's life development, including areas such as self-image, career choices and advancement, family relations, and personal significance. The personal well-being of an individual woman cannot be isolated from the context of being a member of the larger culture of women. Therefore, it is important to address the social transitions women have passed through in recent history.

The U.S. women's rights movement was born during the drive for the abolition of slavery during the nineteenth century and owes much to the publication of Mary Wollstonecraft's *A Vindication of the Rights of Women* in 1792.[25] At that time, women were mostly considered in the context of their husbands or fathers. In almost all instances, only the male head of the household was allowed to own property, borrow money, sign legal documents, initiate divorce, or obtain legal custody of children after a divorce.

U.S. women today owe a great debt of gratitude to political activists Elizabeth Cady Stanton (1815–1902) and Susan B. Anthony (1820–1906), who energized the women's rights movement in the 1800s.[26] Stanton, along with Lucretia Mott (1793–1880) and three other women, organized the first women's rights convention in Seneca Falls, New York, in July 1848. Many sentiments for the cause of women's rights were presented at the convention, but the most controversial was Stanton's call for women's right to vote. Even Mott thought this was asking for too much too soon and encouraged Stanton not to persist. Mott feared that asking for the vote would make the whole convention a laughingstock to the public. But Stanton persisted and after great debate this sentiment was adopted by the convention. At the convention's end women went back to their own communities to advocate for the rights of women, giving birth to the women's suffrage movement.

Stanton met Anthony soon after the Seneca Falls convention, and they began a lifelong friendship and partnership for the cause of women's rights. In the early years of this friendship, Stanton wrote the speeches and stayed home to care for her children while Anthony traveled the country delivering Stanton's eloquent and moving words. Stanton and Anthony were among the first **feminists** in the United States, advocating for equal rights for all persons with a special focus on women's concerns. **Liberal feminism** is a philosophy that sees the oppression of women as a denial of equal rights, representation, and access to opportunities.[27] Stanton and Anthony's initiatives changed laws for women, first in New York and later in other states, helping women to gain the right to own property, hold wages, initiate divorce, and retain custody of their children. They also advocated for a woman's right to equal pay for equal work and a woman's right to vote, but neither lived to see these laws passed. Seventy-two years passed between the time U.S. women organized to ask for the vote in 1848 and the time they eventually received it in 1920.

A second U.S. feminist movement took place during the civil rights era of the 1960s and 1970s. Betty Friedan (1921–2006) was a significant contributor to this women's rights movement.[28] Friedan surveyed classmates from her fifteenth college reunion and asked them to describe their lives since college. From their answers she wrote *The Feminine Mystique,* published in 1963. It was a national best seller. In her book, Friedan suggested that middle-class housewives were not necessarily fulfilled by housework and childbearing. She criticized politicians, health professionals, educators, businesspeople, and social scientists who pressured women to stay at home and play the stereotypic roles of mother and wife. Any inclination by a woman to do otherwise was considered by these professionals to be emotionally abnormal and socially irresponsible. Friedan helped found the National Organization for Women (NOW) in 1966 and served as its president for the first 3 years. She led the organization in its decision in 1967 to support the Equal Rights Amendment (ERA) for women and to support legalized abortion.

The ERA declared, "Equality of rights under the law shall not be denied or abridged by the United States or any State on account of sex." The amendment was approved by the requisite two-thirds vote of the House of Representatives in October 1971 and by the Senate in March 1972. But it ultimately failed to achieve ratification by the required thirty-eight states by the extended deadline of June 30, 1982. Despite its defeat, public support for the ERA never fell below 54 percent, and as late as 1976 support for its passage was included in the platforms of both major political parties. Technically the ERA is still alive and with thirty-five of the required thirty-eight states having already ratified it, the ERA needs only three more states to become an amendment to the Constitution.

Women continued to actively challenge the traditional domestic role assigned to them and rallied for sexual freedom. During this period, lesbians began "stepping out of the closet" and challenging society's bigoted attitudes of heterosexism. The civil rights movement gave birth to women's advocate groups all over the nation as women banded together to promote their cause. The feminist movement is spurred on today by organizations such as the National Organization for Women and the international Feminist Majority Foundation. Many women's advocate groups exist today around the world.

LEGISLATION FOR WOMEN AND MINORITIES

Over the years legislation designed to protect the rights of women and minorities in the United States has been passed, including these major legislative acts:

- The Nineteenth Amendment to the U.S. Constitution passed in 1920 awarded women the right to vote in government elections.
- Title VII of the Civil Rights Act of 1964 prohibits employment discrimination based on race, color, religion, sex, or national origin (for companies with fifteen or more employees).
- The Civil Rights Act amendments of 1991 allow for awarding damages when discrimination is proved.
- The Age Discrimination in Employment Act of 1967 protects individuals who are 40 years of age or older.
- The Equal Pay Act of 1963 requires an employer to pay all employees equally for equal work, regardless of gender.
- Title I and Title V of the Americans with Disabilities Act of 1990 prohibit employment discrimination against qualified individuals with disabilities, in the private sector and in state and local governments.
- Sections 501 and 505 of the Rehabilitation Act of 1973 prohibit discrimination in the federal government against qualified individuals with disabilities.
- The Family and Medical Leave Act of 1992 requires employers of fifty or more employees within a 75-mile area to provide up to 12 weeks of unpaid, job-protected leave for certain family and medical reasons.
- Title IX of the Education Amendments of 1972 prohibits sex discrimination, including sexual

harassment in schools. This act especially opened avenues for women in schools by requiring equal opportunities in education and sports.

- The Violence Against Women Act (VAWA) increased funding for programs and services, and also attempted to improve law enforcement's response to violence. It was sponsored by U.S. Senator Joe Biden and signed into law by President Bill Clinton in 1994. It expired on October 1, 2005 but with the efforts of U.S. Senator Hillary Rodham Clinton (as co-sponsor) it was reauthorized on October 5, 2005.
- Title X of the Public Health Service Act was created in 1970 and is the only federal program solely dedicated to family planning and reproductive health. Title X is administered by the Office of Family Planning, although its budget is located within the Health and Human Services Administration. The program is designed to provide access to contraceptive supplies, family planning information, and preventive health services to all who need them, with a priority given to low-income persons. Preventive health services include patient education and counseling; breast and pelvic examinations; cervical cancer, sexually transmitted disease and HIV screenings; and pregnancy diagnosis and counseling. For many clients, Title X clinics provide the only continuing source of health care and health education.

SEXUAL DISCRIMINATION

Legislation helps to protect the rights of those who might otherwise be exploited. Because of legislation, **sexual discrimination** in wages and salaries became illegal in 1963 and sexual discrimination in employment decisions became illegal in 1964.

The Pregnancy Discrimination Act of 1978 was passed as an amendment to Title VII of the Civil Rights Act of 1964 to protect a woman against discriminatory practices at the workplace because of her pregnancy. A woman could no longer legally be denied employment or be fired because of her pregnancy, and health care coverage for her pregnancy was protected. It states that "women affected by pregnancy, childbirth, or related medical conditions shall be treated the same for all employment related purposes, including receipt of benefits under fringe benefit programs, as other persons not so affected but similar in their ability or inability to work." In 2011, the U.S. Equal Employment Opportunity Commission (EEOC) received 5,797 charges of pregnancy-based discrimination. The EEOC resolved 6482 pregnancy discrimination charges in 2011 and recovered $17.2 million in monetary benefits for charging parties and other aggrieved individuals[29] (not including monetary benefits obtained through litigation) (see *FYI: Pregnancy Discrimination*).

Even with legislation in place designed to protect women from wage and salary discrimination, there remained a

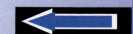

Pregnancy Discrimination

Following are some high profile lawsuits based on pregnancy discrimination that were settled by the U.S. Equal Employment Opportunity Commission (EEOC).

- *Verizon* (February 26, 2002): Under the settlement, thousands of current and former female employees in 13 states and the District of Columbia receive benefits estimated in the millions of dollars that were previously not made available to them because of pregnancy or maternity leave. This is one of the largest EEOC settlements of its kind involving pregnancy-related service credit adjustments.
- *Motherhood Maternity* (January 8, 2007): The Philadelphia-based clothes retailer will pay $375,000 to settle a pregnancy discrimination and retaliation lawsuit for refusing to hire qualified female applicants because they were pregnant and for firing an assistant manager who complained about the practice. Motherhood Maternity is the leading designer, manufacturer, and retailer of maternity fashion in the United States. Charges nationally against the company rose from 3,385 in 1992 to 4,512 in 2005. "It is shocking that a corporation whose market is pregnant women would refuse to employ them and then retaliate against a woman who complained about the practice," commented Nora Curtin, attorney for the EEOC Miami District Office.
- *Wal-Mart* (December 23, 2002): Will pay $220,000 in damages for refusing to hire a female applicant due to her pregnancy in Bentonville, Arkansas. The applicant was told by the assistant manager, "Come back after you have the baby." It took 11 years to settle this suit filed in 1991.
- *Johnson International, Inc.* (December 28, 2004): This global financial services company settled for $450,000 for a discrimination suit based on withdrawing an offer as Executive Vice President to Rae Ann Good after she disclosed that she was pregnant. Chester Bailey, Director of the EEOC's Milwaukee District Office commented, "The problem of women advancing to top executive positions is an ongoing concern of the EEOC. Certainly one of the factors which may contribute to the low numbers of women in such jobs is pregnancy discrimination, which we are committed to combating."

significant gender pay gap in the United States. In 2001 the Department of Labor's Current Population Survey showed that for full-time wage and salary workers, women's weekly earnings were about three-fourths of men's. However, the Department of Labor report stated that this difference did not reflect key factors such as work experience and education that may affect the level of earnings individuals receive, so the U.S. Government Accountability Office published an investigative report in 2003 to try and explain the gender pay gap. According to this report:

[Of] the many factors that account for differences in earnings between men and women. . . . work patterns are key. Specifically women have fewer years of experience, work fewer hours per year, are less likely to work a full-time schedule, and leave the labor force for longer periods of time than men. . . . When we account for differences between male and female work patterns as well as other key factors, women earned, on average, 80 percent of what men earned in 2000. . . . Even after accounting for key factors that affect earnings, our model could not explain all of the differences [in earnings] between men and women.

When the Equal Pay Act was passed in 1963, women made 58 cents for every dollar earned by men and in the year 2002, women were paid 73 cents for every dollar earned by men.[30] On December 1, 2003, the EEOC published a new code of practice on equal pay that explains to employers what they have to do to comply with the equal pay law that was established in 1963. All employers were encouraged to perform an audit to make sure women were being paid equally to the men doing the same job or work of equal value. As a response to the continuing existence of a gender pay gap, on April 19, 2005, the Paycheck Fairness Act was introduced in both houses of Congress by Senator Hillary Rodham Clinton and Representative Rosa DeLauro. This act, if passed, would strengthen enforcement of the Equal Pay Act of 1963. It would work to improve Equal Pay Act remedies, make it easier to bring about class action claims, improve collection of pay information, prohibit employer retaliation, develop voluntary guidelines, increase training and education, and recognize model employers. As of 2012, the Paycheck Fairness Act was still under consideration in the legislative process.

The gender wage gap is still significant, but gradual decreases in the gap are occurring over time. According to the June 2010 report of the U.S. Department of Labor, U.S. Bureau of Labor Statistics, *Highlights of Women's Earnings in 2009*, women who were full-time wage and salary workers had median weekly earnings of $657, or about 80 percent of the $819 median for their male counterparts. After a gradual rise in the 1980s and 1990s, the women's-to-men's earnings ratio peaked at 81 percent in 2005 and 2006. Earnings differences in 2009 between women and men were widest for whites and Asians. White women earned 79 percent as much as their male counterparts in 2009, while Asian women earned 82 percent as much as Asian men. By comparison, Hispanic women had earnings that were 90 percent of those of their male counterparts in 2009, while black women earned 94 percent as much as black men. The ratio of female-to-male earnings varied by place of residence, ranging from 65 percent in Louisiana to 97 percent in the District of Columbia (Washington, D.C.). The differences among states reflect, in part, variation in the occupations and industries found in each state and in the age composition of each state's labor force.

The Organization for Economic Cooperation and Development reported 2009 data for industrialized countries that showed men's median, full-time earnings were on average 17.6 percent higher than women's.[31] The biggest wage gap was in South Korea (38 percent) and Japan (27 percent), where men earn wages much higher than women, and was smallest in Belgium (9 percent), Norway (9 percent), New Zealand (8 percent), and Hungary (4 percent). In the United States, the typical full-time female worker earns 20 percent less than the typical full-time male worker.

Businesses are aware that sexual discrimination is wrong and illegal, yet they do it anyway (see *FYI:* "Sexual Discrimination Leads to Lawsuits"). This is why it

 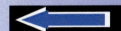

Sexual Discrimination Leads to Lawsuits

Following are high-profile sexual discrimination class action lawsuits. How important is it that women have the right to seek compensation after discrimination at the workplace? Should there be a limit placed on how much compensation can be awarded to plaintiffs?

- Women filed a class action suit against Wal-Mart Stores, Inc., in June 2004 for gender discrimination in salary and promotion practices. As many as 1.6 million current and former female employees were represented, making this the largest civil rights case in U.S. history. In June 2011, the U.S. Supreme Court ruled against the plaintiffs and for Wal-Mart in a 5-to-4 decision along ideological lines on "the basic question in the case—whether the suit satisfied a requirement of the class-action rules that 'there are questions of law or fact common to the class' of female employees. The court's five more- consecutive justices said no, shutting down the suit and limiting the ability of other plaintiffs to band together in large class actions."[32]
- More than 750 women employees filed a class action suit against Costco Wholesale Corporation in August 2004 for gender discrimination in promotion practices. Based on the legal decision in the Wal-Mart case just described, the Costco suit was rejected in 2011 on the basis that it is required that claimants must provide "rigorous analysis" proving Class Members have enough in common to pursue claims in a single class action lawsuit.[33]

Because of the 2011 Supreme Court ruling from the Wal-Mart case, that it must be rigorously proven that plaintiffs show enough commonalities to be included in a class-action lawsuit, it will now be extremely difficult for women to band together to fight discrimination in the workplace. It can be argued that this was the hidden agenda of the Supreme Court justices who ruled in this fashion because it is almost impossible for one person to fight a big corporation, whereas class-action lawsuits made such a fight much more feasible.

is necessary to have a legal system that allows persons to seek help to stop sexual discrimination. However, women's rights and protection come under attack by the legislative and judicial systems that are designed to protect them (see *FYI:* "Rulings and Legislation That Limit Women's Rights and Protection").

Another form of sexual discrimination that is of great concern is the denial of prescription drugs to women for reproductive health concerns (see *Viewpoint:* "Pharmacists Refuse to Fill Prescriptions Related to Reproductive Rights"). Reports of pharmacists refusing to fill legally prescribed prescriptions for birth control, including emergency contraceptives ("morning after" pill), have surfaced in several states, including California, Georgia, Illinois, Louisiana, Massachusetts, Minnesota, Missouri, New Hampshire, New York, North Carolina, Ohio, Texas, Washington, and Wisconsin.[35] These refusals appear to be based on a pharmacist's

personal religious beliefs, not on legitimate medical or professional concerns about safety and the welfare of the customer.

Sexual harassment is recognized as a form of sex discrimination that violates the Civil Rights Act of 1964 (and the 1991 amendments to that act). Sexual harassment is described as unwanted sexual advances, requests for sexual favors, and other verbal or physical conduct of a sexual nature that negatively affects the work environment.

The U.S. Equal Employment Opportunity Commission (EEOC) received 11,364 charges of sexual harassment in 2011, with about 84 percent of those charges filed by women. The EEOC resolved 12,571 sexual harassment charges in 2011 and recovered $52.3 million in monetary benefits for charging parties (not including monetary benefits obtained through litigation). A 2006 telephone poll by Louis Harris and Associates

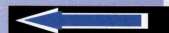

Rulings and Legislation That Limit Women's Rights and Protection

What persons or entities do you believe the following acts and rulings are designed to assist? What do you believe will be the impact of the following acts and ruling?

Partial Birth Abortion Ban Act Passed by Congress in November of 2003 and upheld by the Supreme Court on April 18, 2007. Prohibits midterm abortions regardless of whether the mother's health is at risk or whether the child would be born with ailments.

Class Action Fairness Act of 2005 Signed into law by President Bush, the so-called "Class Action Fairness Act" threatens to unfairly prevent victims of discrimination from seeking legal justice and thus, women's ability to seek redress in a court of law will be severely restricted. The act will allow the removal of almost all state class actions to the federal courts, a process that will most certainly overload the federal courts, delaying the resolution of cases and making it more difficult for federal civil rights cases to be heard. In addition, this act prohibits courts from granting settlements that award a named plaintiff a greater share of relief than is awarded to all other members of the class. In effect, this forces the named plaintiffs to forego full relief and compensation as the price for protecting others in the class. According to the Feminist Majority Foundation, the changes that this act makes in the class action process will seriously affect the marginalized and disadvantaged members of society, including women, as it seeks to deny them access to relief from discrimination and injury.

Deficit Reduction Act Passed by Congress in 2005 It included a little-noticed provision that prohibited a decades-old practice of pharmaceutical companies selling contraceptives to college clinics and clinics serving low-income women at deeply discounted rates. This has resulted in birth control soaring to as high as $50 per month in the year 2008 and making it unaffordable for many women.

Ledbetter v. Goodyear Tire and Rubber Co. The Supreme Court ruled on May 29, 2007 that Lilly Ledbetter, a lone female supervisor at a tire plant in Gadsden, Alabama did not file her lawsuit, claiming 19 years of gender wage discrimination, "in a timely manner." Ledbetter had worked at Goodyear for 20 years before she discovered that men were paid more than she for the same job. The ruling now requires claims to be filed within 180 days of the initial discriminatory salary decision, even if the victim is unaware of the discrimination until much later. This ruling gutted the Civil Rights Act of 1964, which was designed to protect women from wage discrimination. In response to the Ledbetter decision by the Supreme Court, the Fair Pay Restoration Act was presented to the U.S. Senate in April 2008 and is designed to reverse the Supreme Court decision on the Ledbetter case. The Fair Pay Restoration Act was introduced by two Democrats and two Republicans, respectively, Senators Edward M. Kennedy, Hillary Rodham Clinton, Olympia Snowe, and Arlen Specter. The bill was signed into law by President Barack Obama on January 29, 2009, as H.R. 2831: Lilly Ledbetter Fair Pay Act of 2007.

Viewpoint

Pharmacists Refuse to Fill Prescriptions Related to Reproductive Rights[36]

On March 28, 2004, a pharmacist working at a CVS store in the north Texas town of Richland Hills refused to refill a prescription for birth-control pills for a 32-year-old woman. A spokesperson for CVS stated that the pharmacist's actions were not part of store policy. In January 2004, three Eckerd pharmacists in the north Texas town of Denton wouldn't sell the "morning after" emergency contraceptive to a woman identified as a rape victim. The Eckerd pharmacists were later fired. "This could become a serious problem, particularly if it spreads to rural areas where there are fewer drugstores," said Suzanne Martinez, vice president for public policy for the Planned Parenthood Federation of America, the nation's largest supporter of reproductive health. However, the largest professional society of pharmacists, the American Pharmacists Association, supports a "pharmacist's right to exercise conscientious refusal" in not filling certain prescriptions, said spokesperson Michael Stewart. In 22 years at the Texas State Board of Pharmacy, Executive Director Gay Dodson said she had never heard of a pharmacist refusing to fill prescriptions on moral or religious grounds before this year. South Dakota, in 1998, became the first state to adopt a "conscience clause" protecting a pharmacist's right to refuse to fill a prescription in certain cases: if the prescription would cause an abortion, destroy an unborn child as defined by state law, or cause the death of a person by any means of assisted suicide or euthanasia. Several other states are considering similar laws.

Do you think a pharmacist has the right to refuse to fill legal prescriptions related to reproductive health because of personal, moral, or religious beliefs? How does the refusal to fill these prescriptions translate into a denial of rights for women?

The creation of the term "sexual harassment" dates back to 1975, and it gradually evolved into a legal precedent based on several court rulings over time.

In 1975, a forty-five-year-old university secretary named Carmita Wood quit working for a Cornell [University] physicist after the stress of his repeated sexual advances made her physically ill. When Wood filed for unemployment compensation claiming that it was not her fault that she could no longer work, her case was discovered by Lin Farley, who taught a course at Cornell about women being forced to leave their jobs to avoid their boss's unwanted sexual advances. Farley and two of her colleagues coined the term *sexual harassment* to describe the phenomenon. That spring, she accompanied Wood to a feminist "speak out" in Ithaca, where the term *sexual harassment* found its first public airing.[38]

Later that same year, Lin Farley testified at hearings by the New York City Commission on Human Rights on the topic of women in the workplace.

When the *New York Times* ran an article about the hearings titled "Women Begin to Speak Out Against Sexual Harassment at Work," the term entered the national lexicon for the first time.[39]

After the publication of the *Times* article, Lin Farley and her colleagues received a flood of reports from women who had had a similar experience as Carmita Wood. Yet, lacking a legal precedent for sexual harassment, the legal world framed early cases as unemployment insurance or workmen's compensation claims. Gradually, courts began to recognize sexual harassment as a form of sexual discrimination under Title VII of the Civil Rights Act of 1964.[40]

Protection against sexual discrimination and sexual harassment under Title VII of the Civil Rights Act of 1964 was actually a historical accident because the act did not originally include language that would offer protection based on gender. A major opponent of the bill to establish the Civil Rights Act was Virginia congressman Howard Smith, the leader of the southern conservatives who opposed the bill. Smith inserted the word "sex" into the act in hopes that including protection for women in Title VII of the Civil Rights Act would lead to its demise. But the move backfired on Smith and his constituents when the Civil Rights Act passed along with his "sex" amendment.[41]

Because the insertion of the "sex" amendment was actually a ploy meant to sink the Civil Rights Act of 1964, no one in Congress had thought through its potential ramifications. And it would take 12 years for the act that was established in 1964 to be recognized by the courts as a legal protection against sexual harassment. In 1976, two courts rejected sexual harassment as a form of

---

of 782 workers showed that 100 percent of female workers claimed their harasser was a man; and of these female workers 43 percent were harassed by a supervisor, 27 percent were harassed by an employee senior to them, 19 percent were harassed by a coworker at their level, and 8 percent were harassed by a junior employee.[37] This poll revealed that 62 percent of targets of sexual harassment took no action. Thus, the actual number of sexual harassment incidents is likely to be much higher than the number of charges filed with the EEOC.

gender discrimination under Title VII of the Civil Rights Acts of 1964, but one U.S. District Court in Washington, D.C., became the first federal court to hold otherwise, in *Williams v. Saxbe.*

In that case, a woman named Diane Williams was fired from her job with the community relations department of the U.S. Department of Justice after she refused her supervisor's sexual advances. She claimed that this was a violation of Title VII, because she had been denied equal employment opportunities. If she had been a man, she argued, her boss would never have propositioned her. It was her turning down the proposition that led to her firing. . . . The court found that, in firing Williams for refusing to have sex with him, the supervisor had imposed a condition of employment on Williams that he did not impose on other workers, and that he did so because she was a woman. Therefore, the court reasoned it was a violation of Title VII. . . . That precedent stuck, and by 1977 three federal courts of appeals and a number of district courts had held that sexual harassment could be a form of sex discrimination under Title VII.[42]

In 1979 a treatise titled, *Sexual Harassment of the Working Woman* was published by a young law professor at the University of Michigan, Catharine MacKinnon, in which she stipulated that "quid pro quo" harassment, meaning "this for that" (or "put out or get out"), was not the only form of sexual harassment. MacKinnon argued that "subjecting women to a hostile work environment, including repeated exposure to sexually offensive or denigrating material, as a condition of employment could also constitute a violation of Title VII."[43] In 1980 the EEOC issued federal guidelines on sexual harassment in the workplace that incorporated both the "quid pro quo" and "hostile work environment" concepts, and these federal guidelines, though not a binding legal force, "became a benchmark for courts and employers in sorting out what conduct violated Title VII."[44] The EEOC guidelines stated:

Unwelcome sexual advances, requests for sexual favors, and other verbal or physical conduct of a sexual nature constitute sexual harassment when (1) submission to such conduct is made either explicitly or implicitly a condition of an individual's employment, (2) submission to or rejection of such conduct by an individual is used as the basis for employment decisions affecting such individual, or (3) such conduct has the purpose or effect of unreasonably interfering with an individual's work performance or creating an intimidating, hostile, or offensive working environment.[45]

In 2002, Clara Bingham and Laura Leedy Gansler published *Class Action: The Landmark Case That Changed Sexual Harassment Law.* This book describes the true story of Lois Jenson and her female coworkers at Eveleth Mine of Minnesota who experienced repeated acts of sexual harassment in a work environment that was extremely hostile to women—a story that inspired the major motion picture *North Country* (Warner Bros. Pictures, 2005). The book details the 12-year journey, 1987–1999, of the case of *Jenson v. Eveleth* that set the most important precedent of certifying sexual harassment as a class action lawsuit. "That decision elevated sexual harassment from an individual complaint by one, usually a powerless person against another, more powerful one—a complaint that could easily be ignored or swept under the rug—to a significant civil rights issue. . . . *Jenson v. Eveleth* did not eradicate sexual harassment in the work-place. But it made corporate America take real note of it for the first time, and established once and for all that women who are subjected to a hostile work environment need never stand alone."[46]

Considered by the courts as a form of sex discrimination under Title IX of the Education Amendment of 1972, *sexual harassment* is defined as unwanted sexual behavior that interferes with a student's right to receive an equal education. The American Association of University Women (AAUW) published in 2011 the report *Crossing the Line: Sexual Harassment at School,* which showed sexual harassment in schools to be problematic.[47] Sexual harassment is a form of school bullying. The AAUW report presented results from a nationally representative survey of 1965 middle and high school students (grades 7–12) conducted in the 2010–2011 school year that asked students whether they had experienced the following types of sexual harassment:

In Person

- Having someone make unwelcome sexual comments, jokes, or gestures to or about you.
- Being called gay or lesbian in a negative way.
- Being touched in an unwelcome sexual way.
- Having someone flash or expose themselves to you.
- Being shown sexy or sexual pictures that you didn't want to see.
- Being physically intimidated in a sexual way.
- Being forced to do something sexual.

Through Text, E-mail, Facebook, or Other Electronic Means

- Being sent unwelcome sexual comments, jokes, or pictures or having someone post them about you.
- Having someone spread unwelcome sexual rumors about you.
- Being called gay or lesbian in a negative way.

The results of the AAUW survey on sexual harassment at school showed that about half (48 percent) in grades

7–12 experienced some form of sexual harassment at school during the 2010–2011 school year. Girls were more likely than boys to experience sexual harassment (56 percent versus 40 percent). The gender gap was similar for both in-person harassment (52 percent versus 35 percent) and electronic harassment (36 percent versus 24 percent). The most common type of sexual harassment for all students was unwelcome sexual comments, jokes, and gestures, and one-third of students (33 percent) encountered them at least once in school year 2010–2011. The AAUW survey showed girls were more likely than boys to encounter most forms of sexual harassment. "Girls were much more likely to experience unwanted sexual jokes, comments, or gestures (46 percent versus 22 percent). Girls and boys were about equally likely to be called gay or lesbian in a negative way (18 percent of students). Girls were more likely to say that they were shown sexy or sexual pictures that they did not want to see (16 percent of girls versus 10 percent of boys) and that they had been touched in an unwelcome sexual way (13 percent of girls versus 3 percent of boys). Girls were also more likely to say that they had been physically intimidated in a sexual way (9 percent of girls versus 2 percent of boys) and were forced to do something sexual (4 percent of girls versus less than 1 percent of boys). Girls (7 percent) and boys (7 percent) were equally likely to say that someone flashed or exposed him-, or herself to them."[48]

Two additional constructs that are related to discrimination against women are **homophobia** and **heterosexism.** Homophobia is the fear or dislike of a person who is homosexual. Many people in the United States are homophobic, and thus, many homosexual women hide their lesbian orientation to avoid being ostracized or rejected by others (see *Her Story:* "Professional Basketball Star Sheryl Swoopes Comes Out as a Lesbian"). Heterosexism is a belief or attitude that results in bias or discrimination toward anyone who is not heterosexual. Heterosexism is highly prevalent in the United States. Many states have laws that (a) prevent recognition of out-of-state same-sex marriage, (b) prohibit benefits for a state employee's unmarried partner, (c) amend the state's constitution to ban same-sex marriage, or (d) prohibit adoption of children by homosexuals (see *Viewpoint:* "Same-Sex Marriage"). These laws are perceived by many to be unconstitutional yet they exist as legal justification for discrimination against an entire group of U.S. citizens.

Discrimination against homosexuals is a worldwide phenomenon. However, the countries of Canada and Spain have become social justice role models for the rest of the world regarding equal rights for gays and lesbians. In 1996 Canada amended the national Human Rights Act to provide protection from discrimination based on

Her Story

Professional Basketball Star Sheryl Swoopes Comes Out as a Lesbian

High-profile WNBA star Sheryl Swoopes publicly revealed that she was a lesbian in 2005. The story was first reported by *ESPN Magazine* on October 26. Swoopes is a three-time Olympic gold medalist and a four-time WNBA champion with the Houston Comets, where she started as a rookie in 1997, and she led Texas Tech University to a national basketball championship in 1993. In coming out to the public about her relationship with former Comets assistant coach Alisa Scott, which she had kept hidden for 7 years, Swoopes said, "I feel like I've been living a lie. . . . I'm at a place in my life right now where I'm very happy, very content. I'm finally OK with the idea of who I love, who I want to be with. . . . I don't want to have to hide from the world anymore. . . . [My mother] doesn't think it's right. She'll probably never accept it. . . . But she's dealing with it. . . . I worry about the reaction throughout the country, but I really worry about Brownfield [her home town] and Lubbock [the location of her college alma mater]. . . . Because they're both small towns and Sheryl Swoopes is a local hero. Now what? I hope it doesn't change. It's important to me." Swoopes is perhaps the highest-profile active team-sport athlete to come out as a lesbian and the third WNBA player to do so. Sue Wicks of the New York Liberty, who came out shortly before her retirement in 2002, was the first active WNBA player to come out publicly about her sexual orientation.[49]

Does your opinion of celebrities change when they reveal they are gay or lesbian? How much discrimination or distress do you think a gay or lesbian celebrity experiences because of negative public attitudes about homosexuality?

sexual orientation, extend benefits to same-sex partners, allow civil marriage for same-sex couples, and allow foreign partners of its homosexual citizenry to receive residency permits. Spain has a national gay rights law (established in 2005) that bans some antigay discrimination, including for housing, employment, and public and professional services. Spain provides homosexual couples with health care benefits, access to state widowers' pensions, and alimony in the event of a separation. Spain allows same-sex couples the right to marry, adopt children, and inherit each other's property, making their legal status the same as that of heterosexual

Viewpoint

Same-Sex Marriage[50]

On June 16, 2008 at 5:01 P.M., California officials began issuing marriage licenses to same-sex couples. This was made possible by a California Supreme Court ruling one month earlier on May 15. County clerks met a long line of same-sex couples with new forms listing "Partner A" and "Partner B" changed from the previous forms which listed "Bride" and "Groom." The decision made California the second state in the United States, after Massachusetts, to legalize same-sex marriage. Some other states have what are called "civil unions" that are a legal recognition of same-sex relationships, but do not constitute legal marriage. To see what laws support and discriminate against gays and lesbians in the United States, see the Web site for the Human Rights Campaign, www.hrc.org. On November 4, 2008, a majority of the people of California voted "Yes" for Proposition 8, which changed the state constitution to restrict the definition of marriage to a union between a man and a woman. With the passage of Proposition 8, same-sex marriage was no longer legal in California. Thousands of gay rights activists marched through city streets in protest. This fight for social justice continues. What is your view on same-sex marriage? What is your view on same-sex civil unions? What is your view on amendments to state constitutions that ban same-sex marriage or define marriage strictly as between a man and a woman?

couples. The first same-sex marriages took place in the Netherlands on April 1, 2001. As of 2011, same-sex marriage has been adopted by Belgium (2003), Spain (2005), Canada (2005), South Africa (2006), Norway (2009), Sweden (2009), Portugal (2010), Iceland (2010), and Argentina (2010).[51] Argentina was the first Latin American country to approve a same-sex marriage law, this occurring on July 15, 2010.[52]

DISPARITIES IN ACCESS TO HEALTH CARE

The National Healthcare Disparities Report (NHDR) is provided by the U.S. Department of Health and Human Services. According to the NHDR 2010, access to health care means having the timely use of personal health services to achieve the best health outcomes. Attaining good access to care requires three discrete steps:

- Gaining entry into the health care system.
- Getting access to sites of care where patients can receive needed services.

- Finding providers who meet the needs of individual patients and with whom patients can develop a relationship based on mutual communication and trust.

Health care access is measured in several ways, including:

- Structural measures of the presence or absence of specific resources that facilitate health care, such as having health insurance or a usual source of care.
- Assessments by patients of how easily they are able to gain access to health care.
- Utilization measures of the ultimate outcome of good access to care (i.e., the successful receipt of needed services).

Health insurance facilitates entry into the health care system. Uninsured people are less likely to receive medical care and more likely to have poor health status. The NHDR 2010 states the costs of poor health among uninsured people total $65 billion to $130 billion annually. The financial burden of uninsurance is also high for uninsured individuals; almost 50 percent of personal bankruptcy filings are due to medical expenses. Uninsured individuals report more problems getting care, are diagnosed at later disease stages, and get less therapeutic care. They are sicker when hospitalized and more likely to die during their stay. According to the NHDR 2010, those persons less likely to have health insurance are in any of the following groups: poor, less educated, and do not speak English. The NHDR 2010 states that the percentage of people with health insurance was about one-third lower for people with less than a high school education than for people with at least some college education (56.9 percent compared with 89.0 percent). From 1999 to 2008, while the percentage of people with health insurance increased for poor people (from 66.2 percent to 71.0 percent), the percentage worsened for middle-income people (from 86.4 percent to 83.4 percent). In 2008, the percentage of people with health insurance was significantly lower for poor, near-poor, and middle-income people than for high-income people (71.0, 69.4, and 83.4 percent, respectively, compared with 93.8 percent). Overall, there was no significant change from 1999 to 2008 in the percentage of people with health insurance. In 2008, about 83.2 percent of people under age 65 had health insurance. In 2008, Asians under age 65 were more likely than whites to have health insurance (86.1 percent compared with 83.3 percent). American Indians and Alaska Natives under age 65 were less likely than whites to have health insurance (71.6 percent compared with 83.3 percent). In 2008, Hispanics under age 65 were less likely than non-Hispanic whites to have health insurance (66.7 percent compared with

87.5 percent). Overall, females were more likely to have health insurance than males, and females were more likely to have a primary health care provider than males.

The NHDR 2010 states that about one in five Americans lives in a nonmetropolitan area. Compared with their urban counterparts, rural residents are more likely to be older, be poor, and be in fair or poor health, and have chronic conditions. Rural residents are less likely than their urban counterparts to receive recommended preventive services and on average report fewer visits to health care providers. Although 20 percent of Americans live in rural areas, only 9 percent of physicians in America practice in those settings. Other important providers of health care in those settings include nurse practitioners, nurse midwives, and physician assistants. A variety of programs deliver needed services in rural areas, such as the National Health Service Corps Scholarship Program, Indian Health Service, State offices of rural health, rural health clinics, and community health centers. Cost-based Medicare reimbursement incentives are also available for rural health clinics, critical access hospitals, sole community hospitals, and Medicare-dependent hospitals and physicians in health professional shortage areas.[53]

HEALTH ISSUES FOR MINORITY WOMEN

The U.S. Census Bureau reported 156,964,212 females in 2010, or 50.8 percent of the population, of whom about 55 million are members of a racial or ethnic minority group (including Hispanic origin). Detailed population statistics reports are still being generated from the 2010 Census and thus not all demographic data are available at this time, but the U.S. Census estimated that in 2009 the female racial distribution was 79 percent white, 13 percent black or African American, 4.6 percent Asian, 1 percent American Indian and Alaska Native, and 0.18 percent Native Hawaiian and Other Pacific Islander. Additionally, 1.7 percent women reported being a member of two or more races. Hispanic origin is not considered a separate race category by the U.S. Census Bureau, but the number of females who reported being Hispanic was 15 percent. Women of color are nearly a third of all U.S. women. By 2050 it is projected that just under half of females in the United States will be members of racial or ethnic minority groups. The U.S. Census Bureau reported the Hispanic population is the fastest growing minority group, projected to grow from 31.7 million in 1999 (12 percent of the population) to 98.2 million in 2050 (24 percent of the population). Over the same period, the non-Hispanic white population is projected to decrease from 72 percent to 53 percent, and the non- Hispanic black population is projected to increase slightly, from 13 percent to 15 percent of the total population in 2050. What does it mean for the health care system that the population of the United States is becoming more ethnically diverse? Is there adequate representation of diverse health care workers to provide culturally sensitive services for an increasingly diverse population? Is there adequate representation of minority groups in health research?

There is significant variation in health status and health-related behaviors for women of different races and ethnicities. The U.S. Department of Health and Human Services (DHHS) reports that access to health care plays an important role in the quality of health care, the quality and years of healthy life, and the presence or absence of health disparities. Race and ethnicity is one of the key factors that contribute to disparities in health and health care utilization. Following is a discussion of social and cultural factors that affect the health of minority women. More in-depth coverage of health issues and concerns specific to women is provided in later chapters.

Hispanic or Latino Women

DHHS reported the following discoveries from a 2006 study examining access to health care among Hispanic or Latino women in the United States. Lack of access to health care was most prevalent among Hispanic or Latino women who had poor or near poor poverty status, had less than a high school diploma, or were foreign born. In interviews with Hispanic and Latino women it was discovered that 31 percent lacked health insurance coverage at the time of the interview, 20 percent had no usual place to go for medical care during the past year, and 22 percent experienced unmet health care needs during the past year due to cost; in comparing the five subgroups, Mexican women and Central or South American women were more likely than Puerto Rican women and Cuban women to experience these disadvantages. The DHHS study concluded that access to health care varied among subgroups of Hispanic or Latino women; understanding these subgroup differences may help community-based programs improve access to care among these women. Since Hispanic and Latino women originate in Spanish-speaking countries, the language barrier may inhibit access to and quality of care for this group. Also, those who immigrate illegally may be hesitant to access health care services for fear of being noticed by immigration services.

The *Women of Color Data Book, 2006* of the Office of Research on Women's Health (ORWH) of the National Institutes of Health, reports the major health concerns for Hispanic or Latino women living in the United

States. More than 43 percent of poor Hispanic families are headed by females and are likely to face the combined stresses of poverty. When Hispanic women are employed, they tend to hold jobs of low status and low pay. More Hispanics are obese, less physically active, and less likely to participate in lifestyles that promote cardiovascular health than are other populations. As a consequence, some Latinos are more likely to have diabetes than the general U.S. population; the prevalence among Mexican American women is 50 percent higher than among white women. Lack of materials in Spanish explaining the benefits of an active-lifestyle and economic barriers to accessing fitness facilities may contribute to the problem. Also, for many, cultural mores dictate that Hispanics first try home remedies, seek the advice of family and friends, or engage folk healers before getting professional health care. Among the Hispanic community, Puerto Ricans are disproportionately likely to have AIDS. Although less than 10 percent of the U.S. Latino population, Puerto Ricans were 17 percent of the Hispanics in the United States infected with AIDS in 2003. This may be explained by the fact that Puerto Ricans are a very close-knit group culturally and are more likely to have sex with and marry other Puerto Ricans. The AIDS prevalence with this group may also be exacerbated by homogenous needle-sharing networks among Puerto Rican drug users. Cultural factors that contribute to AIDS infection in the Hispanic or Latino communities at large include: the gender role of women precludes they have little to no advanced knowledge about sex and sexuality, machismo among males may dissuade condom use, and there is less material written in Spanish educating Hispanics and Latinos about the dangers of unprotected sex.

The ORWH reported in 2006 that large portions of Hispanic women work in the semiconductor and agriculture industries, both of which have occupational hazards. Workers in the semiconductor industry experience occupational illnesses at three times the rate of workers in other manufacturing industries. Agricultural workers are exposed to pesticides, the use of faulty equipment, and to a range of health problems such as dermatitis, musculoskeletal and soft-tissue problems, communicable diseases, and reproductive disorders, as well as health problems related to climate. Among Hispanic subpopulations Mexican Americans appear to enjoy better health than would be predicted, given their high poverty status and low utilization rates for health care services for both physical and mental conditions. Specifically, Mexican American women are less likely than white or black American women to have hypertension.

African American Women

According to the U.S. Census Bureau, black Americans are a largely urban population (more than 87 percent) and reside in all 50 states. Fifty-four percent of African Americans live in thirteen southern states—Alabama, Arkansas, Florida, Georgia, Kentucky, Louisiana, Maryland, Mississippi, North Carolina, South Carolina, Tennessee, Texas, and Virginia. However, several other non-southern states also have large African-American populations: California, Illinois, Michigan, and New York. The U.S. Centers for Disease Control and Prevention reports morbidity and mortality rates for African Americans from many conditions (cancer, HIV/AIDS, pneumonia, and homicide) exceeding those for whites.

More black women live in poverty in the United States (one-fourth) than any other group of women. In addition, single-parent, female-headed households—which represent 44 percent of all black-family households—were living in poverty to a greater degree than the entire black population. According to the ORWH, in 2006, most black women were employed in service occupations (27 percent), followed closely by administrative support/clerical (23 percent). Inadequate income carries over into other aspects of daily life that impinge upon health. This includes exposure to inadequate housing, which increases exposure risks to communicable diseases, lead poisoning, and other harmful environment agents. Low income contributes to improper nutrition, chronic stress from trying to pay bills, dangerous jobs, violence, and reduced access to medical care. Malnutrition in young black girls may later result in low birth weight babies and high infant mortality when these girls become mothers. African American mothers are more likely than white mothers to live in areas with high levels of air and water pollution. High blood levels of lead are more prevalent in black women and are associated with higher blood pressure levels among blacks. The risk of lung cancer associated with cigarette smoking is significantly greater for black women than for white. African American women make use of health care facilities and services at about the same rate as white women. Despite a similar use of preventive screenings, black breast cancer patients tend to be diagnosed at a more advanced stage than other women, and significantly fewer black women than white women survive 5 years after diagnosis with breast cancer. The ORWH cited several factors identified as barriers to diagnosis, care, and treatment for black women, including: poor access to health care services, lack of education and knowledge about cancer prevention and screening, mistrust of the health care system, fear and fatalism concerning treatment, and dealing with other competing priorities, such as food, shelter, and safety.

The ORWH reported in 2006 that racial discrimination and racism have remained significant operative factors in the health and health care of blacks. Racism creates barriers to getting access to health care and racial insults may contribute to stress-related health problems. Stress related to racism has been linked to the high rates of high blood pressure in blacks. The mortality rate for infants is higher among black women than white women. No one factor explains the higher infant mortality rate for black women or the higher frequency of low birth weight babies, but several factors have been linked to a possible cause: higher incidence of younger mothers; higher incidence of single mothers (and absent fathers); stress due to racism and poverty; lack of access to health care; delaying receiving prenatal care; and shorter intervals between pregnancies.

The ORWH reported in 2006 that African American women account for a growing share of the increasing numbers of AIDS cases in the U.S; black women represented 64 percent of AIDS cases reported among women. Black women are more likely than other women to die from AIDS. AIDS was the leading cause of death for black women ages 25 to 44 and the third leading cause of death for black women ages 35 to 44. A majority (52 percent) of black women in 2004 who were infected with HIV, the human immunodeficiency virus that causes AIDS, could not or did not identify the source of their infection. Intravenous drug use was indicated as the cause of HIV infection for 14 percent of all cases ever reported (1985 through 2004) among black women, while heterosexual contact was indicated as the cause of infection for 45 percent of all cases ever reported among black women.

Asian Women

The U.S. Census Bureau reported the majority of Asian Americans, more than 91 percent, reside in metropolitan areas. The five U.S. cities with the largest Asian population are New York, Los Angeles, San Jose, San Francisco, and Honolulu. The largest Asian American population is Chinese (23 percent) followed by Filipinos (19 percent), and Asian Indians (16 percent). The current fastest growing Asian American population is Koreans (almost 11 percent). The other major Asian American groups include the Japanese (nearly 8 percent) and Southeast Asians (Laotians, Cambodians, Vietnamese, and Hmong). More than 60 percent of all Japanese Americans were born in the United States, making them one of the most acculturated Asian populations, with a stable middle class composed largely of white collar workers and professionals. According to the ORWH, the health problems of Asian Americans are worsened by a complex set of cultural, linguistic, structural, and financial barriers to care. This applies primarily to Asian Americans who are foreign born or whom are less acculturated to the U.S. system. Thirty-seven percent of Asian American women were reported in managerial or professional occupations. More than 33 percent of Asian American females had technical, sales, or administrative support

occupations, while 17 percent had service occupations. Poverty rates are generally low for Asian Americans. Poverty rates for Asian American subgroups were reported as: Hmong, 38 percent; Cambodians, 29 percent; and Filipinos, 6 percent. These high poverty subgroups tend to have less health insurance coverage, higher unemployment rates, and work in lower-wage jobs.

The ORWH reported in 2006 that Asian American women overall exhibit healthful lifestyle behaviors. Health risks that exist vary among Asian American subgroups. The risk of hypertension was highest for Japanese (28 percent), followed by Filipinos (22 percent), Koreans (18 percent), Vietnamese (17 percent), Chinese (16 percent), and South Asians (11 percent). Smoking has a low prevalence among Asian American women (10 percent) as compared to all American women (16 percent); among Asian American subgroups smoking is greatest among Filipino women at (11 percent) followed by Chinese women (6 percent). Tuberculosis is more common among Asian Americans than among all other racial/ethnic groups in the United States, nearly 21 times that of white non-Hispanic Americans.

Lack of knowledge about cancer for some Asian American subgroups contributes to a failure to get regular screening. The ORWH reported in 2006 that in one study of Cambodian and Vietnamese American women in Philadelphia, 71 percent did not know what cancer is. In 2006, the ORWH further reported the results of a survey of Vietnamese women in Seattle that found 39 percent did not think cervical cancer was curable, even if detected early, and 35 percent believed illness was "a matter of Karma or fate." Cervical cancer disproportionately affects certain Asian women, with Vietnamese women having one of the highest incidences of invasive cervical cancer than any other racial/ethnic group in the United States (43 per 100,000). The incidence among Korean American women is 15 per 100,000. Hmong women have a high cervical cancer rate at 33.7 percent per 100,000 and, once diagnosed, are less likely to accept Western medical treatment for cervical cancer. Cervical cancer is the most frequently occurring type of cancer among Laotian women and the second most common cancer among Cambodian women. Despite high incidence rates, Asian women often do not participate in screenings. This is explained by concerns with modesty, as well as concerns about pain and discomfort associated with the test. Breast cancer is the most common cancer among Chinese, Filipino, Japanese, and Korean women, and the second most common cancer for Vietnamese women. Asian American women often do not receive prenatal care. According to the ORWH this is due to a variety of cultural and socioeconomic factors, including lack of knowledge about its importance. Asian Americans often do not utilize mental health facilities or services. Fear of difficulties in communicating, compounded by shame, guilt, anger, depression, and other responses to certain stigmatized conditions such as mental illness and substance abuse, often deter Asian Americans from seeking care promptly. Many Asian Americans would prefer to be treated for physical symptoms, even if they have a psychological origin. Thus, many Asian Americans suffering from stress, trauma, and depression do not receive appropriate treatment.

Native American Indian and Alaskan Native Women

The ORWH reports that Native American Indian and Alaskan Native subgroups are culturally diverse to the extent that it is almost meaningless to classify them together or make comparisons. However, some shared experiences explain, for most members of this minority category, their health care utilization patterns. First, many Native Americans are highly suspicious of authority because of their history with the white government that included forced removal from their ancestral homelands, brutal colonization, and confinement to reservations. Thus, Native people today are strongly autonomous, non-linear thinkers when it comes to time, use indirect communication, and have a suspicion of authority. The U.S. Public Health Service oversees the Indian Health Services (IHS), which provides health care through clinics and hospitals to all who belong to a federally recognized tribe and live on or near the reservations. IHS services in urban areas and in nonreservation rural areas often are very limited and uncoordinated. Forty-six percent of all American Indians/Alaska Natives have no access to IHS facilities.

The forced relocation of Native American Indians/ Alaska Natives placed them in communities in which they confront racism and hostility from non-Native neighbors. The ORWH reported in 2006 that this racism along with a mistrust of the U.S. government has created low self-esteem among many Natives. Racism and discrimination has contributed to the incidence of poverty of individuals: American Indians, 26 percent; Eskimos, 19 percent; Aleutians, 17 percent. Poverty rates for female-headed households is even greater than for individuals in that 33 percent of all Native American Indian/Alaska Native households were female headed, and 38 percent of these households had incomes below the poverty level. More than one-third of all Native American Indian/Alaska Native children under the age of six are estimated to live in poverty. Poverty and unemployment have fostered a welfare dependency and diets that consist of government commodity foods that are high in both fat and calories. Seventy-seven percent of male and 61 percent of female Native American Indians/Alaska Natives are reported to be overweight

and at risk for diabetes. Native American Indians and Alaska Natives have among the highest Type II diabetes rates in the world and these rates are increasing in epidemic proportions. End-stage renal (kidney) disease is 3.5 times as common among Native American Indians/ Alaska Natives as among whites. The ORWH reported in 2006 that a sedentary lifestyle and sharp decreases in hunting and gathering have contributed to the high prevalence of obesity and related health problems and mortality among Native American Indians/Alaska Natives. Of all the Native American Indian/Alaska Native women, 28 percent were hypertensive, 35 percent were current smokers, and 29 percent were obese.

The ORWH reported in 2006 that exposure to dangerous toxins is one source of health risks for Native American Indians/Alaska Natives. Of the more than 1000 open dumps located on Native American Indian/ Alaska Native lands, a third contained hazardous waste or waste that required special handling. Lacking a safe water supply or sewage disposal also places Native American Indians/Alaska Natives at risk of illness and disease. One of every five homes lacks complete plumbing facilities. Fewer than half of homes on reservations are connected to a public sewer system. After heavy rainfalls, waste and sewage can wash back into the community, causing contamination and infection. Forty percent of housing on reservations is considered inadequate, compared to about 6 percent of all homes in the United States.

Family violence is highly problematic for Native American Indians/Alaska Natives as frustrated males, and some females, take their rage out on family members in many forms: child abuse and neglect, elder abuse, intimate partner violence and sexual assault, and sexual abuse of young children. American Indian victims of intimate and family violence are more likely than victims of other races to be injured and need medical attention. Native American Indian/Alaska Native women often cope with victimization (from incest, rape, and other forms of sexual assault) experienced in childhood and adolescence by escaping into alcohol and drugs and doing other high-risk behaviors. Among Native American/ Alaska Native women, death rates associated with alcoholism are much higher than among women of all races. Native American/Alaska Native women who are alcoholics or substance abusers often do not receive hospitalization, detoxification, or counseling for their addictions.

Native Hawaiian or Other Pacific Islander Women

The U.S. Census Bureau estimated in 2009 that 578,000 persons identified themselves as Native Hawaiian and Other Pacific Islander, of which nearly half were women.

Native Hawaiians are the largest subpopulation at 36 percent, followed by Samoans at 23 percent, and Other Pacific Islanders at 19 percent of this population. The ORWH reported in 2006 that the health problems of Native Hawaiians reflect their socioeconomic status with nearly 15 percent living well below the poverty level; this 15 percent makes up the largest portion of the total 20 percent of persons living in poverty in the State of Hawaii. Thirty-five percent of female- headed households had incomes below the poverty level. Poverty among Native Hawaiian women is associated with labor market outcomes. Native Hawaiian and Other Pacific Islander women were 8.3 percent of the females in the civilian labor force, but they were 15.9 percent of the unemployed females in the civilian labor force.

The ORWH reported in 2006 that many Native Hawaiians engage in high-risk behaviors and the group as a whole has poorer health outcomes, such as lower life expectancy than other groups in Hawaii. In one study comparing whites, Japanese, Native Hawaiians, Filipinos, and Chinese in Hawaii, Native Hawaiians ranked highest in behavioral risk factors such as being overweight, smoking, and excessive use of alcohol, but not in risk factors such as physical inactivity. More than 71 percent of Native Hawaiians/Part Hawaiians in Hawaii were reported to be overweight. Twenty-six percent of Hawaiians reported being smokers. Native Hawaiian women (and men) who smoke have a greater risk of developing lung cancer than white women (and men) who smoke. Native Hawaiians often enter medical treatment at late stages of disease, seeking medical treatment only when self-care and traditional practices have not brought sufficient relief. This pattern applies to prenatal care for women. Seventy-eight percent of Hawaiian women began prenatal care in the first trimester compared to 83 percent of all women in the United States who began care early in their pregnancies. Nearly 5 percent of all Native Hawaiian women waited until the third trimester to seek prenatal care or received no prenatal care.

The U.S. Centers for Disease Control and Prevention reported in 2003 that heart disease and cancer are the major causes of death among Native Hawaiians. The hypertension rate for Native Hawaiians was 26.6 percent, greater than the risk for hypertension among the general population of Hawaii. The ORWH reported in 2006 that breast cancer is the most common cancer for Native Hawaiian women. Native Hawaiian women have the highest incidence of breast cancer of all women in Hawaii. According to the ORWH, because the perception of cancer in Hawaiians is bound up with beliefs about shame, guilt, and retribution, Native Hawaiian breast cancer patients often are fatalistic; many feel powerless to control the outcome of the disease. AIDS also affects Native Hawaiian females, but this is less than would be expected, given their share of the population. Between 2000 and 2004, nine cases of AIDS were reported among Native Hawaiian females which represents 12 percent of all AIDS cases reported among females in the state of Hawaii during that period.

Adolescent Females

If one defines the adolescent population as between ages 10 and 19 years, then it accounted for 13.2 percent of the U.S. population in 2009. U.S. Census Bureau statistics reveal that adolescents are a very diverse group. In 2009, 35 percent of all adolescents were members of a racial/ethnic group other than white non-Hispanic, with this expected to grow to 40 by the year 2020. Teenagers of color comprised more than half of all adolescents whose families had incomes in the poverty level. The ORWH reported in 2006 that living in poverty plays a critical role in access to health care services and in shaping health outcomes of adolescents, as it does for adults. Adolescents have low rates of physician contact and of medical examinations. In 2001, nearly 15 percent of females ages 12 to 17 reported they had not had contact with a health care professional in more than a year. Nearly 13 percent of all adolescents ages 12 to 17 were uninsured in 2003; of the uninsured adolescent group this represented: 16 percent black, 24 percent Hispanic, 16 percent Asian, 17 percent Native Hawaiian/Other Pacific Islander, and 18 percent Native American Indian/Alaska Native.

According to the ORWH, adolescent females are about twice as likely as adolescent males to report severe depressive symptoms and to consider or attempt suicide. Young Asian-American women have the highest depression rates for any group in the United States, and the second highest suicidal rate for females ages 15 to 24. Native American Indian/Alaska Native adolescents are more likely than other teens to attempt suicide, at 22 percent. Also, Native American teens are more likely to die as a result of the suicide attempt than adolescents from other ethnic groups. Fifteen percent of Hispanic adolescents attempted suicide in the previous 12 months compared to 10 percent white and 9 percent black. In 2001, nearly 20 percent of females ages 12 to 17 received mental health treatment.

The ORWH reports that adolescents are more likely to participate in behaviors with a high health risk such as: unprotected sexual intercourse, substance use or abuse, and operating a motor vehicle in an unsafe manner. Black adolescent females were most likely to report currently being sexually active (44 percent) with about a third of Hispanic (36 percent) and white (33 percent) adolescent females reporting current sexual activity. High rates of teen pregnancy are found among young Hispanic and black women. Teen pregnancy rates among black adolescents are lower than the rates among

Hispanic adolescents but higher than the rates among white adolescents. Teen females of color made up comparable percentages of HIV/AIDS cases of all women diagnosed, with the largest group of infected teen females being black, followed by Hispanics and a relatively smaller number for other teens of color.

Substance abuse is a common health risk for teens. The ORWH reported in 2006 that adolescent females reporting current cigarette use (defined as smoking on at least one occasion during the past 30 days) included the following portion of their adolescent, female ethnic group: 27 percent of white, 18 percent of Hispanic, and 11 percent of black. Health conditions associated with smoking and marijuana use include: addiction, lung cancer, emphysema, oral cancers, and cervical cancer. Alcohol abuse, prescription drug abuse, and the use of cocaine or crack by teens can also negatively influence present and future health. Adolescent females reporting current alcohol use (within the past 30 days) represent the following portion of their adolescent, female ethnic group: white and Hispanic, both 48 percent; Native American Indian/Alaska Native, 47 percent; black, 37 percent; and Asian/Pacific Islander, 25 percent. Current marijuana use for adolescent females is distributed as the following portions among their age and gender, ethnic group: white and Hispanic, 20 percent; black 18 percent. Driving a motor vehicle in an unsafe manner is also a common health risk for teens. White and black adolescent females have similar unsafe driving patterns. Adolescent females indicating that they had been driving while drinking alcohol represented the following shares of their ethnic group: 10 percent white and 5 percent black; in addition, 30 percent of these same groups reported riding with a driver who had been drinking.

In conclusion, health risk behaviors exist among all adolescents, but certain health risk behaviors are more common among some ethnic groups than others. It is of great concern that female adolescents in all ethnic groups are less likely to visit a physician than any other age group of women. How can we design a health care program that can reach out to female teenagers from diverse cultures, backgrounds, and sometimes different languages? If many teenagers will not go to health care clinics, how can we increase female adolescent usage of health care services and facilities?

Elderly Women

The U.S. Census Bureau reported for 2010 that there were 49,972,181 million persons (or 16.2 percent of the total population) who were age 62 years and over; this is a rise of 21.1 percent since the year 2000. The older population is expected to grow to 72 million by 2030, representing approximately 20 percent of the population, due to the aging baby boom generation. In 2005 older women composed 6.9 percent of the total population, while men composed 5.2 percent. Older women represent a larger portion of the elderly population than men within every age group. Of the elderly, 83 percent were white non-Hispanic, 8 percent were black, 6 percent were Hispanic, and 3 percent were Asian, with the remaining ethnic groups combined making up 1 percent. By the year 2020, these numbers for elderly persons are expected to shift, with white non-Hispanic numbers going down at least 6 percent and Hispanic numbers rising at least 3 percent, while black elderly numbers are expected to rise about 1 percent.

The *Women's Health USA, 2007* of DHHS reported that employment plays a significant role in the lives of many older Americans. In 2006, more than 2.3 million women aged 65 years or older were working, accounting for 11.4 percent of women in this age group. While elderly men are more likely than women to be employed, since 1994 the percentage of employed older adults has increased faster among women than men. Older women who chose to retire cite a variety of reasons, including being required to do so, poor health, wanting to do other things, and wanting to spend time with family. Very few cited not liking work as a reason for retirement.

According to the ORWH 2006 report, elderly women of color share with all elderly women many characteristics that impact their access to health care: They outnumber men in every senior age group and they are more likely to be widowed than men. Also, the health of elderly women of color reflects the cumulative effects of living in a society in which they often face disadvantages because of their gender and their color. These disadvantages include limited resources available throughout their lives to meet health care needs. Lower socioeconomic status, including higher poverty rates, is more prevalent in elderly women of color than white elderly women. This may cause them to have to work longer in their life and may limit their ability to afford health care or medication. Elderly women are likely to be widowed and thus live alone and be heads of households. Among unmarried women 65 years of age and older, black and Hispanic women are more likely than white women to be poor or near poor, that is, 49 percent of unmarried Hispanic elderly women and 42 percent of unmarried black elderly women. Medicare is a federal government program that subsidizes health care costs for the elderly, but Medicare does not cover all of the expenses incurred by the elderly population. When they can afford it, many elderly supplement Medicare benefits with private insurance, Medicaid, or other types of insurance.

Lack of utilization or access to health care may result in a failure to diagnose breast cancer at earlier stages for elderly women. For instance, the ORWH reports that many black women, especially those who live in rural areas, are unaware of their breast cancer risk and the need for a breast cancer screening. The ORWH reports that part of this problem is due to a failure by physicians and health care providers to refer elderly black women for screening. Studies have shown that if a physician or health care worker informs a woman of her cancer risk, she is much more likely to get a mammogram. Some avoid a breast cancer screening due to a sense of fatalism or fear of cancer. Avoidance of breast cancer screening by elderly women is about the same for all ethnic groups: 66 percent for blacks, and 68 percent for both white non-Hispanics and Hispanics.

Functional disabilities, that is, limitations in activities of daily living, are more frequent in elderly people of color. The ORWH reported in 2006 that black and Hispanic elderly women were more likely than white elderly women to rate their health as fair to poor—43, 39, and 24 percent, respectively. Arthritis is especially severe for African American women and prevalent in other women of color. Osteoporosis, often the cause of hip fractures among elderly women, is known to be more common in Asian women than other elderly women of color. Hip fractures in elderly black women occur about half as frequently as in white women. Elderly Native American/Alaska Native women reported a greater incidence of diabetes than all U.S. women. Among black women, diabetes affects 26 percent of those aged 65 to 74 and 20 percent of those 75 and older. Diabetes is a prominent cause of death among African American, Hispanic, and Native American/Alaska Native elders, while hypertension is a major killer of both Asian, Pacific Islander, and African American elders.

Psychosocial stress is higher for elderly people of color because of a higher incidence of low income, minimal education, substandard housing, a general lack of opportunity, and having fewer social and psychological resources available to them. A strong support system can buffer these effects and reduce the risk of mental illness in elderly women.

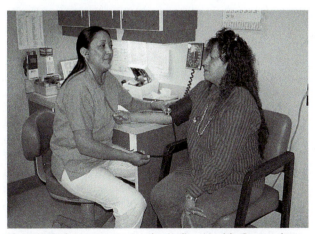

Flora Archuletta, a nurse at the Indian Health Center, has a special interest in Native American women's health issues.

Due to a history of discrimination, especially in southern states, older black women may not turn to the health care system for support and information. And for all elder women, hearing and vision disabilities associated with age may interfere with a desire or ability to travel to health care facilities. Even when they do utilize health care facilities, some elder persons may have difficulty hearing the health care worker or reading health care instructions. Neighborhood, community health clinics and outreach programs have the best chance of providing elderly the services they need. Unfortunately, these programs are too few in number and underfunded, and these facilities lack the specialists required for illnesses common for elder women, such as diabetes, osteoporosis, and hypertension. How would a federal, universal health care program contribute to health care provision for the elderly? What specific issues would this type of program need to address to provide comprehensive coverage for the health care needs of elderly women, including elderly women of color?

ETHNIC, CLASS, AND GENDER BIAS IN HEALTH RESEARCH

Historically, a majority of human health studies have been performed only with white, middle-class, young to middle-aged male subjects. Applications of research outcomes to individuals not represented in a study remain purely hypothetical. A case in point: The National Institutes of Health (NIH) was placed under congressional investigation in 1990 for failing to include female subjects in health studies that dictated diagnostic and prescriptive guidelines for both men *and* women. "The NIH excuse for not using females in such studies—that additional costs and complications are incurred with women subjects because of their numerous physiological differences in comparison with men—is the very reason women should have been included."[54]

Gender bias is common in health research. Some medications prescribed for women have not been tested on women, and some diagnostic and treatment guidelines for women are based on studies performed strictly with male samples.

Ethnic bias is also very present in health research. Studies that do incorporate women as subjects typically limit the subject pool to white, middle-class, young to middle-aged females. Ethnic minorities remain significantly underrepresented in health research.

Socioeconomic bias is prevalent in the health field. The provision of continuous, high-quality health care is often limited to the middle and upper class—that is, to those who have plenty of money or can afford health insurance. Social programs for the underprivileged, such as Social Security, Welfare, Medicaid, and Medicare are limited and frequently targeted by politicians for budget cuts. The poor are often deprived of adequate health care, the middle class can usually manage to at least maintain good health care, and the wealthy can take the greatest advantage of the most up-to-date health information and medical treatment. In addition, even when health care is available, educational efforts about certain health risks or the availability of medical treatment are usually targeted toward the upper and middle class via restricted avenues such as a doctor's office or specialized magazines. Lower-income families may never know that a health service or a health risk exists unless special efforts are made to reach out to this population.

Another cultural issue of concern is geographic differences. The majority of inner-city families are poor, and they are often not aware of health services or cannot afford them. Rural families frequently do not have quick access to hospitals or specialists, and thus adequate health care may not be available when needed. Or the family may have to drive a long distance to receive emergency health care or special services. Urban and suburban families are the most fortunate regarding the availability and affordability of quality health care.

WOMEN'S HEALTH RESEARCH

Historically, women's health research focused on diseases affecting fertility and reproduction—a focus reflective of the value society placed on women, that of primarily being a reproductive organism. Other disease research has focused disproportionately on men. Despite this imbalance, new drug therapies tested on men, once approved, were prescribed to women without comparable trials of clinical safety or efficacy. For example, a 1994 study suggested that aspirin could help prevent heart attacks in men. Women were not included in this study even though heart disease was the number-one killer of U.S. women. Yet aspirin was now recommended to both men and women as a preventive measure for heart attacks. Women have been excluded from medical research for at least two reasons: (1) concerns about pregnancy during a trial and (2) concerns that women's changing hormone levels during menstrual cycles might skew test results. We now know that there are no significant reasons to exclude women in medical research. In most cases, both sexes respond similarly to many therapies; however, there may be exceptions. For example, women may need lower dosages, or therapies may need to be specific to women.

The first comprehensive effort to clinically study health issues for women was the Nurses' Health Study.

The Nurses' Health Study began in 1976, enrolling about 121,000 nurses. In 1989 a second group of 116,000 was enrolled in the Nurses' Health Study II. The groups, designated NHS I and NHS II, were followed by means of a biennial mail questionnaire that inquired about lifestyle and health problems. Results from the Nurses' Health Study were published in *Nursing* and other medical journals over the years.

In response to public criticism of the lack of involvement of women subjects in its medical research, the National Institutes of Health in 1990 established the Office of Research on Women's Health (ORWH). The earliest undertakings of the ORWH included development of a research agenda to identify and address gaps in the biomedical community's knowledge of women's health, and strengthening and revitalizing already-existing NIH guidelines and policies for the inclusion of women and minorities in clinical studies.

The ORWH launched the Women's Health Initiative (WHI) in 1991. The WHI was transferred in October 1997 to the NIH division, the National Heart, Lung, and Blood Institute (NHLBI), where it is conducted as a consortium effort in cooperation with the National Cancer Institute and the National Institute of Arthritis and Musculoskeletal and Skin Diseases.

The WHI is a long-term, national study that focuses on strategies for preventing heart disease, breast and colorectal cancer, and osteoporosis in women, especially postmenopausal women. The WHI is one of the largest studies of its kind ever undertaken in the United States and involves more than forty centers nationwide and 162,000 American women ages 50 to 79, about 18 percent from minority groups. Enrollment in the study began in 1993 and ended in 1998. Some of the first results for the WHI were released in 2005. The WHI conducted three primary clinical studies: hormone replacement therapy, dietary modification, and calcium and vitamin D supplements. Studies and reports can be located at the following Web sites: Women's Health Initiative (http://www.nhlbi.nih.gov/whi/), Women's Health Initiative Scientific Resources (http://www.whiscience.org/), and Women's Health Initiative—Clinical Trials (http://clinicaltrials.gov/show/NCT00000611).

In 1990 the U.S. Department of Health and Human Services released *Healthy People 2000: National Health Promotion and Disease Prevention Objectives*. This document outlined the strategic plan for improving the health of the public and paid special attention to women's health issues. The three primary goals for the nation were (1) to increase the span of healthy life for Americans, (2) to reduce health disparities among Americans, and (3) to achieve access to preventive services for all Americans. An important follow-up document was published in 1996 titled *Healthy People 2000: Midcourse Review and 1995 Revisions*. The revision, *Healthy People*

2010, had two primary goals: (1) to increase quality and years of healthy life and (2) to eliminate health disparities. *Healthy People 2010* "challenges individuals, communities, and professionals—indeed all of us—to take specific steps to ensure that good health, as well as long life, are enjoyed by all." *Healthy People 2020* was released in two phases— the "Education for Health" framework (the vision, mission, goals, focus areas, and criteria for selecting and prioritizing objectives) was released in 2009. In 2010, the *Healthy People 2020* objectives were released along with guidance for achieving the new 10-year targets. It is available from the U.S. Department of Health and Human Services (see the Web site http://www.healthypeople.gov/).

SOCIAL, POLITICAL, AND MEDICAL CONTEXT

Women and men differ in terms of biological makeup, power, status, norms, and roles in society. The WHO stresses that these differences must be acknowledged, analyzed, and addressed through gender analysis and actions.[55] "In May 2007, the World Health Assembly, WHO's supreme decision-making body, adopted resolution WHA60.25, which urges Member States to mainstream gender in any planned health action and requests the WHO Director-General to ensure full implementation of the WHO strategy for integrating gender analysis and actions into the work of WHO. WHO takes action in four strategic directions:

1. Building WHO capacity for gender analysis and planning
2. Bringing gender into the mainstream of WHO's management
3. Promoting the use of sex-disaggregated data and gender analysis
4. Establishing accountability"[56]

According to the then WHO Director-General, Dr. Margaret Chan, "The obstacles that stand in the way of better health for women are not primarily technical or medical in nature. They are social and political, and the two go together."[57] Since 2007, WHO's Gender, Women and Health Network has been piloting and developing practical capacity building materials to assist in the progressive mainstreaming of gender considerations in health sector activities. The WHO report Women and Health: Today's Evidence Tomorrow's Agenda was published in 2009. This is a report on women and health—both women's health needs and their contribution to the health of societies. Women's health has long been a concern for WHO, but today it has become an urgent priority. This report explains why. Using current data, it takes stock of what we know now about the health of women throughout their lives and across the different regions of the world (information on ordering or downloading this report can be found at the website www.who.int/gender/en/). To further facilitate remediation of gender inequities, the *Gender Mainstreaming Manual for Health Managers: A Practical Approach* was published by WHO in 2011 and serves as the core capacity building manual, with a range of tools available to support national teams to identify and address gender and health inequities. According to WHO, without due attention to gender equality, health services, programs, laws, and policies will have limited effects and women will not achieve their full health potential over the life-course.[58]

Women have health needs and concerns that are unique to their gender. Thus, it is important to have a health text dedicated specifically to women. The culture of women has evolved, like all cultures do. Who women are today and the issues they face have developed over time as a result of both positive and negative events throughout history. This text addresses the importance of women's health issues within the context of social, political, and medical arenas. We hope you enjoy using this text as much as we enjoyed writing it. The topic of women's health is vast and we do not suppose that we have covered everything. We do hope that we have addressed most of the major issues. We leave it to you to continue the journey and advocate for greater awareness and attention to the field of women's health.

Chapter Summary

- There are three common types of health action: proactive care, health care maintenance, and reactive care.
- Holistic health care incorporates all that we know about health and utilizes this information to keep the body, mind, and spirit healthy.
- Sexual discrimination affects women in the workplace, in the pharmacy, and in personal lifestyle choices.

- A major cultural bias is the absence of adequate representation of women and ethnic minorities in medical research.
- Women around the globe share many of the same health concerns. However, cultural differences significantly impact the type and severity of these concerns.
- The status of women's health must be examined from cultural, political, and social perspectives.

Review Questions

1. Why do we need a text specific to women's health issues?
2. Can you name and describe three common types of health action?
3. How would you describe holistic health care?
4. Why is cultural sensitivity necessary in health care?
5. Can you name the various types of cultural bias in health care?
6. What are some health issues that are shared by women around the globe?
7. What are some major contributions to the U.S. women's health movement of the 1960s and 1970s?
8. What are some major social and political events in the history of the U.S. women's movement?
9. What is the Nurses' Health Study?
10. What is the Women's Health Initiative?

Resources

Web Sites

American Medical Women's Association
http://www.amwa-doc.org/

Black Women's Health
www.blackwomenshealth.com

Black Women's Health Imperative
http://www.blackwomenshealth.org/site/c.eeJIIWOCIrH/
b.3082485/k.BEBA/Home.htm

Centers for Disease Control and Prevention, Women's Health
www.cdc.gov/women

Feminist.com
www.feminist.com

Feminist Majority Foundation
www.feminist.org

Healthy People 2010
www.healthypeople.gov/

Jacob's Institute of Women's Health
http://www.jiwh.org/

Middle East and Islamic Studies Collection, Cornell University
Library: Women and Gender Issues
www.library.cornell.edu/colldev/mideast/women.htm

Mujer (Hispanic women's organization)
www.mujerinc.net

Mujeres Latinas En Acción (Latina Women in Action; bilingual site)
www.mujereslatinasenacción.org

National Center for Health Statistics
www.cdc.gov/nchs

National Institutes of Health
www.nih.gov

National Organization for Women
www.now.org

National Women's Health Information Center
www.womanshealth.gov

National Women's Health Network
www.nwhn.org

National Women's Health Resource Center
http://www.healthywomen.org/

Native American Women's Health Education Resource Center
www.nativeshop.org

Native Web
www.nativeweb.org

North American Menopause Society
http://www.menopause.org/

Office of Research on Women's Health, National Institutes
of Health
http://orwh.od.nih.gov

Office of Women's Health, Food and Drug Administration
www.fda.gov/womens

Older Women's League
http://www.owl-national.org/

Our Bodies, Ourselves
http://www.ourbodiesourselves.org/

Society for Women's Health Research
http://www.womenshealthresearch.org/site/PageServer

United Nations
www.un.org

United Nations Entity for Gender Equality and the Empowerment
of Women
www.unwomen.org

U.S. Department of Health and Human Services
www.hhs.gov

Women's Human Rights Net
www.whrnet.org

Women in the Middle East—Columbia University Libraries,
Middle East and Islamic Studies
www.library.columbia.edu/indiv/area/mideast.html

World Health Organization, Department of Gender,
Women and Health
www.who.int/gender/en

References

1. Smith-Spark, L. 2004. How did rape become a weapon of war? BBC News. http://news.bbc.co.uk/2hi/4078677.stm, pp. 1–2.
2. Drakulic, S. 2008. Rape as a weapon of war. *New York Times.* http://www.nytimes.com/2008/06/26/opinion/26iht-eddrakulic.1.13013076.html?_r=1, pp. 1–2.
3. May, M. 2006. Sex Trafficking: San Francisco is a major center for international crime networks that smuggle and enslave. http://www.sfgate.com (retrieved September 4, 2008).
4. Chesler, P. 2009, Spring. Are honor killings simply domestic violence? *Middle East Quarterly.* http://www.meforum.org/2067/are-honor-killings-simply-domestic-violence, pp. 1–2.
5. Spencer, R. 2008. Honor killing in Texas. Human Events.com. http://www.humanevents.com.php?id=24329, pp. 1–2.
6. Tuhus-Dubrow, R. 2007. USA: Rites and wrongs: Is outlawing female genital mutilation enough to stop it from happening here? The Female Genital Cutting Education and

Networking Project. http://fgmnetwork.org (retrieved September 4, 2008).

7. Robinson, B. 2008. Female genital mutilation in North American and Europe. http://www.religioustolerance.org (retrieved September 4, 2008).

8. Filkins, D. 2009. Afghan girls, scarred by acid, defy terror, embracing school. *The New York Times*. http://www.nytimes.com/2009/01/14/world/asia/14kandahar.html?r=1, p. 1.

9. Goodwin, L. 2011, March 13. Women in the world summit: A weekend of courageous women. *The Daily Beast*. http://www.thedailybeast.com/articles/2011/02/13/women-in-th-world-summit-a-weekend-of-courageous-women.htm. pp. 1–2.

10. Kennedy Cuomo, K. 2009. Rana Husseini: Honor killings. PBS. http://www.pbs.org/speaktruthtopower/rana.html, p. 1–5.

11. Husseini, R. n.d.. Biography of Rana Husseini. Rana Husseini Website. http://www.ranahusseini.com/Biography2.html, p. 1–4.

12. NPR Staff. 2012, Feb 22. A favored daughter fights for Afghan women. New Hampshire Public Radio. http://www.nhpr.org/post/favored-daughter-fights-afghan-women, pp. 1.

13. *Columbia encyclopedia*. 6th ed. 2003. www.encyclopedia.com (retrieved September 22, 2006).

14. Ibid.

15. Ibid.

16. Ibid.

17. National Women's Hall of Fame. 2003. *Great women*. www.greatwomen.org (retrieved September 22, 2006).

18. Ibid.

19. Ibid.

20. Ibid.

21. *Columbia encyclopedia*.

22. United States Department of Interior, National Register of Historic Places. 2000. *History of frontier nursing*. www.frontiernursing.org/history_of_fsn.htm (retrieved March 17, 2004).

23. Shaw, S., and J. Lee. 2007. *Women's voices, feminist visions*. 3rd. ed. New York: McGraw-Hill.

24. Ibid.

25. Ruth, S. 2001. *Issues in feminism*. 5th ed. Mountain View, CA: Mayfield.

26. Shaw and Lee, *Women's voices*.

27. Kirk, G., and M. Okazawa-Rey. 2007. *Women's lives: Multicultural perspectives*. 4th ed. New York: McGraw-Hill.

28. Shaw and Lee, *Women's voices*.

29. U.S. Equal Employment Opportunity Commission. 2012. Pregnancy discrimination charges EEOC & FEPAs Combined: FY 1997–2011. EEOC website, http://www.eeoc.gov/eeoc/statistics/enforcement/pregnancy.cfm.

30. About Women's Issues. 2006. Gender pay gap—women make less money. *New York Times*. http://womensissues.about.com/od/genderdiscrimination/i/isgendergap.htm (retrieved February 14, 2006).

31. OECD Employment Outlook 2010. OECD Family Database: Gender pay gaps for full-time workers and earnings differentials by educational attainment. http://www.oecd.org/social/family/database, p. 1.

32. Liptak, A. 2011, June 20. Justices rule for Wal-Mart in class-action bias case. *The New York Times*. http://www.nytimes.com/2011/06/21/business/21bizcourt.html?pagewanted=all.

33. Price, S. 2011, Sept. 19. Costco gender discrimination class action partially rejected. LEGAFI. http://legafi.com/lawsuits/news/900-costco-gender-discrimination-class-action-partially-rejected-

34. Wolfe, L. 2007, June 22. Glossary of bills and laws—H.R. 2831—Lilly Ledbetter Fair Pay Act of 2007: Bill to address discriminatory pay practices. About.com: Women in Business. http://womeninbusiness.about.com/od/billsandlaws/a/hr2831-lilly.htm.

35. National Organization for Women. Action alert: Support the Access to Legal Pharmaceuticals Act. 2005. June 23. www.now.org (retrieved February 16, 2006).

36. Jacobson, S., and G. C. Kovach. 2004. Birth-control battleground? *Denton Record-Chronicle*, April 1, p. 3A (originally printed in the *Dallas Morning News*).

37. About Women's Issues. 2006. Sexual harassment statistics in the workplace and in education. *New York Times*. http://womensissues.about.com/cs/sexdiscrimination/a/sexharassstats.htm (retrieved February 14, 2006).

38. Bingham, C., and L. L. Gansler. 2005. *Class action: The landmark case that changed sexual harassment law*. New York: Anchor, p. 70.

39. Ibid., p. 70.

40. Ibid., p. 70.

41. Ibid., p. 71.

42. Ibid., pp. 71–72.

43. Ibid., p. 72.

44. Ibid., p. 72.

45. Equal Employment Opportunity Commission. 2003. Guidelines on discrimination because of sex. 1604.11 Sexual harassment. July 1, p. 186.

46. Bingham and Gansler, p. 382.

47. Hill, C., & Kearl, H. 2011. *Crossing the line: Sexual harassment at school*. Washington, D.C.: American Association of University Women. http://www.aauw.org/learn/research/upload/CrossingTheLine.pdf.

48. Ibid.

49. Associated Press. 2005. WNBA star Swoopes says she's lesbian. *MSNBC.com*. http://msnbc.msn.com/id/9823452 (retrieved September 22, 2006).

50. CNN.com. 2008. Wedding bells chime for California same-sex couples. http://www.cnn.com/2008/US/06/16/samesexmarriage/index.html (retrieved June 16, 2008).

51. Human Rights Watch. March 14, 2011. A decade on, progress on same-sex marriages. http://www.hrw.org./news/2011/03/14/decade-progress-same-sex-marriages.

52. Barrionuevo, A. July 15, 2010. Argentina approves gay marriage, in a first for region. *The New York Times*. http://www.nytimes.com/2010/07/16/world/americas/16argentina.html.

53. U.S. Department of Health and Human Services. 2010. National healthcare disparities report 2010. DHHS. http://www.ahrq.gov/qual/nhdr10/nhdr10.pdf.

54. Chandler, C. 1991. The psychology of women: Approaching the twenty-first century. *Individual Psychology* 47 (4): 487.

55. World Health Organization. 2012. Gender, women and health. http://who.int/gender/en.

56. World Health Organization, Department of Gender, Women and Health. Gender equality is good for health. www.who.int/gender/about/about_gwh_20100526.pdf, p. 1

57. Ibid, p. 2.

58. World Health Organization. 2012. Gender, women and health.

Chapter Two

Becoming a Wise Consumer

CHAPTER OBJECTIVES

When you complete this chapter, you will be able to do the following:

◇ Define consumerism and identify the various components of consumer health

◇ Describe the benefits and practices of intelligent consumer choices

◇ Identify characteristics of effectual and qualified health care providers

◇ Differentiate between quackery and effective alternative healing and treatment methods

◇ Compare and contrast generic and brand-name prescription drugs

◇ Identify the types of information written on drug labels

◇ Explain the difference between prescription and over-the-counter drugs and provide examples of both

◇ Evaluate beauty-enhancing products that claim to be safe and beneficial

◇ Analyze the benefits and risks of beauty-enhancing procedures

◇ Explain the influence that advertising has on the images of and attitudes toward women

◇ Explain the impact of advertising on the financial, emotional, and social aspects of consumer practices

◇ Describe the appropriate actions necessary to become a wise and effective health consumer

CONSUMERISM

Being a wise consumer takes time and energy, but a lack of effective consumer skills and practices can cost you money. We are deluged with consumer information every day from an array of sources, some of which are reliable and others that are not. Included among these are news releases, public service media campaigns, publications for women, their families, and their health care providers, toll-free hotlines, governmental clearinghouse services, and of course, advertisements via various mediums. Consumer information from these varied sources can increase awareness and knowledge, influence attitudes and choices, and promote demands for better consumer services. They have to be credible and proven sources of information; otherwise, the information is of little value.

FYI

Consumer Bill of Rights[1]

I. Information Disclosure
Consumers have the right to receive accurate, easily understood information and some require assistance in making informed health care decisions about their health plans, professionals, and facilities.

II. Choice of Providers and Plans
Consumers have the right to a choice of health care providers that is sufficient to ensure access to appropriate high-quality health care. Access to Qualified Specialists for Women's Health Services: Women should be able to choose a qualified provider offered by a plan—such as gynecologists, certified nurse midwives, and other qualified health care providers—for the provision of covered care necessary to provide routine and preventative women's health care services.

III. Access to Emergency Services
Consumers have the right to access emergency health care services when and where the need arises. Health plans should provide payment when a consumer presents to an emergency department with acute symptoms of sufficient severity—including severe pain—such that a "prudent layperson" could reasonably expect the absence of medical attention to result in placing that consumer's health in serious jeopardy, serious impairment to bodily functions, or serious dysfunction of any bodily organ or part.

IV. Participation in Treatment Decisions
Consumers have the right and responsibility to fully participate in all decisions related to their health care. Consumers who are unable to fully participate in treatment decisions have the right to be represented by parents, guardians, family members, or other conservators.

V. Respect and Nondiscrimination
Consumers have the right to considerate, respectful care from all members of the health care system at all times and under all circumstances. An environment of mutual respect is essential to maintain a quality health care system.

VI. Confidentiality of Health Information
Consumers have the right to communicate with health care providers in confidence and to have the confidentiality of their individually identifiable health care information protected. Consumers also have the right to review and copy their own medical records and request amendments to their records.

VII. Complaints and Appeals
All consumers have the right to a fair and efficient process for resolving differences with their health plans, health care providers, and the institutions that serve them, including a rigorous system of internal review and an independent system of external review.

VIII. Consumer Responsibilities
In a health care system that protects consumers' rights, it is reasonable to expect and encourage consumers to assume reasonable responsibilities. Greater individual involvement by consumers in their care increases the likelihood of achieving the best outcomes and helps support a quality improvement, cost-conscious environment.

Public access to both health information and health misinformation abounds. Americans spend billions of dollars on unproven, worthless, and sometimes dangerous health remedies, with more money spent on "disease-curing" quackery than on research to prevent or cure these same diseases. As women, we often want to attain the body and beauty promised via weight loss gimmicks, miracle potions, or unnecessary elective surgeries. Knowledge about health products and health care personnel, procedures, and facilities is valuable. You can protect both your money and your health by developing and using wise consumer skills. (See *FYI:* "Consumer Bill of Rights.")

As of April 14, 2003, health care providers were required to comply with the requirements of the Health Insurance Portability and Accountability Act of 1996, also known as **HIPAA**. Establishing standards for the privacy of individuals, HIPAA created national standards related to the delivery of health care, health fraud and abuse, insurance portability, and simplification of electronic transmission of claims and privacy of medical records. The Privacy Rule requires (1) that patients receive information about their privacy rights, (2) that privacy procedures are adopted in hospitals and practices, (3) that employees are trained to understand the privacy procedures, (4) that a designated individual be in charge of privacy procedures, and (5) that patient records be secured.

CHOOSING A HEALTH CARE PROVIDER

Selecting your health care providers is an important consumer skill. You will be sharing some of the most intimate concerns of your life with these persons.

Health Tips

Selecting Your Health Care Provider

Upon entering the university, Elizabeth wants to search for a quality health care provider of the same caliber as her family-selected health care providers that she had for a number of years. She has two objectives: to locate two or three reputable physicians and then to determine which one best meets her health care needs. To do this, she will do the following:

To locate a provider

- Ask local friends and relatives for their recommendations.
- Check with the local medical society for suggestions specific to providers' specialty, gender, and age.
- Call local and/or regional women's health groups or organizations for suggestions.
- Call local hospitals to ask professional personnel about specific physicians. Check with the state

medical society or licensing board to determine whether any complaints have been registered about a particular provider.

Once located, to select a provider

- Discuss his or her general health care practices; is he or she a single provider or a member of a group?
- What are the office location, the hours, fees, insurance requirements, and waiting period for appointments?
- Ask about the use of local health care facilities and interaction with other physicians.
- Is the physician an HMO member or in another health care group?
- Request a preliminary interview to determine rapport, mutual respect, treatment approaches, and referrals to specialists.

Qualifications, training, reputation, availability, and patient relation skills of health care providers are important. See *Health Tips:* "Selecting Your Health Care Provider" for suggestions about how to find the right provider for you.

Once you have visited the health care provider, consider the following questions: Do I like this provider? Do I feel respected? Does she or he take the time to answer my questions patiently? Was I able to understand the physician's information and instructions? Would this provider consider my health concerns and opinion as a part of a satisfactory treatment plan?

Health Care Providers

Health care providers include a variety of medical practitioners who have completed training in an accredited medical school and passed a medical examination. They can be divided into three groups[2]:

1. Independent practitioners who have been trained and licensed for all types of medical practices. There are medical and osteopathic physicians.
2. Independent practitioners with restricted practices such as podiatrists, dentists, psychologists, and optometrists.
3. Ancillary practitioners who practice only under the supervision of a medical practitioner. These include nurses, physical therapists, physician assistants, pharmacists, nurse practitioners, occupational therapists, and X-ray and laboratory technicians.

The following information gives a thumbnail sketch of health care providers with differing educational levels, skills, abilities, and responsibilities.

Physician   The process of becoming a medical doctor, or MD, requires a minimum of 3 years of premedical college work for admission to medical school. However, 97 percent of premed students have a baccalaureate degree prior to admission.[3] Of those medical school students admitted in 2002, approximately 49.1 percent were women.[4] Students then spend 4 years in medical school, which should be accredited by a joint committee representing the American Medical Association (AMA) Council on Medical Education and the Association of American Medical Colleges. Following graduation, students must pass state or national board examinations to become licensed practitioners. (See *Women Making a Difference* to learn about a female physician who became surgeon general.)

Ever-changing research outcomes, improved technology, and new medicines create the need for developing medical specialties. Becoming a specialist such as a pediatrician, neurologist, or psychiatrist requires 3 or more years of additional training. Following the course work, the physician engages in additional clinical hours, obtains board certification, which means that the doctor has additional training, and passes a national examination in his or her specialty. A doctor of osteopathy, a DO, is legally equivalent to a medical doctor and is licensed to practice in all states. Prior to admission to an osteopathy school, the student must have 3 years of college work

Women Making a Difference

Antonia C. Novello: Surgeon General of the United States, 1990–1993

Antonia C. Novello was born and educated in Puerto Rico, receiving an MD degree from the University of Puerto Rico School of Medicine at San Juan in 1970. Following a fellowship in the Department of Pediatrics at Georgetown University, she was in private practice until 1978. Dr. Novello then held various positions in public health service at the National Institutes of Health (NIH), rising to the position of Deputy Director of the National Institute of Child Health and Human Development in1986. During her years at NIH, Dr. Novello earned an MPH degree from Johns Hopkins and made major contributions to the drafting and enactment of the Organ Transplantation Procurement Act of 1984, while assigned to the Senate Committee on Labor and Human Resources.

Antonia Novello was appointed surgeon general by President George H. W. Bush in 1990; she was the first Hispanic woman to hold this position. Dr. Novello focused on the health of women, children, and minorities as well as underage drinking, smoking, and AIDS. She helped to launch the Healthy Children Ready to Learn Initiative, and she worked with groups to promote immunization of children and childhood injury prevention. After her tenure as surgeon general, Dr. Novello served as the United Nations Children's Fund (UNICEF) Special Representative for Health and Nutrition from 1993 to 1996. Dr. Novello became commissioner of health for the State of New York in 1999. Antonia Novello has made a world of difference in the lives of women, children, and youth in her various health-related roles at the national level.

FYI

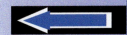

Periodic Checkups and Screening Tests[5]

Your doctor should ask about your . . .

- Family history, personal medical history, and any current medications, if any, that you take
- Dietary habits with special attention to fat, calories, fiber, iron, and calcium
- Exercise habits
- Use of any drugs, including alcohol and tobacco
- Safety practices (seat belt, safety equipment)
- Sexual practices related to disease prevention
- Birth control method (if any)
- What concerns you have about your health

Screening tests for generally healthy women include

- Blood pressure measurement: checked at least once or twice per year and during every doctor visit
- Clinical breast exam: yearly for all women aged 40 and over; every 3 years for women 20–40 years
- Mammography: yearly for women over 40; depending on family history of breast cancer, a physician may adjust these recommendations
- Pap smear: every 1–3 years beginning at age of first intercourse, or age 18
- Colorectal cancer: annual fecal occult blood test forage 50 and over and flexible sigmoidoscopy every 5 years
- Cholesterol screening: check every 5 years beginning at age 18, and more frequently as age increases or risks become prevalent
- Skin examination: every 3 years between 20 and 40 years of age, and every year for age 40 and over

related to the profession. During the 4 years of osteopathic college, the candidate will have over 5000 hours of training, followed by a 1-year rotating internship at an approved hospital. If the DO decides to specialize, which about one-half do, a 2- to 6-year residency follows, depending on the chosen specialty.[6] Osteopathic doctors specialize in such areas as obstetrics, neurology, psychiatry, and anesthesiology. There is very little difference in the training of DOs and MDs. The difference is more in the philosophy of treatment. The American Osteopathic Association states that osteopathic medicine must closely follow the Hippocratic approach to medicine in that the body's musculoskeletal system is central to a person's well-being. Osteopathic medicine, because of its hands-on approach to diagnoses, can provide an alternative to surgery and/or drugs. The profession maintains its independence in order to provide a unique and comprehensive approach to health care.

Ordering a wide range of tests and X-rays, taking blood, poking, prodding, and peering often compose the medical checkup. However, a more comprehensive look at an individual's lifestyle can often provide better quantity and quality of health information. A preventive health exam tailored to the age, risk factors, and life style of the patient can promote an enhanced quality of life and is more predictive of potential disease development. So, what constitutes a good periodic exam? See *FYI:* "Periodic Checkups and Screening Tests."

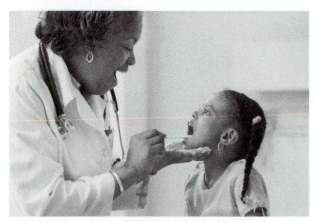

Selecting a health care provider is an important consumer skill.

Physician Assistant

A physician assistant (PA) works in the primary care medical setting under the supervision of a physician. He or she can give physical exams, prescribe drugs or therapies, and offer health counseling. Universities and medical schools that prepare PAs require varying entrance requirements and offer a curriculum that usually takes about 30 months to complete, including clinical training. Students may earn a Master of Physician Assistant Studies and then be a certified physician's assistant by passing an exam from the National Commission on the Certification of Physician Assistants. Because PAs are paid much less than physicians, health care programs often use them to help reduce the cost of health care. Physician assistants can work in private doctors' offices, hospitals, clinics, and other health care settings.

Nurse Practitioner

A nurse practitioner can function as a primary care provider but often performs under a physician's supervision. Training includes additional nursing education, usually at the master's level, beyond the requirements needed to become a registered nurse (RN). Licensed by the state, registered nurses assess patients' physical and emotional needs and assist physicians and patients in prevention and treatment practices. Nurse practitioners are certified through the American Nurses Credentialing Center (ANCC) for work in geriatric, pediatric, and family health care, as well as in elementary and secondary school nursing. Nurse practitioners may also specialize in women's health and work in settings that treat health concerns of women.

Midwife

Midwives are usually RNs who have received additional training and are certified to perform specific health care activities. One to two years of additional training is required from an approved school of midwifery. They can also earn nurse-midwife certification, CNM, which allows them to practice in almost every state by passing an exam from the American College of Nurse-Midwives.[7] Responsibilities include caring for pregnant women, managing labor and delivery, and caring form other and baby after childbirth. A midwife may also be a vital part of the obstetrical team in physicians' offices, clinics, and hospitals. Midwives often are certified in CPR as well as neonatal resuscitation. In some states, midwives are required to obtain continuing education credits to maintain current knowledge in the field. In the past, using midwives for childbirth and after-birth care was disparaged by traditional health care, but recently, trained and qualified midwives have been found to offer effective, lower-cost, and patient-friendly health care. Currently, between 6 and 10 percent of all births in this country are attended by midwives, and some foremost medical schools in the United States offer certified midwife training programs.[8]

Mental Health Therapists

Mental health professionals treat a variety of conditions related to one's mental and emotional well-being. Treatment can range from occasional outpatient counseling with single or group meetings to inpatient confinement using medication. Seeking professional counseling and locating a competent and highly trained therapist are essential when you are concerned about your mental or emotional health. Determining that you may need professional assistance with a mental or emotional health problem, what type of therapist should you seek? A wide range of mental health professionals have special training to work with a variety of issues. The most common types of mental health therapists include:[9]

- Psychiatrists, who have a doctorate in medicine which allows them to prescribe medication for mental health disorders, and includes 6–7 years' training in medicine, psychotherapy techniques, and mental health assessment with an emphasis in mental health pathology
- Psychologists, who have a doctorate in clinical or counseling psychology, which includes 6–7 years' training in psychotherapy techniques and assessment with an emphasis in pathology
- Counselors, who have a master's degree in the field of counseling, clinical or counseling psychology, or marriage and family therapy, which includes 2–3 years of training in psychotherapy techniques and assessment
- Clinical social workers, who have a master's degree in social work that includes 2–3 years' training in psychotherapy techniques and social work

Every mental health practitioner is required to have a license from the state where they practice. This license must be displayed in their office with visible issue and expiration dates. Most mental health practitioners are required to regularly renew their license to practice every 2 years, which includes completion of a certain amount and type of continuing education requirement.

Therapists should be trustworthy, nonjudgmental, empathetic, respectful, sincere, and well trained in their area of therapy. Consider the following criteria when determining the merits of a potential therapist:

- What are the credentials of the therapist?
- Is she or he a licensed therapist?
- Will your insurance cover the costs of this therapy?
- What type of treatment does the therapist use?
- Will he or she prescribe medication?
- How long and how often should you expect to be in treatment?
- Do you know anyone who this therapist has treated for a similar problem? Was the treatment successful?
- Are any complaints about this therapist filed with local medical personnel or professional licensing boards?

There are always "professionals" who will take our money and provide poor quality and even harmful health care. In some states, it is legal to use such titles as "therapists," "counselors," and "sex therapists" without any specific or certified credentials. Be smart! Check for the appropriate credentials before investing time and money with a mental health professional. Locate trusted physicians, and check with family, friends, or coworkers who can recommend competent and qualified professionals to work with you.

Reporting Unprofessional Treatment

Knowing what to do if you have received inadequate, unprofessional, or unethical health care treatment is important. Taking action immediately by contacting proper authorities and providing written statements and any supporting documentation will aid you and other potential patients to avoid unnecessary, painful, incorrect, or even fatal treatment at the hands of a health care provider. To report this concern, write a letter to the hospital or doctor involved and send a copy to any or all of the following: a referring doctor, the administrator or director of the hospital or clinic, the local medical society, the state licensing board, your insurance carrier, and any local health consumer or women's health group. A doctor–patient relationship should be one of equality and mutual respect, with you and your doctor making responsible and health-enhancing decisions together. An online complaint form is found at www.ftc.gov/ftc/consumer.htm.

HEALTH CARE DELIVERY

The socioeconomic circumstances and roles of women continue to evolve and change as they relate to parenting, employment, and relationships. Today, the health care needs of women vary significantly from the time when the "typical" female was a stay-at-home wife and mother and sheltered under her partner's health care plan and the long-time family physician. Meeting the changing needs of women's health care is the responsibility of the health care system, health-related institutions, and women themselves. How do we meet this challenge? There is a need to improve health care delivery for women and to provide for health needs whether women live in the inner city, rural America, or the "burbs." This could be accomplished by having health care clinics near public transport or in inner-city neighborhoods. An awareness of the differing health needs of women could be developed via better training in medical and nursing schools and by fostering an understanding attitude toward the special health needs of women.

Removing barriers to quality health care services is essential if women are to garner the necessary examinations, treatment, and rehabilitation. Barriers may include too little money for health care, lack of insurance, no transportation to and from health facilities, distant travel to health care providers, job-related demands, and no sick leave or time allotted away from the job. (Health insurance concerns are discussed later in this chapter.)

Solutions to effective health care delivery specific to the needs of women must include experts in medical, community, and government factions. All of these factions must identify the problems related to health care for women, determine the various alternatives and the positives and negatives of each, assess the possible solutions, and then act accordingly. A health care delivery system that addresses all women must be accessible, culturally relevant, affordable, and available.

HOME HEALTH TESTS

At-home methods to determine the status of one's health have come a long way from only using scales, thermometers, and taking your pulse. Over-the-counter home health test kits have expanded our access to faster results and vital information related to numerous health concerns. Well over $1 billion is spent annually in markets or online to monitor health conditions in the privacy of one's home. Home health tests can mean lower medical costs, better monitoring of chronic conditions, and earlier detection of health problems. Additionally, home health tests can be an easy-to-use method for providing private information in a brief amount of time. However, over reliance on these various tests (e.g., used as an indicator of diagnosis or cure) or misinterpretation of the results can be dangerous; a wise consumer will not make medical decisions without consulting with a medical professional. The FDA offers suggestions for purchasing home diagnostic tests and general precautions to consider.[10]

There are basically three types of home tests: (1) diagnostic tests (for sexually transmitted infections, ovulation, pregnancy, urinary tract infections), (2) continuous monitoring tests (for blood glucose, blood pressure) that are often recommended by one's physician to assist in overseeing an existing disease, and (3) screening tests to determine if a disease is present even though symptoms are not present, such as cholesterol testing or hepatitis screening The best known are pregnancy tests, whereas the biggest sellers are blood glucose monitors and test strips used by individuals with diabetes. (See *FYI:* "Common Home Health Tests.") Together they account for 90 percent of home health test kits sold nationally.

It has been estimated that one in seven medical tests, including those administered by health professionals, results in false findings. Certainly, the margin for error associated with the general consumer administering a test at home can be even greater. However, many of the use-at-home test kits, when used properly, can provide accurate and cost-effective results. Complete *Assess Yourself:* "Improving Your Chances for Accurate Home Health Test Results" to help improve the effectiveness of your test results.

COMPLEMENTARY AND ALTERNATIVE MEDICINE

Complementary and alternative medicine (CAM), such as herbs, acupuncture, chiropractic care, and massage therapy, increasingly are recognized as having the potential for relief, treatment, and cure of certain diseases. **Complementary medicine** is used *with* conventional medicine, and **alternative medicine** is used *in place of* conventional medicine. CAM has been defined as a group of diverse medical and health care systems, practices, and products that are not presently considered

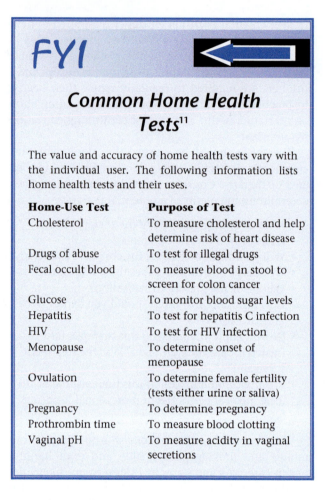

FYI

Common Home Health Tests[11]

The value and accuracy of home health tests vary with the individual user. The following information lists home health tests and their uses.

Home-Use Test	Purpose of Test
Cholesterol	To measure cholesterol and help determine risk of heart disease
Drugs of abuse	To test for illegal drugs
Fecal occult blood	To measure blood in stool to screen for colon cancer
Glucose	To monitor blood sugar levels
Hepatitis	To test for hepatitis C infection
HIV	To test for HIV infection
Menopause	To determine onset of menopause
Ovulation	To determine female fertility (tests either urine or saliva)
Pregnancy	To determine pregnancy
Prothrombin time	To measure blood clotting
Vaginal pH	To measure acidity in vaginal secretions

part of conventional Western medicine.[12] However, this is changing as the federal Committee on the Use of Complementary and Alternative Medicine by the American People recommends that health profession schools, such as schools of medicine and nursing, incorporate sufficient information about CAM into the standard curriculum at the undergraduate, graduate, and postgraduate levels so that licensed professionals can advise their patients about CAM in a competent manner.[13] Currently, 42 percent of U.S. citizens report that they have used at least one CAM therapy, and the number of visits to CAM providers exceeds the number of visits to all primary care physicians. The American public is currently spending over $27 billion a year on various CAM practices.[14] Women, with higher education levels overall, are more likely than men to use CAM therapies, and patterns of use vary among ethnic groups.

The National Institutes of Health now has a National Center for Complementary and Alternative Medicine (NCCAM), which investigates nontraditional healing regimens (see Chapter 5 for a more detailed description of the NCCAM and the use of mind–body medicine to heal and manage stress). Numerous medical schools,

Assess Yourself

Improving Your Chances for Accurate Home Health Test Results

If you have purchased a home health test kit, answer the following questions. This information will assist you in obtaining accurate test results.

Question	Yes	No
1. Has the expiration date expired?	____	____
2. Has the kit been exposed to extreme heat or cold?	____	____
3. Are the directions for using the kit and chemicals clear to you?	____	____
4. Have you read and do you understand the special precautions, if any?	____	____
5. Did you follow the directions exactly as stated?	____	____
6. Did you time the test accurately and precisely as instructed?	____	____
7. Do you understand what the test kit is intended to find?	____	____
8. Do you know what to do when you obtain the results, whether they are positive or negative?	____	____
9. Do you know whom to contact to follow up with the results of the test?	____	____
10. Do you know where to get help administering the test if you are unsure about the directions?	____	____

If you answered eight or more of the questions with a positive response, your health kit test results should be accurate. If you answered less than eight with a positive response, you need to read directions more accurately and discuss the procedures with a medical professional.

---

such as Georgetown University, University of Louisville, and University of Massachusetts in Worcester, offer courses and lectures on CAM medical therapies.[15]

Why has interest in alternative therapies experienced such phenomenal growth? Although we have seen amazing progress in high-tech medical practices, these procedures are often painful, expensive, and even dehumanizing. People began to seek therapies that would take healing a step beyond "treatment." Milestones in the women's movement toward alternative therapy began in the early 1960s which enlightened many women and led to new heights of competence and empowerment. Near this time, yoga, meditation, and macrobiotic diets emerged as the idea of a mind–body connection in illness and wellness found its practitioner sand patients. *Our Bodies, Ourselves,* initially published in 1973, created the desire in many women to take charge of their own well-being through increased knowledge about their own bodies and better education. Women desired a redefinition of the doctor–female patient relationship in which a partnership was formed that enabled them to become part of the decision-making healing process. Books such as *Type A Behavior and Your Heart* (Friedman and Rosenman, 1974), *The Relaxation Response* (Benson, 1975), *Anatomy of an Illness* (Cousins, 1979), and *Psychoneuroimmunology* (Ader, 1981) discussed the connection among our mind, our emotions, and our health. This literature led us to believe that, with effective training, we could become partners in our own level of health. Visiting a bookstore today, you will find an uncanny array of books related to alternative health–related practices. An important step is to find the "right" type of alternative approach and the "right" practitioner to aid in the ability to control pain, reduce stress, and improve well-being.

Unfortunately, in some instances the results have not been positive. Women were/are too often the victims of scam artists or quacks; their money is taken, but the results are less than desirable, even worse, harmful or deadly. However, there are certainly reputable alternative practitioners, medicines, and methodologies that offer, in some instances, more favorable results than conventional medicine. Let us look at a number of alternative therapies and find out what they are, how they "work," and possible risks and benefits of each.

Herbalism

Herbs could be called alternative "drugs" that promote the premise that many disorders or injuries can be treated with a plant or parts of a plant. Herbal medicine was practiced in ancient Rome, Greece, and Babylon and is still used throughout the world, especially in less developed countries. Historically, plants such as myrrh, oil of cloves, peppermint, and caraway were used to treat a range of disorders, including sexually transmitted diseases, inflammation, and heart disease. Patent medicines (nonprescription drugs, protected by a trademark) contained a variety of plants such as ginger root, castor oil, juniper bush, and alfalfa. Herbalists found that drinks made of herbs soothe the nerves, aloe can soothe the skin, leaves from foxglove contain digitalis, and so on.

It only takes a visit to a "health food" market to realize that herbs and products containing herbs are widely available. In fact, in the quest for a more "natural" approach to healing, Americans spend billions of dollars each year on herbal medicines, bulk herbs, and other herbal products. Brochures, books, and pamphlets espouse the benefits of available herbal "medicines," yet researchers state that we need to be wary of some of these medicines. Concerns about herbal medicines include lack of scientific "proof" that they indeed treat and heal health problems; most reports of herbal healing abilities are based on unfounded claims from folklore and some outdated reports. Herbs can be dangerous, even deadly in fact, and some herbs have been banned from sale, whereas others carry a warning on their labels. Herbs contain many hundreds of chemicals, and their reaction in the body can be unknown: perhaps helpful, but perhaps harmful. An excellent resource for herbal information is the Natural Medicines Comprehensive Database, which is available online.[16] Herbal medicines are not controlled by the **Food and Drug Administration** (FDA) and certain strengths of the herb can vary from product to product. Safe and effective medicines are available to treat conditions for which they are known to work (see *FYI:* "Herbs and Their Uses"). Purchasing and using unproven and potentially dangerous herbal medicines is not wise. It appears that it would be advantageous for Western researchers to continue to research and examine the benefits and risks of herbs.

Acupuncture

In its 5000-year history, acupuncture has been used by more people than any other form of alternative medicine. Acupuncture claims to restore balance (Qi) to promote healing and functioning through inserting needles at precise points on the body. Heat may be applied to the acupuncture point to promote the healing process. The premise is that meridians, channels of energy, run like energy throughout the body. When blockage in one part of a channel occurs, it impedes the flow to others. Acupuncture claims to remove the blockage and allow the usual flow through the meridians, restoring Qi and aiding the bodily organs with imbalances. The World Health

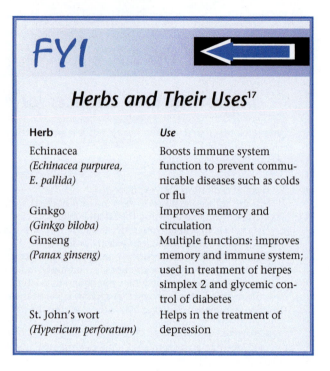

Herbs and Their Uses[17]

Herb	Use
Echinacea (*Echinacea purpurea, E. pallida*)	Boosts immune system function to prevent communicable diseases such as colds or flu
Ginkgo (*Ginkgo biloba*)	Improves memory and circulation
Ginseng (*Panax ginseng*)	Multiple functions: improves memory and immune system; used in treatment of herpes simplex 2 and glycemic control of diabetes
St. John's wort (*Hypericum perforatum*)	Helps in the treatment of depression

Organization acknowledges acupuncture treatment for digestive and respiratory disorders, neurological and muscular ailments, and urinary, menstrual, and reproductive problems. It appears to be especially helpful for physical difficulties related to stress and tension.

Data from the Department of Health and Human Services 2004 survey found that 4 percent of the American public had tried acupuncture and that it is a more popular complementary medicine than homeopathy, naturopathy, and ayurveda.[18] The National Commission for the Certification of Acupuncturists is the certifying agency in this country. Acupuncturists have submitted scientific evidence to the FDA that shows that the needles used in acupuncture do have the ability to heal. If the FDA decides to recognize the tools of acupuncture as bona fide medical instruments, then certain acupuncture treatments could be reimbursed by Medicare, Medicaid, and private insurers.

Women find relief with acupuncture for a variety of ailments: menstrual cramps, headaches, nausea, backaches, and depression. (See *Her Story:* "Ping: Acupuncture for Emotional Relief" and *Health Tips:* "Acupuncture: Use Caution.") Pain relief is the most common and well-documented use of acupuncture. With a certified acupuncturist using sterile equipment, this form of therapy has almost no side effects or risk of complication. However, it is important to remember that using acupuncture does not preclude seeing a physician and using medicinal drugs in conjunction with this type of alternative medicine.

Her Story

Ping: Acupuncture for Emotional Relief

Ping found that she continued to have more and more frequent bouts of anxiety and emotional outbursts close to her menstrual period. After she had consulted with three physicians and tried several tranquilizers, a co-worker recommended acupuncture. Ping was open to, but skeptical of, the suggested treatment. However, she located a reputable acupuncturist and began a series of treatments with needles inserted at points along her back, arms, and legs. After 6 weeks of treatments, she was less anxious not only during premenstrual days but the rest of the time as well.

- Based on Ping's experience, would you be willing to try acupuncture yourself?
- What are the advantages of acupuncture? The disadvantages?
- How can you find a certified acupuncturist?

Health Tips

Acupuncture: Use Caution[22]

Consider the following when contemplating the use of acupuncture as alternative therapy:

- Although complications from acupuncture are few, serious complications can occur because it is an invasive procedure.
- No scientific data exist that prove acupuncture is successful in treating or reducing the risks of organic diseases.
- Acupuncture most often is used for pain relief, but the relief, if there is any, is usually brief.
- Training for acupuncture practitioners is often inadequate or unsupervised, and practitioners may use unscientific methods that are, at the least, not beneficial, or at most, harmful.

Chiropractic Care

Reports of spinal manipulation appear in written records of ancient China and Greece. Indians in early America had family members walk on and maneuver their backbones to reduce problems with their spine. Another form of spinal manipulation, chiropractic, was founded around 1895 by Daniel David Palmer, a grocer and "magnetic healer" in Iowa.[19] After a number of battles with the AMA and other medical and political groups, chiropractic medicine became recognized as a method to treat disorders, with some degree of success, which chiropractors attribute to spinal manipulation.

There are over 50,000 licensed chiropractors in this country, and they make up the third largest group of health care practitioners, after physicians and dentists.[20] Chiropractors must complete 4200 hours of study over a 4-year period and take both national and state board examinations to be a licensed practitioner. Although chiropractic is practiced in all fifty states, a chiropractor must pass the state board exam to be able to treat patients in certain states.[21] In many instances, chiropractic services are reimbursed through private as well as state and federal insurance providers.

Chiropractic medicine is nonscientific medical practices based on the belief that good health depends on the proper functioning of nerve impulse transmission through the nervous system. Therefore, when nerve impulse transmission encounters any type of interference, such as an ill-aligned spine, the person develops an illness. Chiropractic medicine claims that restoring the flow of nerve impulses through proper spinal manipulation can return the person to good health.

The medical science community is concerned about the claims of chiropractors because the claim that interference of nerve impulses is a cause of disease has not been proven scientifically. Additionally, the anatomical structure of the body does not lend itself to the healing and pain relief claims made by chiropractors. However, there does seem to be evidence that chiropractic medicine can be helpful in treating certain musculoskeletal ailments and relieving menstrual pain, which has a back-related component. There are also claims that manipulating and stretching muscles in the back of the head can be beneficial for migraine and tension headaches.

Concerns arise about chiropractic care when chiropractors use treatment modalities for which they have no specific training such as physical therapy, "sports chiropractic," acupuncture, and sometimes nutritional and homeopathic medicine. Conventional medical practitioners worry that spinal manipulation may do more harm than good, especially if the pain has been long lasting or if a tumor or fracture is present. Additionally, some unethical chiropractors keep patients returning for unnecessary treatments and X-rays.

There is movement in chiropractic medicine to focus on a scientific approach to musculoskeletal problems and eliminate procedures for which chiropractors have little or no training. Should you and your physician determine that you have a condition for which chiropractic medicine may be beneficial, such as low-back

Health Tips

When to See a Chiropractor[23]

1. See your physician to determine the reason for your condition.
2. Select a chiropractor who is referred by the National Association for Chiropractic Medicine (www.chiromed.org).
3. Call first to find out about the kind of treatment offered:

   - Does the chiropractor primarily treat musculo-skeletal problems?
   - Will he or she cooperate with your medical doc-tor to reach the best treatment for you?
   - How long and how often should you expect to be in treatment?
   - What are the charges and financial expectations?
   - To which professional associations does the chiropractor belong?
   - Can the chiropractor be reimbursed by your insurance company?

FYI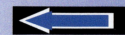

Assessing the Chiropractor[26]

Avoid the chiropractor who engages in the following practices:

- Takes repeated or full-spine X rays
- Does not attempt to assess the nature of the problem in a professional manner
- Claims that benefits to organ systems, immune function, or even a cure will result
- Offers vitamins or nutritional and/or homeopathic treatment
- Asks you to sign a contract for long-term care
- States that you will be kept healthy by regular checkups and manipulations
- Solicits other family members from you for treatment

pain, refer to *Health Tips:* "When to See a Chiropractor" and *FYI:* "Assessing the Chiropractor."

Massage

Massage, in addition to feeling good, appears to offer healthful benefits for the promotion of healing of disease and injuries. Recent research confirms that massage therapy is an effective treatment for low back pain, helps breast cancer survivors both emotionally and physically, helps to ease pain after surgery, and boosts the immune system functions.[24] The same research found that children receiving a nightly massage also experience less anxiety and depression and have lower stress hormone levels. Researchers believe that massage helps to counteract the body's stress response, thereby reducing the ill effects stress hormones can have on the body.

Many active women, such as athletes, have experienced some relief from soreness, injury, and pain due to the use of massage therapy. This approach may eliminate the use of drugs and/or surgery to realize these benefits.

Trigger-point massage promotes the healing of muscle sprains, chronic tendonitis, and chronic muscle spasms, and **cross-fiber friction massage** assists in breaking up adhesions and stretches and realigns scar tissues with healthy muscle fiber.[25] Massages can also help to reduce fatigue and soreness in muscles by promoting muscle relaxation, increasing blood flow to muscles, and reducing inflammation and swelling.

Thirty-three states offer massage licenses, and the requirements to receive a license vary according to the state in which it is issued. Other states allow massage certification of individuals who acquire training and pass written and practical exams; these criteria vary according to state requirements. Either ask someone who has had a positive outcome using a masseur, or contact the American Massage Therapy Association at www.amtamassage.com for the name of the nearest licensed masseur. Time of massage sessions may be anywhere from 15 to 60 minutes and range in cost from $20 to $80 or more. Be sure the masseur you choose treats you in a respectful and professional manner. If not, as with any other practitioner, she or he should be reported to their professional association as well as to local authorities. Using massage, or any other alternative healing method, in lieu of determining the exact cause of the injury or pain through scientifically proven tests is not being a wise consumer.

Holistic Medicine

Holistic, or wholistic, medicine had its origin in ancient times and is derived from the Greek term *holo*, which means "whole." The whole person, which includes the physical, mental, emotional, social, and spiritual dimensions, is considered in the treatment and healing process. Although certain components of holistic medicine can be beneficial, other components embraced by holistic healers lend themselves to questionable medical practices. Of the major concerns related to holistic medicine, the potential for use of nonscientific medical

Viewpoint

Holistic Medicine Practices

Here are some characteristics of holistic medicine practices. Which ones do you consider to be worthwhile, and which ones lend themselves to questionable practices? Explain your position for each one.

- Uses nonscientific approaches to diagnose and treat medical problems
- Uses laypeople and other professionals in the treatment process
- Examines the lifestyle of the individual: nutrition, exercise practices, environment, emotions, use of chemicals, social interactions, and/or spirituality
- Encourages the woman's participation in all aspects of diagnosis and treatment
- Views illness as a means to evaluate and change one's lifestyle
- Emphasizes health as promotion of a healthy lifestyle rather than the absence of disease
- Emphasizes self-care rather than treatment and dependence on medical personnel
- Desires to reduce dependence on medicines, surgery, and treatment
- Promotes healing through meeting the needs of mind, body, and spirit of the individual

to stimulate peak functioning of body systems. Massaging certain areas of the body to promote healing or pain reduction is the major premise of *craniosacral therapy*—skull, spine, and sacrum areas; *myofascial* and *Rolfing* massage connective tissue for pain relief and to promote structural integration; myotherapists manipulate trigger points in elbows, knuckles, and fingers to relieve pain and tension. *Yoga* attempts to integrate body, mind, and spirit with the universe through movement, relaxation, breathing techniques, and music. Aromatherapy is a practice in which aromatic oils are used in warm baths, massage oils, and other products. They can also be massaged into the body or inhaled for treatment of common disorders and to influence mind and emotions. Aromas may be used in a birthing environment to promote tranquility during the birthing process.

Using the best of Western medicine (orthodox health care) and the best of alternative health care practices may be a wise approach to obtaining the best health care possible. Although surgery, medicine, and physical therapy are essential treatments for the injured or critically ill woman, preventing major disease, promoting well-being, and providing the opportunity for partnership in health care have an important place. Medication and diagnostic tools for acute health problems combined with healing touch, needles, and herbs for tension, pain, and relaxation can be effective.

practices and for practitioners to provide useless, harmful, or even deadly care (for a large fee) is of greatest concern. Two long-time professionals who concerned themselves with the holistic healing movement believed it to be "a pabulum of common sense and nonsense offered by cranks and quacks and failed pedants who share an attachment to magic and an animosity to reason."[27] (See *Viewpoint:* "Holistic Medicine Practices.")

There is promise of effective treatment in many holistic health care practices, but until more funding is available for research to determine scientific proof of positive results, this concept of alternative health care will continue to be just that—an alternative.

Other Types of Alternative Health Care

Consider the following brief descriptions of various other alternative health care practices and you will see why the consumer needs information and guidelines to make wise choices.

Naturopathic medicine promotes the concept of the body's own natural healing ability through use of herbal medicine, nutrition, relaxation exercises, and acupuncture. *Reflexologists* use foot massage as a means

Health Quackery

In the search for "hope" when no other was offered or a "quick and painless fix" to any ailment or problem from wrinkle reduction cream to weight loss plans, U.S. citizens spend over $15 billion annually on a variety of products that purport to address these concerns.[28] When there is a health-related concern, there will often be some gimmick, potion, or practitioner available—for a price—to remedy the concern. These products promise that we can eat all we want and still lose weight, build a bigger bust line, melt away cellulite, or increase our libido. The FDA defines health **quackery** as the promotion of a medical remedy that doesn't work and is known to be false or unproven.[29]

PRESCRIPTION DRUGS

Currently, the FDA has approved more than 2500 prescription drugs, all of which are intended to prevent, treat, or cure various types of illnesses. Prescription drugs are made of natural and/or synthetic chemicals and can be obtained only with a physician's written authorization. Prescription drugs are potent, but when used as directed, they can produce positive results for treatment and healing. The FDA regulates prescription drugs for form, strength, safety, purity, effectiveness, and method of administration. More than 2.3 billion prescriptions are filled each year, including 1.02 billion refills and 1.29 billion new prescriptions.[30]

Prescription drugs have three names: the generic name, the chemical name, and the brand name. Generic names pertain to the kind of drug and also describe the drug, such as penicillin. Although generic drugs are identical in their chemical compounds with the same brand-name drug, generic drugs may not be equivalent in therapeutic effect. Legally, drugs are identified by their generic names and are listed by that name in the **United States Pharmacopoeia (USP)**. The USP is responsible for conferring the official standards of identity, purity, and effectiveness for all prescription drugs. In laboratories, drugs are called by their **chemical name**, which usually refers to the chemicals from which the drugs have been developed. The **brand name**, under the control of the FDA, is patented by the pharmaceutical company, which develops, manufactures, and distributes the drug to pharmacies. The company that develops and tests the drug has exclusive rights to produce it for 17 years. Once the patent expires, other pharmaceutical companies are then permitted to manufacture the drug under another brand name or under its generic name. Table 2.1 provides a few examples of brand and generic names of commonly prescribed drugs.

Pharmacists can dispense generic drugs instead of brand-name products with a doctor's approval in almost all states. Brand-name drugs can be 30–50 percent more expensive than their generic counterparts, and approximately 400 different generic drugs can presently be substituted for brand-name drugs.[31] The equivalent effectiveness of generic and brand-name drugs is determined by scientists who measure the time it takes the generic drug to reach the blood stream. The rate of

TABLE 2.1 Generic and Brand Names of Commonly Prescribed Drugs*	
BRAND NAME	**GENERIC NAME**
Zovirax	acyclovir
Xanax	alprazolam
Valium	diazepam
Tylenol	acetaminophen

*Brand names are Capitalized; generic names are lowercased.

absorption, called **bioavailability**, is then compared to the rate for the brand-name drug. If it is found that the generic and brand-name versions deliver the same amount of active ingredients into a patient's bloodstream with equal absorption rates, the two drugs are considered to be equivalent. The FDA ensures the equivalency of generic and brand-name drugs. However, even if drugs are therapeutically equivalent, they may not produce the same effects in all women.

Understanding Drug Labels

Carefully following the directions on a prescription label enables the consumer to receive the most effective results when taking a drug. A prescription label provides the patient's name and the physician's name as well as the name, address, and phone number of the pharmacy dispensing the drug. Drug-related information includes the name of the drug, the dosage form (liquid, capsule, tablet), and the strength of the drug, in either milligrams (mg) or ounces. How much, how often, and when to take the drug are indicated along with any special instructions and refill information. Essential information

Journal Activity

Questions to Ask When Purchasing Medications

Try this activity the next time you visit a pharmacy: Ask the pharmacist the questions in *Health Tips:* "Questions to Ask When Taking Prescription Medicine." You can do this activity when obtaining prescription medicine or purchasing an over-the-counter medication. Consider the following:

- Did the pharmacist answer your questions in language that you could understand?
- If you were unsure of the information, did you ask the pharmacist to provide additional information?
- Did the pharmacist treat you with respect and consideration?
- Did you feel comfortable with your interaction with this health professional?
- How was this activity beneficial to you regarding your own health care?

FIGURE 2.1 Looking at prescription drug labels. Components of a prescription for a sleep-aid, *traZODONE,* one to three tablets at bedtime.

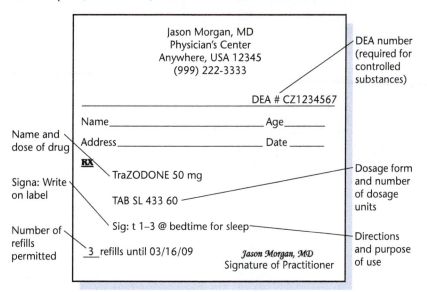

Jason Morgan, MD
Physician's Center
Anywhere, USA 12345
(999) 222-3333

DEA # CZ1234567 — DEA number (required for controlled substances)

Name_____ Age_____

Name and dose of drug — Address_____ Date_____

RX

Signa: Write on label — TraZODONE 50 mg — Dosage form and number of dosage units

TAB SL 433 60

Number of refills permitted — Sig: t 1–3 @ bedtime for sleep — Directions and purpose of use

3 refills until 03/16/09

Jason Morgan, MD
Signature of Practitioner

regarding warnings about drug–drug or food–drug interactions is also provided.[32] (See Figure 2.1.)

Almost half of all prescription drugs will fail to produce the desired effects because of incorrect use. Patients do such things as take too much or too little of a drug, take it too often or not often enough, skip doses, take it with food when directions say without food, drink alcohol when they're taking the drug, or use expired drugs. A woman needs to ask her physician and/or pharmacist critical questions and seek information that will permit her to use the medication safely and effectively. She should tell her physician about any previous allergic reactions to foods or medicines, any medication (including over-the-counter) being taken on a regular basis, any physical conditions for which she is being treated by other physicians, and if she is pregnant or breast-feeding. *Journal Activity:* "Questions to Ask When Taking Prescription Medicine" lists questions women should ask their physicians about prescription drug use.

Commonly Prescribed Drugs

Two-thirds of the women who visit a doctor's office will have a written prescription in their hands when they leave the office. Between 1994 and 2005, the number of prescriptions have increased 71 percent, from 2.1 billion to 3.6 billion.[33] Substances that assist in weight management are among the most commonly prescribed drugs for women. Antidepressants, sedative hypnotics, and hormone regulation substances are also among the most commonly prescribed drugs for women. These medications will be discussed further in later chapters.

Using Prescription Drugs Safely

Our bodies are chemical-laden machines. When we add chemicals such as prescription drugs, we may be brewing a chemical mix in our bodies that could result in undesirable, uncomfortable, and in some instances, unsafe side effects. Side effects often result from using the drug incorrectly, such as skipping a dose, taking too much, taking it at the wrong time, taking it with beverages other than water, or taking it with or without food when directions suggest differently. However, most side effects can be reduced or, even better, eliminated.

Health Tips

Questions to Ask When Taking Prescription Medicine

Asking basic questions and seeking information from your physician or pharmacist can assist you in receiving the proper medication for your health, as well as result in the most effective use of your consumer dollars.

- What is the purpose of this medicine?
- What are the possible side effects?
- What foods, beverages, or other medication should I avoid while taking this medicine?
- Exactly when and how do I take the medication?
- What should I do if I experience side effects?
- How long should I take this medication?

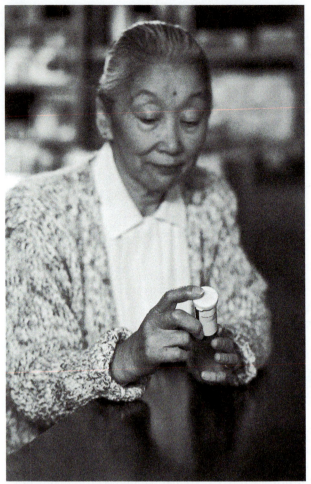

Reading prescription labels carefully is important for being a healthy and informed consumer.

Weight, age, gender, health status, and/or diet can affect how drugs react when used by women.

Health Tips: "Guidelines When Taking Medications" provides guidelines to follow when taking medications. Getting the most out of the medication you have been prescribed is as important as taking it correctly. *Assess Yourself:* "Safety Tips When Taking Medications" is a checklist to determine it you are using medicines safely.

The benefits resulting from using drugs that prevent, treat, and heal diseases correctly outweigh any risks one might encounter. Although medicines are powerful drugs, wise and careful use does eliminate most complications. (See *Health Tips:* "Caution: Watch for Tampering.")

OVER-THE-COUNTER (OTC) DRUGS

More than 80 therapeutic categories with more than 100,000 drug products of over-the-counter (OTC) drugs are available without prescription in markets across the

Health Tips

Guidelines When Taking Medications

Following safe guidelines can help enhance drug effectiveness and safety:

- Take the prescribed dosage; do not take more or less than instructed.
- Follow the directions on the label; modify only as your physician specifies.
- Ask the pharmacist or physician about directions if you are unsure about using the medication properly.
- Finish the prescription even after you are feeling better; women often relapse when they fail to finish all their medication.
- Seek a second opinion if you are concerned about taking the drug.
- Notify your physician immediately if you have any unusual or serious side effects.

country today.[34] These include such categories as analgesics, antihistamines, stimulants, laxatives, topical analgesics, antacids, and others. Are these drugs safe and effective? The 1962 Kefauver-Harris Act required scientific evidence to prove that OTC drugs were safe and

Assess Yourself

Safety Tips When Taking Medications

Do you	Yes	No
Alert all your physicians to all medications you are currently taking?	____	____
Refuse to share your medications with friends and family?	____	____
Store medication properly and away from light, heat, and moisture?	____	____
Use nonmedical treatment for occasional illnesses?	____	____
Review with your physician any medications used on a long-term basis?	____	____
Dispose of any medications that are expired or that you are no longer using?	____	____

Health Tips

Caution: Watch for Tampering

Although prescription and over-the-counter drugs are considered to be packaged safely in the United States, manufacturers cannot make a tamper-proof package. It is important to know how to protect yourself from possible tampering and contaminating of medicines. You can protect yourself by doing the following:

- Inspect the outer package for tears, cuts, or punctures.
- Inspect the medicine and look for discoloration or damage.
- Look for tablets or capsules that appear to be different from others in the package.
- Never take medicine in the dark.
- Pay attention to the safety features provided by the manufacturer.
- Use time and care, and good common sense. It is your own best safety feature!

FYI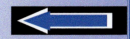

How a Prescription Drug Becomes an OTC Drug

Manufacturers who own a patent for a prescription drug must apply to the FDA for permission to reconstruct the formula for the drug to be sold as an OTC drug. Usually, the active ingredients are made less concentrated and safer to use without a doctor's prescription. Products do retain their prescription brand name. Once approval is given by the FDA, the former prescription drug can be marketed and sold as an OTC medicine. Examples of such products include Aleve for premenstrual discomfort, Monistat and Gyne-Lotrimin, which are creams to treat vaginal infection, and ibuprofen (Advil, Motrin, etc.) for headaches.

effective. A regulatory program was developed by the FDA in 1972 in which active ingredients of OTC drugs were assigned to one of three categories: GRAS (Generally Recognized as Safe),GRAE (Generally Recognized as Effective), and GRAHL (Generally Recognized as Honestly Labeled). These categories with their FDA-developed acronyms are used to effectively describe the safety of the ingredients found in OTC drugs. (See Table 2.2.)

In 1992 the U.S. General Accounting Office reported that the FDA is unable to determine the exact number of OTC products that are marketed each year, and that all of them may not be safe and effective. The Center for Drug Evaluation and Research (CDER) oversees OTC drugs, as well as prescription drugs, to ensure they are labeled properly and that the benefits outweigh the risks. OTC drugs usually have the following characteristics:

- Their benefits outweigh their risks.
- The potential for misuse and abuse is low.
- Consumers can use them for self-diagnosed conditions.
- They are properly labeled.
- Health practitioners are not needed for safe, effective use of the product.[35]

However, as more prescription drugs become OTC drugs, these OTC drugs are becoming safer and more effective. *FYI:* "How a Prescription Drug Becomes an OTC Drug" explains how this is done.

OTC Drugs Used by Women

Rising medical care costs are a major concern for those women who have little, if any, money for professional health care. Thus, self-diagnosis of illness is on the increase, which leads to frequent purchase of OTC drugs. Hundreds of thousands of OTC drugs are purchased each year simply by consumer choice. Therefore, consumers must be informed about the advantages and the potential hazards of those medicines purchased without benefit of a physician's consultation or prescription.

To help reduce the misuse of OTC medicines, labeling and package inserts are provided with each drug and

TABLE 2.2 FDA Categories for OTC Drug Ingredients	
Category I	Ingredient is *GRAS* and *GRAE*.
Category II	Ingredient is either not *GRAS* and/or not *GRAE* and would be removed from stores within 6 months if the manufacturer did not prove its safety and effectiveness.
Category III	Insufficient data to determine the ingredient's safety and/or effectiveness. If the manufacturer cannot prove *GRAS* within one year, the drug becomes a Category II rather than a Category I drug.*

*Only drugs that have been proven safe and effective are now placed in the OTC market.

have become more reliable since the FDA assumed control over OTC medicines. FDA regulations mandate that labels on all OTC medication list information in the same order, arranged in a simple, eye-catching, consistent style, and use understandable terms. The following information is required on all OTC drug labels:[36]

- *Active ingredient:* the type of therapeutic substance and the amount of active ingredient per unit
- *Uses:* diseases, disorders, or symptoms the medication will treat or prevent
- *Warnings:* suggestions for safe use of the product, including when not to use, when to see a physician, possible interactions or side effects, use related to pregnancy or breast-feeding, keep out of reach of children
- *Inactive ingredients:* other substances in the product (colors, flavors)
- *Purpose:* product action or category (such as antacid, cough suppressant, painkiller)
- *Directions:* specific age categories, how to use, how much, how often, and how long to take the medication
- *Other information:* how to store properly and information about other ingredients

Other information found on labels includes the expiration date; the lot or batch number to help identify the product; the name and address of the manufacturer, packer, or distributor; the net quantity of contents; and what to do if an overdose occurs. By reading the information on each label, women should not have any problem in determining the purpose of the drug and the safe and effective way to take it.

Prescription and OTC Drug Use during Pregnancy

Rubin and colleagues[37] analyzed the drug use of more than 2700 pregnant females and found that 68 percent used at least one drug during their pregnancy. The average intake of drugs was 1.2 drugs per female while pregnant. Educated, married, white women with higher than average incomes were more likely to use legal drugs, especially OTC products, while pregnant.

The majority of these women gave birth to normal infants. However, women must be aware that each pregnancy is unique, and the best approach is to avoid exposing the fetus to unnecessary drugs. Therefore, it is strongly recommended that women avoid all medication, both prescription and OTC, if possible during pregnancy. Communication between pregnant women and their physicians, and strict adherence to the warnings about taking any drugs during pregnancy, must be a priority. (See *Journal Activity:* "Recording the Medicines You Take.")

Journal Activity

Recording the Medicines You Take

Find all the medications that you take on a regular basis. Divide them into prescription and OTC drugs, and use this chart to record essential information. This information can be useful when visiting your physician.

Date	Name of Medicine	Amount Taken	When Taken	Purpose	Refills
Example	Hurt-No-More Pain Pills	1–2 tabs 400 mg	3 times a day with meals	Headaches	2

Adapted from *Use medicine wisely.* Washington, DC: Food and Drug Administration.

BEAUTY-ENHANCING PRODUCTS AND PROCEDURES

Products

Women, and sometimes men, elect to use products to improve the way we look and feel about ourselves. Cosmetics of all descriptions, creams, lotions, hair products, and fragrances are developed and sold, for large profits, because there is a demand for them. As purchasers of these products, we need to be knowledgeable and aware in order to select products that meet our needs and desires.

Cosmetics   Cosmetics as defined by the U.S. Food, Drug, and Cosmetic Act are "articles intended to be rubbed, poured, sprinkled, or sprayed on, introduced into, or otherwise applied to the human body . . . for cleansing, beautifying, promoting attractiveness, or altering the appearance."[38] Strangely enough, premarket approval is not required by the FDA for cosmetics. However, if a product proves to be harmful once it is on the market, the FDA can take legal action to obtain the manufacturer's safety data. Cosmetics are classified into thirteen categories: deodorants, eye makeup, skin care, fragrances, makeup other than eye (lipsticks, for example), hair coloring preparations, shampoos and other hair products, manicure products, shaving products, baby products, bath products, mouthwashes, and sunscreens.[39] Cosmetics containing poisonous or harmful substances may not, by law, be placed on the market. With the exception of color additives and a few prohibited ingredients, any ingredient or raw material may be used in the manufacture of cosmetics. See *Health Tips: "Safety Tips for Beauty-Enhancing Products"* for tips to protect yourself after you purchase cosmetics.

Cosmetic manufacturers must do the following to market their products: work in a sanitary environment and allow no filthy, putrid, or decomposed substances in the product; test for color additives and obtain FDA approval for their use in products; list ingredients on labels in descending order of predominance; and avoid the use of prohibited ingredients such as mercury compounds, chloroform, or vinyl chloride. If a manufacturer chooses to do so, it may register its manufacturing plant, cosmetic formulas, and report adverse reactions with the FDA. An increase in the demand for ethnic cosmetics has the manufacturers of products scrambling to meet this demand. An increase in the Latino and African American populations, as well as an increase in economic status of both groups, has been credited with this new market component. The youth of these particular groups appear to have boosted ethnic cosmetic sales.[40]

Health Tips

Safety Tips for Beauty-Enhancing Products

Protect yourself by following these guidelines to use cosmetics safely:

- When not in use, keep containers closed tightly.
- Store products, especially liquids, in a cool, dry place.
- Keep products away from sunlight, as ingredients may degrade.
- Never moisten dry cosmetics or applicators with saliva.
- Toss out any cosmetics that smell strange, separate into layers, or have different colors or consistencies than when purchased.
- Do not share cosmetics or applicators or use in-store samples and applicators.
- Do not use cosmetics if you have an eye or skin infection.
- Be sure to wash cosmetic sponges and brushes with warm water and soap frequently; throw them away if they degrade or lose bristles.

Skin Care Products   Our skin continually renews itself by producing new cells deep within the skin layers and sloughing off dead cells on the skin's surface. Skin layers contain water and oil, but as we age less oil is produced within the skin and skin loses water faster, becomes dry, cracks, and develops fine wrinkles. When we attempt to replenish water and oil in our skin with moisturizers, we only moisturize the top layer of the skin. Because this is the skin layer that dries out, moisturizers need only to moisturize this layer. That can occur in two ways: use an occlusive type product that physically blocks moisture from leaving the skin (e.g., petroleum jelly) or use a "humectant" type product that attracts moisture from the skin and air and slows down the rate of water loss.[41] Most skin care products have both types of ingredients as well as water. If a product is intended to be used for a drier type of skin, it will have more oil; for oily skin types, the product should have more or only humectants.

Ingredients in addition to oil and water add benefits, but may make the moisturizer more expensive. Ingredients found in today's moisturizers may include (1) sunscreen to reduce the damage caused by exposure to sun, (2) alpha-hydroxy acids which help rid the skin of dead cells, (3) tretinoin to help replace dead skin cells with new skin, and (4) petrolatum, which reduces scaling of skin and helps retain moisture.[42]

Moisturizers for the body and the face work similarly, but we tend to pay more attention to our face.

Therefore, the advertiser more often promotes moisturizers for the face, and the consumer will find that face moisturizers are more expensive than those for the body. A comparison chart found on the Consumer Search Web site offers limited information about different type of moisturizers.[43]

Procedures

In attempting to obtain the image of women publicized by print and electronic media, women undergo intrusive and sometimes painful and disfiguring procedures. The demand for breast augmentation, face-lifts, chemical peels, tummy tucks, and liposuctions has increased. Why do women elect to go through these unpleasant and expensive procedures? (See *FYI:* "Reasons for Beauty-Enhancing Procedures.")

Cosmetic Surgery   Cosmetic surgery is more prevalent than ever in our society, and we are more aware of the improved technology to achieve the image we desire. Television shows such as Extreme Makeover have brought the many possibilities of cosmetic surgery into almost every living room in America and created an awareness of beauty-enhancing procedures more than at any time in the past. Cosmetic surgeons now advertise their practice and provide "in-office" operating rooms and financing. What is the difference between a "cosmetic" and a "plastic" surgeon? A cosmetic surgeon specializes in procedures that enhance appearance such as face-lifts, breast reduction/augmentation, or "nose jobs." A plastic surgeon is trained in reconstructive surgery and performs procedures such as facial reconstruction, skin grafts, or hand surgery as well as cosmetic surgery. In selecting a cosmetic or plastic surgeon, look for the following: board certified in the area of surgical specialty; experience in the procedure you desire; recommendation from someone you trust who has had a procedure done by the surgeon; remains current with new procedures; communicates with you about the positives and negatives of the procedure and your motivation for having the surgical procedure; and has privileges at area hospitals.

Types of Cosmetic Procedures   Many types of cosmetic procedures are available to accomplish a variety of desirable changes in one's appearance. The following list provides the common and medical procedural term and briefly explains the purpose of the procedures:

- Eyelid lift (*blepharoplasty*) corrects sagging or droopy lids above the eyes and/or bags below the eyes.
- Neck/face-lift (*rhytidectomy*) lifts the lower two-thirds of the face and improves sagging skin, jowls, double chin, and aging neck.
- Forehead or brow lift is accomplished with an ear-to-ear incision and removal of extra skin to reduce forehead and frown lines and to raise sagging eyebrows.
- Liposuction uses small tubes attached to a type of vacuum to remove pounds of fatty tissue from buttocks, upper arms, stomach, hips, or face.
- Chin (*mentoplasty*) or cheek (*malar*) augmentation provides for a more pleasing face contour by adding cheekbones and a stronger, more prominent chin line.
- Nose job (*rhinoplasty*) reshapes the nose by changing nostrils, building or removing the bridge, recontouring the tip, or cutting or adding bone or cartilage. This procedure may improve breathing (insurance may apply in this instance).
- Botulinum toxin injections (BOTOX) are biological toxins transformed into a therapeutic agent and are used to treat frown lines, crow's feet, and lines and wrinkles in many areas of the face, BOTOX smoothes wrinkles that contract during facial expressions. These injections are a temporary solution and last about 3–4 months, therefore requiring repeated treatments. Side effects such as facial numbness, swelling, or bruising may result from this treatment. Women may feel a burning sensation during the injection.[45]
- Chemical peel (*phenol*) helps to remove, erase, or fade fine facial wrinkles, acne scars, or sun damage by use of certain types of acid such as phenol or trichloroacetic acid or use of certain types of laser.
- Dermabrasion scrapes top layers of the skin to help remove fine wrinkles and marred skin so that new and smoother skin will be produced.
- Collagen or fat injections help to fill out skin to reduce wrinkling or scar tissue, "plump" up lips, or

FYI

Reasons for Beauty-Enhancing Procedures[44]

- Anxiety over appearance based on a societal prejudice against aging females
- To increase feelings of worthiness, often dependent upon childhood development situations
- To maintain positive feelings about appearance
- To fulfill a personal desire to achieve the best appearance possible
- To attain an unconscious obligation to be a youthful and attractive member of society

smooth the back of the hands. Each of these procedures can have very positive benefits, but each can also be harmful and produce unexpected outcomes. The importance of utilizing a board-certified, experienced, and highly qualified surgeon is essential to avoid such side effects as infection, pooling of blood under the skin, nerve damage, numbness, scarring, or ill-positioned or hardening of implants. Side effects, such as bruising, swelling, redness, throbbing, numbness, tightness, and stiffness, can be expected, but they are usually temporary.

Breast Augmentation

Breast implants appeared on the market in 1962; in 2003 alone over 323,000 breast augmentation and reconstructive surgeries were performed.[46]

Prior to April 1995, **silicone gel–filled** and **saline implants** were available to any woman who could afford the procedure. However, continuing problems related to silicone gel–filled implants created a need for valid and reliable clinical research to determine the safety and long-term effects of these products. Hardening of the breast because of scar tissue shrink age around the implant, possibility of negative effects on the immune system, risks of cancer development, and potential interference with mammogram readings all contributed to the investigation and eventual restrictions of silicone gel–filled implants. After being off the market for more than a decade, the FDA Advisory Committee has recommended that the restrictions on silicone breast implants be lifted. Multiple reasons are the foundation for this reversal, but the truth is that not much more is known about silicone implants than a decade ago.[47] However, in November 2006, the FDA stated that silicone implants from two manufacturers, Allergan and Mentor, are approved for breast augmentation in women aged 22 years and older and for breast reconstruction in women of any age.[48]

Of the women who get breast implants, the vast majority do so to increase the size of their breast, called **breast augmentation**. Saline pouches, filled with a saltwater solution, fill the inflatable implants and then are placed between breast tissue and the chest wall. These types of implants are presently available even though the safety of saline implants has not been proven. Concerns regarding saline implants relate to deflation due to leak-age or rupture, which can require additional surgery to correct. Calcium deposits often develop, causing difficulty in reading and interpreting mammograms. Seepage of saline solution into the body may occur, creating a risk of developing an autoimmune disease.

Another breast augmentation procedure, called breast augmentation mammoplasty, is applied by injection (BAMBI). In this procedure, excess fat is suctioned from the buttocks, thighs, or abdomen and injected between the breast and the chest wall. The surgeon who developed this procedure, Dr. Gerald Johnson, claims that it can permanently increase the breast by one-half a cupsize.[49] However, other cosmetic surgeons claim that the injected fat either breaks down and is absorbed into the body or develops a hard calcium mass that can mask or mimic breast cancer. Dr. Johnson, although no longer performing this procedure, claims that it is a safe and effective operation.[50] Perhaps with further study this procedure will be used again in future breast augmentation surgeries.

What do you think about breast augmentation? Answer the questions in *Viewpoint:* "Should Silicone Gel–Filled Breast Implants Be Available?" Women who have any type of breast implants are reminded to have regular checkups, especially if experiencing a change in size, shape, or consistency or feeling any discomfort. *Health Tips:* "Breast Augmentation Guidelines" provides guidelines that women should diligently follow.

Although information about different types of and precautions about cosmetic surgery is important if women choose to have any type of cosmetic surgical procedure, perhaps the more important questions are: Why are we seeing such an increase in the number of women who desire a "beauty-enhancing procedure" that carries so many risks? Shouldn't women be able to appreciate their "natural" qualities without feeling the need to undergo risky surgery, painful recovery, and undue expense for cosmetic procedures that may or may not yield positive results? Reading the next section about advertising and the media's portrayal of women may assist us in understanding the desire to enhance our physical being, even at the potential risk of experiencing negative health consequences.

EFFECTS OF ADVERTISING

We see the beautiful, slim bodies of attractive people having an exciting and fun time in a lovely environment many times every day through the magic of television or the turn of a page in a popular magazine. Everyone and everything appears to be just right! Whether it's wrinkle cream, beer, exercise equipment, or the latest weight control product, it's the advertiser's job to persuade people to buy products and services. Too often consumers must follow the concept of **caveat emptor**, a phrase that means "Let the buyer beware." In other words, it is the consumer's problem to determine if the advertisement is misleading, and she must make the decision to purchase at her own discretion or risk. Not fair! Consumers should be able to trust that the information presented by advertisements is accurate and truthful. There have been strides toward truth in advertising and the products that are promoted. The Federal Trade Commission (FTC) was established in 1914 to protect citizens

Viewpoint

Should Silicone Gel–Filled Breast Implants Be Available?

The consequences of silicone gel–filled implants are not totally known, but it has been documented that implants should not be expected to last a lifetime; all implants leak silicone through their outer envelope; the health effects of this leakage are not truly clear; the percentage of silicone gel–filled implant ruptures is not known; the connection between silicone gel–filled breast implants and cancer, immune system disorders, and interference with mammogram readings, and the formation of calcium deposits is not clear. Because we do not have definitive answers to some of these possible health effects, should women still have the choice to have silicone gel–filled implants placed in their breasts if they so desire?

There appear to be some psychological benefits for women who elect to have their breasts enlarged. Women have reported feeling more attractive, more confident, and better about themselves. Do you think women who choose to take the unknown risks related to this surgery should be denied the right to make this choice? Why or why not?

Health Tips

Breast Augmentation Guidelines

Follow these guidelines to prevent any potential danger from breast implants:

- Have regular breast exams by a qualified physician.
- Perform monthly breast self-exams.
- Have screening mammograms at intervals prescribed for your age group.
- Stay in contact with your regular physician as well as the cosmetic surgeon who performed the surgery.

from unfair business practices. Congress expanded the responsibilities of the FTC with the 1938 Wheeler-Lea Amendment, which protects consumers against individuals or companies engaged in false advertisements of cosmetics, foods, drugs, and devices. The Fair Packing and Labeling Act of 1966 requires the labels on products involving foods, drugs, cosmetics, and medical devices to honestly inform consumers what they are buying and how it is to be used effectively.

Even with protective laws and agencies, consumers must still be aware, informed, and conscientious in regard to purchasing health-related products promoted by advertisers. The advertiser's objective is to sell a product; our objective is to purchase a product that is safe and effective for our needs. We hope the following information will be beneficial in assisting you, the female consumer, in selecting products that meet your needs and do not adversely affect your pocketbook.

Types of Advertising Techniques

Strategies for promoting health-related products (as well as other types of products) range from humorous and glitzy to sophisticated and ethereal. When purchasing a product to meet your needs, keep in mind a number of questions that will aid in your decision: How does it compare to other products? What is the evidence that the product works? Can any product really do what this product claims to do? Am I buying the product or trying to purchase the image that is portrayed by the advertisement?

Advertisers do an outstanding job of product promotion. Some advertisements are beneficial in helping us make a decision; other products are almost camouflaged as to their real purpose due to the hype (music, lighting, gorgeous people, celebrities, good times) used to promote the product. Awareness plays a significant part in making an informed decision about consumer issues. *FYI:* "Advertising Techniques for Health-Related Products" lists the techniques used by advertisers to sell their products. Which do you recognize in products you have purchased? Have any of these techniques persuaded you to purchase a cosmetic, drug, or device?

Through beautiful people, funny phrases, setting a mood, and testimonials, we are exposed to claims about products that are appealing and believable. Complete *Journal Activity:* "Analyzing Advertisements" to help you "see" beyond the image and glitz to find the real message, if there is one, about the product. Then determine if the product meets your needs.

Unrealistic Portrayals of Women

When advertisers promote products to women, the message is often that the product is necessary for us to be thinner, more attractive, or more youthful, or that it will improve our lifestyle. Promoting products in this manner sends the message that women are not thin, attractive, or young enough and that our situation in life can be improved by purchasing and using a particular product. Dissatisfaction with one's physique contributes to being vulnerable to advertisements that feature thin, young women who represent the "norm" of feminine beauty. Often the heart of female-directed advertisements plays to the lack of belief in one's self-worth

FYI

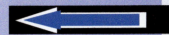

Advertising Techniques for Health-Related Products[51]

Technique	What You Hear	What You Can Ask
Bandwagon	Used by majority of hospitals/doctors; people rely on . . .	Does everyone use this? If so how do other companies stay in business?
Testimonials	By celebrities (sports, actors), by medical personnel	Do they know more than others? How much are they being paid to promote this product? Do they use the product?
Nonverbal/visuals	Music, colors, beautiful scenes and people, animation	What does this have to do with the effectiveness of products?
Humor, slogans	Jokes, silly costumes, phrases, songs,	Helps to sell, but what does it mean? Is a product better because its ad is funny?
Power words	Works wonders, famous, revolutionary natural, amazing	What is the truth? What makes this product amazing or revolutionary or natural?
Scientific evidence	Studies say; doctors recommend; clinical trials indicate; scientists say . . .	What test, research, or clinical trials? What doctors? Which scientists?
Superiority	Leading brand, more effective, stronger, no other, best	Are differences significant? Who says it's more effective?
Emotions and attitudes	Relieves tension, improves mood; you'll feel sexier, feel better about self, feel good all over	How was this determined? Where is the evidence?

Journal Activity

Analyzing Advertisements

Select advertisements from television and women's journals and answer the following questions related to the techniques presented in the FYI box on advertising techniques.

1. Does the person (celebrity or otherwise) have the credentials to know about the product he or she is promoting?
2. Can the product, in reality, do all the things it claims it can do?
3. Where is the scientific evidence that this product can produce the results for my well-being that it claims?
4. How do I know that the clinical trials produced the outcomes that the advertisement claims occurred?
5. Does the scenery or music or imagery in this advertisement make this product better than another in a less-appealing advertisement? As a result of this type of advertisement, will the cost of the product be higher than that of similar products?
6. Does the product claim to be painless, miraculous, fast and effective, FDA-approved, or guaranteed?
7. Does the product claim to work while you sleep, cure serious disease, retard aging, reduce fat without exercise, or improve your sex life?
8. Does the product claim that it can improve your social life, make you popular, or make you more appealing to other people?
9. Does the product claim to be an effective foreign product?
10. Is the cost of this product in accord with other brands of this type?

or attractiveness. Women of today are programmed to believe they should be able to do and have it all—challenging careers, children and partners, and attractive, thin, and fit bodies. Therefore, if we don't achieve this "ideal," we often feel deficient and unworthy. Thus, advertisements often portray women who use certain products as attractive and successful in all areas of their lives. Examples of these include a young, thin, fit mother riding a bike with her son; a beautiful young woman with thick, blond hair sitting on the beach promoting shampoo; a woman displaying devices that can be worn to provide a face-lift effect without surgery; a gorgeous, young woman with long, thick dark hair promoting a hair conditioner; a beautiful, young Asian woman with no wrinkles selling moisturizer; and a thin, young woman draped only in soft, see-through fabric and floating in a carefree position promoting a "soothing" line of hair products.

What about women who are of average to over average weight, are over 40 years of age, and may not have wrinkle-free complexions—are there no products for this group? Do only beautiful, thin, young, energetic women purchase products? No! Do these advertisements mean that we, of average looks and bodies, are not worthy of health-promoting and lifestyle-enhancing products? Is there some place for reality in advertising?

Advertisements also portray women as frivolous and preoccupied with self. In 1992, Quebec's Council for the Status of Women studied women in advertisements in 3,000 prime-time television shows reviewed over a 7-week period. The study determined that women were depicted as frivolous, superficial, ignorant, and incapable of doing difficult tasks.[52] Magazine advertisements directed at female consumers, unfortunately, depicted women in a similar manner. A Canadian writer reported that upon reviewing women's magazines, she observed an inordinate amount of information about dressing, eating, loving, shampooing, or exercising.[53] It can be disconcerting to be the gender viewed as superficial and perceived as having only a decorative contribution to make to society.

Is the mental and physical health of women negatively impacted when only thin and attractive models, implied as the cultural norm, are used in advertisements, or when women are portrayed as self-absorbed and frivolous? Advertisements that stereotype gender have been a major concern of feminist leaders. Has the image of women portrayed in the media been partially responsible for creating and maintaining limited social roles for women? In an analysis of research studies about women in advertisements from the 1950s through the 1980s, Bushy and Leichty[54] found that although there were not as many advertisements showing women in home or family settings, an increased number of advertisements showed women as decorative or in "alluring" roles in the ads.

Realistic Portrayals of Women

How about another view? A number of advertisements are beginning to portray women as decision makers who are financially independent. A phone company owned and operated by women, an automobile advertisement with a woman making the purchase decision, and a mortgage company showing a woman in the role of home buyer are examples of an enlightened and inclusive advertisement model. Another new approach finds advertisers seeking to find a neutral position; the trend is away from either-or images but, instead, seeks an image balanced between career and home.[55] Advertisers must place more emphasis on portraying women as capable, confident, and caring—as individuals who want factual information about products and services, not as individuals preoccupied by looks and images. An accurate and representative portrayal of women in advertisements can only be "healthful" for women, especially for women who are searching for their physical and psychological identities. (See *Journal Activity:* "Forming Your Own Opinion.")

As women continue to have a major financial impact on the marketplace, we will see advertisers present a more realistic image of women—one of an intelligent, pragmatic, attentive, concerned, and financially stable individual—because it is justified. (See *FYI:* "What Is Direct-to-Consumer Advertising?")

FINANCIAL CONSIDERATIONS

Health Insurance

All aspects of health care, ranging from prevention to treatment to cure, are essential to the health and well-being of all people. The continuing exponential growth of health care costs too often leaves individuals without the benefit of this vital care, especially the uninsured. Health insurance is a contract between an individual and/or a group and an insurance company, and it can assist individuals in meeting the demands and needs of paying for their health care. What types of health insurance plans are available, and how do we select one that meets our health needs and financial ability? (See *FYI:* "The Three Basic Health Insurance Plans.")

Health insurance plans vary according to the types of services offered and the price for coverage. *Basic health insurance* covers hospital, surgical, and medical expenses, and individual health plans differ according to the company and the contract. Major medical insurance (or catastrophic coverage) assists with any major and/or long-term illness, such as heart disease or cancer, and is usually a supplement to basic health insurance. *Comprehensive major medical insurance* combines basic health and major medical insurance plans to provide for the majority of

Journal Activity

Forming Your Own Opinion

Complete the following activity to help you form your own opinion and develop perceptions about the portrayal of women in advertising. Monitor the media (television, radio, magazines, etc.) for their portrayal of women. Then answer these questions:

- Do you find evidence of traditional roles for women in the media?
- Is there evidence of sexism?
- Do you find advertisements in which women are portrayed as capable decision makers?
- Do you find women portrayed with a "Barbie doll" image?
- In advertisements including men and women, what is the implicit message about women?
- Do advertisers have a responsibility to portray both genders in a manner that promotes the well-being of the individual?

health care needs. There is usually a deductible, often of $500 or more, which must be paid by the insuree before the insurance company is required to pay anything.

Not only do too many people not have health insurance, but people continue to lose the coverage they have—tens of thousands lose their health insurance each month, and more than 46 million Americans do not have any health insurance.[56]

 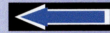

What Is Direct-to-Consumer Advertising?[57]

For decades, physicians or pharmacists have been expected to provide and interpret information, provided by pharmaceutical companies, about medications to their patients. However, as an increasing number of patients have become more involved in making their own health care decisions, some manufacturers have begun to create medical-related ads direct to consumers. In the past 20 years, direct-to-consumer (DTC) advertising has become increasingly popular.

These advertisements fall under the jurisdiction of the FDA, which helps to ensure that prescription drug information provided by drug firms is truthful, balanced, and accurately communicated. By surveying physicians and consumers, the FDA can determine if advertising rules need to be altered to help consumers better understand the benefits and risks of various medications.

Women and children are disproportionately represented among all uninsured individuals, with more than 23 million U.S. women uninsured. In addition, millions of women who are insured have difficulty accessing health care due to health coverage gaps, including noncoverage of essential services (medical screenings, dental care) and high deductibles or co-pays.[58] Uninsured women often postpone necessary health care, have limited access to preventive screenings such as a Pap test or cancer screenings, have delayed diagnoses of serious illness, often at incurable stages, receive less therapeutic care, and die at an earlier age or earlier in the disease process.[59] Uninsured or under insured women usually have no regular doctor, do not fill needed prescriptions, and often use emergency rooms as their health care facility, which is more expensive and often less effective. Disparities exist between women of color and white women: Hispanic and African American women are two to three times more likely to be uninsured than are white women.

A comprehensive health insurance plan that meets the specific needs of women, especially low-income women, should (1) provide universal access—especially for women who work part-time or are seasonal, or who move in and out of the workforce; (2) be affordable—especially because women have average earnings that are 25 percent less than men's; (3) allow reimbursement for a range of providers—midwives, nurse practitioners, and other medical personnel who are effective but less expensive than physicians; (4) be nondiscriminatory; (5) have equal rating factors—adopt a community rating and prohibit the insurance industry from using gender as a rating factor; (6) require a minimum benefits package with preventive care, reproductive care (family planning, abortion, infertility), mental health benefits, drug abuse care, long-term health care, HIV AIDS treatment, and care for battered women. When considering health care

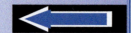

FYI

The Three Basic Health Insurance Plans

The type of health insurance plan a woman has will determine the type of medical services, procedures, and practitioners she will be able to use. Here is a brief look at three basic types of plans.

- *Private, fee-for-service plan:* The individual or employer pays a certain amount each month that ensures that a woman can receive health care on a fee-for-service basis. A deductible, paid by the patient, must be met and then the insurance pays a major portion, usually 80 percent, after the deductible is met. To lower costs of insurance, **preferred provider organizations (PPOs),** which are composed of private medical practitioners, provide services at a lower rate to a particular insurance company. Use of the PPO physicians produces lower health care fees; use of non-PPO physicians costs more.
- *Prepaid group insurance:* **Health maintenance organizations (HMOs)** are composed of various medical personnel who provide a wide range of medical services (e.g., specialists, lab work) for a prepaid amount that is usually deducted from each paycheck. There is often a co-pay (usually a minimal amount such as $15–$20) each time an HMO service is used. The HMO is usually associated with a hospital and provides care from a limited group of medical practitioners.
- *Government-financed insurance:* For women of certain ages and socioeconomic levels, the local, state, and/or federal government provides health care insurance under various types of plans. Briefly, two types of government insurance plans are (1) Medicare, which is paid from Social Security benefits for people 65 and older and for individuals with specific health concerns, and (2) Medicaid, which provides some health care coverage for individuals who meet certain financial criteria. These two types of coverage are discussed in greater detail in the text.

insurance, assess the quality of the provisions by comparing these components to the policy components.

Medicare and Medicaid

Medicare, provided by the federal government Social Security Act, is a government health insurance program that provides health care benefits for individuals 65 years of age and older. Disabled women under 65 may also be eligible for Medicare. Medicare consists of two parts: *Part A* is the Hospital Insurance and *Part B*

is Supplementary Medical Insurance. Part A helps to pay for inpatient care while in a hospital, or a skilled nursing facility, for home health care, and for hospice care. Medicare is a mandatory hospital insurance plan financed by federal Social Security taxes, but paid for by employers paying into Social Security on their employees' behalf and by self-employed persons. Part B helps to pay for physician services, outpatient care, lab tests, and other medical services and supplies. Monthly premiums paid by enrollees and from federal general revenues finance Part B Medicare. To enroll for Medicare, contact the Social Security Administration office found in the government section of your local phone book.[60]

Medicaid is a medical assistance program jointly financed by state and federal governments to help provide health care for low-income women with no health care. Eligible recipients include low-income women and those who cannot work; blind, elderly, and/or disabled individuals; low-income families with dependent children; and others with special circumstances. In 2004, 12.8 percent of the non-elderly population had health coverage through the use of Medicaid.[61] Of the Medicaid population recipients, women make up nearly 70 percent over the age of 15; women are twice as likely as men to qualify for Medicaid.[62] Even though states have expanded Medicaid coverage, 17.7 percent of women between the ages of 18 and 64 still do not have health insurance.[63] Federally mandated Medicaid services of significance to women include inpatient and outpatient hospital, physician, midwife, and certified nurse practitioner; laboratory and X ray; nursing home and home health care; rural health clinics; family planning; and early and periodic screening, diagnosis, and treatment for children under age 21. States have varying eligibility requirements, and the services are administered out of the county or state Human Services office. Women can contact this office for assistance.

In 2007, 50 million Americans were covered by Medicaid. In times of economic hardship, more people require economic assistance and have to turn to government programs such as Medicaid for health care insurance coverage. In 2008, the United States faced a severe economic recession and the number requiring Medicaid assistance soared, placing the Medicaid program officially in crisis. With Medicaid already the largest or second largest expense in every state's budget, increases on Medicaid rolls placed such a financial strain on the program that many states had to cut back Medicaid services, depriving millions of needed health care. Following are news reports from 2008 describing the Medicaid crisis.

Nineteen states—including Maryland and Virginia and the District of Columbia—have lowered payments to hospitals and nursing homes, eliminated coverage for some treatments, and forced some recipients out of the insurance program. Many are halting payments for healthcare services not required by the federal government, such as physical therapy, eyeglasses, hearing aids and hospice care. A few states are requiring poor patients to chip in more toward their care. . . All but one [of these 19 states], plus six other states, are drafting deeper reductions for the coming fiscal year that they hope to avoid.[64]

In late 2008, Florida's Medicaid officials handed the governor a blueprint for a 10 percent reduction; this would eliminate coverage for 7800 18- and 19-year-olds and 6800 pregnant women. In July 2008, California slashed its Medicaid program, known there as Medi-Cal, by 10 percent for the rates it pays hospitals, nursing homes, speech pathologists and other providers of health care in just one year, 2008, in Washington, D.C., the Medicaid rolls rose by 5000 to reach a total of nearly 150,000 people on the program in that area; to cope, the District adjusted the provision of program services by $20 million. In Maryland, Medicaid enrollment jumped 8 percent in 2008 and the state had to pare out $82 million from the program. In late 2008, Virginia proposed a $245 million cut from the nearly $3.3 billion that the state devotes to Medicaid, including reduced payments to hospitals and new limits on home health care. Rhode Island's approach was the most far-reaching in that the state chose to "forfeit its [federal] Medicaid entitlement and accept a total of $12 billion in federal money over the next five years. In exchange, Rhode Island would win uncommon freedom from federal rules, allowing it to enroll all its Medicaid patients in managed care, cover less treatment and expand care for elderly patients at home, instead of in more-expensive nursing homes."[65] In South Carolina officials made three rounds of cuts in 2008 that effectively will stop paying for dental care for adults, eliminate nutritional supplements, cut home delivered meals from fourteen a week to seven, curtail mental health counseling, stop building wheel-chair ramps and pay for fewer breast and cervical cancer screenings.

> Edna McClain, founder of Hospice Care of Tri-County in Columbia, S.C., helped coax state health officials to expand Medicaid to cover nursing care and other support for dying patients in the mid-1990s. She was stunned this month [December, 2008] when an e-mail arrived from South Carolina's Department of Health and Human Services informing her that as of January 1, Medicaid no longer would pay for new hospice patients. And after March 31, it would stop covering most people on Medicaid already in hospice care.[66]

When an economy is in such distress that state assistance programs are unable to provide many health services for the poor, what will happen to those who do not receive their much needed health care?

Social Security

Social Security (SS) is a protective program that provides benefits to workers and their families who have financial and health care needs. The program began in 1935 as a way to assist retired workers, most of whom were men, and the families of deceased workers. In the 1930s only a very small percentage of women worked in jobs outside the home; however, today about 60 percent of all women are employed outside the home and earn credit toward their retirement.[67] Women earn SS protection for themselves and their children, but also earn assistance if they become disabled and cannot work, and survivor benefits if they should die. Married women who choose not to work outside the home, or who enter the workforce for only a few years, may have Social Security benefits if their spouse retires, becomes disabled, or dies.

Retirement Benefits Retirement benefits vary according to age of the retiree. A woman can be eligible for benefits by age 62, but the payments will be permanently reduced because she will be receiving payments for a longer period of time than if she had waited until age 65. A woman will be eligible for full retirement benefits if she waits until she is 65 years of age to retire. In the future, the age in which full benefits are payable will be gradually increased—by the year 2027, a woman will need to be 67 years old to receive full retirement benefits.

If you are married, you can receive retirement payments on your husband's as well as your own employment record. There are often special circumstances related to SS retirement benefits, including age, former and current marital status, and the work history of both partners.

Special situations such as never being employed, self-employment, household worker, or service in the military have some unique aspects. Information related to these and other considerations can be obtained from the Social Security Administration office at www.ssa.org or from the local SS office. Social Security benefits related to remarriage, being widowed, and being divorced are multifaceted and sometimes complex.

To contact a representative from the local, state, or national Social Security office, see the Web site: www.ssa.gov.

TAKING ACTION AS A CONSUMER

Agencies

The Food and Drug Administration (FDA) has the responsibility to regulate the following products (with examples): foods (labeling, safety), drugs (approval, advertising), cosmetics (safety, purity), biological products (blood banks, human vaccines), medical devices (registration, approval), radiological devices (microwave, X-ray equipment), and veterinary products (pet foods, vet drugs) sold in interstate commerce. States enforce regulations on products that do not cross state lines. The states are also responsible for licensing health professionals such as dentists, physicians, and pharmacists as well as inspection and regulation of restaurants and health clubs.

The FDA offers a variety of services to assist the consumer with questions or concerns related to any product under its regulatory control. Consumer Affairs Officers (COAs) are located throughout the United States to answer questions and provide informational literature, either by print or through media. These officers (often referred to as public affairs specialists) will also speak to groups on specific topics related to drugs, fraud, safety, and many other topics of interest to consumers. Your local COA can be found under the Food and Drug Administration in the federal government section of the local phone book. The Consumer Inquiries Staff, located in Washington, D.C., has the responsibility of answering consumers' questions of any type. This staff has the ability to utilize the expertise of a variety of federal agencies to find the answer to inquiries, about 2500 each month. See the Resources at the end of this chapter for additional consumer resources.

Credit Reports

Reports of your credit history may be requested when you seek to purchase items such as an automobile, a home, or a large appliance. Credit bureaus collect and maintain great volumes of information on an individual's financial activities, including your buying and paying history. If a company wants to assess your creditworthiness, it can obtain a copy of your credit report from a number of credit agencies. Because of the increase in identity theft, it is essential to check your credit report regularly to determine if someone else is using any of your credit cards or bank accounts without your knowledge. You can obtain a copy of your credit report by contacting one of three national credit report agencies: Equifax, Trans Union, and Experian. Each year, you can order one free credit report from one of these agencies. Check carefully to see if there are any inaccuracies or questionable listings of debts. All three agencies can be accessed via the Web site, www.majorcreditreports.com.

Knowing what to do if inaccuracies appear in your credit report is an important consumer skill. If you find inaccuracies, write to the credit bureau that issued the report and report which credit listing is inaccurate. The credit report agency must, by law, reverify the information within a reasonable amount of time (usually 30–35 days) or the credit listing must be removed from your file. Information that is inaccurate or cannot be verified must be corrected or removed from your report. If you have some negative information on your report that is accurate, you may elect to write a brief explanation (about 100 words) to the credit bureaus and explain why the negative credit incident occurred. This may be helpful in obtaining credit even though the negative report usually must stay in your file for 7 years. Bankruptcy information is kept for 10 years. If this information appeared on one credit bureau report, it may appear on others. Therefore, it is a good idea to review all three major credit report agencies. Be sure to establish credit for yourself and not rely on your partner's credit line. There may be situations in which you will need to have established a credit rating for yourself.

Righting a Wrong

Even if we are wise consumers, there are times when we may be taken advantage of by an individual or a company or we may have purchased a faulty product. Knowing what to do and how to rectify this situation can be helpful and save time and money. Purchase-related paperwork of a product that is intended to last for a period of time should be saved in an organized file with other product-related information. If a problem occurs, contact the business (or person) that sold you the product and describe the problem and how you would like for it to be resolved. For example, do you want the product repaired or your money back? Keep a record of calls and/or letters to and from the company and include when and with whom you spoke. If the problem has not been resolved within a reasonable amount of time, then it is time to contact the company headquarters. Look on the packaging for a toll-free 800 number or call the toll-free 800 operator at 800-555-1212 to locate the number of the company. Most local libraries have a directory of 800 numbers, or you can get this information online (http://inter800.com or www.anywho.com.tt.html).

Many companies require a complaint to be in writing; therefore, knowing where to write and what to say can be valuable. Look for the address of the product manufacturer on the packaging of the product. If it is not there, or you do not have the packaging, go to the reference section in your local library and search for the company address in one of the following books: *Standard & Poor's Register of Corporations, Directors and Executives;* the *Standard Directory of Advertisers;* the *Trade Names Directory;* or the *Dun & Bradstreet Directory.* The *Thomas Register of American Manufacturers* can provide you with a list of manufacturers of thousands of products. After locating the address of the company, it is important to write a concise and reasonable, but not threatening, letter explaining what is wrong with their product and how you have attempted to resolve the problem. (See Figure 2.2.) Include your name, address, work or home phone numbers, and your company account number, if you have one. Provide the company with place and date of product purchase, and serial or model number of the product, and include copies, not originals, of all documentation. If, after a reasonable time, usually 2–4 weeks, you have not received satisfaction, file a complaint, along with a copy of your letter, with the local or state consumer protection agency that pertains to the nature of your concern. Addresses and phone numbers for agencies that govern banking, hospitals, insurance, products, and utilities can usually be found in the government pages of the telephone directory. Addresses for more specific agencies and companies are found in the *Consumer Action Handbook*.[68]

WHAT SHOULD BE THE PUBLIC'S PRIORITY: CORPORATE PROFIT OR CONSUMER SAFETY?

Corporations in the United States have a dual obligation: one, to make a profit so as to stay in business and two, to uphold the integrity of their product to maintain consumer safety. To enhance profit, companies have moved the production of most U.S. pharmaceuticals and medical devices outside of the United States to where there is an abundance of cheap labor, but an absence of appropriate oversight.

FIGURE 2.2 Sample complaint letter.[69]

Your street address
Your city, state, zip code
Date

(Name of contact person if available)
(Title, if available)
(Company name)
(Consumer complaint division, if you have no contact person)
(Street address)
(City, state, zip code)

Dear (contact person):

Re: (account number, if applicable)

　　On (date), I (bought, leased, rented, or had repaired) a (name of product with serial or model number or service performed) at (location, date, and other important details of the transaction).
　　Unfortunately, your product (or service) has not performed well (or service was inadequate) because (state the problem). I am disappointed because (explain the problem: for example, the product does not work properly, the service was not performed correctly, I was billed the wrong amount, something was not disclosed clearly or was misrepresented, etc.).
　　To resolve the problem, I would appreciate your (state the specific action you want— money back, charge card credit, repair, exchange, etc.). Enclosed are copies (do not send originals) of my records (include receipts, guarantees, warranties, canceled checks, contracts, model and serial numbers, and any other documentation).
　　I look forward to your reply and a resolution to my problem, and will wait until (set a time limit) before seeking help from consumer protection or the Better Business Bureau. Please contact me at the above address or by phone at (home or other number with area code).

Sincerely,

(Your name)

Enclosure(s)

cc: (who you are sending a copy of this letter, if anyone)

India and China, countries where the Food and Drug Administration rarely conducts quality-control inspections, have become major suppliers of low-cost drugs and drug ingredients to American consumers. Analysts say their products are becoming pervasive in the generic and over-the-counter marketplace. . . 'As the manufacturing goes to China and India, the risk to human health is growing exponentially,' said Brant Zell, past chairman of the Bulk Pharmaceuticals Task Force. . . 'The low level there' of follow-up inspections, 'combined with the huge amount of importing, greatly increases the potential that consumers will get products that have impurities or ineffective ingredients.'[70]

According to Gardiner Harris, Science Reporter for the New York Times,

The general perception is that the FDA is broken, and it's gotten there over decades of neglect on the part of Congress and on the part of presidents going back to Jimmy Carter's time. I think everybody thinks that the biggest

problem is the FDA's poor oversight of imported goods. Thirty years ago most of what you consumed, food-wise, drug-wise, medical device-wise, were made here. In the years since, obviously, there has been a wave of imports, so that now about 80 percent of the drugs that you take are imported, most of the medical devices, and obviously around 20-odd percent of the food. And the FDA just simply has gone nowhere in terms of its inspectional oversight of that flood. So the consequence is that at its present pace, the FDA would need about 27 years to inspect all foreign medical device plants, about 13 years to inspect all drug plants, and about 1900 years to inspect all food plants. It's obviously a situation that has to change and Congress knows it.[71]

Sidney Wolfe, director of the Health Research Group at Public Citizen and editor of WorstPills.org, states,

[I]ts own Science Board–Subcommittee of the FDA Science Board basically said, past reports have said, if you don't do this, there's going to be a crisis. They said the

FYI

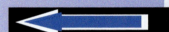

Products Protected from Damage Claims

During his term of office, from 2000 to 2008, President George W. Bush added language to FDA regulations that would pre-empt product-liability litigation. This would save corporations millions of dollars by not having to pay persons awards for damages from unsafe products. Below is a list of some of the products affected.

FOOD AND DRUG ADMINISTRATION REGULATIONS

Physician labeling rules	Noncarcinogenic sweeteners	Raw fruits, vegetables, fish
OTC nasal medication	Calcium	Nutrient content claims
OTC dandruff products	OTC laxatives	Dietary sweeteners
OTC contraceptives	Skin protection drug products	Soluble fiber
Skin bleaching products	OTC drugs in trial size packages	OTC analgesics
Sunscreen products	Fatty acids	Pregnancy and lactation labeling

NATIONAL HIGHWAY TRAFFIC SAFETY ADMINISTRATION REGULATIONS

Door locks	Head restraints	Tire pressure monitoring
Occupant crash protection	Side impact protection	Power operated windows
Lamps and reflective devices	School bus passenger seating	Roof crush resistance
Rearview mirrors	Electric-powered vehicles	Brake hoses
Child restraint systems	Motorcycle helmets	Motorcycle brakes

How can corporations make enough profit to stay in business and still sufficiently protect consumers? Corporate officers in the United States typically receive multi-million dollar salaries and year-end bonuses. Should these corporate officers be expected to defer a portion of such large incomes and redirect funds toward efforts to enhance consumer safety? Pharmaceutical companies make annual earnings in the billions but they say this is necessary to finance research for new drugs. Should pharmaceutical and other medical companies contribute a percentage of their profits to finance adequate inspection of drugs and medical devices, especially those imported from outside the United States?

crisis is here now, and they talked both about funding and the need to have better leadership and attract better scientists there. The FDA has unfortunately lost a lot of scientists there because they've not been treated very well during their stay.[72]

A willingness by corporations to increase profit at the expense of consumer safety can be directly enabled by political leanings. President George W. Bush's administration, 2000–2008, applied a heavy emphasis on increasing corporate profit at the expense of personal safety. Up until the last days of his presidency, Bush placed language into many FDA regulations that would preempt product-liability litigation, and thereby prevent persons from obtaining financial retribution for damages caused by unsafe products.[73] With little likelihood of penalty or punishment for inferior products, corporations were given a green light to cut corners where consumer safety is concerned. Bush basically obliterated a person's right to civil justice and provided corporations immunity for negligence (see *FYI:* "Products Protected from Damage Claims"). An example is a rule issued by Bush on October 8, 2008 at the

> Department of Transportation that limits the number of seatbelts car makers can be forced to install and prohibits suits by injured passengers who didn't get to wear one. These new rules can't quickly be undone by order of the next president. Federal rules usually must go through lengthy review processes before they are changed. Rulemaking at the Food and Drug Administration, where most of the new preemption rules have appeared, can take a year or more.[74]

The Bush administration further sided with corporate profit over personal safety by imposing a new rule inhibiting regulation of workplace hazards by the Occupational Safety and Health Administration (OSHA).[75] This Bush ruling prevents OSHA from fulfilling the primary reason it was created. Furthermore, the Bush administration rulings have interfered with the Environmental Protection Agency's (EPA) ability to perform its duties. For instance, the Bush administration has made it possible for oil and mining companies to infringe upon lands without concern for detrimental impact on air, water, animals, or people. Normally, environmental impact studies would be required, but no longer with Bush's rulings.

While it is clear that the FDA, OSHA, and EPA were designed to protect individuals and the environment, it is also clear that their ability to perform the purpose for which they were created has been greatly impaired by institutional neglect, reduction of staff and finances, and implication of rules that contradict or impede the true mission of the agency.

AFFORDABLE CARE ACT

One of the greatest political victories of U.S. President Barack Obama was the passage of his health care bill, which he signed into law as the Affordable Care Act on March 23, 2010. This sweeping overhaul of the U.S. health care system moved the country closer to universal health care than it has ever been before by ensuring health coverage for 95% of Americans. The Affordable Care Act is expected to have a profound impact on health and economic well-being of American families, businesses, and the economy. Some of the key provisions of the legislation were designed to:

- Ensure that all Americans have access to quality, affordable health care.
- Create a new, regulated marketplace where consumers can purchase affordable health care.
- Extend much needed relief to small businesses.
- Improve Medicare by helping seniors and people with disabilities afford their prescription drugs.
- Prohibit denials of coverage based on pre-existing conditions.
- Limit out-of-pocket costs so that Americans have security and peace of mind.
- Help young adults by requiring insurers to allow all dependents to remain on their parents plan until age 26.
- Provide sliding-scale subsidies to make insurance premiums affordable.
- Hold insurance companies accountable for how our health care dollars are spent.
- Clamp down on insurance company abuses.
- Invest in preventive care.

The Affordable Care Act cracks down on some of the most egregious practices of the insurance industry while providing the stability and the flexibility that families and businesses need to make the choices that work best for them. On June 22, 2010, the Departments of Health and Human Services, Labor, and Treasury issued regulations to implement a new Patient's Bill of Rights under the Affordable Care Act—which will help children, and eventually all Americans, with pre-existing conditions gain coverage and keep it, protect all Americans' choice of doctors and end lifetime limits on the care consumers may receive.[76] You can learn more about the Affordable Care Act at the government sponsored websites: Health Reform in Action (www.whitehouse.gov/HealthReform); My Care (www.HealthCare.gov); and A New Patient's Bill of Rights (www.whitehouse.gov/files/documents/healthcare-fact-sheets/patients-bill-rights.pdf).

The Affordable Care Act was far from controversial narrowly passing with a March 22, 2010 vote of 219–212 in the U.S. House of Representatives.[77] President Obama signed the bill into law the next day, and merely seven minutes after the bill was signed the attorneys general of thirteen U.S. States filed a lawsuit against the federal government claiming that legislating healthcare was unconstitutional—"The Constitution nowhere authorizes the United States to mandate . . . that all citizens and legal residents have qualifying health care coverage."[78]

BEING A CONSUMER ADVOCATE

While being a wise consumer is important to your health, equally important is being an ever watchful consumer advocate for individual and environmental health and safety. The Internet is a great resource for tracking current legislative activity; for example see the Web site "Reg Watch" at www.ombwatch.org, sponsored by OMB watch, a consumer group that monitors the federal Office of Management and Budget. The Internet is also a handy tool for sending a quick e-mail to your congress persons informing them of your stance on pending legislative actions on the state and federal level. Take a moment now to look up who your state and federal representatives are and find their Web sites on the Internet. The following websites are designed to help you to identify and contact your federal senators and representatives: http://www.senate.gov and https://writerep.house.gov/writerep/welcome.shtml.

Chapter Summary

- Effective consumer skills include having an awareness and knowledge of health products and services, making informed choices, and knowing how to obtain better consumer services.
- There are important guidelines that can be utilized when locating and selecting a health care provider.
- A variety of health care practitioners provide special and specific services that can be beneficial to women's health.
- Alternative health care offers options to conventional medicine but as a rule is not taught in U.S. medical schools. Many of these alternative practices have not been scientifically proven to be medically beneficial.
- Fraudulent health care costs American citizens more than $10 billion annually; therefore, it is essential to recognize and report acts of fraudulent behavior.
- Prescription and over-the-counter (OTC) drugs can cause physical and psychological addiction as well as tolerance and withdrawal symptoms.
- Prescription drugs are legal drugs used to treat and/or cure diseases and may be obtained in generic or brand-name forms.
- OTC drugs are purchased without a physician's prescription and can be used to treat various common ailments.
- Reading labels, following instructions, and consulting a physician as needed are important precautions to remember when taking OTC drugs.

- The physician's instructions should be strictly followed by pregnant women who use prescriptions and OTC drugs.
- An unrealistic portrayal of women has been created in order to promote the perception that certain types of products need to be purchased.
- Cosmetics, skin-care products, and facial and body cosmetic surgery are all products/procedures that can be expensive and risky; women can learn important guidelines for better selection of these products and procedures.
- Advertising is a major influence in the purchase of healthrelated products, and the media use a variety of techniques to sell these commodities.
- Women have specific needs in health insurance coverage yet are too often without important insurance coverage for themselves and their children.
- Information regarding health insurance, Social Security benefits, and retirement plans is needed by women in order to make health- and life-enhancing financial decisions.
- Medicare and Medicaid are government health insurance programs that provide health care benefits for women and children who meet specific criteria.
- Government and citizen consumer protection agencies provide avenues by which women can learn how to report problems with products/people/procedures and find assistance in correcting the problems.

Review Questions

1. What is the Consumer Bill of Rights, and what is its purpose?
2. What are the processes for locating and selecting a health care provider?
3. What are the advantages and disadvantages of using home health tests? Which are designed specifically for women?
4. Why are more women turning to alternative health care? What are some of the advantages and disadvantages of alternative health care?
5. How can you protect yourself from health care fraud?
6. What is the difference between brand-name and generic drugs?

7. What information is available on prescription and OTC drug labels, and what are the benefits of knowing this information?
8. What three federal laws were passed to help protect the consumer from poor-quality health products and inadequate health care?
9. How can women use medicinal drugs safely?
10. What are the pros and cons of purchasing an OTC drug? Which are purchased specifically by women?
11. What are some safety measures that women can take when selecting and purchasing cosmetics?
12. What are some of the concerns about cosmetic surgery? Why do many women elect to have these beauty-enhancing procedures?
13. What criteria should a woman use when selecting a cosmetic surgeon?

14. What is the purpose of the various advertising techniques used by companies to sell their products?
15. What techniques do advertisers use in promoting their products? Provide an example of a product for each of these techniques.
16. Why should women be concerned about how they are portrayed in advertisements?
17. What is the difference between basic, major medical, and comprehensive major medical insurance coverage?
18. Why are women and their children disproportionately uninsured in this country?
19. What health care benefits are provided by Medicare and Medicaid?
20. What elements should be included when writing a letter of complaint about a product, a professional, an agency, or a facility?

Resources

Agency for Healthcare Research and Quality
    www.ahcpr.gov/consumer
American Society of Plastic Surgeons
    www.plasticsurgery.org
Better Business Bureau
    www.bbb.org
Consumer Health Sourcebook
    www.chsourcebook.com
ConsumerLab.com
    www.consumerlab.com
FDA Office of Women's Health
    www.fda.gov/womens
Federal Citizen Information Center
    www.pueblo.gsa.gov
Federal Trade Commission
    www.ftc.gov/bcp/consumer.shtm
FirstGov for Consumers
    www.consumer.gov/index.htm
Food and Drug Administration
    www.fda.gov
Medline Plus

www.medlineplus.gov
National Association for Chiropractic Medicine
    www.chiromed.org
National Center for Complementary and Alternative Medicine
    nccam.nih.gov
National Council Against Health Fraud
    www.ncahf.org
National Women's Law Center
    capwiz.com/nwlc/home
Natural Medicines Comprehensive Database
    www.naturaldatabase.com
Quackwatch
    www.quackwatch.com
Social Security Online
    www.ssa.gov
U.S. Consumer Product Safety Commission
    www.cpsc.gov

References

1. Consumer Advisory Commission on Consumer Protection and Quality in the Health Care Industry. 1997. *Final report, consumer bill of rights & responsibilities.* www.hcqualitycommission.gov/cborr (retrieved September 15, 2006).
2. Barrett, S., W. London, R. Baratz, and M. Kroger. 2007. *Consumer health: A guide to intelligent decisions.* 8th ed. New York: McGraw-Hill.
3. Ibid.
4. Barzansky, B., and S. I. Etzel. 2003. Education programs in US medical schools, 2002–2003. *Journal of the American Medical Association* 290:1190–96.
5. Smith, M. 2002. The screening test you need. *WebMD Medical News.* http://aolsvc.health.webmd.aol.com/content/article/54/65232.htm (retrieved September 15, 2006).
6. Barrett et al., *Consumer health.*
7. American College of Nurse-Midwives. *A career in midwifery.* www.midwife.org (retrieved September 15, 2006).

8. Payne, H., D. B. Hahn, and E. Lucus. 2007. *Understanding your health.* 9th ed. New York: McGraw-Hill.

9. 4therapy.com. 2000. *Understanding therapists' professional degrees.* www.4therapy.com/consumer/about_therapy/item.php?uniqueid=4936&categoryid=402& (retrieved September 15, 2006).

10. U.S. Food and Drug Administration. 2003. *Buying diagnostic tests from the Internet: Buyer beware.* www.fda.gov/cdrh/consumer/ buyerbeware.html (retrieved September 15, 2006).

11. U.S. Food and Drug Administration: Office of In Vitro Diagnostic Device and Evaluation and Safety. *Home-use tests.* www.fda.gov/cdrh/oivd.consumer-homeuse.html (retrieved January 12, 2006).

12. National Institutes of Health: National Center for Complementary and Alternative Medicine. 2002. *What is complementary and alternative medicine (CAM)?* http://nccam.nih.gov/health/whatiscam (retrieved September 15, 2006).

13. Institute of Medicine, Committee on the Use of Complementary and Alternative Medicine by the American Public. 2005. *Complementary and alternative medicine in the United States.* Washington, DC: National Academies Press.

14. Ibid.

15. Barasch, D. S. 1994. The mainstreaming of alternative medicine. *Good Health* (October 4): 6–9, 36, 38.

16. Natural Medicine Comprehensive Database. 2003. www.naturaldatabase.com (retrieved September 15, 2006).

17. Common herbs. 2006. www.herbalgram.org/default.asp?c=common_herbs (retrieved September 15, 2006).

18. National Center for Complementary and Alternative Medicine. *Get the facts: Acupuncture.* http://nccam.nih.gov/health/acupuncture/(retrieved September 15, 2006).

19. Chiropractors. 1994. *Consumer Reports* 59 (6): 383–90.

20. Barrett et al., *Consumer health.*

21. American Chiropractic Association. 2003. *What is chiropractic?* www.amerchiro.org/level2_css.cfm?T1ID=13&T2ID=61 (retrieved September 15, 2006).

22. Barrett et al., *Consumer health.*

23. Chiropractors. *Consumer Reports.*

24. American Massage Therapists Association. 2005. *Research confirms massage therapy enhances health.* (retrieved on January 10, 2006).

25. Witherell, M. 1995. Massage: De-stress in minutes. *American Health* (September): 70.

26. Chiropractors. *Consumer Reports.*

27. Stalker, D., and O. Glymour. 1983. Engineers, cranks, physicians, magicians. *New England Journal of Medicine* 308:60–64.

28. Barrett et al. *Consumer health,* p. 37.

29. Ibid.

30. Carroll, C. R. 2000. *Drugs in modern society.* 5th ed. New York: McGraw-Hill, p. 280.

31. Barrett, et al., *Consumer health,* p. 410.

32. Food and Drug Administration. 2000. Requirements on content and format of labeling for human prescription drugs and biologics: Requirements for prescription drug product labels; proposed rule. *Federal Register* 65: 81081–131.

33. Prescription Kaiser Family Foundation. 2006. *Prescription drug trends.* www.kff.org/rxdrugs/upload/13057-05.pdf (retrieved May 1, 2007).

34. Food and Drug Administration: Center for Drug Evaluation and Research. 2003. *Nonprescription products: What we do.* www.fda.gov/cder/Offices/OTC/whatwedo.htm. (retrieved September 16, 2006).

35. Center for Drug Evaluation and Research. 2003. *Nonprescription products.* www.fda.gov/cder/Offices/OTC/default.htm (retrieved September 16, 2006).

36. Center for Drug Education and Research. 2002. *The new over-the-counter medicine label: Take a look.* www.fda.gov/cder/Offices/OTC/default.htm (retrieved September 16, 2006).

37. Rubin, J. P., C. Ferencz, and C. Loffredo. 1993. Use of prescription & non-prescription drugs in pregnancy. *Clinical Epidemiology* 46 (6): 581–89.

38. U.S. Food and Drug Administration. 2002. *Is it a cosmetic, a drug or both? (or soap)?* www.cfsan.fda.gov/~dms-cos-218.html (retrieved September 16, 2006).

39. Ibid.

40. Cavanaugh, T. 1995. Ethics expand. *Chemical Marketing Reporter* 2 (17): SR 21–22.

41. Moisturizers. 1994. *Consumer Reports* 59 (9): 577–81.

42. Columbia University: Go Ask Alice. 2003. *Moisturizers.* www.goaskalice.columbia.edu/2408.html (retrieved September 15, 2006).

43. Consumer Search. 2004. *Moisturizer comparison chart.* www.consumersearch.com/www/family/facial_moisturizers/comparisonchart.html (retrieved September 16, 2006).

44. Goodman, M. 1994. Social, psychological & developmental factors in women's receptivity to cosmetic surgery. *Journal of Aging Studies* 8 (4): 375–96.

45. The American Society for Aesthetic Plastic Surgery. 2003. *Botulinum toxin injections.* www.surgery.org/public/procedures-injectables.php. (retrieved September 15, 2006).

46. U.S. Food and Drug Administration. 2004. *Making an informed decision about breast implants.* www.fda.gov/fdac/features/2004/504_implants.html (retrieved May 1, 2007).

47. Jacobson, N. 2003. No clearer than it was before. *Washington Post,* October 26.

48. Food and Drug Administration. 2006. *Breast implants.* www.fda.gov/cdrh/breastimplants/qa2006.html#s1 (retrieved March 3, 2007).

49. Margolis, D. 1993. Fat chance: Rearrange the unwanted mass. *American Health* (March): 12, 18.

50. Ibid.

51. Barrett et al. *Consumer health.*

52. Shier, M. 1995. On being a boy toy. *Canada and the World Backgrounder* 60 (4): 8–10.

53. Ibid.

54. Bushy, J., and G. Leichty. 1993. Feminism & advertising in traditional and nontraditional women's magazine, 1950s–1980s. *Journalism Quarterly* 70 (2): 247–64.

55. Kanner, B. 1995. Advertisers take aim at women at home. *New York Times.*

56. National Coalition on Health Care. 2004. *Health insurance coverage.* www.nchc.org/facts/coverage.shtml (retrieved March 3, 2007).

57. Lewis, C. 2003. The impact of direct-to-consumer advertising. *FDA Consumer Magazine* online. (March/April). www.fda.gov/fdac/features/2003/203_dtc.html (retrieved September 16, 2006).

58. National Women's Law Center. 2005. *Women and health insurance.* www.nwlc.org/details.cfm?id=2186&section=health (retrieved March 3, 2007).

59. Ibid.

60. *Medicare.* 2007. The Official U.S. Government Site for People with Medicare. www.medicare.gov/Coverage/Home.asp (retrieved May 1, 2007).

61. Employee Benefit Research Institute. 2004. *Sources of health insurance and characteristics of the uninsured, analysis of the March 2004 Current Population Survey.* Issue brief #276.

62. National Women's Law Center. 2004. *Women and Medicaid.* http://nwlc.org/WomenMedicaidUpdate.June2004.pdf (retrieved January 27, 2006).

63. Ibid.

64. Goldstein, A. 2008. States cut Medicaid coverage further, p. 1. http://www.washingtospost.com (retrieved January 8, 2009.

65. Ibid., p. 2.

66. Ibid., p. 2.

67. Social Security Administration. 2003. *Social Security . . . what every woman should know.* SSA Publication No. 05-10127, ICN 480067. www.ssa.gov/pubs/10127.html#part6 (retrieved September 16, 2006).

68. *Consumer Action Handbook.* 2003. Washington, DC: U.S. Office of Consumer Affairs. www.consumeraction.gov (retrieved September 16, 2006). You can also request this handbook by calling the federal Consumer Information Center at 1-800-878-3256.

69. Consumer Action Webpage. 2007. *2007 Consumer action handbook.* http//www.consumeraction.gov/pdfs/2007revisedCAH.pdf (retrieved May 1, 2007).

70. Kaufman, M. 2007. FDA scrutiny scant in India, China as drugs pour into U.S.: Board oversees checks called too costly.

71. Harris, G. December, 22, 2008. Transcript, *The Diane Rehm Show: FDA,* pp. 5–6. National Public Radio: American University Radio (WAMU).

72. Wolfe, S. Transcript, *The Diane Rehm Show: FDA,* p. 6.

73. Fuson, J. 2008. Midnight regulation watch: Bush adminis tration gives gift that keeps on giving—Corporate immunity for negligence American Association for Justice (retrieved December 21, 2008).

74. Mundy, A. 2008. Bush rule changes could block product-safety suits. *The Wall Street Journal,* p. 1 http://online .wsj.com/article/SB122403828537735379.html (retrieved December 21, 2008).

75. Schwartz E. 2008. The Bush administration's midnight regulations: Critics say proposed rules would hurt consumers, environment, safety. *ABC News,* p. 1 http://abcnews.go.com/print?id=6146929 (retrieved December 21, 2008).

76. HealthCare.gov. June 22, 2010. Fact sheet: The Affordable Care Act's new patient's bill of rights. http://healthreform .gov/newsroom/new_patients_bill_of_rithgs.html.

77. Tumulty, K. March 23, 2010. Making history: House passes health care reform. *Time.* http://www.time.com/time/politics/article/0,8599,1973989,00.html.

78. Associated Press. March 23, 2010. Quotes of the day. *Time.* http://www.time.com/time/quotes/0,26174,1974701,00 .html.

(retrieved December 12, 2008). http://www.washingtonpost .com/wp-dyn/ content/article/2007/06/16/AR2007061601295.

Chapter Three

Developing a Healthy Lifestyle

CHAPTER OBJECTIVES

When you complete this chapter, you will be able to do the following:

◇ Define the dimensions of wellness with regard to the whole person concept

◇ Describe the health continuum, from wellness to illness, and appropriate intervention strategies

◇ Describe theories of learning and models of behavior change

◇ Plan a lifestyle change using the following: behavioral assessment, goal setting, behavioral contracting, initiation of behavior change, and periodic evaluation of progress

WHAT IS HEALTHY?

Do you consider yourself to be healthy? What do you compare yourself with to decide that you are healthy? How old do you feel? How long do you expect to live? These are not easy questions to answer primarily because living is a very complex process. Your health is dependent upon your personal lifestyle choices as well as upon uncontrollable elements, such as genetics, environmental conditions, the technological development of your country, your gender, your ethnicity, cultural issues, age-specific risks, and the potential for accidents.

This whole book serves as a guide for lifestyle assessment and enhancement for women. The ideas introduced in this chapter are meant to prepare you for the material presented in later chapters. And although much of the information in this chapter may be applied to anyone, you can use this information to help you understand how you, personally, make lifestyle choices. Think of this chapter as a presentation of the basic philosophies of health and behavior change.

Some people live to be over 100 years old and some die in infancy. Many factors must be considered in determining just how long you will actually live. Life expectancy figures are important in that they provide researchers with overall, statistical averages for tracking health concerns, but statistical averages do not consider the individual. The most important consideration for you is what you are doing to achieve a lifestyle that is enjoyable for you and that will prolong your enjoyment as much as possible.

This chapter presents average life expectancy figures and describes established models for healthy living. These health models serve as a basis for you to understand your own personal life concerns and can aid in the design of a lifestyle that suits you best.

Life Expectancy

On October 17, 2006, the population of the United States reached 300 million, making it the third most populous country behind China and India.[1] The United States claimed 100 million in 1915 and 200 million in 1967. According to the Census Bureau, one reason the population continues to rise is that births, one every 7 seconds, outnumber deaths, one every 13 seconds. Immigration also plays a role. The Census Bureau estimates that a migrant enters the country every 31 seconds. The fastest growing immigrant populations today are Asian and Hispanic, whose numbers are projected to double between 2000 and 2050. The U.S. growth rate is larger than that of any other industrialized country in the world, but it remains slower than that of developing countries, including India and China. According to the U.S. Population Reference Bureau,

> [T]he country's burgeoning population is having an adverse effect on the environment. Land is being developed at twice the rate of population growth, and some of the nation's fastest-growing regions are in the Western dry areas, which affects water resources. Air pollution is a problem in larger cities . . . and poor air quality may contribute to increased health problems among children and the elderly. Energy is also a concern; the United States consumes a quarter of the world's energy and is the single largest emitter of carbon dioxide in the world.[2]

On the morning of April 27, 2012, the U.S. population clock was 313,439,277 and the world population clock was 7,009,720,886 (for the latest numbers go to the U.S. Census Bureau web site, www.census.gov/main/www/popclock.html). The National Center for Health Statistics reported the following information on life expectancy.[3] Expectation of life at birth for all persons in the United States in the year 2010 was an average of 78.7 years; by gender this was 81.1 years for females and 76.2 years for males. Life expectancy in 2010 for white women was 81.3 years, which was 4.8 years more than white men. Life expectancy in the same year for black women was only 78.0 years, which was 6.2 years more than black men. Life expectancy in 2010 for Hispanic women was 83.8 years, which was 5.0 years more than Hispanic men.

According to a 2009 report by the Organization for Economic Co-operation and Development (OECD), the U.S. ranked near the bottom in life expectancy among wealthy nations despite spending more than double per person on health care than the industrialized world's average. The OECD report suggested the United States was not getting great value for its health spending in terms of life expectancy. The United States far outspent the next biggest health care spenders, Norway and Switzerland, despite the fact that those countries' life expectancies were 2–4 years longer, according to the report. The OECD reported life expectancy in years from birth in selected technologically developed countries. The top 14 highest life expectancy rankings for women reported by the OECD in the year 2007 were Japan (86.0), France (84.4), Switzerland (84.4), Spain (84.3), Australia (83.7), Finland (83.1), Sweden (83.0), Austria (82.9), Iceland (82.9), Norway (82.9), Germany (82.7), Republic of Korea (South Korea) (82.7), Belgium (82.6), and the Netherlands (82.3). The United States (80.4) was ranked 21st by the OECD for years of life expectancy for women in 2007 out of 29 industrialized

countries listed. The United Nations also compiled life expectancy rankings from birth examining data from 194 countries across the years 2005–2010; in the United Nations data the United States is ranked 38th overall (see Table 3.1, United Nations Life Expectancy Rankings). Women outlive men in almost every country and, on average, are expected to live 4 years longer than men.

Life expectancy refers to the number of years we are expected to live from birth. Although there is no way to predict how long each person is going to live at the time they are born, we can take an average of how long people have lived, which provides an indication of how long a certain cross section of a population might live. Life expectancy seems to be directly tied to income. The countries with the largest increase in life expectancy were also among the countries with the most rapid increase in their income per capita. There are big differences between regions. Africa has the lowest life expectancy. The HIV/AIDS epidemic is rampant in Africa. Among the obvious life-threatening health problems specific to women around the world is maternal mortality. The United Nations estimated in 2005 that each year about 600,000 women die of complications related to childbirth. With better maternal health care and education, this figure could change dramatically. Other factors that dramatically affect life expectancy are prolonged periods of war, civil strife, and genocide in a country or region. Examine Table 3.1 and then research what might be contributing to a high or low life expectancy for women in various countries. For example, the countries of North and South Korea are geographically similar and located next to one another, but North Korean women have a life expectancy much lower than South Korean women. This is a tremendous gap in years of life expectancy. Consider how different political and social climates in each of these countries might impact life expectancy. Japan has the greatest overall life expectancy for women. Several factors go into making Japan number one in the rankings, including a low rate of heart disease, which is associated with their traditional low fat and high soy and fish diet, and, until recently, limited use of tobacco.

More and more people are living longer, healthier lives. In the United States it is estimated that 76 million baby boomers will start retiring in the year 2010. The nation is about to experience a great demographic shock. Between 2010 and 2030 the over-65 population is expected to rise more than 70 percent while the population paying payroll taxes to support the elderly will rise less than 4 percent. While seniors can place a financial burden on a country, they can also serve as an incredible resource of knowledge and wisdom,

TABLE 3.1 United Nations Life Expectancy Rankings (2005–2010)

RANK	COUNTRY (TERRITORY)	OVERALL	MALE	FEMALE
1	Japan	82.6	79.0	86.1
2	Hong Kong	82.2	79.4	85.1
3	Switzerland	82.1	80.0	84.2
4	Israel	82.0	80.0	84.0
5	Iceland	81.8	80.2	83.3
6	Australia	81.2	78.9	83.6
7	Singapore	81.0	79.0	83.0
8	Spain	80.9	77.7	84.2
9	Sweden	80.9	78.7	83.0
10	Macau	80.7	78.5	82.8
11	France	80.7	77.1	84.1
12	Canada	80.7	78.3	82.9
13	Italy	80.5	77.5	83.5
13	New Zealand	80.2	78.2	82.2
15	Norway	80.2	77.8	82.5
16	Austria	79.8	76.9	82.6
16	Netherlands	79.8	77.5	81.9
18	Martinique	79.5	76.5	82.3
18	Greece	79.5	77.1	81.9
20	Belgium	79.4	76.5	82.3
20	Malta	79.4	77.3	81.3
20	United Kingdom	79.4	77.2	81.6
20	Germany	79.4	76.5	82.1
20	Virgin Islands	79.4	75.5	83.3
25	Finland	79.3	76.1	82.4
26	Guadeloupe	79.2	76.0	82.2
27	Channel Islands	79.0	76.6	81.5
27	Cyprus	79.0	76.5	81.6
29	Ireland	78.9	76.5	81.3
30	Costa Rica	78.8	76.5	81.2
31	Puerto Rico	78.7	74.7	82.7
31	Luxembourg	78.7	75.7	81.6
31	United Arab Emirates	78.7	77.2	81.5
34	South Korea	78.6	75.0	82.2
34	Chile	78.6	75.5	81.5
36	Denmark	78.3	76.0	80.6
36	Cuba	78.3	76.2	80.4
38	United States	78.2	75.6	80.8
39	Portugal	78.1	75.0	81.2
40	Slovenia	77.9	74.1	81.5
41	Kuwait	77.6	76.0	79.9
42	Barbados	77.3	74.4	79.8

43	Brunei	77.1	75.0	79.7
44	Czech Republic	76.5	73.4	79.5
45	Réunion	76.4	72.3	80.5
45	Albania	76.4	73.4	79.7
45	Uruguay	76.4	72.8	79.9
48	Mexico	76.2	73.7	78.6
49	Belize	76.1	73.3	79.2
49	New Caledonia	76.1	72.8	79.7
51	French Guiana	75.9	72.5	79.9
52	Croatia	75.7	72.3	79.2
53	Oman	75.6	74.2	77.5
53	Bahrain	75.6	74.3	77.5
53	Qatar	75.6	75.2	76.4
53	Poland	75.6	71.3	79.8
57	Panama	75.5	73.0	78.2
58	Guam	75.5	73.3	77.9
59	Argentina	75.3	71.6	79.1
60	Netherlands Antilles	75.1	71.3	78.8
61	Ecuador	75.0	72.1	78.0
62	Bosnia & Herzegovina	74.9	72.2	77.4
63	Slovakia	74.7	70.7	78.5
64	Montenegro	74.5	72.4	76.8
65	Vietnam	74.2	72.3	76.2
65	Malaysia	74.2	72.0	76.7
65	Aruba	74.2	71.3	77.1
65	Macedonia	74.2	71.8	76.6
69	Syria	74.1	72.3	76.1
69	French Polynesia	74.1	71.7	76.8
71	Serbia	74.0	71.7	76.3
71	Libya	74.0	71.7	76.9
73	Tunisia	73.9	71.9	76.0
	10% above World Average	73.9		
74	Venezuela	73.7	70.9	76.8
74	Saint Lucia	73.7	70.9	75.6
76	Bahamas	73.5	70.6	76.3
77	Palestinian Territories	73.4	71.8	75.0
78	Hungary	73.3	69.2	77.4
78	Tonga	73.3	72.3	74.3
80	Bulgaria	73.0	69.5	76.7
80	Lithuania	73.0	71.3	74.8
80	China (mainland)	73.0	71.3	74.8
83	Nicaragua	72.9	69.9	76.0
83	Colombia	72.9	69.2	76.6
85	Mauritius	72.8	69.5	76.2

(continued)

TABLE 3.1 *(continued)*

85	Saudi Arabia	72.8	70.9	75.3
87	Latvia	72.7	67.3	77.7
88	Jamaica	72.6	70.0	75.2
89	Jordan	72.5	70.8	74.5
89	Romania	72.5	69.0	76.1
91	Sri Lanka	72.4	68.8	76.2
91	Brazil	72.4	68.8	76.1
93	Algeria	72.3	70.9	73.7
94	Dominican Republic	72.2	69.3	75.5
95	Lebanon	72.0	69.9	74.2
95	Armenia	72.0	68.4	75.1
97	El Salvador	71.9	68.8	74.9
98	Turkey	71.8	69.4	74.3
98	Paraguay	71.8	69.7	73.9
100	Philippines	71.7	69.5	73.9
100	Cape Verde	71.7	68.3	74.5
102	Saint Vincent & the Grenadines	71.6	69.5	73.8
103	Samoa	71.5	68.5	74.8
104	Peru	71.4	68.9	74.0
104	Estonia	71.4	65.9	76.8
106	Egypt	71.3	69.1	73.6
107	Morocco	71.2	69.0	73.4
108	Georgia	71.0	67.1	74.8
108	Iran	71.0	69.4	72.6
110	Indonesia	70.7	68.7	72.7
111	Thailand	70.6	66.5	75.0
112	Russia	70.3	64.3	76.4
113	Guatemala	70.3	66.7	73.8
114	Suriname	70.2	67.0	73.6
115	Honduras	70.2	66.9	73.7
116	Vanuatu	70.0	68.3	72.1
117	Trinidad and Tobago	69.8	67.8	71.8
118	Belarus	69.0	63.1	75.2
119	Moldova	68.9	65.1	72.5
120	Fiji	68.8	66.6	71.1
121	Grenada	68.7	67.0	70.3
122	Micronesia	68.5	67.7	69.3
123	Maldives	68.5	67.6	69.5
124	Ukraine	67.9	62.1	73.8
125	Azerbaijan	67.5	63.8	71.2
126	North Korea	67.3	65.1	69.3
127	Uzbekistan	67.2	65.0	69.5
	World Average	67.2	65.0	69.5
128	Kazakhstan	67.0	61.6	72.4

129	Guyana	66.8	64.2	69.9
130	Mongolia	66.8	63.9	69.9
131	Tajikistan	66.7	64.1	69.4
132	Western Sahara	65.9	64.3	68.1
133	Kyrgyzstan	65.9	62.0	69.9
134	Bhutan	65.6	64.0	67.5
135	Bolivia	65.6	63.4	67.7
136	São Tomé & Príncipe	65.5	63.6	67.4
137	Pakistan	65.5	65.2	65.8
138	Comoros	65.2	63.0	67.4
139	India	64.7	63.2	66.4
140	Laos	64.4	63.0	65.8
141	Mauritania	64.2	62.4	66.0
142	Bangladesh	64.1	63.2	65.0
143	Nepal	63.8	63.2	64.2
144	Solomon Islands	63.6	62.7	64.5
145	Turkmenistan	63.2	59.0	67.5
146	Senegal	63.1	61.0	65.1
147	Yemen	62.7	61.1	64.3
148	Myanmar	62.1	59.0	65.3
149	Haiti	60.9	59.1	65.3
150	East Timor	60.8	60.0	61.7
	10% below World Average	60.8		
151	Ghana	60.0	59.6	60.5
152	Cambodia	59.7	57.3	61.9
153	Iraq	59.5	57.8	61.5
154	Gambia	59.4	58.6	60.3
155	Madagascar	59.4	57.7	61.3
156	Sudan	58.6	57.1	60.1
157	Togo	58.4	56.7	60.1
158	Eritrea	58.0	55.6	60.3
159	Papua New Guinea	57.2	54.6	60.4
160	Niger	56.9	57.8	56.0
161	Gabon	56.7	56.4	56.6
161	Benin	56.7	55.6	57.8
163	Guinea	56.0	54.4	57.6
164	Republic of the Congo	55.3	54.0	56.6
165	Djibouti	54.8	53.6	56.0
166	Mali	54.5	52.1	56.6
167	Kenya	54.1	53.0	55.2
	20% below World Average	54.1		
168	Ethiopia	52.9	51.7	54.3
168	Namibia	52.9	53.5	53.1
170	Tanzania	52.5	51.4	53.6
171	Burkina Faso	52.3	50.7	53.8

(continued)

TABLE 3.1 *(continued)*

172	Equatorial Guinea	51.6	50.4	52.8
173	Uganda	51.5	50.8	52.2
174	Botswana	50.7	50.5	50.7
175	Chad	50.6	49.3	52.0
176	Cameroon	50.4	50.0	50.8
177	Burundi	49.6	48.1	51.0
178	South Africa	49.3	48.8	49.7
179	Côte d'Ivoire	48.3	47.5	49.3
179	Malawi	48.3	48.1	48.4
181	Somalia	48.2	46.9	49.4
182	Nigeria	46.9	46.4	47.3
	30% below World Average	46.9		
183	Democratic Republic of the Congo	46.5	45.2	47.7
184	Guinea-Bissau	46.4	44.9	47.9
185	Rwanda	46.2	44.6	47.8
186	Liberia	45.7	44.8	46.6
187	Central African Republic	44.7	43.3	46.1
188	Afghanistan	43.8	43.9	43.8
189	Zimbabwe	43.5	44.1	42.6
190	Lesotho	42.6	42.9	42.3
190	Sierra Leone	42.6	41.0	44.1
192	Zambia	42.4	42.1	42.5
193	Swaziland	39.6	39.8	39.4
	40% below World Average	39.6		
194	Mozambique	39.2	38.3	39.0

giving much to enrich a community. Take, for example, the case of Maggie Kuhn who at the age of 65 organized senior citizens to protest the Vietnam War in 1970. The group was named the Gray Panthers. Kuhn and the Gray Panthers successfully addressed numerous issues in the community, especially those that stereotyped or discriminated against the elderly. (See *Women Making a Difference:* "Maggie Kuhn: Senior Activist.")

People living to be over 100 years old fascinate most of us. Those reaching 100 years or more are called centenarians. The United Nations World Population Revision released in 2000 included for the first time the numbers of octogenarians (ages 80–89), nonagenarians (ages 90–99), and centenarians (ages 100 and older). In 1998 around 135,000 persons in the world were estimated to be aged 100 years or older. The number of centenarians is projected to increase 16-fold by the year 2050

to reach 2.2 million. (See *Her Story:* "Portraits of Two Centenarians.")

Leading Causes of Death

The Centers for Disease Control and Prevention (CDC) reported the leading causes of death for U.S. females in 2007 as:

1. Heart disease (25.1 percent)
2. Cancer (22.1 percent)
3. Stroke (6.7 percent)
4. Chronic lower respiratory diseases (5.5 percent)
5. Alzheimer's disease (4.3 percent)
6. Unintentional injuries (3.6 percent)
7. Diabetes (2.9 percent)
8. Influenza and pneumonia (2.3 percent)
9. Kidney disease (2.0 percent)
10. Septicemia (1.6 percent)

Women Making a Difference

Maggie Kuhn: Senior Activist[4]

Maggie Kuhn was one of the founders of the Gray Panthers. She led a full and interesting life. She was born in Buffalo, New York, on August 31, 1905, in her grandmother's front bedroom; grew up in Cleveland; and graduated with honors from high school in 1922 and from college in 1926. She was sexually active with her boyfriend and utilized a diaphragm to prevent pregnancy. After college, she worked at the YWCA in Cleveland, Philadelphia, and later in New York, where she organized programs for working women, started classes on marriage and human sexuality, and provided programming for women workers assisting in the World War II effort. In 1950 she went to work for the Presbyterian Church, for which she traveled extensively to teach social justice issues to clergy and laity; however, her salary was thousands less than that of men who had equal or lesser jobs. By age 41, she had had two mastectomies. In 1958 she secured a mortgage and bought her own home in Philadelphia during a time when single women were not readily given loans because they were considered to be "undesirable risks." She commuted to work in New York City. In the 1960s, she developed a special interest in the problems of the elderly. During this period, the Presbyterian Church enforced its mandatory retirement policy upon her when she was 65 years old even though she did not yet desire retirement.

In 1970 Kuhn and five other active professional women who were facing retirement founded the Gray Panthers to protest the Vietnam War and later to address numerous social issues specific to the elderly. These issues included minority discrimination by the Social Security system, discrimination of lending policies by banks, nursing home reform, health care policies and concerns, home health care advocacy, and combating the myths and stereotypes of old age. In 1976 she was diagnosed with uterine cancer and had a radical hysterectomy. In 1977 she was attacked by a man in a hotel corridor and forced into her hotel room where she was physically assaulted and robbed. She refused to let the mugging incident keep her from her work or her travels, but she never walked down a hotel corridor alone again. She had a number of romances, but chose to never marry or have children. She remained sexually active through her senior years and promoted the premise of sexual activity for the elderly. She remained active in social causes until she died in 1995.

- How well do you know the seniors in your life?
- Are you missing out on some really good life stories, and perhaps life lessons, by not taking more time to listen to the elder persons in your life?

Her Story

Portraits of Two Centenarians

Jeanne Calment died in 1997 at the age of 122. She was born in France in 1875, before the Eiffel Tower was built. She remembered when a Dutch painter named Vincent van Gogh visited her hometown, Arles, in the south of France in 1888. She recalled that he was "very ugly, ungracious, impolite, crazy. I forgive him. They called him 'the Nut.'" Now both she and van Gogh are very famous people.[5]

Cruz Hernandez was a Salvadoran woman believed to be 128 years old and possibly the world's oldest person at the time of her death in 2007. National birth records show she was born on May 3, 1878, in central El Salvador. Ms. Hernandez gave birth to 13 children and ended up with 60 grandchildren, 80 great-grandchildren and 25 great-great grandchildren. Many who know her attributed her longevity to her favorite drink of a beer

with two raw eggs in it. She served as a midwife until she was 100 years old. Ms. Hernandez died peacefully in her sleep at her home in San Agustin. The evening before she had been feeling poorly and after eating a tamale and drinking some milk she went to sleep and never woke up. About 200 guests had celebrated her 128th birthday the previous May.[6]

A "supercentenarian" is a validated centenarian who has obtained the age of 110 years or more. To discover more supercentenarians see the Official Tables from the International Committee on Supercentenarians at http://www.grg.org/Adams/Tables.htm.

- Do you know any centenarians?
- Have you asked them to recall events in history from their point of view?

Cultural factors such as gender, age, and race/ethnicity may influence trends, and it is often necessary to look at data more closely in order to have an accurate perspective. It takes several years for the CDC to compile comprehensive data comparing multiple variables such as gender, age, and race/ethnicity and this data is presented in Table 3.2. In examining the data from the U.S. CDC for the year 2007, HIV was the fourth leading cause of death for black females aged 25–34, and the third leading cause of death for black females aged 35–44. In contrast, HIV disease as a cause of death for white females was tenth for ages 25–34, and did not break the top ten for any other white, female age groups. Thus, HIV disease was a much more prevalent cause of death for black females than for white females. A very different profile is demonstrated for suicide as a cause of death for females. As a cause of death for white females in the United States in 2007, suicide was ranked second for age groups 15–19 and 20–24, ranked third for white females aged 25–34, ranked fourth for age group 35–44, ranked fifth for age group 45–54, and ranked tenth for white females aged 55–64. In contrast for black females, suicide was ranked sixth for age group 10–14 years, fifth for age group 15–19 years, seventh for age group 20–24 years, and ninth for age group 25–34 years. Thus, suicide was somewhat more prevalent for white females than black females. Awareness about differences in cause of death related to gender, age, and race or ethnicity is vital for targeting health education and resources where they are needed most.

The leading causes of death for people in economically advanced countries may be very different from those for people in impoverished, developing countries. Lack of education, income, nutrition, and access to adequate health care are major contributors to diseases and deaths in poor countries. The lack of food can be most perilous for young children since it retards their physical and mental development. Food crises are a result of several contributing factors including declining agricultural productivity, drought, growing populations, economic failures, and conflicts.

The United Nations reported in 2005 that each year almost 11 million children worldwide die before the age of 5 (or 30,000 children per day), and most of these children live in developing countries. Most of these deaths are from diseases that are easily preventable with vaccines or conditions that can be successfully treated with proper attention and medication. Five diseases, including AIDS, account for half of all deaths in children under the age of 5. Among diseases that can be eradicated through immunization, measles is the leading cause of death for children. Measles strikes 30 million children a year, killing 540,000 and leaving many others blind or deaf.

The World Health Organization (WHO) reported the top ten leading causes of death in 2004 for women worldwide who were of reproductive age as:

1. HIV/AIDS (19.2 percent)
2. Maternal conditions (14.6 percent)
3. Tuberculosis (6.4 percent)
4. Self-inflicted injuries [suicide] (4.7 percent)
5. Road traffic accidents (3.7 percent)
6. Lower respiratory infections (2.9 percent)
7. Heart disease (2.9 percent)
8. Fires (2.9 percent)
9. Stroke (2.2 percent)
10. Violence (1.7 percent)

According to the WHO report, complications during pregnancy and childbirth were the second leading cause of death in 2004 among women of reproductive age worldwide. The WHO reported that HIV/AIDS was the leading cause of death in 2004 for women worldwide who were of reproductive age. Nearly two-thirds of HIV-infected persons live in sub-Saharan Africa. Slowing the spread of HIV/AIDS is a major goal of the WHO.

Globally, the epidemic shows no signs of slowing, with an estimated 4.9 million people becoming infected with HIV in the year 2004 and 3.1 million deaths due to AIDS this same year (500,000 of these deaths among children under 15 years of age). Nearly half of all people living with HIV are females, and as the epidemic worsens, the share of infected women and girls is growing. In sub-Saharan Africa, 57 percent of those infected with HIV are female.

We live in a global society and it is important to consider the health of women not only in the country in which we live but in other countries as well. Worldwide poverty and disease place a strain on the global economy. Economic and social services from countries that are relatively better off are sent as assistance to countries that lack the resources to combat poverty and disease. When certain countries are in despair, in some ways the whole world is impacted by the pain and suffering. We must remain ever diligent in our pursuit of health and wellness for women worldwide.

WHOLE PERSON CONCEPT

Your health status is not limited to the physical realm because you also have emotions, thoughts, and spirit. These all work together to bring about your state of well-being. Each of these interacts with the other, so, if you are affected in one area, the other areas will also be impacted. When examining your lifestyle, it is important to look at the whole picture of your health.

TABLE 3.2 Leading Causes of Death for U.S. Females by Age and Race [8]

All races	%	White	%	Black	%	Asian/Pacific Is.	%	American Indian	%
All races, all ages	%	*White, all ages*	%	*Black, all ages*	%	*Asian/Pacific Is., all ages*	%	*American Indian, all ages*	%
Diseases of heart	25.1	Diseases of heart	25.2	Diseases of heart	27.2	Malignant neoplasms	27.2	Malignant neoplasms	18.8
Malignant neoplasms	22.1	Malignant neoplasms	21.9	Malignant neoplasms	23.3	Diseases of heart	23.3	Diseases of heart	17.4
Cerebrovascular diseases	6.7	Cerebrovascular diseases	6.7	Cerebrovascular diseases	9.2	Cerebrovascular diseases	9.2	Accidents	8.8
Respiratory diseases	5.5	Respiratory diseases	5.9	Diabetes mellitus	4.1	Diabetes mellitus	4.1	Diabetes mellitus	6.3
Alzheimer's disease	4.3	Alzheimer's disease	4.6	Kidney diseases	3.8	Accidents	3.3	Cerebrovascular diseases	4.9
All races, 1–4 yrs.	%	*White, 1–4 yrs.*	%	*Black, 1–4 yrs.*	%	*Asian/Pacific Is., 1–4 yrs.*	%	*American Indian, 1–4 yrs.*	%
Accidents	29.6	Accidents	29.9	Accidents	26.4	Accidents	20.5	Accidents	48.5
Congenital defects	12.6	Congenital defects	12.8	Assault (homicide)	15.3	Congenital defects	15.1	Congenital defects	7.5
Malignant neoplasms	8.9	Malignant neoplasms	9.8	Congenital defects	11.8	Malignant neoplasms	12.3	Assault (homicide)	5.0
Assault (homicide)	8.9	Assault (homicide)	6.9	Malignant neoplasms	9.3	Diseases of heart	12.3	Diseases of heart	5.0
Diseases of heart	4.4	Diseases of heart	4.5	Respiratory diseases	3.3	Assault (homicide)	5.5	Malignant neoplasms	2.5
All races, 5–9 yrs.	%	*White, 5–9 yrs.*	%	*Black, 5–9 yrs.*	%	*Asian/Pacific Is., 5–9 yrs.*	%	*American Indian, 5–9 yrs.*	%
Accidents	33.0	Accidents	32.4	Accidents	35.0	Accidents	26.2	Accidents	53.3
Malignant neoplasms	18.9	Malignant neoplasms	20.8	Malignant neoplasms	13.4	Malignant neoplasms	14.3	All other causes	20.0
Congenital defects	8.3	Congenital defects	8.0	Congenital defects	8.5	Congenital defects	9.5	Malignant neoplasms	6.7
Assault (homicide)	5.6	Assault (homicide)	5.6	Assault (homicide)	6.5	Diseases of heart	7.1	Congenital defects	20.0
Diseases of heart	3.9	Diseases of heart	4.2	Respiratory diseases	3.3	Cerebrovascular diseases	7.1		
All races, 10–14 yrs.	%	*White, 10–14 yrs.*	%	*Black, 10–14 yrs.*	%	*Asian/Pacific Is., 10–14 yrs.*	%	*American Indian, 10–14 yrs.*	%
Accidents	33.2	Accidents	33.7	Accidents	31.2	Accidents	32.0	Accidents	44.0
Malignant neoplasms	17.2	Malignant neoplasms	18.7	Malignant neoplasms	12.6	Malignant neoplasms	18.0	Suicide	16.7
Congenital defects	5.9	Congenital defects	5.8	Assault (homicide)	9.3	Congenital defects	8.0	Septicemia	5.6
Assault (homicide)	5.0	Assault (homicide)	4.0	Diseases of heart	7.0	Suicide	8.0	Malignant neoplasms	5.6
Diseases of heart	4.5	Diseases of heart	3.9	Congenital defects	6.3	Cerebrovascular diseases	4.0	Benign neoplasms	5.6
All races, 15–19 yrs.	%	*White, 15–19 yrs.*	%	*Black, 15–19 yrs.*	%	*Asian/Pacific Is., 15–19 yrs.*	%	*American Indian, 15–19 yrs.*	%
Accidents	52.2	Accidents	58.5	Accidents	42.2	Accidents	41.2	Accidents	50.6
Assault (homicide)	7.8	Suicide	7.4	Assault (homicide)	14.4	Malignant neoplasms	11.2	Suicide	14.5
Suicide	7.4	Malignant neoplasms	7.2	Malignant neoplasms	10.0	Suicide	6.9	Assault (homicide)	6.0
Malignant neoplasms	7.0	Assault (homicide)	5.6	Diseases of heart	5.6	Assault (homicide)	2.9	Malignant neoplasms	4.8
Diseases of heart	3.1	Diseases of heart	2.8	Suicide	3.3	Congenital defects	1.3	Pregnancy/childbirth	4.8
All races, 20–24 yrs.	%	*White, 20–24 yrs.*	%	*Black, 20–24 yrs.*	%	*Asian/Pacific Is., 20–24 yrs.*	%	*American Indian, 20–24 yrs.*	%
Accidents	41.4	Accidents	45.4	Accidents	25.0	Accidents	41.5	Accidents	54.1
Assault (homicide)	8.7	Suicide	8.9	Assault (homicide)	17.9	Suicide	19.0	Suicide	11.2
Suicide	8.1	Malignant neoplasms	8.2	Diseases of heart	8.2	Malignant neoplasms	11.3	Assault (homicide)	7.1
Malignant neoplasms	7.9	Assault (homicide)	6.4	Malignant neoplasms	6.8	Assault (homicide)	6.3	Diseases of heart	6.1
Diseases of heart	5.4	Diseases of heart	4.9	Pregnancy/childbirth	5.0	Diseases of heart	1.4	Malignant neoplasms	2.0

(continued)

TABLE 3.2 (continued)

All races, 25–34 yrs.

Cause	%
Accidents	28.1
Malignant neoplasms	13.9
Diseases of heart	8.2
Suicide	7.8
Assault (homicide)	5.8

All races, 35–44 yrs.

Cause	%
Malignant neoplasms	25.9
Accidents	16.6
Diseases of heart	11.8
Suicide	5.3
HIV disease	3.6

All races, 45–54 yrs.

Cause	%
Malignant neoplasms	35.3
Diseases of heart	15.0
Accidents	7.0
Cerebrovascular diseases	4.1
Liver disease/cirrhosis	3.5

All races, 55–64 yrs.

Cause	%
Malignant neoplasms	41.1
Diseases of heart	17.6
Respiratory diseases	5.3
Diabetes mellitus	4.1
Cerebrovascular diseases	4.0

All races, 65+ yrs.

Cause	%
Diseases of heart	28.0
Malignant neoplasms	19.4
Cerebrovascular diseases	7.5
Respiratory diseases	6.0
Alzheimer's disease	5.4

White, 25–34 yrs.

Cause	%
Accidents	32.9
Diseases of heart	14.5
Malignant neoplasms	9.2
Suicide	4.6
Assault (homicide)	7.0

White, 35–44 yrs.

Cause	%
Malignant neoplasms	26.9
Accidents	19.3
Diseases of heart	10.9
Suicide	6.6
Liver disease/cirrhosis	3.3

White, 45–54 yrs.

Cause	%
Malignant neoplasms	36.9
Diseases of heart	13.8
Accidents	10.0
Cerebrovascular diseases	3.8
Suicide	3.5

White, 55–64 yrs.

Cause	%
Malignant neoplasms	42.6
Diseases of heart	16.5
Respiratory diseases	6.0
Diabetes mellitus	3.6
Accidents	3.6

White, 65+ yrs.

Cause	%
Diseases of heart	27.9
Malignant neoplasms	19.3
Cerebrovascular diseases	7.5
Respiratory diseases	6.4
Alzheimer's disease	5.6

Black, 25–34 yrs.

Cause	%
Accidents	13.6
Diseases of heart	12.1
Malignant neoplasms	11.8
HIV disease	10.9
Assault (homicide)	9.2

Black, 35–44 yrs.

Cause	%
Malignant neoplasms	21.2
Diseases of heart	15.1
HIV disease	11.3
Accidents	8.0
Cerebrovascular diseases	4.6

Black, 45–54 yrs.

Cause	%
Malignant neoplasms	29.1
Diseases of heart	19.9
Cerebrovascular diseases	6.1
Accidents	5.3
HIV disease	5.1

Black, 55–64 yrs.

Cause	%
Malignant neoplasms	33.7
Diseases of heart	23.2
Diabetes mellitus	6.1
Cerebrovascular diseases	5.6
Kidney diseases	3.4

Black, 65+ yrs.

Cause	%
Diseases of heart	29.3
Malignant neoplasms	19.9
Cerebrovascular diseases	7.9
Diabetes mellitus	5.3
Alzheimer's disease	3.8

Asian/Pacific Is., 25–34 yrs.

Cause	%
Malignant neoplasms	21.3
Accidents	18.0
Suicide	16.4
Assault (homicide)	6.6
Diseases of heart	6.6

Asian/Pacific Is., 35–44 yrs.

Cause	%
Malignant neoplasms	43.8
Accidents	10.1
Suicide	8.3
Diseases of heart	8.0
Cerebrovascular diseases	6.4

Asian/Pacific Is., 45–54 yrs.

Cause	%
Malignant neoplasms	51.4
Diseases of heart	8.9
Cerebrovascular diseases	7.3
Accidents	5.8
Suicide	2.9

Asian/Pacific Is., 55–64 yrs.

Cause	%
Malignant neoplasms	49.3
Diseases of heart	14.2
Cerebrovascular diseases	7.7
Diabetes mellitus	4.3
Accidents	3.8

Asian/Pacific Is., 65+ yrs.

Cause	%
Diseases of heart	26.7
Malignant neoplasms	22.1
Cerebrovascular diseases	10.3
Diabetes mellitus	4.5
Influenza and pneumonia	3.6

American Indian, 25–34 yrs.

Cause	%
Accidents	43.8
Diseases of heart	7.8
Suicide	7.8
Liver disease/cirrhosis	6.9
Assault (homicide)	6.0

American Indian, 35–44 yrs.

Cause	%
Accidents	23.4
Liver disease/cirrhosis	12.4
Malignant neoplasms	10.3
Diseases of heart	10.6
Diabetes mellitus	3.6

American Indian, 45–54 yrs.

Cause	%
Malignant neoplasms	21.8
Liver disease/cirrhosis	13.9
Accidents	13.5
Diseases of heart	10.6
Diabetes mellitus	4.2

American Indian, 55–64 yrs.

Cause	%
Malignant neoplasms	27.4
Diseases of heart	15.7
Diabetes mellitus	7.5
Liver disease/cirrhosis	7.4
Accidents	5.5

American Indian, 65+ yrs.

Cause	%
Diseases of heart	22.5
Malignant neoplasms	19.8
Diabetes mellitus	7.8
Cerebrovascular diseases	6.7
Respiratory diseases	6.3

Mind, Body, and Spirit

One comprehensive conceptual model of individual health involves all three of the following elements: psyche, soma, and spirit (mind, body, and spirit).[9] The psyche involves your emotional, attitudinal, and mental state. Soma, or body, refers to your physical status. Spiritual health is your philosophy about living for yourself and living with others. Have you thought about yourself in these three different ways?

Two major categories of factors influence your status as a whole person: endogenous factors and exogenous factors. **Endogenous factors** are those events that occur within you. Examples are the presence or absence of illness, a positive or negative attitude, ability to have intimacy, and so on. **Exogenous factors** are external events that influence you, such as the type of personal relationships you have, the weather, stressful events, and so on. Endogenous and exogenous events interact to create an impact on your whole person. Can you think of some things occurring within and around you that impact your health? (To assess your current health habits, see *Assess Yourself:* "Personal Health Inventory.")

Assess Yourself

Personal Health Inventory[10]

Circle the number for each item that best describes you.

Cigarette Smoking

Note: If you never smoke, enter a score of 10 for this section and go to the next section on Alcohol and Drugs.

	Almost Always	Sometimes	Almost Never
1. I avoid smoking cigarettes.	1	0	
2. I smoke only low tar and nicotine cigarettes or I smoke a pipe or cigars.	2	1	0

Cigarette Smoking Score: _____

Alcohol and Drugs

	Almost Always	Sometimes	Almost Never
1. I avoid drinking alcoholic beverages or I drink no more than 1 or 2 drinks a day.	4	1	0
2. I avoid using alcohol or other drugs (especially illegal drugs) as a way of handling stressful situations or the problems in my life.	2	1	0
3. I am careful not to drink alcohol when taking certain medicines (for example, medicine for sleeping, pain, colds, and allergies) or when pregnant.	2	1	0
4. I read and follow the label directions when using prescribed and over-the-counter drugs.	2	1	0

Alcohol and Drug Score: _____

	Almost Always	Sometimes	Almost Never
Eating Habits			
1. I eat a variety of food each day, such as fruits and vegetables, whole-grain breads and cereals, lean meats, dairy products, dry peas and beans, and nuts and seeds.	4	1	0
2. I limit the amount of fat, saturated fat, and cholesterol I eat (including fat on meats, eggs, butter, cream, shortenings, and organ meats such as liver).	2	1	0
3. I limit the amount of salt I eat by cooking with only small amounts, not adding salt at the table, and avoiding salty snacks.	2	1	0
4. I avoid eating too much sugar (especially frequent snacks of sticky candy or soft drinks).	2	1	0

Eating Habits Score: _____

	Almost Always	Sometimes	Almost Never
Exercise/Fitness			
1. I maintain a desired weight, avoid being overweight or underweight.	3	1	0
2. I do vigorous exercise for 15–30 minutes at least 3 times a week (examples include running, swimming, brisk walking).	3	1	0
3. I do exercises that enhance my muscle tone for 15–30 minutes at least 3 times a week (examples include yoga and calisthenics).	2	1	0
4. I use part of my leisure time participating in individual, family, or team activities that increase my level of fitness (such as gardening, bowling, golf, and baseball).	2	1	0

Exercise/Fitness Score: _____

Stress Control

1. I have a job or do other work that I enjoy.	2	1	0
2. I find it easy to relax and express my feelings freely.	2	1	0
3. I recognize early, and prepare for, events or situations likely to be stressful for me.	2	1	0
4. I have close friends, relatives, or others to whom I can talk about personal matters and call on for help when needed.	2	1	0
5. I participate in group activities (such as church and community organizations) or hobbies that I enjoy.	2	1	0

Stress Control Score: _____

Safety

1. I wear a seat belt while riding in a car.	2	1	0
2. I avoid driving while under the influence of alcohol and other drugs.	2	1	0
3. I obey traffic rules and the speed limit when driving.	2	1	0
4. I am careful when using potentially harmful products or substances (such as household cleaners, poisons, and electrical devices).	2	1	0
5. I avoid smoking in bed.	2	1	0

Safety Score: _____

Interpretation: There is no total score for this inventory. Compare your individual scores for each topic with the scales below.

9–10   Excellent! Your answers show that you are aware of the importance of this area to your health.

6–8   Your health practices in this area are good, but there is room for improvement.

3–5   Your health risks are showing! You should seek out information on changing your behaviors in this area.

0–2   Your answers show that you may be taking serious and unnecessary risks with your health in this area. It is definitely time to take the steps to change your behaviors. Seek out information and assistance about behavior change.

Dimensions of Wellness

Wellness has been described as consisting of six major dimensions: physical, emotional, social, occupational, intellectual, and spiritual.[11] Do you think it is possible to pay attention to all six dimensions in your life? Some feel that this may be one ultimate goal of wellness. You may not be able to pay attention to all six at once, but you can take turns on each one at different times in your life, depending on which is most important to you at the time. (See *FYI:* "Descriptions of Wellness.")

Holistic Wellness Model

Another way to conceptualize health is as five primary dimensions of wellness—physical, emotional, social, occupational, and intellectual—and two basic components within each dimension, a personal component and a spiritual component (see Figure 3.1).[12] The personal component is striving for the satisfaction of your own personal needs, such as nutrition, exercise, shelter, income, relaxation, recreation, education, and personal achievement. The spiritual component is striving for a relationship or connection with other persons and things, such as family, friends, community, country, world, and higher power. This includes enhanced awareness, knowledge, and love of others. Sometimes an issue or event is not clearly in one area but rather may coexist in more than one wellness dimension and in more than one component, spiritual or personal, at a time.

Developing a healthy lifestyle is a process. It is a goal worth working toward, but it can often be a life goal. Total attention to all wellness dimensions at the same time is very difficult to achieve. Thus, the holistic wellness model is not a mandate, but it is a guide for living.

ACHIEVING OPTIMUM WELLNESS

You must decide for yourself how you want to design your lifestyle. Life events and demands may pull you in one direction or another, and balance may not be possible until the events and demands are worked through. As a woman, your style of living is going to look different from that of a man. In fact, everyone's lifestyle is different. Wellness models can be used to assess your lifestyle based on an ideal. However, it is ultimately up to you to decide how you want your life to be the same or to be different. (See *Journal Activity:* "Your Personal Wellness Guide.")

Even if you currently have an illness or disorder, you can still achieve the optimum level of wellness that is right for you. Design a lifestyle that maximizes your own health potential and contributes to your longevity.

WORLD WELLNESS

There are six primary environmental issues for world wellness: air, water, energy, food, toxins, and

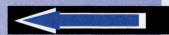

FYI

Descriptions of Wellness[13]

- *Physical wellness* is the willingness to take time each week to pursue activities that increase physical flexibility and endurance. A physically well person understands and employs the relationship between nutrition and body functioning.
- *Emotional wellness* is an awareness and acceptance of a wide range of feelings for oneself and others. It includes an ability to freely express and manage feelings effectively. An emotionally well person functions autonomously, yet is aware of personal limitations and the value of seeking interpersonal support and assistance.
- *Social wellness* is the willingness to actively participate in and contribute to efforts that promote the common welfare of one's community. A socially well person lives in harmony with fellow human beings, seeks positive interdependent relationships with others, develops healthy sexual behaviors, and works for mutual respect and cooperation among community members.

- *Occupational wellness* is the personal satisfaction and enrichment one experiences through work. The occupationally well person has integrated a commitment to work into a total lifestyle and seeks to express personal values through involvement in paid and unpaid activities that are rewarding to the individual and valuable to the community.
- *Intellectual wellness* is self-directed behavior that includes continuous acquisition, development, creative application and articulation of critical thinking, expressive and intuitive skills, and abilities toward the achievement of a more satisfying existence.
- *Spiritual wellness* is the willingness to seek meaning and purpose in human existence, to question everything, and to appreciate the intangibles that cannot be explained or understood readily. A spiritually well person seeks harmony between that which lies within the individual and the forces that come from outside the individual.

FIGURE 3.1 Holistic wellness model. The spiritual component starts from deep within ourselves (center dark circle) and extends outward (dark lines), influencing our personal component (outer white circle) and connecting us with our community.

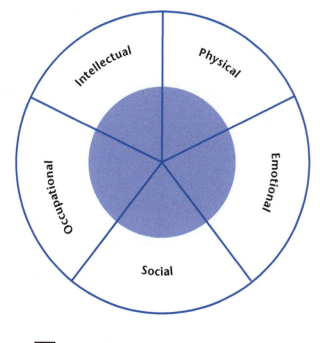

☐ Personal component
☐ Spiritual component

nature.[14] These are described further as air quality, water quality, sustainable energy and recycling, sustainable agriculture, hazardous material and waste management, and protection of wilderness areas and rain forests. The basic essentials of life include air, water, food, physical activity, and sexual activity. Because the earth sustains us, the world must be kept in good shape in order for humans to continue to survive.

In the area of environmental health, many questions remain to be answered. For example, should action be taken to reduce the possible risks of exposure to residential electric and magnetic fields? Should an alternative to water chlorination be found to reduce the chlorination by-product cancer risk in drinking water? Should policies be developed to reduce greenhouse gas emissions to prevent global warming? People who advocate precautionary measures believe we should act now. Those who adopt a more conservative approach prefer that we wait until clear evidence supports the existence of the problem. There are many factors to consider in the environmental decision-making process.[15]

It is vital that we attend to the issues of world health in addition to individual health. What does world wellness have to do with women's health? Well, the world is often referred to as *Mother Earth,* and she does nurture our survival. The Mother Earth concept is perhaps the earliest and strongest female archetype that exists for women. (See *Health Tips:* "Enhancing World Wellness"; *Journal Activity:* "Your World Wellness Guide." *FYI:* "Politics Can Damage World Wellness;" and *Assess Yourself:* "What Is Your EnviroQ?")

Journal Activity

Your Personal Wellness Guide

Use the following guide to become more aware of your own personal wellness. Read the questions and record your ideas. A few examples have been provided to get you started. Some of the dimensions and components may overlap. You may want to include behaviors for both a personal component (a focus more on yourself) and a spiritual component (a focus more on other). See Figure 3.1 as a guide.

- How do you participate in physical wellness?
  Examples:

Personal Component	*Spiritual Component*
nutrition, vitamins	volunteer at a food bank
regular exercise	charity walk-a-thon
get a massage	support a sick friend

- How do you participate in emotional wellness?
  Examples:

Personal Component	*Spiritual Component*
have a positive attitude	avoid blaming others
seek personal therapy	listen and be supportive
express your needs	respect needs of others

- How do you participate in social wellness?
  Examples:

Personal Component	*Spiritual Component*
ask to be included	invite others along
ask for honesty and respect	be honest and respectful
receive community assistance	be a community volunteer

- How do you participate in occupational wellness?
  Examples:

Personal Component	*Spiritual Component*
be in a job you like	help others get a job
develop your skills further	teach job skills to others
invest *your* money	recycle products

- How do you participate in intellectual wellness?
  Examples:

Personal Component	*Spiritual Component*
learn	teach
be creative or artistic	encourage creativity
broaden your experience	share your experience

Health Tips

Enhancing World Wellness

It is very easy to participate in world wellness. You can do small things every day that can have a big impact. Here are some ideas to get you started.

- Turn out the lights in every room you are not using and use energy-efficient light bulbs.
- Do not throw litter on the ground.
- Join a community litter cleanup group.
- Recycle newspaper, paper, plastic, bottles, and aluminum.
- Use biodegradable soaps and detergents; many of these are available in your local grocery store or health food store.
- Plant a garden and grow food.
- Plant and care for a tree.
- Drive environmentally safer vehicles having low exhaust output and safer air-conditioning systems.
- Share a ride or carpool.
- Take short showers, and don't fill the tub all the way when taking a bath.
- Fix water drips and leaks as soon as possible. Water is more precious than gold.
- Use less water in your toilet tank with each flush by setting the water level lower.
- Do not purchase products from companies that regularly violate environmental protection laws.

WORLD WELLNESS FOR WOMEN

The United Nations Fourth World Conference on Women, held in Beijing in 1995, made an important contribution to the global wellness of women. The Platform for Action for this conference was an agenda for women's empowerment and reaffirms the fundamental principle set forth in the World Health Organization's 1994 Vienna Declaration and Program of Action adopted by the World Conference on Human Rights: "[T]he human rights of women and of the girl child are an inalienable, integral and indivisible part of universal human rights."[16] Critical areas of concern for the Beijing conference were

- The burden of poverty on women
- Unequal access to education and training

- Unequal access to health care
- Violence against women
- The effects of armed or other kinds of conflict on women, including those living under foreign occupation
- Inequality in economic structures and policies
- Inequality in the sharing of power and decision making
- Insufficient mechanisms to promote the advancement of women
- Lack of respect for and inadequate promotion and protection of the human rights of women
- Stereotyping of women and inequality in women's access to and participation in all communication systems, especially in the media
- Gender inequalities in the management of natural resources and in safeguarding of the environment
- Persistent discrimination against and violation of the rights of the girl child

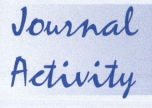

Journal Activity

Your World Wellness Guide

How are you contributing to world wellness in each of these six areas?

- Maintaining and/or improving air quality
- Maintaining and/or improving water quality
- Saving energy and/or recycling
- Growing and/or saving food
- Preventing and/or reducing toxins and pollutants
- Preserving and/or enhancing nature

FYI

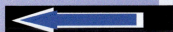

Politics Can Damage World Wellness

Agencies and legislation in place to protect the environment can be handcuffed by political cronyism that is motivated by greed.

Under the Bush administration [2000–2008], the EPA [Environmental Protection Agency] became overly politicized, sided with corporate polluters, and often ignored findings and recommendations by its own scientists . . . [T]he agency charged with safeguarding the nation's health and environment systematically eroded its mission over the years. In the most glaring example, the EPA backed off a finding that said climate change was a risk to public welfare. The findings would have led to the nation's first mandatory global-warming regulations. Instead, EPA Administrator [and Bush appointee] Stephen L. Johnston watered-down the final report, which delayed action to combat global warming. . . More broadly, under [President] Bush the EPA's funding was slashed, scientific findings censored, and enforcement de-emphasized.[17]

The Environmental Protection Agency's pursuit of criminal cases against polluters has dropped off sharply during the Bush administration, with the number of prosecutions, new investigations and total convictions all down by more than a third. Critics of the agency say its flagging efforts have emboldened polluters to flout U.S. environmental laws, threatening progress in cleaning the air, protecting wildlife, eliminating hazardous material, and countless other endeavors overseen by the EPA.[18]

In another glaring example of Bush's interference, EPA officials "tried to set a lower seasonal limit on ozone to protect wildlife, parks and farmland, as required under the law. . . Bush overruled EPA officials and ordered the agency to increase the limit. 'It is unprecedented and an unlawful act of political interference for the president personally to override a decision that the Clean Air Act leaves exclusively to EPA's expert scientific judgment,' said John Walke, clean-air director for the Natural Resources Defense Council [NRDC]."[19]

If you look at NRDC's website you'll see over 400 major environmental roll backs that are listed there that have been implemented or proposed by this administration over the past four years as part of a deliberate concerted effort to eviscerate 30 years of environmental law.[20]

This is the worst environmental president we've had in American history," said Robert F. Kennedy, Jr.[21]

What motivates politicians to reduce or neglect environmental protection? In the long run, does the motivation serve the greater good, helping the most people?

Assess Yourself

What Is Your Enviroq?

1. How many tons of road salt are used each year in the United States?
   a. 500 thousand
   b. 2 million
   c. 11 million
   d. 97 million

2. What percent of U.S. waste materials is potential compost?
   a. 11 percent
   b. 23 percent
   c. 47 percent
   d. 72 percent

3. What type of trash takes up the most space in U.S. landfills?
   a. Plastic
   b. Metal
   c. Paper
   d. Yard waste

4. Transportation consumes about what percent of the total energy used in the United States?
   a. 10 percent
   b. 25 percent
   c. 33 percent
   d. 50 percent

5. Water-efficient fixtures can save how much water per home annually?
   a. 1500 gallons
   b. 9300 gallons
   c. 54,000 gallons
   d. 99,000 gallons

6. Which creates more pollution, the average car or the average home?
   a. Average car
   b. Average home
   c. About the same
   d. Neither

7. What's the number one trash item found on beaches?
   a. Cigarette filters
   b. Plastic bottles
   c. Seaweed
   d. Food bags

8. A typical light bulb wastes what percent of electricity?
   a. 5 percent
   b. 30 percent
   c. 65 percent
   d. 90 percent

9. Recycling aluminum cans saves how much energy, compared to making new aluminum?
   a. 35 percent
   b. 55 percent
   c. 75 percent
   d. 95 percent

10. The average home can accumulate how many pounds of hazardous waste in one year?
    a. 10 pounds
    b. 50 pounds
    c. 100 pounds
    d. 500 pounds

(Answers: 1-c, 2-b, 3-c, 4-b, 5-c, 6-b, 7-a, 8-d, 9-d, 10-c)

(Source: Environmental Protection Agency.)

The twenty-third special session of the United Nations General Assembly on Women 2000: Gender Equality, Development and Peace for the Twenty-First Century took place in June 2000 and adopted a political declaration and outcome document titled "Further Actions and Initiatives to Implement the Beijing Declaration and Platform for Action." This special session of the General Assembly was convened to review current status in the implementation of the plans set forth at the Beijing Conference.[22] The progress of the Beijing Platform is monitored by the United Nations departments of the Division for the Advancement of Women and the Bureau on the Status of Women.

The fiftieth session of the United Nations Commission on the Status of Women was held in February–March 2006. The main themes of this session were (1) enhanced participation of women in development: to create an enabling environment for achieving gender equality and the advancement of women, taking into account the fields of education, health and work; and (2) equal participation of women and men in decision-making processes at all levels. Reports of the sessions of the United Nations Commission on the Status of Women are available from the United Nations Entity for Gender Equity and the Empowerment of Women (see www.unwomen.org).

WELLNESS VERSUS ILLNESS

Health is viewed along a continuum of wellness to illness with myriad possibilities in between. **Health intervention** is defined as the act or fact of interfering so as to modify.[23] Health interventions fall into at least

FIGURE 3.2 Maslow's hierarchy of needs.

Education	Prevention	Treatment
(Primary prevention)	(Secondary prevention)	(Tertiary prevention)

◄ - ►

Wellness Healthy Comfort Discomfort Illness Disease

three categories: education, prevention, and treatment. (See Figure 3.2.)

Education

Health education involves research and study in the causes, prevention, and treatment of disorders and diseases. It also involves the publication and distribution of this information to the public. Paramount to education is the concept of health promotion. **Health promotion** efforts include

- Dissemination through literature and workshops of information regarding healthy lifestyles, enhancement of life quality, and illness prevention
- Provision of information about early warning signs of disorders and diseases
- Provision of information regarding community services for assessment, such as health checkups
- Assistance in the development of personal health programs in each of the wellness dimensions

The American Cancer Society has an extensive education program. They publish pamphlets about the warning signs of breast cancer, posters of women using breast self-examination, and even poems written by and about survivors of breast cancer.

Prevention

Preventive health action is defined as measures serving to avert the occurrence of illness or disease.[24] According to the public health service model for prevention, services may be directed toward the individual (host), toward the source (agent), and toward the environment that encourages and supports, or sustains, the source. This is referred to as the epidemiological model. **Epidemiology** is the study of the relationships of the various factors determining the frequency and distribution of diseases in a human community.[25] For example, let us consider three preventive measures regarding the health risks of drinking alcohol for pregnant women. First, an educational campaign is directed toward women explaining the increased risk to the woman and to her fetus from alcohol consumption while she is pregnant. This preventive action is directed at the individual or host. This educational campaign can take

many forms, such as information provided by physicians or other health care providers, educational materials distributed at prenatal care clinics, and information articles in popular women's magazines or other publications. Second, a legislative bill requires that alcohol products manufacturers and distributors place a statement on their product containers warning that use of that product while pregnant may cause a health hazard. This preventive action is directed at the source or agent. Third, advertisers of these products are required to include on any printed advertisement of their product the warning of the health hazards of drinking alcohol while pregnant. This preventive measure is directed at an environment that may support alcohol consumption, in this case, the advertising industry.

Prevention efforts can be divided into three types: primary, secondary, and tertiary. **Primary prevention** is an extension of health education. Based on what we know, we can take steps to enhance the quality of life and prevent the development of illness. Primary interventions include efforts that assist with the prevention of most discomfort, disorders, diseases, and premature death. This prevention can be accomplished by sufficient attention to those things that keep us healthy—such as proper diet, regular exercise, a positive attitude, stress management and relaxation, fostering relationships, avoidance of toxins and pollutants, avoidance of the abuse of drugs and alcohol, avoidance of tobacco, and looking both ways before crossing the street. The bottom line is to live smart and be well.

In spite of your best efforts, you could possibly still experience some degree of discomfort, disorder, or disease in your life. **Secondary prevention** identifies persons who are in the early stages of "unhealth," which may lead to the development of disorders or illnesses. Secondary prevention attempts are interventions used to stop unhealthy behaviors and seek any necessary treatment.

Tertiary prevention is the application of an intervention to treat an existing disorder or illness. This is for the purpose of preventing the disorder or illness from getting worse. Tertiary prevention can also involve rehabilitation efforts, which attempt to facilitate recovery to the highest degree of health possible for an individual.

Treatment

Treatment interventions are applied to halt the progress of a discomfort, disorder, or disease and, if possible, move the individual away from discomfort and toward increased health. A woman who has entered menopause may experience extreme discomfort that accompanies this phase, such as hot flashes and mood swings. She may want to seek the assistance of a health provider for the purpose of considering hormone replacement therapy, or instead she may want to seek the advice of an herbologist for herbs that can reduce the discomforts of menopause.

Health treatment can involve intervention by a mental health provider, a physical health provider, or both. Examples of mental health providers include mental health counselors, social workers, psychologists, drug and alcohol counselors, marriage and family therapists, and psychiatrists. Examples of physical health providers include physicians, nurse practitioners, nurses, dentists, rehabilitation therapists, osteopaths, chiropractors, herbalists, massage therapists, and physical therapists.

It is up to you to decide from whom you would like to seek treatment and what type of treatment you wish to receive. It is best to act as an educated consumer and be as familiar as possible with the current and most effective treatment or treatments for your condition. It is also advisable to seek an opinion from more than one health professional, whenever appropriate, to explore additional possibilities regarding diagnosis and treatment.

LEARNING AND BEHAVIOR

In considering learning behavior you must understand the role of primary reinforcers: positive, negative, and punishment.[26] A **positive reinforcer** is rewarding.

If your behavior is followed by something perceived by you as rewarding, then you will more likely repeat that behavior. If you exercise and feel better, then you may be more likely to exercise more. A **negative reinforcer** is the removal of something uncomfortable, and this too can be rewarding; thus, if your behavior is followed by the removal of something uncomfortable to you, then the likelihood that you will repeat that behavior increases. For example, if telling an individual to stop criticizing you unnecessarily results in a positive outcome, you are more likely to assert yourself again. **Punishment** involves the presentation of something uncomfortable. Thus, when your behavior is followed by punishment, the likelihood of that behavior being repeated by you decreases. For example, if you drink too much alcohol and become very sick, you will be less likely to drink so much again.

The concept of learned behaviors is basically simple. However, how would you explain resistance to change even with the presentation of reinforcers? Resistance to change is often a result of the existence of secondary reinforcers. A **secondary reinforcer** is much less obvious but still has some influence over behavior. If you are experiencing difficulty in changing your behavior, then consider less obvious reasons that may be holding you back, such as an interfering belief or value. (See *Her Story:* "Danette: Resistance to Change.")

Her Story

Danette: Resistance to Change

Danette came into therapy complaining of extreme stress in her life. She played a major role as a caretaker to her children, spouse, and peers. She left no time for herself. She had anxiety and extreme headaches. The counselor suggested that she reprioritize her life, learn and use assertiveness skills, and incorporate time and stress management techniques. These skills and techniques were recommended to her by the therapist because they are known to be documented, effective strategies for assisting with Danette's kind of problem. However, Danette persisted in her complaints without trying the techniques even though she seemed to understand that they would in fact help her situation. The counselor suspected that Danette might have less obvious motives contributing to her resistance to change (secondary reinforcers), motives that Danette herself might not be completely aware of. Through continued exploration of Danette's values and belief systems, the counselor discovered that Danette believed she was not a worthwhile person unless she sacrificed herself for others. It was further discovered that this was a very old belief that Danette learned as a child from her mother: "To be a good person you must always sacrifice yourself for others, otherwise you are a selfish person." This belief became integrated into Danette's lifestyle when she was rewarded with praise in childhood whenever she acted accordingly. When Danette realized that this old belief was creating difficulty for her, she decided to put it aside in certain situations so that she could make healthier choices in her life.

- How can Danette determine when the act of putting another's needs before her own is too much sacrifice?
- In what other ways can Danette be assured that the needs of others are being met without always having to be the one who meets the needs of these others?

Hierarchy of Needs

The importance placed on a reinforcer is dependent upon the value that you give it. This can vary greatly from person to person. However, the "Hierarchy of Needs" is a way of exploring the motivating potential of a reinforcer.[27] At least five sets of goals, usually referred to as basic needs, are common to all persons: physiological, safety, love, esteem, and self-actualization. These needs contribute to motivating actions or behavior. Maslow summarizes the Hierarchy of Needs as shown in Figure 3.3.

Physiological needs, the lowest level on the hierarchy, refer to such things as freedom from hunger, sufficient oxygen, adequate water, sufficient sleep, freedom of movement, and sexual activity. Safety needs refer to such things as protection from danger, nonisolation, sufficient trust to build relationships, freedom from fear, and freedom from deprivation. Love needs are composed of such things as love, affection, and belongingness. Esteem needs refer to such things as the desire for respect from others, self-respect, self-esteem, achievement, adequacy, confidence, and independence. Self-actualization needs, the highest level on the hierarchy, are the need or desire to become everything one is capable of becoming, to strive for ideals, and to strive for success or life satisfaction.

Typically, you do not move up the Hierarchy of Needs until your lower needs are met sufficiently. However, there may be instances when upper-level needs take precedence over lower-level needs. (See *Her Story:* "Charlene: Hierarchy of Needs.")

FIGURE 3.3 Maslow's hierarchy of needs.

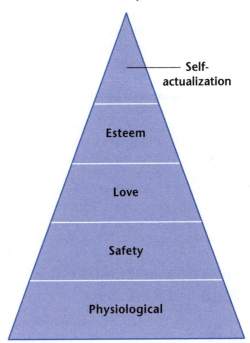

THEORIES AND MODELS OF BEHAVIOR CHANGE

There are many models and theories that suggest ways to change health behaviors. Some of these were developed many years ago but still present ideas that are very relevant today.

Her Story

Charlene: Hierarchy of Needs

Charlene, an 18-year-old college student, was diagnosed with an eating disorder called anorexia nervosa. Charlene was a member of the gymnastics team, and she felt she needed to make her weight as low as possible to stay on the team. She was literally starving herself to death because of her belief that she was overweight and her fear that she would get kicked off the team. Her body weight became dangerously low and, starved for nutrition, it began to rob her muscles and organs of vital nutrients. Her situation had become life threatening. In this case, Charlene placed a higher priority on esteem needs than

on physiological needs. Thus, she was motivated to behavior based on the area of her life in which she believed there was the greatest need. Charlene's belief was not well grounded in reality, because she was an anorexic who was willing to starve her body in an effort to feel better about herself.

- How can education and counseling about the concept of the hierarchy of needs be used to help Charlene?
- How can you relate each level in the hierarchy of needs to your own life and the decisions you have made about your health and well-being?

The Transtheoretical Model

The transtheoretical model of change, sometimes referred to as the multicomponent stage model, suggests that you will experience several stages as you attempt to change your health behavior over time.[28] The first stage is precontemplation, the time when you are not seriously thinking about changing during the next 6 months. The second stage is contemplation, when you are seriously thinking about behavior change during the next 6 months. The third stage is action, the 6-month period following an overt modification of a behavior. The fourth stage is maintenance, the period after action until the unwanted behavior is permanently modified or terminated. The final stage is termination, when you are no longer tempted by the unwanted behavior, and you feel confident in your ability to resist relapse.

Theories of Reasoned Action and Planned Action

The theory of reasoned action promotes three primary concepts that affect behavior change: your attitude toward performing the behavior, standard beliefs about what relevant others think you should do, and your motivation to comply with those others.[29] In other words, sometimes you may do certain things because other people who are important to you or have power over you think that you should do them. This concept is often referred to as the subjective norm. Doing things because others think you should can work in both positive and negative ways. For example, if Charlene's coach keeps encouraging her to lose more and more weight, then the coach may actually reinforce Charlene to be anorexic. However, if Charlene's coach encourages the athletes to maintain a proper, nutritious diet, then Charlene will be less likely to engage in unhealthy eating behavior. The theory of planned action is similar to the theory of reasoned action with one addition. The theory of planned action adds the concept of perceived behavioral control. The perceived ease or difficulty of performing the behavior is assumed to reflect past experience as well as anticipated obstacles and impediments. The more favorable the attitude and subjective norm with respect to behavior, and the greater the perceived behavioral control, the stronger should be the individual's intentions to perform the behavior under consideration.[30]

Self-Efficacy

The perception of potential benefits of action is related to the concept of self-efficacy. **Self-efficacy** is the conviction that one can successfully execute the behavior or behaviors required to produce desired outcomes.[31] Let's say that you were, in fact, significantly overweight. Your ability to design and stick to a plan of behavior change would depend on your belief that you could do it. Self-efficacy suggests that people's beliefs in their ability to perform specific behaviors influence the following:[32]

- Choice of behavior and the situations that will be avoided or attempted
- Effort expended in a specific task
- How long one will persist with a task even when facing difficulties
- Emotional reactions such as positive emotions with perceived success or negative emotions with perceived lack of success

A strong sense of self-efficacy is essential for the promotion of healthy behavior change.

Now that you have reviewed the various models and theories that suggest how behavior is changed, it is time to consider how you can develop your own individualized plan of action.

PLANNING YOUR LIFESTYLE CHANGE

You can manage many lifestyle changes through a self-help plan of action. This involves three primary steps: take a personal inventory, maintain a helpful attitude, and develop a plan of action. The plan should be realistic and developed with an attitude of appreciation for even the smallest of movements toward the goal. Patience is also a major key when persevering a lifestyle change.

Personal Inventory

The first step in a self-help plan is to take a personal inventory. This involves an evaluation of personal health habits and practices. (See *Journal Activity:* "Your Personal Health Behavior Inventory.")

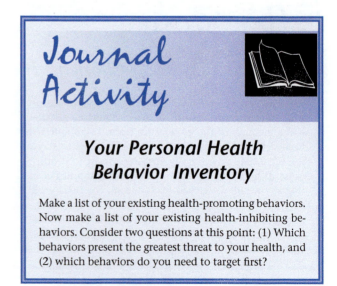

Journal Activity

Your Personal Health Behavior Inventory

Make a list of your existing health-promoting behaviors. Now make a list of your existing health-inhibiting behaviors. Consider two questions at this point: (1) Which behaviors present the greatest threat to your health, and (2) which behaviors do you need to target first?

Helpful Attitude

A realistic and positive attitude is paramount to successful behavior change. It is important not to set goals too high nor expect outcomes too quickly. Both of these attitudes can lead to discouragement and even termination of effort. It is also important to view behavior change as a lifestyle change rather than just a temporary goal. Otherwise, success that is achieved may be short-lived. Avoid an attitude of denial or deprivation; these can result in preoccupations of thought or impulsive actions that worsen the targeted behavior. Instead, find healthy substitutes for the things that you are reducing or eliminating from your life.

Plan of Action

Essential principles of lifestyle management when structuring a plan of action include (1) assessing behavior, (2) setting specific and realistic goals, (3) formulating intervention strategies, and (4) evaluating progress.[33]

Assessment of current behaviors involves the process of counting, recording, measuring, observing, and describing. Assessment tools are usually daily logs, journals, and diaries. The assessment phase is completed when there is sufficient information to form a behavior profile, state specific goals, and customize a program that matches your unique circumstances and personality.

FIGURE 3.4 Behavior change contract.

BEHAVIOR CHANGE CONTRACT

Name: _____ Date of Contract: _____

Identified health area for change: _____

_____

Long-term goal: _____

_____

Intermediate goals: _____

_____

_____

_____

Estimated time to achieve each intermediate goal: _____

_____

_____

_____

Rewards for achieving intermediate goals: _____

_____

_____

_____

Support network (persons and facilities): _____

_____

_____

_____

_____   _____
Signature of Participant   **Signature of Witness**

Goal setting involves establishing specific and realistic goals for behavior change. Specific goals are concrete, observable, and measurable. Realistic goals are reasonable and relate to personal circumstances. Goal setting should start off small to facilitate initial successes that will provide further motivation for continued participation in the personal lifestyle change program.

Intervention strategies should be personalized to fit your needs. Common intervention strategies include the use of stimulus control, healthy positive reinforcers, and positive behavior substitution and behavioral contracts. Stimulus control includes the reduction or elimination of the stimulus that encourages the original unhealthy behavior. For example, to help you stop smoking cigarettes, you might use nicotine patches that have gradually lower dosages of nicotine. The presentation of healthy positive reinforcers or rewards will increase the potential for healthy behaviors to be reported. For example, if you are attempting to overcome procrastination, you can reward yourself with an activity you enjoy, such as a bike ride, after you complete a chore. Positive behavior substitution is the incorporation of a healthy behavior that is incompatible with the unhealthy behavior, such as walking instead of watching television or chewing gum instead of smoking.

A **behavior change contract** is a written agreement in a behavior change program. Most contracts state long-range and intermediate goals, target dates for completion, rewards, intervention strategies, names of friends and resources to serve as a support network, and witnesses to the agreement who serve as sources for encouragement. (See Figure 3.3 for a sample behavior change contract, and then complete *Journal Activity:* "Behavior Change Contract.")

Journal Activity

Behavior Change Contract

Write a behavior change contract in your journal. Keep a record in your journal of your activities related to the contract. Assess your progress periodically. Remember to reward yourself in healthy ways for demonstrating progress toward your goals. Don't forget to frequently seek out encouragement and guidance from your support system.

To evaluate your progress, you must regularly monitor goal-related activities. Consistent monitoring provides information necessary for determining progress toward your goal. Periodic monitoring (weekly or monthly) is better than daily monitoring. Monitoring can be done in the form of charts, graphs, or lists or descriptions of behaviors and attitudes.

The information and activities in this chapter encourage you to understand and, if needed, change your lifestyle. The remaining chapters have additional information and activities to help you with your own personal health journey, including recommended resources by well-known authors that you may find useful (see *Women Making a Difference:* "Marci Shimoff").

Women Making a Difference

Marci Shimoff

Marci Shimoff is the woman's face of the biggest self-help book phenomenon in history, *Chicken Soup for the Soul.* Her six bestselling titles, including *Chicken Soup for the Woman's Soul* and *Chicken Soup for the Mother's Soul,* have met with stunning success, selling more than 13 million copies worldwide in thirty-three languages. They have been on the *New York Times* bestseller list for a total of 108 weeks (#1 for 12 weeks) and have also been #1 on the *USA Today* and *Publishers Weekly* lists. Marci is one of the bestselling female nonfiction authors of all time. Her newest book, *Happy for No Reason,* [was] published by Simon and Schuster in December 2007. Marci is a featured teacher in the hit movie phenomenon and #1 bestselling book, *The Secret.* The film and book, which focus on the powerful use of the Law of Attraction, have been watched and read by millions of people around the world. A savvy and engaging media personality, Marci has been on more than 500 national and regional television and radio shows. She has been interviewed for over 100 newspaper articles nationwide and her writing has appeared in national women's magazines, including *Ladies Home Journal* and *Woman's World.*[34]

Chapter Summary

- Wellness encompasses the whole person concept including the following dimensions of health: physical, emotional, social, occupational, intellectual, and spiritual.
- The primary dimensions of world wellness are air, water, energy, food, toxins, and nature.
- The three primary health-related intervention strategies are education (primary prevention), prevention (secondary prevention), and treatment (tertiary prevention).

- The basic hierarchy of needs for humans are physiological, safety, love, esteem, and self-actualization.
- A self-help plan involves three primary steps: taking a personal inventory, having the right attitude, and developing a plan of action.
- A plan of action involves the following steps: assessment, goal setting, intervention strategies, and evaluating progress.

Review Questions

1. Can you name and describe the six dimensions of wellness?
2. What are the environmental issues for world wellness?
3. What are the three types of interventions utilized in the health services?
4. What are reinforcers?
5. Can you describe the hierarchy of needs?
6. Can you describe the transtheoretical model for change?
7. Can you describe the theory of reasoned action and the theory of planned action?
8. What is self-efficacy?
9. Can you devise a self-help plan for behavior change?

Resources

American Hospital Association
 www.aha.org
American Medical Association
 www.ama-assn.org
American Nurses Association
 www.nursingworld.org
Black Women for Wellness
 www.bwwla.com/index.php
Centers for Disease Control and Prevention
 www.cdc.gov
Health Resources and Services Administration Rural Health
 www.hrsa.gov/ruralhealth/
National Institute of Environmental Health Sciences
 www.niehs.nih.gov

Natural Healers
 www.naturalhealers.com
United Nations Entity for Gender Equity and the Empowerment of Women
 www.unwomen.org
United Nations, Statistics Division
 http://unstats.un.org/unsd/default.htm
U.S. Census Bureau
 www.census.gov
U.S. Environmental Protection Agency
 www.epa.gov
WebMd, Women's Health
 women.webmd.com

References

1. CNN. 2006. U.S. population now 300 million and growing, p. 1. http://wwww.cnn.com/2006/US/10/17/300.million .over/index.html (retrieved January 10, 2009).
2. Ibid., p. 2.
3. Centers for Disease Control and Prevention, National Center for Health Statistics. January 11, 2012. *National vital statistics reports, volume 60, number 4*. www.cdc.gov/nchs/data/nvsr/ nvsr60/nvsr60_04.pdf.
4. Kuhn, M., C. Long, and L. Quinn. 1991. *No stone unturned: The life and times of Maggie Kuhn*. New York: Ballantine Books.
5. Wagner, C. 1999. The centarians are coming. *Futurist*, May, pp. 16–23.
6. *Sidney Morning Herald*. 2007. World's oldest woman dies peacefully at 128. http://www.smh.com.au/news/world/ worlds-oldest-woman-dies-peacefully-at-128/2007/03 (retrieved January 10, 2009).

7. Centers for Disease Control and Prevention. August 26, 2011. *National vital statistics reports, volume 59, number 8*. www.cdc .gov/nchs/data/nvsr/nvsr59/nvsr59_08.pdf.
8. Ibid.
9. Allen, R., and R. Yarian. 1981. The domain of health. *Health Education* 12 (4): 3–5.
10. Assessment adapted from *Health style: A self test*. U.S. Department of Health and Human Services (PHS) 81-50155.
11. Hettler, W. 1979. *Six dimensions of wellness*. Stevens Point, WI: National Wellness Institute, University of Wisconsin; Hettler, W. 1990. Six dimensions of wellness. *Guidepost: American Counseling Association* 33 (September): 1.
12. Chandler, C., J. Holden, and C. Kolander. 1992. Counseling for spiritual wellness: Theory and practice. *Journal of Counseling and Development* 71 (2): 168–75.

13. Opatz, J. 1986. Stevens Point: A long-standing program for students at a midwestern university. *American Journal of Health Promotion* 1 (1): 60–67.

14. Hettler, W. 1991. Environmental issues for world wellness. *Guidepost: American Counseling Association* 33 (17): 17.

15. Tong, S., and Y. Lu. (July, 1999). Major issues in the environmental health decision-making process. *Journal of Environmental Health* 62 (1): 33–35.

16. United Nations. (1995). Fourth World Conference on Women: Platform for action. www.un.org/womenwatch/daw/beijing/platform/plat1.htm (retrieved September 22, 2006).

17. Editor. 2008. A Bush legacy, p. 1. *Philadelphia Inquirer* http://www.philly.com/inquirer/opinion/20081210_Editorial_A_Bush_Legacy.html (retrieved January 12, 2009).

18. Soloman, J. and J. Eilperin. 2007. Bush's EPA is pursuing fewer polluters, p. 1. *Washington Post* http://www.washingpost.com/wp-dyn/content/article/2007/09/29/AR2007092901759 (retrieved January 12, 2009).

19. Eilperin, J. 2008. Ozone rules weakened at Bush's behest. *Washington Post* http://www.washingtonpost.com/wp-dyn/content/article/2008/03/13/AR200801304175 (retrieved January 12, 2009).

20. Source Watch 2008. Bush regime environmental record, p. 1. http://www.sourcewatch.org/index.php?title=Bush_regime_environmental_record (retrieved January 12, 2009).

21. Ibid.

22. United Nations. (2000). Beijing + 5: Process and beyond. www.un.org/womenwatch/daw/followup/bfbeyond.htm (retrieved September 22, 2006).

23. *Mosby's medical, nursing and allied health directory.* 4th ed. 1994. St. Louis: Mosby.

24. Ibid.

25. Ibid.

26. Skinner, B. F. 1953. *Science and human behavior.* New York: Macmillan.

27. Maslow, A. H. 1943. A theory of human motivation. *Psychological Review* 50 (July): 370–96.

28. Prochaska, J., and C. DiClemente. 1992. Stages of change in the modification of problem behaviors. *Progress in Behavior Modification* 28: 183–218.

29. Fishbein, M., and I. Ajzen. 1975. *Belief, attitude, intention and behavior: An introduction to theory and research.* Reading, MA: Addison-Wesley.

30. Ajzen, I. 1988. *Attitudes, personality and behavior.* Chicago: Dorsey Press.

31. Bandura, A. 1986. *Social foundations of thought and action.* Englewood Cliffs, NJ: Prentice-Hall.

32. Lyn, L., and K. R. McLeroy. 1986. Self-efficacy and health education. *Journal of School Health* 56 (2): 317–21; Schunck, D. H., and J. P. Carbonari. 1984. Self-efficacy models. In J. D. Malarazzo and others, *Behavioral health: A handbook of health enhancement and disease prevention,* pp. 230–47. New York: John Wiley & Sons.

33. Anspaugh, D. J., M. H. Hamrick, and F. D. Rosato. 2006. *Wellness: Concepts and applications.* 6th ed. New York: McGraw-Hill.

34. Women's Wellness Society. Women that win: Marci Shimoff http://www.womenswellnesssociety.com (retrieved January 12, 2009).

Mental and Emotional Wellness

Part Two

Chapter Four

Enhancing Emotional Well-Being

CHAPTER OBJECTIVES

When you complete this chapter, you will be able to do the following:

◇ Describe self-in-relation theory

◇ Demonstrate assertive communication and effective listening skills

◇ Delineate the steps for effective problem solving

◇ Describe activities for enhancing self-image and self-esteem

◇ Identify the types of eating disorders

◇ Describe the natural stages of the grief process

◇ Identify the types of depression

THE EMERGING SELF

How is it that you become the person that you are? How do you develop your values, beliefs, feelings, thoughts, and ideas about yourself, others, and the world around you? How does your personality emerge, and what contributes to the happiness and unhappiness in your life? How do you decide when it is time to change, and to think, feel, believe, or behave differently about something or someone? Whom do you decide to include in your social support system as persons who influence you and help you? These are important questions to consider as you explore your personal development and your emotional health.

THEORIES OF DEVELOPMENT

Until 1979 when psychologist Carol Gilligan began to challenge the views of earlier male psychologists,[1] the psychology profession generally supported the long-held societal belief that women were inferior to men. For example, in 1905, Sigmund Freud, who is considered to be the father of psychology, designed the theory of psychosexual development around the experiences of the male child, depicting women as envying that which they lacked, such as a penis, and being "driven" largely by a highly "irrational" and oftentimes "hysterical" portion of female anatomy, the uterus. From Freud's view, differences between men and women resulted from women's developmental failure to meet the male standard.[2] As a physician, Freud relied heavily on traditional medical training and terminology to describe the emotional conditions of his patients. Women who presented as emotionally distraught were referred to by physicians of this era as "hysterical." The origin of the word *hysteria* derived from the Greek *hystera*, meaning "the womb." Thus, an emotionally distraught, or hysterical, woman was considered one whose behavior originated from the womb. Taking into consideration nineteenth-century medicine's general view of the inferior anatomy of women as compared to men's anatomy, a common cure for women's emotional distress in the late 1800s was a hysterectomy, that is, removal of the uterus. Many unnecessary hysterectomies were performed throughout the late 1800s and across much of the 1900s because of a biased view toward women and women's anatomy. Up until the women's rights movement in the 1960s and 1970s, little consideration was given, by the medical profession at large, to the possibility that much of nineteenth- and twentieth-century women's emotional distress could have been the result of the prevalent oppression of women who were forced into social and political positions inferior to men.

Jean Piaget did not acknowledge the value of the female pattern in his theory of cognitive development in 1932. Piaget equated normal child development with male development and considered females to be far less developed in capacities that would allow them to deal adequately with the realities of adult life. Piaget based his assumption on his observations of adolescent children playing games. Boys focused more on a resolution of conflicts by following established rules to the letter, whereas girls were more tolerant in their attitudes, more easily reconciled to innovative solutions, and more willing to make exceptions if the rules did not seem to result in fair outcomes relative to the situation. Piaget determined that the female pattern of conflict resolution lacked the necessary legal sense that was essential to moral development; thus, he determined that girls were inferior to boys.[3] Piaget failed to recognize that the approach that girls took to conflict resolution, although different from that of boys, was an equal or sometimes more favorable approach to resolving the conflict depending upon the circumstances of the particular situation.

Lawrence Kohlberg, in 1969, derived his theory of moral development without considering the potential benefits of gender differences.[4] Kohlberg explains that gender differences develop because girls play games that are less likely to involve strict rules, such as hopscotch and jump rope. And, he observed, when conflicts over rules do develop in girls' games, the games often end. Rather than elaborating a set of rules to settle the dispute, girls subordinate the continuation of the game in favor of the continuation of relationships. This type of solution to conflict resolution was considered inferior by Kohlberg. Thus, when Kohlberg developed a scale to measure moral development, he utilized an exclusively male subject group; so, when measured by Kohlberg's scale, women are consistently found to be deficient in moral development.

In 1968 another prominent psychologist, Erik Erikson, did recognize gender differences by noting that in males the ability to develop an identity precedes intimacy development, but the development of intimacy occurs along with identity development in females. This tendency for women to identify themselves through their relationships with others remains strong for most women throughout their life. Despite Erikson's observation of gender differences, his life-cycle stages consistently depicted the male pattern as the standard for healthy psychosocial development.[5]

As a response to gender bias within the psychology profession, Gilligan proposed to the profession that a new psychology for women be developed that was independent of comparisons to male standards and that encouraged women to trust their own judgments about themselves. The psychology profession gradually began to respond to Gilligan's suggestion, and sensitivity to women's issues continues to evolve within the field. In fact, the American Psychological Association has a subdivision dedicated entirely to the psychology of women.

Women's Relational Model of Development

Traditional male models of development emphasize the separation and individuation process as primary for psychological well-being, but women demonstrate a very different process. The self-concept of a woman, her identity and self-esteem, is strongly associated with her relationship to others. The ability to relate to others is a woman's strength, and it enhances her process of empathy. This tendency of girls and women to relate self to others, and to even sacrifice self-achievement in order to preserve a relationship, was observed by early psychologists, such as Piaget, Kohlberg, and Erikson, but they erroneously dismissed this demonstration as inferior to the male process. A woman tends to foster and encourage relationships as an integral part of her self-identity. This relational approach to psychological understanding was initially called "self-in-relation theory," and it was primarily developed by women psychologists and their associates working together at the Stone Center at Wellesley College in the late 1980s and early 1990s.[6]

What began as self-in-relation theory has emerged to be referred to as **gender-relations theory,** and it is a response to traditional Western psychology that emphasizes separation and individuation but neglects the intricacies of human interconnection. Men tend to identify themselves mostly through their work and competition; this is the model of normal human development espoused by Western psychology. Women tend to identify themselves mostly through persons and relationships; this is largely ignored by Western psychology. Gender-relations theory espouses that the primacy of responsive relationships is a powerful determinant of women's psychological reality—women mostly develop their sense of self through their connections with others, whereas men mostly develop their sense of self through separating from others. Maintaining a healthy sense of self, while in relation with others, is a key to self-worth and self-esteem for women. In many cases, the primary problem for a woman in therapy is "how to be the kind of self she wants to be, a being-in-relationship, now able to value the very valuable parts of herself, along with her own perceptions and desires—and to find others who will be with her in that way."[7] A woman's sense of self can be annihilated due to her tendency to give up self in order to maintain a relation with another. "Women tend to define power as having the strength to care for and give to others, which is very different from the way men have defined power."[8]

To encourage a woman to separate and individuate completely from another is asking her not to be a woman. Truly, some women become too enmeshed with others, as in the case of a woman who repeatedly returns to an abusive partner. When dysfunctional relationships occur, the goal is not to get a woman to stop her relational aspect of self but instead to channel it in a healthier way. A tendency women must watch out for is giving too much of themselves to others. A woman who spends all of her time fostering others and not enough time nurturing her own needs and desires can begin to feel lost and empty. The Stone Center relational model emphasizes the centrality of connection in women's lives. Understanding this is core in helping a woman find fulfillment.

Sociocultural Influences

Sociocultural influences (SCIs) may significantly impact your emotional health. Examples of SCIs include, but may not be limited to, family members, family history, family values, religious doctrine, media, school activities and personnel, community events, national events, world events, historical events, friends, famous persons, and significant others. These SCIs can affect you in many different ways. As you experience them in your life you will choose, either consciously or unconsciously, to integrate them into your self in some meaningful way. Once integrated, these SCIs can guide and direct your thinking, feeling, believing, and behaving. The influence of these SCIs in your life can lead to life satisfaction and the pursuit or achievement of wellness, or they can lead you to some points of dissatisfaction or dysfunction. In fact, some SCIs may have a positive impact early on in your life but will eventually lose their usefulness as you grow and change and thus may eventually begin to have negative consequences in your life. It is important to be in touch with yourself, the impact that SCIs have on you, and when and how you need to alter your course to maintain or achieve greater degrees of life satisfaction and wellness.

Mindful Self-Exploration and Integration

There are many things to be happy about in life, but there can also be varying degrees of unhappiness. It is important to understand how you developed happiness about yourself, other people, and things so that you can maintain and continue to add to your happiness.

It is equally important to understand how you might have developed unhappiness about yourself, other people, and things so you can change what led to that unhappiness.

Some SCIs are appropriate for some persons and inappropriate for others. You must decide for yourself which ones are best for you and in what ways you need to integrate their meaningfulness into your life in order to lead a more satisfactory and functional life. There are many possibilities for life dissatisfaction and dysfunction, but just a few warning signs might be low self-esteem, a poor self-concept, relationship conflict, prolonged unhappiness, depression, an eating disorder, dissatisfaction about your body, drug or alcohol abuse, and so on.

The integration of SCIs into yourself with a state of ongoing mindfulness can result in greater satisfaction and functioning and less dissatisfaction and dysfunction in your life. **Ongoing mindfulness** is the process of exploring your inner self and the influence that SCIs have on you. You are then more mindful, or consciously aware, of how you are integrating, and did integrate in your past, certain SCIs that led to particular beliefs, thoughts, feelings, and actions in your life. When dissatisfaction or dysfunction is discovered through this process of self-exploration, you can reorganize the meaningfulness of the SCIs and their impact on you. You can then reintegrate new beliefs, thoughts, feelings, or actions that can provide you with greater satisfaction and wellness. The reorganization of the effects of certain SCIs may involve taking the relevant SCI and discarding all or part of it from your life, or transforming its meaning into something different that may be more helpful to you. (See Figure 4.1.)

Without mindful integration of SCIs, these can dictate your development and state of emotional well-being in ways not completely appropriate for who you are and thus lead to your unhappiness. It is important to maintain, or regain when it is not present, a state of mindfulness about past and present SCIs and their impact on you. You can then discard inappropriate ones in order to lead a more satisfied and functional life.

Resistance to self-exploration and change can often be a result of your fear of trying something unfamiliar to you. You may also be afraid of appearing to be disloyal to your family, friends, or familiar institutions (for example, your religious affiliation) because you want to be different from them. You may fear rejection by those important to you if you change the way you are. You may be uncomfortable with change and fear harm, failure, or destruction if you change. When your resistance to change gets in the way so that you find it too difficult to self-explore and reorganize yourself on your own, then you may want to seek assistance from someone else to help you, such as a mental health professional.

FIGURE 4.1 The impact of sociocultural influences (SCIs).

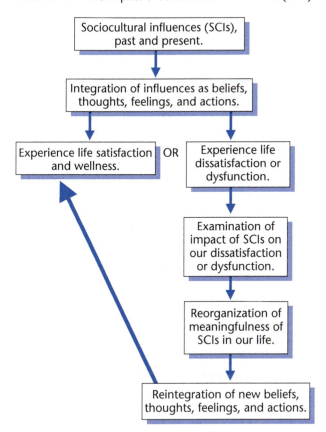

THE COUNSELING OPTION

There might be times in your life when you or someone you know needs counseling to assist with a mental or emotional concern. A mental health counselor can be very effective at facilitating the recovery process either through therapy or by recommending available resources.

The therapeutic orientation of the counselor may make no difference in how effective the counselor is with a client; however, one therapeutic approach is designed specifically to assist women. **Feminist therapy,** also referred to as gender equity therapy, empowers women through an egalitarian (equity-based) relationship with the therapist. Women are so frequently abused, attacked, or discriminated against in society that their self-concept and sense of self-worth may be depleted. Feminist therapy assists in rebuilding and reinforcing a woman's inner strength and ability to survive, overcome, and succeed in the face of emotional burdens.

Feminist therapists often respond to a client's issues or problems by understanding the impact of societal gender-role expectations on the client. Feminist theory examines issues such as how men and women are similar and different in their moral decision making, the way they relate to others, and how they contribute to and confront abuse and violence.[9]

A feminist therapy approach can be combined with any style of counseling. What is meant by style of counseling? A mental health counselor typically bases client conceptualization, meaning understanding a client's presenting problem, on a particular **counseling model** in which they have been trained. A counselor's model for counseling is further beneficial in assisting the counselor to establish with the client appropriate treatment goals and a treatment plan for client recovery. In addition, a mental health counselor may utilize with a client various counseling techniques (intervention strategies) that are consistent with the counselor's model or style of counseling. Existing models for counseling may sometimes be adapted or new counseling models developed as the needs of groups of people change or evolve over time. A brief description of some of the more common counseling models follows.

Person-centered counseling is a nondirective approach whereby the mental health counselor utilizes reflection and clarification of clients' verbal and nonverbal communications to enhance insight and move clients toward greater self-acceptance.[10] Person-centered counselors do not manage or conduct a session nor do they take responsibility for the client; rather, they help clients to feel safe and open by being congruent, authentic, genuine, caring, accepting, warm and empathic. With this counseling experience, referred to as *unconditional positive regard,* clients increasingly trust themselves and move in the direction of being more self-actualized. Clients free themselves from the past, distort less in the here and now, and experience greater self acceptance as they progress through person-centered therapy.[11]

A primary focus of **cognitive behavioral therapy** is on identifying and challenging irrational client beliefs that contribute to maladaptive feelings and behaviors.[12] Cognitive-behavioral methods involve identifying and challenging irrational thoughts, changing communication style, modeling and role playing new behaviors, and completing cognitive homework. Cognitive-behavioral counselors are viewed primarily as teachers and practice partners for clients to challenge self-defeating beliefs, thoughts, and behaviors and to learn and integrate new ways of believing, feeling, and behaving.

Behavioral counseling is a goal-focused method with the intent of altering behavior which restricts clients' social, occupational, and other important activities, thereby improving their quality of life.[13] Behavioral counseling involves continual assessment and measurement of client progression toward goals. The role of mental health counselors is to teach clients new skills by providing instructions, modeling new behaviors, designing opportunities for behavioral rehearsal, and providing feedback on client performance.[14] Within this role, mental health counselors assign homework and self-monitoring in order to assist clients to generalize and transfer what they learn during therapy sessions to outside situations.[15]

The **Adlerian counseling** view of human nature is that humans are motivated primarily by social relatedness; that is, *inferiority feelings* motivate individuals to *strive for significance (superiority)* within family and community.[16] Each individual develops a unique life plan for achieving a sense of social belonging and achievement, and behavior is purposefully enacted to achieve these goals. Striving for social significance and superiority can be manifest in functional or dysfunctional ways depending upon an individual's perception of life events. Healthy striving moves a person toward greater social connectedness, while unhealthy striving moves a person away from social connectedness. Perceived frustrations or failures within a social system can result in discouragement, which may compound movement away from *social interest*. The Adlerian counselor assists clients in understanding and adapting the *private logic* that drives their life style in order to achieve greater social success and satisfaction in the life tasks of *work, love, and friendship*. The counselor may focus on client perceptions of childhood experiences and interpretations in order to illustrate private logic and empower clients to modify beliefs and reorient their approach to life in a manner that is more satisfying and functional.[17]

Freudian psychoanalytic theory postulates a deterministic view of human nature in that unconscious biological and instinctual drives may result in irrational motivations as the individual evolves through key psychosexual stages in the early years of life. Freud proclaimed that a person's internal psyche is composed of the id (innate, instinctual personality at birth), ego (mediator between internal instincts and reality of the external world), and superego (social code, traditional values, and ideas) that vie for control over the person's psychic energy.[18] According to Freud's psychoanalytic theory, people are mostly unaware of why they feel or act the way they do and when dysfunction occurs it is usually because either neurotic or moral anxiety has threatened to throw the balance of power more toward the id or the superego. Through psychoanalytic counseling, clients can gain conscious awareness of the unconscious patterns of their thinking, which enables them to work through their trauma and relieve internal pressure.[19] To return a client's internal world to a state of balance, psychoanalytic counselors assist the client to bring unconscious processes into conscious awareness so that they may rely on logic instead of being influenced by anxiety. Psychoanalysis is a long-term process whereby clients are encouraged to free associate about whatever comes to mind: about their feelings, fantasies, experiences, memories, and so forth.[20]

A major premise of **gestalt counseling** is that unexpressed feelings result in *unfinished business*, which detracts from feeling whole and interferes with personal growth.[21] Clients may reach an *impasse*, or a stuck point that interferes with life satisfaction or functioning. In the counseling process, it is necessary for clients to fully explore an impasse, accept life circumstances, and become fully present and aware in the here and now. Gestalt counselors help clients to develop awareness regarding language patterns that are incongruent with feelings and experiences; in essence, clients become free to see things more completely through a genuine, authentic counseling relationship. Gaining more complete images of the here and now is to subjectively fill in the "blank spaces" to effect *closure* through the Gestalt concept of *figure and ground*. Gestalt counseling often involves a number of exercises and experiments that create opportunities for clients to move toward self-determined goals.[22]

A primary goal of **existential counseling** is to assist clients to recognize the ways in which they are not living fully authentic lives and to make choices that will lead to becoming what they are capable of being.[23] From an existential perspective, feelings of anxiety, guilt, dread, despair, and unsettledness are responses to the reality of human living. However, individuals try to avoid these uncomfortable experiences by pretending they do not exist via a process referred to as *inauthentic living*. This is problematic because at the heart of self-deception is a denial of personal freedom and responsibility. It is through acknowledgment of the whole life experience that persons can *live authentically* and make the most of their life experiences. Clients are encouraged to accept their freedom to make choices, take personal responsibility for these choices, and decide what fears, feelings, and anxieties they will explore. The existential approach of *logotherapy* hypothesizes that when clients experience a deep sense of anxiety (fear), emptiness, depression, or neurosis it is because they have become lost in their pursuit of finding meaning in their lives. Their meaninglessness is created when they have become aware that there is no predesigned direction or pre-approved plan for their life.[24]

The view of human nature from a **choice theory and reality therapy** perspective is that humans are born with four genetically coded needs designed for their survival: "*love and belonging, power, freedom, and fun*."[25] According to choice theory, individuals have a special place in their brains called the *quality world* in which energy toward our relationships with honored individuals of importance are emphasized. The *quality world* is the core of our lives, and the most important component of our quality world is people. According to choice theory, all behavior is chosen and purposeful, and individuals work to satisfy needs through *total behavior* (i.e., "*acting, thinking, feeling, and physiology*").[26] Reality therapy, which is the implementation of choice theory, emphasizes client choice and responsibility for choosing behaviors that meet their needs.

Solution-focused therapy (SFT) views humans as competent with a therapeutic focus on what is possible.[27] A main goal of SFT involves helping clients shift from talking about problems to focusing on finding solutions. "SFT counselors believe that it is more useful for clients to understand and elaborate these solutions rather than dwell on the problems of the past. Clients are encouraged to believe that positive changes are always possible."[28] Counselors encourage clients to focus on what is going right in their lives, what needs to happen to make things better in their lives, and thereafter plan the next steps to take action. The therapeutic relationship is terminated once clients arrive at their solution.[29]

Factors for Successful Counseling Outcome

Meta-analytical researchers have concluded that a *counselor's model and techniques* account for 15 percent of successful therapeutic outcome, meaning client change.[30,31] This same research reported that *relationship factors* (the client's experience of respect, collaboration, acceptance, and validation from the counselor) account for 30 percent of successful client change. Thus, while implementing a

counseling model effectively is an important contributor to successful therapeutic outcome, an even more important factor is establishing and maintaining a **positive therapeutic relationship** with the client. Trust is a very important component of an effective therapeutic relationship and counselors are bound by law and ethics to maintain client privacy and confidentiality of all client information, including name and identity. There are only a few exceptions to this, that include counselors' obligation to protect self and others (including the client) in the face of threat of harm or a crime.[32] The remaining factors that determine successful therapeutic outcome are *client factors*, accounting for 40 percent of client change (everything that the client brings to counseling—strengths, interests, perceptions, values, social supports, resilience, and other resources), and *hope factors*, accounting for 15 percent of client change (the client's positive expectancy and anticipation of change).[33,34]

When looking for a mental health professional, it is wise to get a referral from someone who has knowledge about the capabilities and expertise of a particular counselor that might be helpful for you. This referral might come from a family member, a friend, a physician, a teacher, or a spiritual counselor. If a referral is not possible, the telephone yellow pages can suggest several possibilities, though the expertise and training of a counselor cannot be guaranteed this way.

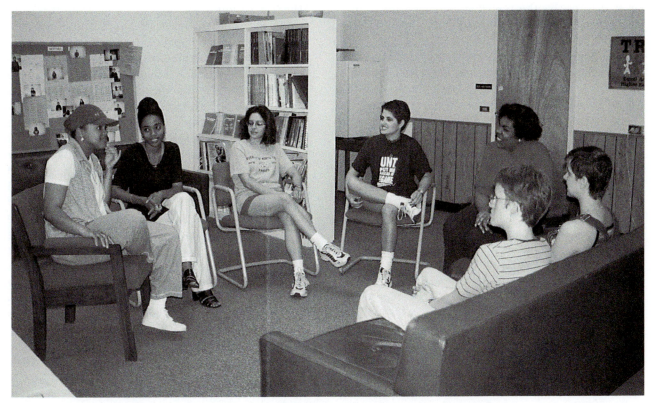

A personal growth group is a good outlet for sharing concerns and getting support from peers.

LIFE SKILL DEVELOPMENT

Certain life skills make it easier to cope with life demands. Examples of helpful life skills for emotional health include emotional intelligence, assertiveness training, effective communication, problem solving, and having good self-esteem. Life skills can be taught to any age group, including very young children. When children do not learn life skills early on, they may have a rougher time growing up emotionally healthy or staying emotionally healthy throughout their life span. It is never too late to learn helpful life skills. Many very good self-help books are on the market to assist with this process. In addition, schools, community organizations, and mental health counselors and agencies commonly offer one or more life skill building programs to the public.

Emotional Intelligence

Emotional intelligence is the ability to recognize your emotions and those of the people around you and have the competence to work with those emotions to resolve problems, especially problems in the workplace. The classic two-step approach to emotional intelligence involves becoming aware of your own emotions and developing an action plan. Sometimes you may have more than one emotion regarding a person or a situation. A thorough self-examination of these emotions will help you be better prepared to devise a plan. An action plan is used to resolve the troubling emotions, and it may require changing the way you speak to someone or developing better listening skills.

Emotional intelligence includes self-awareness and impulse control, persistence, zeal and self-motivation, empathy, and social deftness.[35] These are the qualities of people who excel in life, whose intimate relationships flourish, who are stars in the workplace. These are also fundamental to having good character, self-discipline, altruism, and compassion. The personal costs of deficits in emotional intelligence can range from relationship dysfunction to poor physical health. Children who lack emotional intelligence are prone to high-risk behavior that may result in depression, eating disorders, unwanted pregnancy, aggressiveness, and violent crime. Emotional intelligence is not fixed at birth and can be taught in life skills education programs and through supportive counseling.[36]

Assertiveness Training

Assertiveness training is one of the most common personal improvement programs currently offered. Many health educators and mental health professionals have some experience and knowledge in training assertion skills to individuals and groups. Assertiveness

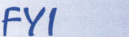 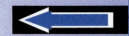

What Is Assertiveness?

Assertiveness, or assertion, is standing up for personal rights and expressing thoughts, feelings, and beliefs in direct, honest, and appropriate ways that do not violate another person's rights. Assertiveness involves the use of "I" messages, for example: "This is what *I* think." "This is what *I* feel." "This is how *I* see the situation." These types of messages express "who the person is" and are said without dominating, humiliating, or degrading the other person.

"Assertiveness involves respect—not deference. Deference is acting in a subservient manner as though the other person is right or better simply because the other person is older, more powerful, experienced, knowledgeable, or is of a different sex or race. Deference is present when people express themselves in ways that are self-effacing, appeasing, or overly apologetic."[37] With assertion, one must communicate respect for self and for others.

training teaches the differences between assertive, aggressive, and nonassertive behavior and increases experience in applying responsible assertive behavior. *FYI:* "What Is Assertiveness?" explains what assertiveness is.

A need for assertiveness training is more prevalent for women than for men because many messages from American society tend to encourage boys to be aggressive career professionals while encouraging girls to be passive caregivers and homemakers. Assertive behavior is more common in working women than in homemakers. In a study regarding women's views about leisure time, homemakers were less likely than working women to feel assertive, competent, or independent during their leisure. They felt more constrained by lack of skills and opportunity, poor self-image, fear, personal values, and the belief that some leisure activities are only for men.[38]

Adventure-based activities can have a positive influence on assertiveness enhancement for women. Ropes course training is one such activity. Women must overcome obstacles, usually constructed in an outdoor wilderness area, that include crossing rivers on rope ladders, scaling high walls, swinging across chasms on ropes, rock climbing, or rappelling down cliffs. Adventure-based courses have produced positive changes in women participants, such as increases in women's abilities to take risks, to practice assertive leadership, to solve problems effectively, and to feel more competent in general.[39] Participants in adventure-based courses for women report that feelings of power and achievement emerge in this setting.

In spite of the positive impact that assertiveness can have in your life, such as enhancing your success in a career and increasing your ability to meet your needs and the needs of significant others, there is some pressure exerted by society for women to not be assertive. For example, one study of 122 men between the ages of 17 and 25 years rated women described as independent and assertive as less physically attractive than women described as affectionate and compassionate.[40] What is especially significant about this study is that the two groups of women had been rated as equally physically attractive by a separate sample of men when no personality characteristics were described. It was only with the addition of the differentiating personality characteristics that men now found one group, the independent and assertive women, less physically attractive than the other group.

Sending assertive messages is an important step for getting your needs met. *Health Tips:* "When Do You Need to Be Assertive?" and *FYI:* "Types of Assertive Messages" provide examples of when and how to be assertive. Being an effective communicator is also important in creating positive and productive interactions.

Effective Communication

The components of **effective listening** and **effective communication** are appropriate body language, encouraging responses, paraphrasing, clarification, and

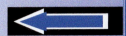

FYI

Types of Assertive Messages[42]

There are six basic types of assertive messages: *I want* statements help to clarify to both yourself and others what you really want. For example, "I want you to call when you are going to be late." *I feel* statements help express your feelings without attacking the other person. For example, "I feel embarrassed when you criticize my clothes in front of my friends." *Mixed feelings* statements name more than one feeling and explain where each is coming from. For example, "I enjoy going out and doing things with you, yet I feel it is unfair that you frequently do not bring enough money and ask me to pay for you." *Empathic assertion* presents some sensitive understanding about the other person and then expresses how you feel. For example, "I know you said that you are angry and do not want to talk about it. However, I feel we need to talk about it when you feel ready." *Confrontive assertion* is necessary when there are contradictions such as differences between what a person says and what she or he does. For example, "I know you said you would teach the newer students some of the beginning information as part of your internship, yet you consistently put them off or do not show up for appointments. I want you to be more responsible and follow through on the tasks that you agreed to do." *I language assertion* is useful for expressing difficult negative feelings. For example, "When you cancel a weekend event with me because you say you are busy working and then I find out you went out with someone else, I feel rejected and humiliated. I need for you to be honest with me about why you do things or it could damage our friendship."

Health Tips

When Do You Need to Be Assertive?

Applying assertive behavior may be required in many situations in order to get your needs met in a healthy manner. Here are just a few examples in which you may need to be assertive:[41]

- Maintaining assertion in the face of someone's aggression and personal attack
- Being assertive with repair people who overcharge or do not properly do the work
- Giving supervisory criticism
- Presenting yourself at a task meeting where others ignore, discount, or put down your ideas
- Negotiating salary increases, and dealing with changes in job title or job function
- Being assertive with colleagues who make sexist, racist, or condescending remarks
- Expressing feelings of hurt, anger, and disappointment with people who are close to you

summarization. Effective listening begins with appropriate body language. When someone is talking, be attentive. Watch the person's his face and, when appropriate, make eye contact. From time to time, make brief encouraging responses (one to three words only) to let the person know you are listening, for example, "I see" or "I hear you." Sometimes a brief nod is appropriate. The purpose of encouraging responses is to let the individual know you are listening without implying agreement at this point. When the individual pauses, attempt to paraphrase what has been said; that is, in one or two sentences, restate in your own words what has been told to you.

Occasionally, effective listening involves a need for clarification if you are having difficulty understanding the person talking. Clarification can be achieved through brief exploratory statements and open-ended questions. An exploratory statement is an attempt to request further information without disrupting the flow of communication by the other person. An example exploratory statement would be, "Tell me more about your need for space." Another example of an exploratory statement would be, "Please give me more details about how you see our relationship evolving." An example of an open-ended question would be, "When you said my being late for meetings causes a disruption, could you tell me in what ways so that I might better understand your concern?" Open-ended questions usually ask what, when, where, or how.

When the individual stops talking, briefly summarize the main contents of what you think was communicated and then ask the person if he or she feels you understood. This effective listening process can then be followed by communication from you to the other person regarding your thoughts, ideas, or needs. Assertive communication can be useful at this point. The goal of effective listening is that each party be heard and understood. Then, via assertive communication, attempts can be made at caregiving, problem solving, conflict resolution, or negotiation and compromise. (Complete *Journal Activity:* "Practice Assertive 'I' Messages.")

Rosenberg's *Nonviolent Communication: A Language of Compassion* describes an approach to communication that enhances both personal and other awareness of needs and desires that may contaminate our communication. Expressing from the heart with compassion is a key to healthy communication. The types of communication that block compassion include *moralistic judgments, making comparisons,* and *denial of responsibility.* Using a *language of compassion* involves being able *to observe another's communication without evaluating, to identify and express your feelings honestly but with empathy for the other, to take responsibility for your own feelings, to request that which would enrich your life,* and *to receive communication empathically* (trying to understand where the other is coming from). Rosenberg's "NVC process" teaches how to create personal and professional relationships grounded in mutual respect, compassion, and emotional safety.[43]

Effective Problem Solving

Everyone appreciates the love, warmth, and potential companionship that can come from a relationship. Most people do not consider or adequately prepare for the disagreements or conflicts that will inevitably arise in any type of relationship, be it family, friends, relationship partner, or colleagues at work. Some individuals have misconceptions about conflict and disagreements that can impair adequate resolution. Many people incorrectly believe that a conflict must automatically be their fault, or that they must win a conflict, or that they should be able to handle a conflict so well that the problem never recurs.[44] Here are some other similar kinds of misconceptions to avoid: a compromise means losing and being less powerful than the other person; conflict should be avoided at any cost; your solution is the only worthwhile one; all conflicts must be resolved; and one party must be right and one must be wrong in any conflict.

Successful **problem solving** is a step-by-step approach of planning and negotiating and involves all parties to be affected. A common model for problem solving and negotiation involves six basic steps: defining the problem, generating possible solutions, evaluating the solutions, making the decision, determining how to implement the decision, and assessing the success of the solution.[45] After assessing success, some adjustments might have to be made, but it is important that all involved parties have a say in any adjustments to the original agreement.

Self-Esteem Enhancement

Self-esteem is based on the distance between the perceived self and the ideal self. The perceived self is how you currently see yourself. The ideal self is how you believe you "should" be. The greater the distance between the perceived self and the ideal self, the lower your self-esteem.

Self-esteem enhancement is the process of reducing the distance between the perceived self and the ideal self. In cases of low self-esteem, typically the ideal self is too unrealistic. Thus, the process here would be to bring

---

Journal Activity

Practice Assertive "I" Messages

Practice writing assertive *I messages* to someone you would like to communicate with assertively. Here is a template for writing I statements:

I feel (emotion) when (behavior) and would like (behavioral request).

Now, let's look at some examples containing I messages:

I feel (irritated) when (dirty clothes are left on the floor), and I would like (you to pick up your dirty clothes each day).
I feel (glad) when (I see you have taken the trash out), and I would like (to thank you).

the ideal self into reality, to make the view of the ideal self more realistic and less perfectionistic. Once the ideal self is more realistic, then you can have a healthier opinion about yourself and greater self-esteem. When you desire to make some changes, having good self-esteem is prerequisite to making healthier and more realistic decisions about change.

Individuals who have low self-esteem are often discouraged persons. Activities that help to instill a belief in oneself can raise self-esteem, bring the ideal self into a healthier perspective, and build success and confidence. Participation in adventure programs, sports, music and arts, and community service are just a few examples of activities that enhance self-esteem through the experience of success while having fun.

Low self-esteem can originate from discouraging messages we received from our parents. Parents serve as primary role models and message senders. For a woman, the most common primary role model is her mother. The presence of critical messages or the absence of encouraging messages from a woman's mother can create severe doubt in a woman's own judgment and ability throughout her life span.

> If we feel trapped by unfulfilled needs that arose out of childhood experiences, we first need to understand them as best we can. In terms of the self-concept, it is helpful to understand how much of any belief about ourselves is an accurate reflection of us and how much is the product of circumstance or other people's misperceptions.[46]

At some point in their life women have to ask, "Whom are we to believe?" An integral part of moving on is learning to trust our own judgments as much as or more than our parents'.

Not only is it important to feel good about yourself, but it also may be important to let others know this. Characters who were boastful or positive about themselves were rated by undergraduate college students as being more competent than characters who made negative statements about themselves.[47] Thus, bragging about yourself may enhance the opinion that others have about you.

The process of maintaining or enhancing self-esteem in women may vary across cultures. Conditions that impact self-esteem were compared for young Asian, black, and white women in America.[48] The best predictors of good self-esteem among Asian women included having children, having nonconflicting social networks, and experiencing positive life events. For black women, the best predictors of good self-esteem included having educational opportunities and nonconflicting social networks. For white women, the best predictors of good self-esteem included the absence of negative life events, the presence of nonconflicting social networks, and a good income. (See *Health Tips:* "Understanding and Enhancing Self-Esteem in Women.")

BODY IMAGE AND EATING DISORDERS

A positive image of self is central to feeling good and being successful. A key element to building and maintaining a positive self-image is to focus on being what you want to be—that is, building an image from the inside out instead of trying to be what others want you to be.

Society presents many messages about the supposed "ideal image." This is a myth; there is no such thing as the "ideal woman." Every woman has something unique to offer on an emotional, physical, mental, social, occupational, and spiritual level. It is the differences you present that help to make the world diverse and complete.

To enhance your self-image, start by loving yourself and accepting yourself as you are right now at this very moment. If you can do this, then any changes you want to make in yourself can be much more fun instead of seeming so difficult and laborious.

A preoccupation with body image can reach elevations significant enough to be considered clinical in nature. **Body dysmorphic disorder (BDD)** is the classification of body-image disturbance reserved for the non—eating disorder population. BDD is a preoccupation with an imagined defect in appearance that results in distress in social or other important areas of life functioning.[49] Preliminary evidence suggests that BDD is diagnosed with approximately equal frequency in women and in men. BDD behaviors include frequent mirror checking or avoidance of mirrors, frequent comparisons to others, and excessive grooming behavior. Dysmorphophobia is the label the Europeans have assigned to BDD and the term used by the World Health Organization and the *International Classification of Diseases* diagnostic reference.

Body Image and the Media

Glamorous images projected in the media have contributed to harsh self-criticism by women regarding their own body image. Television, movies, and magazines present images of women that seem real but are, in fact, impossible to compete with. Many models and actresses have what is considered to be an ideal body image, but they also have all of the best clothes designers, hair dressers, and makeup staff. These professionals spend many hours sculpting a woman into a form that is, supposedly, "ideal" but that is pretty unrealistic most of the time. What they have created is an image of a woman that does not occur naturally in the world. One example is the glamorization of Barbara Stanwyck, a well-known actress in the United States in the mid-1940s, 1950s, and 1960s. Ms. Stanwyck had a "figure fault" by Hollywood standards; her hips were considered to be too low in the back and thought to look odd when she was walking.

Health Tips

Understanding and Enhancing Self-Esteem in Women

IMPAIRED COMPETENCE DEVELOPMENT

- Self-esteem is based on competence, and competence means having a sense of control over our self and mastery of our environment.
- Acquiring self-competence is more difficult for female children (and female adults) because males are more highly valued in our society, females have more limits placed on them from childhood through adulthood, and females are more susceptible to discrimination and violence than males in childhood and adulthood.

HINDRANCES TO SELF-ESTEEM DEVELOPMENT AND MAINTENANCE

- Women are stereotyped to play the role of caregiver and servant: good mother, good wife, good woman—to sacrifice herself for others.
- Prominent health and mental health care models are designed and maintained mostly by men and thus are sorely lacking in a proper understanding of and attention to women's issues.
- There is a tendency to medicate a woman who is anxious and depressed instead of fostering a sense of her personal power through therapy.

TEN TIPS FOR SELF-ESTEEM ENHANCEMENT

- Identify and challenge negative feelings and thoughts you have about yourself and other women. Women

with low self-esteem often are critical of other women, thereby contributing to the problem in a larger sense.
- Examine and challenge critical self-messages (and the origins of these messages, most likely from a critical parent).
- Build up a large repertoire of positive feelings and thoughts about yourself and repeat them daily (even if you do not believe them yet).
- Practice assertive behavior.
- Learn to set limits and boundaries on what you will and will not do, what you will not tolerate from others, and what you expect from others.
- Enhance your ability to practice effective communication.
- Enhance your problem-solving and decision-making abilities.
- Learn to filter out or ignore stereotypical messages from other persons and the media about body-image preferences and gender-role expectations.
- Avoid the temptation to be a "martyr"; learn to delegate responsibility so that you have more time for yourself.
- Participate in activities that challenge you to grow and contribute to a sense of self-competency and personal power.

A famous designer in Hollywood at the time created a new design for Ms. Stanwyck to hide this "flaw." The design created by Edith Head was a dress with a high midriff, as opposed to a well-defined waistline that would accentuate the hips. This new design resulted in a taller, sleeker-looking Barbara. The dress design was incorporated into Ms. Stanwyck's wardrobe and was presented in the 1941 movie *The Lady Eve.* After this, Barbara Stanwyck had a career boost and played more glamorous roles. Edith Head's high midriff dress design, known as "The Lady Eve dress," was copied by many designers and purchased in abundance by women all over the country who wanted to camouflage their waistline or hips.[50] This type of camouflaging of a woman's natural image can be seen throughout history. More public efforts have been put into hiding a woman's natural image than in accepting the nature of a woman's uniqueness.

There have been instances where the media industry has been beneficial to the image of women. For example, the movie wardrobe of Marlene Dietrich, a famous actress of the 1930s, 1940s, and 1950s, made wearing pants more socially acceptable for women at a time when

dresses had been socially demanded.[51] It is important to remember that in the movie and fashion industry, what is "in" one day may be "out" the next. This should add emphasis to the point that diversity and uniqueness enable us to be individuals and still fit in.

For the most part, the media have contributed more to the fictional "ideal woman" image than to the healthy "real woman" concept. In the 1990 movie *Pretty Woman*, Julia Roberts was portrayed as having a beautiful and desirable perfect body type. What the general public did not know was that several models were used as stand-ins. When Ms. Roberts's body was supposedly revealed, it was actually one of these body doubles that was being shown.[52] Thus, the "pretty woman" was not considered pretty enough for Hollywood standards. In fact, on the movie poster to advertise the film, Julia Roberts's head was superimposed on another woman's body. The unsuspecting public was led to believe that the woman on this poster was actually Julia Roberts. Another example of how the media promotes a fictionalized presentation of how women "should be" is the cover girl on a 1990s modeling magazine who was actually computer generated. Different parts of different women, including different facial features, were put together to create a whole new woman. An unsuspecting public can be easily misled by media magic tricks.

The **glamorization** of women, or basing the desirability of a woman on her body shape, mainly thinness in the arms, legs, face, and waist, and largeness of breasts and hips (the hourglass figure), is thought to have begun in the 1830s when the camera was invented.[53] This type of woman's figure was additionally popularized in the late 1800s by male artist Charles Gibson, who created the "Gibson girl" in a series of his paintings, which presented the supposed ideal woman.[54] Gibson's fictional depictions became very popular, and women strived to model after them.

Modern media technology is now reaching newly developing countries, and these societies are being exposed to fictionalized presentations of the ideal woman's body image. As this media technology is made more available in these countries, we have seen the instigation and rise of eating disorders and other emotional distresses that accompany striving to become the fictional ideal woman.[55]

There are ethnic differences in how women view body-image satisfaction. White women in the United States report greater levels of disordered eating and dieting behaviors and attitudes and greater body dissatisfaction than Asian Americans and African Americans.[56] Low self-esteem and high public self-consciousness are associated with greater levels of problematic eating behaviors and attitudes and body dissatisfaction.

There are some differences in how men and women view their own body. Women reportedly have lower body-image satisfaction than men, and self-esteem is linked to body-image attitudes more for women than for men.[57] These differences are evident as early as adolescence, in that adolescent males are found to feel more positive about their bodies than are adolescent females.[58]

Most women do not actually have unattractive and unacceptable bodies. It is more likely that society has been generating unfair messages to women about how they "should" and "should not" look so that most women feel that they may have unattractive bodies or features. The reality is that most women's sense of unattractiveness has been created by media bias. It is difficult to turn around a pattern of thinking that has endured for such a long time. Some progress has been made in countering the fictional images of a woman's body. However, society has a long way to go. In the meantime, the image of women will sustain harsh criticism as it continues to be based on biased and unrealistic thinking.

Eating Disorders

Poor body image has been identified as the central factor in the development of eating disorders. Ninety percent of people with an eating disorder are female.[59] Eating disorders include **anorexia nervosa, bulimia nervosa,** and **binge eating disorder.**[60] Anorexia nervosa is starving oneself, sometimes even to death, because of a personal belief that one is unattractive or unlovable. Bulimia nervosa is eating and then vomiting soon afterward or using a laxative to get rid of the food in order to avoid weight gain. Binge eating disorder involves binge eating but not purging (vomiting and laxative abuse) afterward. People with anorexia nervosa were found to have a sixfold increase in mortality compared to the general population. Reasons for death include starvation, substance abuse, and suicide. The elevated mortality risks for bulimia nervosa and eating disorder not otherwise specified were similar to those for anorexia nervosa. Mortality rates were estimated to be 4.0 percent for anorexia nervosa, 3.9 percent for bulimia nervosa, and 5.2 percent for eating disorder not otherwise specified. A high suicide rate is also found for bulimia nervosa. Eating disorders have the highest mortality rate of all psychiatric disorders.[61]

About 3.5 percent of all women have binge eating disorder.[62] About 10–15 percent of people who are mildly obese and who try to lose weight on their own or through commercial weight-loss programs have binge eating disorder. The disorder is even more common in people who are severely obese, and it occurs more frequently in adults than adolescents.

Bulimics are at risk for a number of serious health problems. The use of laxatives eventually creates a dependency upon them for normal bowel function. The constant vomiting causes teeth to erode and salivary glands to enlarge due to the effects of acidic stomach fluids that pass through the mouth. About 0.5 percent of women have bulimia nervosa.[63]

Many of the deaths of anorexics are sudden and are probably due to irregular heartbeats or coma induced by low blood sugar. Chances of death are highest in anorectic women who lose more than 30 percent of their original weight and in those who rely on purging to enhance their weight loss.

Approximately 0.9 percent of women have anorexia nervosa.[64] Onset is typically between the ages of 14 and 18 years, with almost all cases starting between the ages of 11 and 22. Approximately 1 to 3 percent of adolescent and college-age women have bulimia.[65] In addition, persons who miss a diagnosis of anorexia or bulimia by only one criterion are diagnosed with the clinical condition **EDNOS (Eating Disorder Not Otherwise Specified).** The prevalence of EDNOS is twice that of anorexia and twice that of bulimia at 2 to 6 percent of the population.[66] Many therapists who treat eating disorders suggest the criteria for anorexia and bulimia are too restrictive because they exclude so many persons on the basis of just one criterion. For example, if a client exhibits all criteria required for anorexia except she still has her menstrual period or she has an inconsistent menstrual period, then she does not qualify for the diagnosis of anorexia because the required criterion is for her to have a complete absence of a menstrual period for three consecutive months, a criterion that is usually only present once the anorexia has progressed to a later, and potentially life-threatening, stage. Exclusion from an eating disorder category on the basis of one criterion is problematic in that one, it significantly dilutes the statistics for the number of persons struggling with a serious eating disorder (EDNOS is typically not reported by databases), and two, insurance companies are less likely to reimburse clients for EDNOS because of a mistaken belief that EDNOS is less serious, and three, significantly less research is performed on EDNOS even though it is much more prevalent than anorexia or bulimia. Also, it is important to note that women who do not quite meet the criteria for a clinical eating disorder may suffer from a number of subclinical eating disorders. For example, many women who diet obsessively use some similar techniques such as bingeing, vomiting, or abusing laxatives, diet pills, and diuretics to keep their weight under control.

It is more difficult for women to lose weight because women's bodies are designed to retain fat so that the population can survive during times of famine with women still able to breast feed from fat stores. A healthy woman has as much as 20 to 30 percent body fat, whereas a healthy man has only about 10 to 15 percent.

Results of a survey of teenage girls reported that 90 percent of white girls were dissatisfied with their bodies and that 62 percent had dieted within the past year.[67] This contrasted sharply with results among black teenage girls: 70 percent were satisfied with their bodies,

and 64 percent said that it was better to be a little overweight than underweight.

The Centers for Disease Control reports that eating disorders are a serious problem among adolescents, particularly among girls in their teenage years. In 1999, 36.4 percent of female high school students perceived themselves to be overweight. Although some of these students may truly be overweight, many are not. More than 12 percent of the students reported not eating in the 24 hours preceding the CDC survey to lose weight or to avoid gaining weight; 7.6 percent reported taking diet pills, powders, or liquids without a doctor's advice to lose weight or to avoid gaining weight; and 4.8 percent reported having vomited or taken laxatives to lose weight or to avoid gaining weight. These behaviors were consistently more prevalent among females.

Women who suffer from an eating disorder frequently have a poor self-concept. The treatment for eating disorders requires a combination of personal mental health counseling and nutritional guidance. (See *Women Making a Difference:* "Celebrities Support National Eating Disorders Association," *FYI:* "Treatment for Eating Disorders," and *FYI:* "The Prevalence of Eating Disorders.")

GRIEF AND BEREAVEMENT

During your life, you will lose someone or something very important to you. This will probably happen many times in your lifetime. Losing someone or something meaningful is very painful. Understanding the grief

Women Making a Difference

Celebrities Support National Eating Disorders Association[68]

National Eating Disorders Association Ambassadors include:

Elizabeth Showers—celebrity jewelry designer and recovered anorexic

Emme—supermodel, TV personality, author, lecturer, clothing designer, and women's advocate

Jenni Schaefer—motivational speaker and author. Books include *Goodbye Ed, Hello Me: Recover from Your Eating Disorder and Fall in Love with Life* and *Life Without Ed: How One Woman Declared Independence from Her Eating Disorder and How You Can Too.*

Jessica Weiner—Jessica Weiner is an "actionist," author, motivational speaker, and advice columnist for *Seventeen* magazine. She has written three books: *A Very Hungry Girl, Life Doesn't Begin 5 Pounds from Now* and *Do I Look Fat in This?* She is also a global ambassador for the DOVE Self-Esteem Fund.

Kristen Moeller—personal life coach with a masters in counseling, Web talk show host of "What Are You Waiting For?" (which highlights extraordinary people making a difference) on RealCoachingRadio.com and author of *Waiting for Jack* and a recovered bulimic.

The National Eating Disorders Association (NEDA), headquartered in Seattle, Washington, a not-for-profit organization, supports individuals and families affected by eating disorders and advocates for prevention, treatment and research funding for eating disorders. Since the inception of its Helpline in 1999, NEDA has referred more than 50,000 people to treatment and tallies more than 40 million hits annually on its Web site. For more information on eating disorders contact NEDA's helpline at telephone 800-931-2237 or visit the NEDA Web site www.NationalEatingDisorders.org.

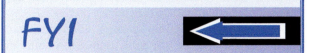

Treatment for Eating Disorders[69]

Common issues for persons with an eating disorder include

- Perfectionism.
- Dichotomous thinking.
- Diminished awareness of internal standards.
- Overreliance on external reinforcement.
- Desire to please and caretake others.
- Sense of helplessness and being out of control.
- Avoidance of emotions.

The most common approach to the treatment of an eating disorder is

- Appropriate assessment and diagnosis.
- Treatment focused on having a realistic body image and resolving personal issues that impair one's ability to do this.
- Multidisciplinary approach involving a mental health therapist, a physician, and a nutritionist.
- Medication: none for anorexia; some antidepressants are helpful with bulimia (such as fluoxetine, known as Prozac) in combination with mental health therapy.

Family therapy is the treatment of choice for anorexia. Cognitive-behavioral therapy is the treatment of choice for bulimia. A combination of individual and group treatment can be effective for both anorexia and bulimia. Inpatient hospitalization may be necessary for anorexics whose body weight causes medical complications or drops dangerously low. Inpatient hospitalization may be required for bulimics who are unresponsive to psychological treatment. Day treatment programs for eating disorders are rapidly rising in popularity because insurance companies are more often choosing not to reimburse for hospital treatment.

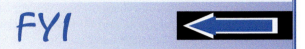

The Prevalence of Eating Disorders[70]

According to the National Eating Disorders Association (NEDA), in the United States as many as 10 million females and 1 million males are fighting a life and death battle with an eating disorder such as anorexia or bulimia. Approximately 25 million more are struggling with binge eating disorder. Because of the secretiveness and shame associated with eating disorders, many cases are probably not reported. In addition, many individuals struggle with body dissatisfaction and subclinical disordered eating attitudes and behaviors. For example, it has been shown that 80 percent of American women are dissatisfied with their appearance. For females between 15 and 24 years old who suffer from anorexia nervosa, the mortality rate associated with the illness is twelve times higher than the death rate of all other causes of death." Even though the prevalence of and mortality rate for eating disorders is very high, the NEDA reports that there is a disproportionate amount of research dollars dedicated to the treatment of eating disorders by the National Institutes of Health:

Illness	Prevalence	NIH Research Funds (2005)
Eating disorders	10 million	$ 12,000,000*
Alzheimer's disease	4.5 million	$647,000,000
Schizophrenia	2.2 million	$350,000,000

*The reported research funds are for anorexia nervosa only. No estimated funding is reported for bulimia nervosa or eating disorders not otherwise specified.

resolution process is an important life skill for coping with the pain accompanied by loss.

Grief is the emotional experience of loss, whereas **mourning** is the actual expression of loss, those behaviors that take place as a result of the grief experience.[71] An actual loss or some memory of a previous loss can serve as a trigger to experience the emotions of grief. These emotions then result in behaviors to mourn the loss. It is important to mourn the loss to reconcile the emotions of grief. Unreconciled or poorly reconciled grief experiences can lead to unhealthy behaviors.

Grief is a normal response to loss. It does not matter what or who has been lost. The more meaningful the thing or person that is lost, the more intense will be the sense of loss. People mourn in various ways. Some seek support, and others mourn silently and alone. Some

recover quickly whereas others mourn for a very long time. There is no one right way to mourn. However, the grief process must not consume your life to the degree that you become dysfunctional and risk losing additional things that are important and necessary, such as relationships and employment.

The support of close friends and family is helpful during bereavement (mourning). Sometimes it may become necessary to seek the assistance of a mental health professional experienced in facilitating the grief recovery process. Grief support groups are common. Individuals who participate in a community grief support group or professional grief counseling often recover more quickly from their bereavement. People tend to work through loss in healthier ways and integrate loss more effectively when assistance from others and a variety of resources are readily available. Resources form the basis of a **support network** consisting of three systems that focus on (1) clarifying how you derive meaning from life through your beliefs and values, (2) how you access support from those around you, and (3) how you draw upon your own personal strengths and abilities.[72]

Recovering from loss does not necessarily mean that you will no longer experience any pain from the memory of the loss. It does mean that you will regain a sense of being okay and going on with your life. Recovery means that you are no longer consumed by the loss and can incorporate new beginnings and new ways of thinking into your life. The first 6 months after a loss are usually the most difficult. The formal bereavement or grieving process typically takes about 2 years, although the sense of pain usually subsides gradually over this 2-year period. Even after the 2-year period, you may find certain dates related to the loss just as difficult, for example, the birthday of a deceased child or the anniversary of the death of a spouse or relationship partner.

Some commonalities have been discovered in the **grief process.** One grief process model describes grief from the loss of a loved one as having three phases, each with its own set of characteristics, challenges, and choices: early mourning, mid-mourning, and late mourning.[73] The early mourning phase lasts from the time you first hear about the loss to the final disposition of the body and personal belongings of the deceased. This phase can last as long as 3 to 6 weeks after the funeral. Challenges to face include getting through the funeral, dealing with funeral details, notifying family and friends, settling estate arrangements, and preparing for the transitions to come.

Mid-mourning is the phase of having to face the harsh reality of the loss. As others begin to get on with their lives, you will find it difficult to do so. You may suffer deep separation feelings, pain, or anxiety. You may have difficulty distinguishing fact from fantasy, and physical symptoms may develop such as sleep disturbance, reduced appetite, anxiety attacks, headaches, stomachaches, and shortness of breath. Your health may be fragile during this phase, and it is extremely important, difficult as it may be, to exercise and eat a nutritious diet. During this phase there can be a flood of emotions, intense sadness, and loneliness as well as feelings of guilt, depression, powerlessness, abandonment, anger and rage, fear, and panic. You may choose to be alone in order to grieve completely. However, it is also important to seek out and maintain a support system during this vulnerable time.

The late mourning phase focuses on getting on with your life. Your feelings will focus less on grief, although anger and sadness may still be prevalent, and more on attitudes and perceptions as they relate to moving on with your life. An attitude of acceptance has gradually evolved, and an integration of the loss into your life scheme has occurred.

Another grief process model involves **five stages of grief:** denial, anger, sorrow/despair/depression, bargaining, and acceptance.[74] These stages can be experienced in any order and more than once in the grieving process.

Denial is often the initial reaction, although it can be experienced again at any time. Denial is a buffer of protection against the shock and trauma of the loss. It allows us time to adjust to the event. This stage is accompanied by a feeling of numbness and disbelief. As is the case with each of these stages, it is important to work through the denial. From there, one must regain and maintain a presence of mind as soon as possible so that one can function in the world realistically. Seeking and receiving support and understanding from others is very important during this time.

When you have lost someone or something important to you, you can become very angry. You may want to lash out and hurt others with your words and deeds. It is important to remember that what you are angry about is the loss, and you should not become destructive toward yourself or others as a result. Anger can be worked through by talking with others. Anger is a natural part of the grief process, and it needs to be expressed, but in a healthy manner.

Sorrow, despair, and depression are natural and healthy ways to express sadness from a loss. Crying is useful for releasing the sadness. Ritualistic ceremonies, such as funerals, wakes, and memorial services, are often held to facilitate opportunities for expressing sadness with others who are also feeling the loss or wish to support you in your loss. These ceremonies can assist with the transitions that are necessary from one stage to another in the grieving process.

Bargaining is a desperate attempt to stay in control. This stage is accompanied by our attempts to second-guess the situation or try to reverse the loss. We might say things like "If only I had done this or that, then this would not have happened" or "If I promise this thing or that thing, everything will be okay again." Although the bargaining stage does not necessarily have many healthy aspects, it is still a very common experience during bereavement. The persistent and gentle assurance and reassurance by those close to you that "there is nothing you could have done" or "there is nothing you can do now" will help you through this potentially destructive stage.

Acceptance is the final stage of grief, although it is possible to recycle through the previous stages again. Acceptance is the final goal of the grief process. In this stage, we come to accept the loss that has occurred. We come to terms with reality. We understand that our life will always be different having been impacted by the loss, but that we can and will go on. We can let go of our doubts and anger and lift our sadness. We can go on and live our lives fully again.

Another approach to understanding bereavement identifies grief not as a succession of phases through which a person passes with little or no control, but as four tasks for the bereaved person: accepting the reality of the loss, working through the pain of grief, adjusting to an environment in which the deceased is missing, and emotionally relocating the deceased and moving on with life.[75] In accepting the reality of the loss, individuals must talk about the death and funeral of the deceased. In working through the pain of grief, individuals must allow themselves to indulge in the pain, to feel it and know that one day it will pass. In adjusting to an environment in which the deceased is missing, individuals must reform schedules and responsibilities that once required attention to the deceased when they were living, and create meaningful rituals like a special memorial, keeping a journal, or writing poetry to process the meaning the deceased held. Emotionally relocating the deceased and moving on with life involves changing and maintaining their relationship with the deceased; it is normal to have an ongoing relationship with the deceased through memories and mental life. Failure to accomplish any one of these four tasks may result in complications during the grief process.[76]

Complicated grief is a delayed or incomplete adaptation to loss. "In complicated grief, there is a failure to return, over time, to pre-loss levels of functioning, or to the previous state of emotional well-being. Grief may be more difficult in younger parents, women, and persons with limited social support, thus increasing their risk for complicated grief."[77] Factors that may interfere with the grief process include: avoiding emotions, overactivity leading to exhaustion, use of alcohol or other drugs, unrealistic promises made to the deceased, unresolved grief from a previous loss, judgmental relationships, and resentment of those who try to help.[78] The experience of complicated grief may necessitate professional counseling from the clergy or a mental health professional.

Complicated grief (CG) occurs when an individual experiences prolonged, unabated grief. A breakthrough research study has provided insight into a possible physiological basis for CG.[79] The neural mechanisms distinguishing complicated grief (CG) from noncomplicated grief (NCG) are unclear, but hypothesized mechanisms include both pain-related activity (related to the social pain of loss) and reward-related activity (related to attachment behavior). In this research, bereaved women (11 CG and 12 NCG) who had lost a mother or sister to breast cancer participated in a functional magnetic resonance imaging scan (fMRI) while being shown pictures and words that reminded them of their deceased loved one. Analyses revealed that whereas both CG and NCG participants showed pain-related neural activity in response to reminders of the deceased, only those with CG showed reward-related activity in the nucleus accumbens (NA), a forebrain area most commonly associated with reward. This NA cluster was positively correlated with self-reported yearning, but not with time since death, participant age, or positive/negative affect.

This study supports the hypothesis that attachment activates reward pathways. When someone we love dies our brains have to adapt to the idea that cues associated with our loved one no longer predict a reward experience. But for those with CG, reminders of the deceased still activate neural reward activity, which may interfere with adapting to the loss in the present.[80]

Women's Grief

Death of a Relationship Partner Bereavement research consistently shows that men who lose their relationship partner to death (widowers) have a greater incidence of depression, health problems, and mortality than women who lose their relationship partner to death (widows); these findings apply to both heterosexual and homosexual couples.[81] However, when ethnicity was considered as a factor, African American widows fared worse than African American widowers, "possibly because Black men are more likely to receive high levels of support from family and friends compared to Black women."[82] In general, a likely reason why most men fare worse than women after losing a relationship partner is that men tend to rely on their partner as their primary confidant and when their partner dies, men lose their primary source for social support. Research shows that in general, women, including widows, receive more social support than men. Also, research shows that "the ways in which women cope are superior to those of men because men tend to use more avoidant methods of coping and are therefore less likely to work through their grief" while "women are much more likely to use emotion-focused strategies for coping, such as talking to someone about their feelings."[83]

Death of a Child Grieving parents say that their grief is a lifelong process, "a process in that [they] try to take and keep some meaning from the loss and life without the [child]."[84] The child who died is considered a gift to the parents and family; the parents also see their child as a gift to others. Thus, these "parents seek to find ways to continue to love, honor, and value the lives of their children, and to make the child's presence known and felt in the lives of family and friends. Bereaved parents often try to live their lives more fully and generously because of this painful experience."[85] Gender differences in parental grief have been demonstrated by research. Grieving mothers scored significantly higher than grieving fathers on an instrument that measured: despair, anger/hostility, guilt, loss of control, rumination, depersonalization, somatization, loss of vigor, and physical symptoms. This research found no significant gender differences in denial, social desirability, social isolation, death anxiety, or loss of appetite.[86]

Miscarriage is an unexpected, unplanned pregnancy loss prior to the point of fetal viability. Research studies describe the impact of miscarriage on women that include feelings of shock, grief, lack of control, the need to be supported and listened to, disappointment in those responding to loss with indifference, and fears related to subsequent pregnancy outcomes.[87] Investigators have also found that after miscarriage women may experience a variety of emotions ranging from disappointment to fear and anxiety and from relief to intense pain and grief; but the majority of studies point to the presence of significant psychological distress and depressive symptoms in females lasting from weeks to months.[88] Women at highest risk for depressive symptoms following miscarriage were those with less emotional strength and who ascribed high personal significance to their miscarriage, lacked social support, felt less emotionally strong, had lower incomes, and did not conceive again or give birth by a year after loss.[89] Gender differences also exist in the grief response after miscarriage in that women were significantly more depressed after their miscarriage than their male partners.[90]

Divorce and Grief Research has shown that women are more likely to face adjustment difficulties prior to the decision to divorce, but they have been found to have better post-divorce adjustment compared to men.[91] Women tend to report a greater number of reasons for divorce and tend to give reasons that are related to the quality of their relationships, such as feeling unloved or belittled by their spouse; whereas men tend to report their partners are neglectful of their needs, inattentive, or having incompatible interests. "Despite poorer economic outcomes among divorced women in general, women have been found to be more satisfied with their divorce settlements, and they were more likely to feel in control and empowered by their divorce settlements (but not by child support awards) compared to men. Some of the predictors of women's adjustment to separation and divorce are the women's age; length of the marriage; the presence, number, and age of children; sex role attitudes; relationships with the ex-spouse; and social and emotional support received from family and social networks."[92]

Infertility and Grief Infertility is defined as the inability to conceive after a minimum of 12 months of regular intercourse without contraception.[93] Infertility can be due to many causes, but studies have shown that a little more than half of cases of infertility are a result of female conditions. Most types of infertility are treatable and in some cases in vitro fertilization and other lab procedures may be used to ensure fertilization, and special care or medication may be required to enable the pregnancy to come to term. "Women who seek treatment for infertility are likely to spend at least 3 years trying to have a child without a guaranteed positive outcome. In addition to the tremendous costs associated with most

fertility treatments, there are additional stressors of an emotional, physical, and social nature. The affective consequences of infertility that are most often cited include sadness, frustration and hostility, helplessness and powerlessness, shame, poor self-esteem, and isolation. These affective reactions are similar to grief reactions experienced with other significant losses, such as death."[94]

Job Loss and Grief The negative consequences of job loss are well documented. "Like their male colleagues, women who are unemployed are more likely to suffer from loss of self-esteem, depression and suicide, alcohol and substance abuse, and other psychological and physical consequences (including increased mortality) compared to employed women and men. Some research has shown that unemployed women have higher rates of depression and anxiety compared to unemployed men."[95] Counselors can "help validate women's experiences of the effects of a job loss and facilitate their efforts toward regaining a sense of mastery, control, and self-esteem through activities that are most meaningful to them. These activities can involve enhancing job search and interviewing techniques, cognitive reframing of the job loss to enhance self-esteem, increasing stress management skills, and seeking social support and professional support networks."[96]

DEPRESSION

A common emotional health concern for women is the presence of symptoms associated with depression. **Depression** is an emotional state of persistent dejection that may range from mild discouragement to feelings of extreme despair. These feelings are usually accompanied by loss of motivation, loss of energy, insomnia, loss of appetite, and difficulty in concentrating and making decisions.[97] *FYI:* "Prevalence of Depression." A chemical imbalance in the brain, primarily that of the neurotransmitter serotonin, is thought to be a precursor to depression. The causes of this imbalance may include the experience of stress or trauma or a genetic predisposition toward depression.

Types of Depression

Individuals may have just a few characteristics associated with depression, or they may have more severe symptoms indicative of a clinical depression. Women are twice as likely as men to be diagnosed with a clinical depression, and thus the cost of depression is borne disproportionately by women.[98,99] Most research suggests that women are at greater risk for depression because of interplay between environmental factors (such as social stressors), biological factors (such as hormones), and genetic factors (such as family history).[100]

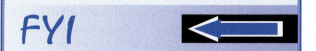

Prevalence of Depression

The U.S. Centers for Disease Control and Prevention CDC reported 6.7% of U.S. adults experienced a major depressive episode in the past 12 months, based on a face-to-face household survey conducted in 2005. According to the CDC, significantly greater percentages of lifetime major depression have been reported among women (11.7%) than men (5.6%). Regarding ethnic differences, lifetime percentages of depression are reported as 6.52% among whites, 4.57% among blacks, and 5.17% among Hispanics. According to the World Health Organization, unipolar depression was the third most important cause of disease burden in 2004. Unipolar depression was in eighth place in low-income countries, but at first place in middle- and high-income countries. The U.S. National Institute of Mental Health estimates that between 17 and 20 million Americans develop depression each year. One of every five adults may experience depression at some time in their lives, but less than half of the people suffering from depression receive treatment. Twice as many women as men suffer from depression, although everybody, including children, can develop the illness. Have you ever been depressed or known anyone who was depressed? If so, what resources did you find most helpful with managing or treating the depression?

Common Types of Clinical Depression[102]

Major depressive episode involves the presence of at least five of the following symptoms for most of the day for at least a 2-week period:

- Feelings of sadness or emptiness
- Diminished interest or pleasure
- Weight loss
- Insomnia
- Feelings of worthlessness or inappropriate guilt
- Diminished ability to think or concentrate
- Recurrent thoughts of death or suicide

Dysthymic disorder involves the presence of at least two of the following symptoms for most of the day for at least 2 years (1 year for adolescents and children):

- Poor appetite or overeating
- Insomnia
- Low energy or fatigue
- Low self-esteem
- Poor concentration or difficulty making decisions
- Feelings of hopelessness

Major depressive disorder is typically the reccurrence of a major depressive episode (two or more within two consecutive months).

Bipolar disorder is a mixture of major depressive episodes and manic episodes. Manic episodes are a distinct period of persistently elevated, expansive, or irritable mood lasting at least 4 days, and that is clearly different from the usual nondepressed mood. If numerous periods of depressive symptoms and numerous periods of manic symptoms occur, the individual may be diagnosed as having **cyclothymic disorder** (a chronic fluctuating mood disturbance involving numerous periods of mania and depression)

Clinical depression usually requires intervention by a trained mental health professional. The most common types of clinical depression are major depressive episode, dysthymic disorder, major depressive disorder, and bipolar disorder (also referred to as manic depression). In any given community, it is estimated that between 10 and 25 percent of women will develop a major depressive disorder sometime in their lifetime.[101] These prevalence rates for major depressive disorder seem to be unrelated to ethnicity, education, income, or marital status. (See *FYI:* "Common Types of Clinical Depression.")

Psychosocial Stressors and Depression

Some researchers believe that the higher incidence of depression in women is because they respond to depressing life events differently than men. Men tend to cut off the depression before it has serious consequences, whereas women tend to remain focused on their depressed mood in ways that prolong its duration and intensify its effects (this is referred to as rumination).[103]

Research has shown that women have better emotional memories than men and there is speculation that

this might contribute to greater incidences of depression in women.[104] Researchers used brain MRI (magnetic resonance imaging) to track the activity of the brain while recalling emotional stimuli, and what they found was that women's brains seem to be wired both to feel and recall emotions more keenly than men's brains. A risk factor in depression is rumination, or dwelling on a memory and reviewing it time after time. This study illuminates a possible biological basis for rumination and suggests another reason depression is more prevalent in women.

Researchers believe that women have higher incidences of depression than men because they experience more stress and discrimination. Women are subject to unique psychosocial stressors that can initiate depression and impede recovery. Examples include conflict between domestic and job demands, gender discrimination in financial and political venues, and pressure by society to maintain a prescribed body image. Body-image dissatisfaction has been linked to low self-esteem and higher rates of depression.[105]

Perceived lower social support for women as compared to men is linked with higher rates of depression for women.[106] Also, significantly more women than men are living in poverty, and poor women have more frequent and uncontrollable adverse life events (danger, violence, crime, etc.) than men.[107]

Research links depression in women with the experience of a higher number of life stressors and negative life events as compared to men.[108,109] Negative life events include serious illness or injury of self or a close family member, relationship discord or divorce, loss of a job, loss of a parent, and death of a family member. Severe adverse life events over which women feel little to no sense of control has been determined to be a major risk factor for women.[110] In one study, a depressive episode in response to adverse life events was found to be three times more likely in women than in men.[111] In another study, women who developed depression following a severely threatening event were more likely to reflect feelings of humiliation and being trapped as compared to women who had not developed depression following such an event.[112]

Women's higher rates of traumatic stressors are shown to be significant contributors to gender differences in major depression. Traumatic stressors such as sexual assault, sexual harassment, relationship partner violence, and childhood sexual abuse have all been linked to depression in women.[113,114,115]

The interpersonal and psychological functioning of women can be significantly impaired from the experience of childhood trauma. Childhood physical abuse, incest, and parental alcoholism have each been associated with higher rates of depression, higher sexual assault rates, lower self-esteem, and greater involvement with a chemically dependent partner.[116]

Women who had experienced childhood abuse and/or adult abuse were studied over 8 years by researchers who discovered that childhood and adult abuse were both independently related to chronic or recurrent depression in these women.[117] Women college undergraduates who reported exposure to abuse between their parents (parental partner abuse) during their childhood were described as having depression and low self-esteem.[118]

The Reproductive System and Depression

Research on the influence of biological factors on depression is somewhat inconclusive. Fluctuations in female hormones and other biochemicals may influence the frequency of depression in women. It is known that gonadal and adrenal steroids affect neurotransmitters, which play a role in regulating mood and behavior and neuroendocrine physiology.[119] The hormones of progesterone and estrogen both affect the neuroendocrine, neurotransmitter, and circadian systems, which affect the synthesis and release of both serotonin and norepinephrine, which in turn influence the development of depression.[120,121] However, most research does not support a definitive relationship between depression and normal fluctuations in ovarian hormones except for the few women who may have had some underlying emotional or social vulnerability during the hormonal fluctuation or who have a family history of depression.[122,123] Further research is needed to clarify the impact and role that endocrinology plays in the onset of depression.

Menstruation and Depression Severe premenstrual mood changes have been associated with a lifetime history of major depression. Premenstrual symptoms appear to have their highest prevalence in women in their late twenties and thirties. Approximately 80 percent of women report mild to minimal mood or somatic (physical) changes premenstrually, and an estimated 5 percent of women experience severe premenstrual symptoms.[124] Common premenstrual symptoms include depressed mood; irritability; hostility; anxiety; changes in sleep, appetite, energy, and libido; and somatic symptoms. (See *Assess Yourself:* "Premenstrual Dysphoric Disorder (PMDD).")

Depression Related to Pregnancy and Childbirth Many women experience some negative emotions after childbirth.[125] Between 50 and 80 percent of women experience a mild postpartum dysphoria, or "the blues." This typically occurs the third or fourth day after delivery and lasts 1–2 weeks. Women giving birth to their first child are more susceptible to postpartum dysphoria and may experience it up to 8 weeks postpartum. Between 12 percent and 16 percent of women experience a major depressive episode in the postpartum period.[126] The more severe condition of postpartum depression occurs in 10 percent of all women after delivery, and it has a greater duration.[127] The onset may occur from 6 weeks to 4 months after delivery and last from 6 months to a year. These women may have any of the following complications: depression, mania, delirium, or psychosis. Postpartum psychosis is a rare condition and is often dangerous. Approximately 2 of 1000 new mothers (about 3500 women each year in the United States) develop postpartum psychosis.[128] (See *Her Story:* "Andrea Yates: Postpartum Depression and Psychosis" and *FYI:* "Risk Factors for Postpartum Depression").

Typically, pregnancy is associated with a low incidence of psychiatric disorders. But for women with a history of even mild emotional problems, pregnancy and childbirth can result in worsened or new psychiatric disorders, sometimes severe enough to endanger a woman's life or her baby's.[129] Mood changes in pregnancy most often occur in women who are predisposed to emotional problems; the rapidly changing hormonal levels during pregnancy exacerbate the condition. Major elevations of steroid hormones occur during pregnancy, yet in contrast to their effect on mood during the menstrual cycle, these steroid elevations usually do not contribute to severe mood changes during pregnancy. It is thought that a change in gonadal steroid receptors during pregnancy may modify the impact of elevated steroid levels,[133] but further research is required to substantiate this.

Antepartum (before labor) and postpartum (after delivery) depression can be made worse with the presence of major life stressors. Among financially impoverished inner-city women, antepartum depression was found among 27.6 percent and postpartum depression was found among 23.4 percent.[134] These rates were about double those found for middle-class women. African American and European American women did not differ in their rates of depression. The larger incidence of antepartum and postpartum depression in the impoverished inner-city women was most likely due to the stress of their financial plight.

 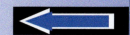

FYI

Risk Factors and Treatment for Postpartum Depression[131]

Major Factors
History of postpartum depression
History of depression
Family history of depression
Depression during pregnancy

Contributing Factors
Poor social support
Adverse life events
Marital instability
Younger maternal age
  (14–18 years)
Infants with health problems or
  perceived poor temperaments
Unwanted or unplanned pregnancy
Being a victim of violence or abuse
Low self-esteem
Low socioeconomic status

Mental health counseling is the first line of treatment for mild to moderate postpartum depression or when a patient refuses pharmacotherapy; this may include individual, group, couple and/or family counseling. Mental health counseling should be used as adjunctive treatments to pharmacotherapy.

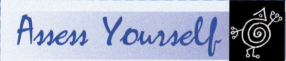

Assess Yourself

Premenstrual Dysphoric Disorder (PMDD)

The most severe type of menstruation-related mood distress is **premenstrual dysphoric disorder (PMDD)**. The criterion for diagnosing this condition is that for most of the menstrual periods over the past year the woman must have experienced at least five or more of the following eleven categories of symptoms:

1. Depressed mood or self-deprecating thoughts
2. Anxiety or tension
3. Sudden feelings of sadness or tearfulness
4. Persistent anger, irritability, or interpersonal conflicts
5. Decreased interest in usual activities (work, school, and so forth)
6. Difficulty concentrating
7. Lethargy or easy to fatigue
8. Marked change in appetite, overeating, or food cravings
9. Hypersomnia or insomnia
10. Feeling of being overwhelmed or out of control
11. Other physical symptoms, such as breast tenderness or swelling, headaches, joint or muscle pain, a sensation of bloating or weight gain.[130]

Menopausal Depression The severe hormonal shifts associated with menopause may incite depression. A survey of working, postmenopausal women reported that at least 40 percent of those surveyed faced difficulties in the work environment due to menopausal symptoms, including weight gain, hot flashes, irritability, depression, bloating, and mood changes.[135]

Infertility and Depression Research on the relation of infertility to depression is based on clinical observations and the self-report of women. Infertility patients tend to report feeling damaged, defective, guilty, less attractive, less desirable, and lacking in capability. Almost half of all women seeking assistance at fertility clinics exhibit some symptoms of depression: 40 percent demonstrate moderate symptoms and 7 percent exhibit severe symptoms.[136] Depression in fertile women has been shown to increase when their partners are diagnosed as being infertile. Attempts to

Her Story

Andrea Yates: Postpartum Depression and Psychosis

On June 20, 2001, 36-year-old Andrea Yates, a Texas mother of five, methodically drowned all of her children, ages 6 months to 7 years. Andrea Yates had been treated for postpartum depression since the birth of her 2-year-old. She had been on medication and had attempted to kill herself in 1999 shortly after childbirth. She cited her reason for attempted suicide as being afraid she would hurt someone. Her depression was compounded by episodes of dissociative thought and psychosis. Even with this emotional instability, her husband insisted she continue to home-school all of the children. Andrea Yates was indicted for murder and pleaded "not guilty by reason of insanity." She was found guilty of murder and sentenced to life in prison. She most likely avoided the death penalty because of her emotional condition.

On January 5, 2005, Yates's murder convictions were overturned because a key witness, who depicted her as knowing right from wrong, had given erroneous testimony. While she waited for her new trial, she stayed in the prison psychiatric ward where she continued to receive treatment. On July 26, 2006, Andrea Yates was found "not guilty by reason of insanity." The ruling was based on the determination that Yates had suffered from severe postpartum psychosis and, in a delusional state, believed Satan was inside her and that she killed her children because she was trying to save them from hell. She was committed to a mental health facility, and mental health experts say she may be there for the rest of her life. Each time she gets better with treatment,

she realizes what she did and descends again into a state of severe emotional distress or psychosis.

- Do you think Andrea Yates should be held responsible for the deaths of her children?
- If Ms. Yates became pregnant again, would her future children be at risk?
- What responsibility did Andrea's husband bear for the safety and welfare of his wife and children?
- Should women be assessed for signs of postpartum depression when they receive their 6-week postpartum checkup? What is the role of the medical community in ensuring that women receive proper diagnosis and treatment for postpartum depression?

Postpartum psychotic depression is sometimes associated with chronic mood disorders, especially untreated depression. The most prevalent psychotic features include paranoid delusions that incorporate the newborn. Hallucinations are rare. A woman with postpartum depression is at a heightened risk for suicide and/or infanticide and is considered a medical emergency that requires immediate hospitalization and treatment to ensure the safety of the infant and the ill mother. When the mother is hospitalized, visitation between the mother and infant should be restricted, particularly if the infant's presence precipitates anxiety in the mother. The goal of hospitalization is to achieve symptom remission and stability in the mother so that bonding and attachment can occur. Maternal-infant bonding is difficult, if not impossible, if the mother is out of touch with reality.[132]

become pregnant can give rise to intense mood swings, anxiety, irritability, emotional liability, and depressive symptoms.

Abortion and Depression   The emotional impact of abortion is not yet fully understood. Mediating social factors such as the woman's religious beliefs and her family value system may negatively or positively impact postabortion mood. Also, women who have a history of emotional vulnerability may be more susceptible to a melancholic postabortion mood.

The scientific literature does not support the idea that severe guilt and depression often follow from a legal abortion. In fact, the predominant response is one of relief. Guilt and depression, when reported, are typically mild and transitory and do not affect the ability of the woman to function socially. Most women report the greatest distress prior to the abortion. The positive psychological effects of abortion have not been fully

assessed, but some studies indicate that women feel more self-directed and more independent and have greater self-efficacy after an abortion.[137]

Do not be fooled by something called "post abortion stress syndrome" (PASS). It sounds scientific, but it is a fictitious condition invented by conservative religious groups to frighten women. There is no clinical evidence to support the existence of PASS, and it is not recognized by any professional medical or mental health organization.

Depression and Genetic Liability

Normal stress hormonal changes may serve as triggers for psychiatric illness in genetically vulnerable women. Research with female twins determined that there is a genetic liability for the onset of major depression in women who experience stressful events.[138] Thus, the tendency to develop depression may be inherited.

Major depressive disorder is 1.5 to 3 times more common among first-degree biological relatives of persons with this disorder than among the general population.

Developmental Issues and Depression

There are no consistent gender differences in rates of depression among prepubescent children. However, by midadolescence, ages 13–15, girls show significantly higher rates of depressive disorders and depressive symptoms than boys.[139] Major depressive disorder is twice as common in adolescent and adult females as in adolescent and adult males.[140] Although not overlooking the biological differences of males and females that become more prevalent during adolescence, additional possible explanations for the emerging differences in the rates of depression exist. First, girls enter early adolescence responding to frustration and distress with a style that is less effective and action-oriented than boys. Second, girls begin to face uncontrollable stressors in early adolescence to a greater extent than boys.[141] Data suggest that girls exhibit more passive and introspective coping styles, which are associated with longer and more severe depressive symptoms; girls undergo biological changes that are less favored by society, and girls and women face more negative life events and social conditions such as sexual abuse and stronger parental and peer expectations.

The most likely age for women to develop depression is in their twenties and thirties.[142] However, a woman in her mid-forties and fifties is also vulnerable to the onset of depression. It is not yet clear whether menopause in midlife by itself predisposes women to depression, but many major life events that occur around this time of life may contribute to depression. Facing the social stigma that devalues the worth and beauty of middle-aged and older women can also be demoralizing. Older women, in their sixties and beyond, face increased medical problems and concern over the limited number of years left in their life. Their physical condition may put limitations on their activity level, and many friends and family have died. These issues can contribute to feelings of depression for the older woman.

Family of Origin Issues and Depression

Many research studies demonstrate the influence of familial factors on depression, especially for persons who have experienced adverse or threatening life events. Chronic depression in women has been associated with family of origin experiences reflecting severe losses, including neglect, rejection, abandonment, and physical,

sexual and emotional abuse.[143] Persons who came from a loving family but still developed depression have reported they lacked an empathic caretaker who could soothe emotional reactions to traumatic losses during critical periods of childhood.[144] Research suggests that "chronically depressed women have often adapted as best they could to an environment that discouraged appropriate mourning by assuming a cognitive-emotional mask, unconsciously defending themselves against expressing or even experiencing the painful emotions generated by their losses. As a result, unresolved mourning typically lies at the root of long-term depressive patterns, especially for women who adapted to their unfortunate childhood circumstances by using a placating approach to secure relationship with significant others."[145] In other words, many women who develop depression did not have the emotional support in childhood necessary to cope effectively with trauma and traumatic loss. Parents may have discouraged and suppressed emotional expression by family members and even encouraged masking and denial of negative emotions thereby leaving significant emotional wounds unattended. Motivations for parents to suppress emotional expression by family members range from a need to keep family "secrets" (such as incest, child abuse, domestic violence, alcoholism/drug abuse) to a simple desire to present the family image to the community in the most favorable light.

Multicultural Issues of Depression and Suicide

African American women may experience racism as an additional stressor that may contribute to depression. Female status, lower social class, and downward social mobility are all related to greater depression.[146] Racism itself can be a factor in whether a black woman is properly diagnosed with or treated for depression. Black female psychiatric patients were diagnosed with depression at a rate 42 percent higher than that of white women, and more black women were more likely to receive drug therapy than white women. It is unclear whether this reflects a discriminatory attitude or is an accurate reflection of the condition of these patients.

Hispanic women and Latinas in the United States may experience economic deprivation, migration, and political discrimination as risk factors for depression. Hispanic women who experienced discrimination, gender-role conflicts, and concern about starting a family in a preceding 3-month period had significantly higher rates of depression than Hispanic women who did not experience these circumstances.[147] Also, many migrant Hispanic women experience gender-role conflicts within their own traditionally male-dominated culture.

Some Asian women have an economic situation as favorable as that of white women in the United States, but immigrant women who had completed eight or fewer years of education were at a high risk for racial and social discrimination.[148] This was most common in immigrant women from Vietnam, China, Guam, the Philippines, Samoa, and Korea. Gender-related risk factors such as low self-esteem are significant problems for many Asian women and may contribute to depression.

Native American women (including Alaskan Natives) are among the least visible and least researched groups in the United States. Compared with other U.S. women, the death rate for Native American women is much higher for alcoholism and cirrhosis and liver diseases, as well as suicide.[149] Risk factors associated with depression for Native Americans include poverty, lack of education, and larger numbers of children.

The CDC reported in 2008 that for youth between the ages of 10 and 24, suicide is the third leading cause of death. It results in approximately 4500 lives lost each year. The top three methods used in suicides of young people include firearms (46 percent), suffocation (39 percent), and poisoning (8 percent). Deaths from youth suicide are only part of the problem. More young people survive suicide attempts than actually die. The CDC sponsored a nationwide survey of youth in grades 9–12 in public and private schools in the United States and found that 15 percent of students reported seriously considering suicide, 11 percent reported creating a plan, and 7 percent reported trying to take their own life in the 12 months preceding the survey. Each year, approximately 149,000 youth between the ages of 10 and 24 receive medical care for self-inflicted injuries at emergency departments across the United States. Suicide affects all youth, but some groups are at higher risk than others. Boys are more likely than girls to die from suicide. Of the reported suicides in the 10 to 24 age group, 83 percent of the deaths were males and 17 percent were females. Girls, however, are more likely to report attempting suicide than boys. Cultural variations in suicide rates also exist, with Native American/Alaskan Native, Hispanic, and Asian/Pacific Islander youth having the highest rates of suicide-related fatalities. A nationwide survey of youth in grades 9–12 in public and private schools in the United States found that Hispanic youth were more likely to report attempting suicide than their black and white, non-Hispanic peers. Several factors can put a young person at risk for suicide. However, having these risk factors does not always mean that suicide will occur. These risk factors are:

- Depression
- Aggressive or disruptive behaviors
- History of previous suicide attempts

- Family history of suicide
- History of depression or other mental illness
- Alcohol or drug abuse
- Stressful life event or loss
- Easy access to lethal methods
- Exposure to the suicidal behavior of others
- Incarceration

Low parental support is a significant predictor for adolescent depression as is low self-esteem; low levels of attachment to either parents or peers, or both; underinvolved parents or authoritarian parents; and depressed parents.[150] An unstable family life was a major factor in 50–80 percent of all adolescent suicides. Lesbian and gay youth are two to three times more likely to commit suicide than other youths, and 30 percent of all completed youth suicides are related to the issue of sexual identity.[151] The single largest predictor of mental health in this group was self-acceptance. A general sense of self-worth, with a positive view of their sexual orientation, appears to be critical for good mental health.

More men than women die by suicide with a ratio of 4:1 (males:females). More women than men report a history of attempted suicide, with a gender ratio of 3:1 (females:males). The strongest risk factors for attempted suicide in adults are depression, alcohol abuse, drug abuse, and separation or divorce. (See Table 4.1.)

In the *World Health Report 2001,* the WHO examined suicide trends across the globe for the past 20 years. These rates vary considerably. For example, suicide rates are up in Mexico, India, Brazil, and Russia, but down in the United States, Japan, and China. It is very difficult, if not impossible, to find a common explanation for this variation. However, alcohol consumption and easy access to firearms seem to be positively correlated with suicide across all industrialized and developing countries.

For women who are beaten or sexually assaulted, the emotional and physical strain can lead to suicide. The WHO research suggests that abused women endure enormous psychological suffering because of violence. Many are severely depressed and display symptoms of posttraumatic stress disorder. They may be chronically fatigued but unable to sleep; they may have nightmares and use alcohol and drugs to numb their pain; or they may become isolated and withdrawn. In one study in Leon, Nicaragua, researchers found that abused women were six times more likely to be diagnosed with mental distress than were nonabused women. Likewise, in the United States women battered by their partners have been found to be between four and five times more likely to be depressed than are nonabused women.

TABLE 4.1 Suicide Rank as Leading Cause of Death for Females by Age and Race in 2007[152]

ALL RACES	
10–14 yrs.	6th
15–19 yrs.	4th
20–24 yrs.	3rd
25–34 yrs.	4th
35–44 yrs.	4th
45–54 yrs.	8th
55–64 yrs.	not in top ten
White	
10–14 yrs.	6th
15–19 yrs.	2nd
20–24 yrs.	2nd
25–34 yrs.	3rd
35–44 yrs.	4th
45–54 yrs.	5th
55–64 yrs.	10th
Black	
10–14 yrs.	6th
15–19 yrs.	5th
20–24 yrs.	7th
25–34 yrs.	9th
35–44 yrs.	not in top ten
45–54 yrs.	not in top ten
55–64 yrs.	not in top ten
American Indian or Alaska Native	
10–14 yrs.	2nd
15–19 yrs.	2nd
20–24 yrs.	2nd
25–34 yrs.	2nd (tied)
35–44 yrs.	6th
45–54 yrs.	9th
55–64 yrs.	not in top ten
Asian or Pacific Islander	
10–14 yrs.	3rd
15–19 yrs.	3rd
20–24 yrs.	2nd
25–34 yrs.	3rd
35–44 yrs.	3rd
45–54 yrs.	5th
55–64 yrs.	7th
Hispanic origin (may be of any race)	
10–14 yrs.	6th
15–19 yrs.	4th
20–24 yrs.	4th
25–34 yrs.	4th
35–44 yrs.	7th
45–54 yrs.	10th
55–64 yrs.	not in top ten

Medication for Depression

Most antidepressant drugs work by selectively raising levels in the brain of the neurotransmitters thought to be most responsible for regulating moods. These medications are classified as SSRIs (selective serotonin reuptake inhibitors) and SSNRIs (selective serotonin and norepinephrine reuptake inhibitors). They allow these neurotransmitters to linger longer in the synaptic cleft (space between neurons), thereby increasing the amount available for absorption by receiving neurons along the neuronal pathway (see *FYI*: "Antidepressant Medication Use" and *FYI*: "Antidepressant Medications").

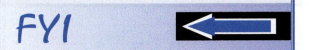

FYI

Antidepressant Medication Use in the United States (for persons aged 12 and over)[153]

Antidepressants were the third most common prescription drug taken by Americans of all ages in 2005–2008 and the most frequently used by persons aged 18–44 years. From 1998 to 2008, the rate of antidepressant use in the U.S. among all ages increased nearly 400 percent. Overall, females are 2.5 times as likely to take antidepressant medications as males; however, there is no difference by gender in rates of antidepressant use among persons aged 12–17 years. Twenty-three percent of women aged 40–59 take antidepressants, more than any other age-gender group. Among both males and females, those aged 40 and over are more likely to take antidepressants than those in younger groups. Non-Hispanic white persons are more likely to take antidepressant medication than persons of other races and ethnicities. Fourteen percent of non-Hispanic white persons take antidepressant medications compared with 4 percent of non-Hispanic black and 3 percent of Mexican-American persons. There is no difference by income in the prevalence of antidepressant usage.

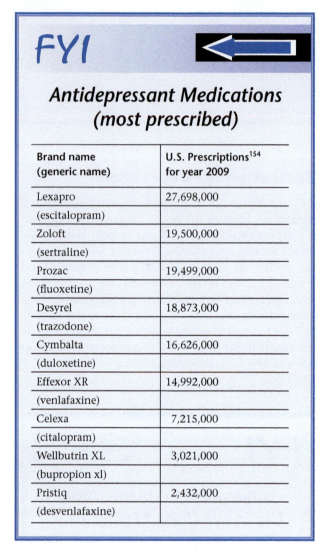

Antidepressant Medications (most prescribed)

Brand name (generic name)	U.S. Prescriptions[154] for year 2009
Lexapro (escitalopram)	27,698,000
Zoloft (sertraline)	19,500,000
Prozac (fluoxetine)	19,499,000
Desyrel (trazodone)	18,873,000
Cymbalta (duloxetine)	16,626,000
Effexor XR (venlafaxine)	14,992,000
Celexa (citalopram)	7,215,000
Wellbutrin XL (bupropion xl)	3,021,000
Pristiq (desvenlafaxine)	2,432,000

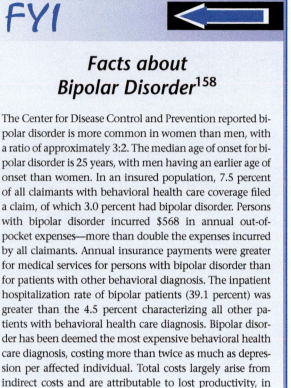

Facts about Bipolar Disorder[158]

The Center for Disease Control and Prevention reported bipolar disorder is more common in women than men, with a ratio of approximately 3:2. The median age of onset for bipolar disorder is 25 years, with men having an earlier age of onset than women. In an insured population, 7.5 percent of all claimants with behavioral health care coverage filed a claim, of which 3.0 percent had bipolar disorder. Persons with bipolar disorder incurred $568 in annual out-of-pocket expenses—more than double the expenses incurred by all claimants. Annual insurance payments were greater for medical services for persons with bipolar disorder than for patients with other behavioral diagnosis. The inpatient hospitalization rate of bipolar patients (39.1 percent) was greater than the 4.5 percent characterizing all other patients with behavioral health care diagnosis. Bipolar disorder has been deemed the most expensive behavioral health care diagnosis, costing more than twice as much as depression per affected individual. Total costs largely arise from indirect costs and are attributable to lost productivity, in turn arising from absenteeism and presenteeism.

Risperdal (risperidone), Abilify (aripiprazole), Zyprexa (olanzapine), and Geodon (ziprasidone)[157] (see *FYI: Facts about Bipolar disorder*).

BIPOLAR DISORDER

Manic-depressive disorder, referred to clinically as bipolar disorder, is a condition in which an individual cycles through episodes of mania and depression.[155] During manic episodes the person may exhibit euphoria, irritability, recklessness, and wild or belligerent behavior. During the depressive episodes the person is extremely sad with feelings of hopelessness. Between manic and depressive episodes, individuals can function normally. Bipolar disorder typically begins in adolescence or early adulthood and continues throughout a person's life. Bipolar disorder affects almost 2 million Americans and puts grave stress on a person, which can result in job loss, divorce, or even suicide. In men, the first episode is most likely to be a manic episode, whereas in women the first episode is more likely to be a depressive episode.[156]

Bipolar disorder can be controlled through medication. The most prescribed medications for the treatment of bipolar disorder in 2009 were: Seroquel (quetiapine),

ANXIETY

Anxiety is the body's natural "fight-or-flight" response gone out of control. (See more about the fight-or-flight response in Chapter 5.) Several broad categories of anxiety disorders are recognized by the psychiatric profession, including generalized anxiety disorder, panic attacks, panic disorder, phobias, obsessive-compulsive disorder, and posttraumatic stress disorder.[159] Generalized anxiety affects about twice as many women as men.[160] About a third of all people who have it eventually recover, although men seem to have a slightly better recovery rate than women. Multiple symptoms may occur during anxiety, including heart palpitations, trembling, shaking, sweating, shortness of breath, nervous stomach, tight throat, goose bumps, flushing, dry mouth, dizziness, tightness or pains in the chest, diarrhea, heartburn, and belching. Prolonged anxiety can lead to headaches, sleep problems, and chronic fatigue. Anxiety is treated with medications such Xanax (alprazolam), Lexapro (escitalopram), Ativan (lorazepam),

Zoloft (sertraline), Prozac (fluoxetine), Desyrel (trazodone), Cymbalta (duloxetine), Effexor XR (venlafaxine), Valium (diazepam), Vistaril (hydroxyzine), Celexa (citalopram), and Buspar (buspirone).[161] Treatment recommendations for anxiety disorders often consider a combination of medication and mental health counseling. (See *Viewpoint:* "Are We Overmedicating but Undertreating Depression and Anxiety?")

Viewpoint

Are We Overmedicating but Undertreating Depression and Anxiety?

In our fast-paced society there is a tendency for depressed or anxious persons to ask for a quick fix from their physician who too often complies with a prescription for the client's condition without consultation with or referral to a mental health provider. While there exist many effective medications for depression and anxiety, medications treat only the resulting physical symptom and do not affect the initial cause of the depression or anxiety. In other words, much anxiety and depression is a result of experiencing pain and suffering from a negative or traumatic life event. Mental health counseling is the treatment of choice for resolving personal issues and healing emotional wounds created from life experience. Medication in combination with mental health therapy can be very helpful in the early stages of treatment because the medication may allow severely impaired individuals to receive greater benefits from the counseling. However, medication without mental health treatment can actually mask the lingering effects of a psychosocial stressor that needs to be attended and prolong the negative impact of the stressor. For example, a woman who is having anxiety attacks and who has a verbally abusive relationship partner needs mental health treatment, and medication alone will not resolve her discomfort. Or, a woman who feels depressed because her relationship partner cheated on her needs to attend to her feelings of anger and betrayal and resolve the impact of this event on her relationship and herself, and not just try to numb her pain by taking medication. Do you agree that many medications are prescribed for depression and anxiety without an accompanying recommendation for mental health therapy? Do you think that every initial prescription for anxiety and depression should be accompanied by a recommended referral to a mental health provider for at least an evaluation and possible counseling? Do you think there is a tendency to medicate a woman who is depressed or anxious instead of empowering her through mental health therapy?

Positive Experiences and Mental Health

Women who have positive experiences can enhance their self-esteem and decrease depression. Studies confirm a negative relationship between depression and the sense of humor in that as humor increases, depression decreases.[162] Support has been found for a positive relationship between achieving the dream of life success and mental health for midlife women.[163] In addition, women who indicated low self-esteem and a negative evaluation of self showed marked improvements in esteem and self-evaluation over a 7-year period due to positive life changes such as increased quality of personal relationships and work status.[164]

SEASONAL AFFECTIVE DISORDER

Seasonal affective disorder (SAD) is a cyclic, seasonal condition, meaning that signs and symptoms come and go at the same times every year. Symptoms may start out mild but become more severe as the season progresses. The Mayo Clinic describes three categories of SAD with their accompanying symptoms: **fall and winter SAD** (depression, hopelessness, anxiety, loss of energy, social withdrawal, oversleeping, loss of interest in activities once enjoyed, appetite changes—especially craving foods high in carbohydrates, weight gain, and difficulty concentrating and processing information), **spring and summer SAD** (anxiety, insomnia, irritability, agitation, weight loss, poor appetite, and increased sex drive), and **reverse SAD** (persistently elevated mood, increased social activity, hyperactivity, and unbridled enthusiasm out of proportion to the situation).[165] For a diagnosis to qualify as SAD it must meet four criteria: depressive episodes at a particular time of the year; remissions or mania/hypomania also at a characteristic time of the year; these patterns must have lasted 2 years with no nonseasonal major depressive episodes during that same period; and these seasonal depressive episodes outnumber other depressive episodes throughout the person's lifetime.[166] About 70–80 percent of those with SAD are women. The most common age of onset is in one's thirties, but cases of childhood SAD have been reported. Specific causes of SAD are unknown but suspected factors may include: disruption of the body's natural circadian rhythm (the internal clock for sleeping and waking) from changes in the amount of sunlight, increases in melatonin (a sleep-related hormone) during long nights of winter, or reduced serotonin (a brain neurotransmitter) from reduced sunlight.[167] Risk factors for SAD include living in northern locations and a family history of SAD. Treatment recommendations may include light therapy, counseling, and medication—specifically, bupropion (Wellbutrin XL), paroxetine (Paxil), sertraline (Zoloft), fluoxetine (Prozac), and venlafaxine (Effexor).[168]

SELF-INJURY

According to the National Institute of Mental Health, self-injury, self-inflicted violence, self-injurious behavior or self-mutilation is a deliberate injury to one's own body that causes tissue damage or leaves marks for more than a few minutes, which is done to cope with an overwhelming or distressing situation. Although cutting is one of the most common and well-documented forms of self-injury, several forms have been documented and include: intentional carving or cutting of the skin, burning or branding of the skin, picking or scratching at the skin, ripping or pulling hair or skin, hitting and self-bruising, bone breaking, head-banging, and swallowing toxic substances. About two million people in the United States are self injurers. Multiple studies show that females are more likely to self-injure than males, but other studies show that males are just as likely to self-injure as females, though males are more likely to choose a form of self-battery to self-injure.[169] Self-injurers report some common reasons for self-injury which are: to regulate strong emotions, to distract from emotional pain, to express things that cannot be put into words, to exert a sense of control over their body. Self-injury can also be a self-soothing behavior for someone who does not otherwise know a healthy way to relieve anxiety. Some people who self-injure have a childhood history of physical, sexual, and emotional abuse.[170] Self-injury is also linked to eating disorders, substance abuse, posttraumatic stress disorder, borderline personality disorder, depression, and anxiety disorders.[171]

EMOTIONS AND HEALTH

Sometimes people talk about good emotions and bad emotions, or healthy emotions and unhealthy emotions. However, it is not the emotion itself that is good or bad, nor is it necessarily the emotion that is healthy or unhealthy. Emotions are natural states that result from the perceived impact of an event or the memory of an event. Emotions serve as guideposts to help you understand just what kind of an impact something has on you. Emotions are designed to direct your behavior for life development and life survival. It is the choice of behavior that follows an emotion that can be judged as good or bad, appropriate or inappropriate, or healthy or unhealthy.

Keeping your emotions pinned up inside you can be very detrimental to your health. Suppressing your feelings can cause escalating tension in the body. Releasing your feelings and thoughts on a regular basis by talking to someone, laughing, or crying can help relieve the pressure that is building inside you. Without regular release, the pressure can rise to the point where you explode, and you say or do things that are harmful to yourself or to others.

Confiding in others appears to protect the body against damaging internal stresses and seems to have long-term health benefits.[172] Whenever possible, confide in friends or family members whom you trust. When this is not sufficient to get you through a stressful time, seek out the services of a professional mental health provider. What you feel and think is important, and sharing your feelings and thoughts with someone else in confidence can be good for you.

Life is a challenge and it helps to have guidance from significant others, teachers, and role models. It also helps to have life skills that help you to cope with the demands that life presents. The greater the personal support system you have and the more life skills you learn and practice, then the higher the likelihood that more of your emotions will be happy ones instead of sad ones, or that the sad ones that you do have will not linger as long. However, remember that emotional health is not determined by how many happy feelings you have versus how many sad feelings. Both happy and sad feelings are normal and natural responses to life's challenges. If you have a good support system and well-developed life skills, the many challenges that life presents can be more enjoyable and perhaps less harsh than they otherwise would be.

Chapter Summary

- Being aware of the various social influences that impact your development can enhance your potential life satisfaction.
- Assertiveness training is a life skill that can enhance self-confidence and result in improvements in relationships and performance.

- Effective listening is required to facilitate healthy communication.
- When conflicts or problems arise, effective problem solving is a useful tool to reach resolution. This involves a step-by-step process: defining the problem, generating solutions, evaluating solutions, making a decision, and implementing the decision.

- Building and maintaining a positive self-image is paramount to feeling good about yourself and achieving successes.
- Similar to self-image, self-esteem involves being realistic about who you think you should be, and loving and accepting who you already are.
- The journey through life will include the loss of loved ones along the way. The grief process is a normal response to loss.

- When life's challenges become too great, depression may arise. If you feel lost and alone, you need to reach out to others for support.
- Sometimes seeking out personal therapy is necessary to facilitate growth when you feel stuck in an uncomfortable emotional state.

Review Questions

1. Can you briefly describe the primary premise of self-in-relation theory, also known as gender-relations theory?
2. What are some of the social and cultural influences that can impact the development of the self?
3. Can you describe the focus of feminist therapy?
4. What is emotional intelligence?
5. What are some situations in which one may need to be assertive?
6. What are the six basic types of assertive messages? Give examples.
7. What are the basic components of effective listening? Give examples.
8. What are some misconceptions about conflict and problem solving?
9. What are the six basic steps to problem solving? Can you describe what is involved with each of these steps?
10. What is a key element to building and maintaining self-image?
11. What are three types of eating disorders?
12. Can you define self-esteem?
13. What is the process of self-esteem enhancement?
14. What are the three phases of mourning, the five stages of the grief process, and the four tasks for the bereaved?
15. Can you name and describe the various types of clinical depression?
16. What are some common predictors of suicide?
17. What is seasonal affective disorder (SAD)?
18. What are some reasons people self-injure?

Resources

American Association for Marriage and Family Therapy
www.aamft.org.
American Counseling Association
www.counseling.org
American Psychiatric Association
www.psychiatry.org
American Psychological Association
www.apa.org
Eating Disorders Resource Catalog
www.bulimia.com/index.cfm

National Eating Disorders Association
www.nationaleatingdisorders.org
National Institute of Mental Health
www.nimh.nih.gov
Mental Health America
www.nmha.org
Screening for Mental Health
www.mentalhealthscreening.org
World Psychiatric Association
www.wpanet.org

References

1. Gilligan, C. 1979. Women's place in man's life cycle *Harvard Educational Review* 49 (4): 431–46.
2. Gilligan, C. 1982. *In a different voice: Psychological theory and women's development*. Cambridge, MA: Harvard University Press.
3. Ibid.
4. Ibid.
5. Ibid.
6. Jordan, J. (Ed.) 1977. *Women's growth in diversity,* New York: Guilford.
7. Ibid., pp. 24–30.
8. Ibid., pp. 24–30.
9. Sharf, R. S. 2006. Feminist therapy. In *Theories of psychotherapy and counseling*. 3rd ed. Albany, NY: Brooks/Cole.
10. Tudor, K. and M. Worrall. 2006. *Person-centered therapy: A clinical philosophy*. New York: Routledge.
11. Ibid.
12. McMullin, R. E. 1986. *Handbook of cognitive therapy techniques*. New York: W. W. Norton.
13. Marks, I. M. 1986. *Behavioural psychotherapy*. Bristol, UK: Wright.
14. Wilson, D. B., D. C. Gottfredson, and S. S. Najakal. 2001. School based prevention of problem behaviors: A meta-analysis. *Journal of Quantitative Criminology* 17 (3): 247–72.
15. Ibid.
16. Dreikurs, R. 1950. *Fundamentals of Adlerian psychology*. Chicago: Alfred Adler Institute.
17. Kottman, T. 2003. *Partners in play: An Adlerian approach to play therapy*. 2nd ed. Alexandria, VA: American Counseling Association.
18. Hall, C. 1954. *A primer of Freudian psychology*. New York: World Publishing.

19. Singer, J. 1973. *Boundaries of the soul: The practice of Jung's psychology*. Garden City, NY: Anchor Press.

20. Hall, *A primer of Freudian psychology*.

21. Perls, F. S., R. F. Hefferline, and P. Goodman. 1980. *Gestalt therapy*. New York: Bantam Books.

22. Ibid.

23. Cooper, M. 2003. *Existential therapies*. Thousand Oaks, CA: Sage.

24. Yalom, I. D. 1980. *Existential psychotherapy*. New York: Basic Books.

25. Glasser, W. 1999. *Choice theory: A new psychology of personal freedom*. New York: Harper/Perennial, p. 28.

26. Ibid., p. 72.

27. Macdonald, A. 2007. *Solution-focused therapy: Theory, research & practice*. Los Angeles: Sage.

28. Fernando, D. M. 2007. Existential theory and solution-focused strategies: Integration and application. *Journal of Mental Health Counseling* 29: 226–41.

29. Macdonald, 2007.

30. Asay, T. P., and M. J. Lambert. 1999. The empirical case for the common factors in therapy: Quantitative findings. In M. A. Hubble, S. D. Miller, and B. L. Duncan (eds.), *The heart and soul of change: What works in therapy*, pp. 33–55. Washington, DC: American Psychological Association.

31. Lambert, M. J., and B. Ogles. 2004. The efficacy and effectiveness of psychotherapy. In M. J. Lambert (ed.), *Bergin and Garfield's handbook of psychotherapy and behavior change*, 5th ed., pp. 39–193. New York: Wiley.

32. American Counseling Association. 2005. *ACA Code of Ethics*. Author. www.counseling.org retrieved March 15, 2009.

33. Asay and Lambert, 1999.

34. Lambert and Ogles, The efficacy and effectiveness of psychotherapy.

35. Goleman, D. 2006. *Emotional intelligence: Why it can matter more than IQ. 10th anniversary edition*. New York: Bantam.

36. Ibid.

37. Lange, J., and P. Jakubowski. 1976. *Responsible assertive behavior*. Champaign, IL: Research Press, pp. 7, 218–20.

38. Harrington, M. 1995. Who has it best? Women's labor force participation, perceptions of leisure and constraints to enjoyment of leisure. *Journal of Leisure Research* 27 (1): 4–24.

39. Hart, L., and L. Silka. 1994. Building self-efficacy through women-centered ropes course experiences. Special issue: Wilderness therapy for women: The power of adventure. *Women and Therapy* 15 (3–4): 111–27; Aubrey, A., and M. MacLeod. 1994. So . . . What does rock climbing have to do with career planning? Special Issue: Wilderness therapy for women: The power of adventure. *Women and Therapy* 15 (3–4): 205–16.

40. Keisling, B., and M. Gynther. 1993. Male perceptions of female attractiveness: The effects of targets' personal attributes and subjects' degree of masculinity. *Journal of Clinical Psychology* 49 (2): 190–95.

41. Lange and Jakubowski, *Responsible assertive behavior*.

42. Jakubowski, P., and A. Lange. 1978. *The assertive option*. Champaign, IL: Research Press, pp. 157–69.

43. Rosenberg, M. 2003. *Nonviolent communication: A language of compassion*. Encinitas, CA: PuddleDancer Press.

44. Jakubowski and Lange, *The assertive option*.

45. Gordon, J. 1974. *Teacher effectiveness training*. New York: Wyden Books.

46. Sanford, L., and M. Donovan. 1988. *Women and self-esteem: Understanding and improving the way we think and feel about ourselves*. New York: Penguin, pp. 97, 101.

47. Miller, L., L. Cooke, J. Tsang, and F. Morgan. 1992. Should I brag? Nature and impact of positive and boastful disclosures for women and men. *Human Communication Research* 18 (3): 364–99.

48. Woods, N., M. Lentz, E. Mitchell, and L. Oakley. 1994. Depressed mood and self-esteem in young Asian, black, and white women in America. *Health Care for Women International* 15 (3): 243–62.

49. American Psychiatric Association. 2000. *Diagnostic and statistical manual of mental disorders*. 4th ed. text revision *(DSM-IV-TR)*. Washington, DC: APA.

50. American Movie Channel (AMC). *The Hollywood fashion machine*. AMC television broadcast March 2, 1996.

51. Ibid.

52. Kilborne, J. 1995. *Slim hopes: Advertising and obsession with thinness*. Video. Northampton, MA: Media Education Foundation.

53. Cohen, B. 1986. *The Snow White syndrome*. New York: Macmillan; Wolf, N. 1991. *The beauty myth*. New York: Anchor/Doubleday; Fallon, A. 1990. Culture in the mirror: Sociocultural determinants of body image. In T. Cash and T. Pruzinsky, *Body images: Development, deviance and change*. New York: Guilford.

54. Zimmerman, J. 1997. An image to heal. *Humanist* 57 (January/February) (1): 20.

55. Lee, A., and S. Lee. 1996. Disordered eating and its psychosocial correlates among Chinese adolescent females in Hong Kong. *International Journal of Eating Disorders* 20 (2): 177–83; Ben-Tovim, D. 1996. Is big still beautiful in Polynesia? *Lancet* 348: 1047–48.

56. Akan, G., and C. Gril. 1995. Sociocultural influences on eating attitudes and behaviors, body image, and psychological functioning: A comparison of African-American, Asian-American, and Caucasian college women. *International Journal of Eating Disorders* 18 (2): 181–87.

57. Furnham, A., and N. Greaves. 1994. Gender and locus of control correlates of body image dissatisfaction. *European Journal of Personality* 8 (3): 183–200.

58. Koff, E., J. Rierdan, and M. Stubbs. 1990. Gender, body image, and self-concept in early adolescence. *Journal of Early Adolescence* 10 (1): 56–68.

59. Probst, M., W. Vandereycken, H. Van Coppenolle, and G. Pieter. 1995. Body size estimation in eating disorder patients: Testing the video distortion method on a life-size screen. *Behaviour Therapy and Research* 33 (8): 985–90.

60. National Eating Disorders Association. 2005. What is an eating disorder? Some basic facts. www.NationalEatingDisorders.org.

61. Kaye, W. 2010. Mortality and eating disorders. National Eating Disorders Association. www.NationalEatingDisorders.org.

62. Insel, T. 2012. Spotlight on eating disorders. National Institute of Mental Health. http://www.nimh.nih.gov/about/director/2012/spotlight-on-eating-disorders.shtml.

63. Ibid.

64. Ibid.

65. Carlson, K. J., S. A. Eisenstat, and T. Ziporyn. 1997. *The women's concise guide to emotional well-being*. Cambridge, MA: Harvard University Press.

66. Ibid.

67. Ibid.

68. National Eating Disorders Association. 2009. National Eating Disorders Awareness Week. www.nationaleatingdisorders.org (retrieved March 15, 2009).

69. Kolander, C. R., and J. L. Delucia-Waack, 2003. Theory and research on eating disorders and disturbances in women. In M. Kopala and M. Keitel (eds.), *Handbook of counseling women,* pp. 506–32. Thousand Oaks, CA: Sage.

70. National Eating Disorders Association. 2005. Statistics: Eating Disorders and their Precursors. www.nationaleatingdisorders.org (retrieved March 15, 2009).

71. Wolfelt, A. D. 1997. *The journey through grief: Reflections on healing.* Fort Collins, CO: Center for Loss and Life Transition.

72. Hundley, M. 1993. *Awaken to good mourning.* Arlington, TX: Crocker Associates, p. 83.

73. Ibid.

74. Kübler-Ross, E. 1969. *On death and dying.* New York: Macmillan.

75. Worden, J. W. 2002. *Grief counseling and grief therapy: A handbook for the mental health practitioner.* 3rd ed. New York: Springer.

76. Ibid.

77. National Sudden and Unexpected Infant/Child Death and Pregnancy Loss Resource Center. 2005. *The death of a child, the grief of the parents: A lifetime journey.* Author. www.sidscenter.org/Bereavement/LifetimeJourney.html (retrieved March 16, 2009).

78. Ibid. p. 3.

79. O'Connor, M., D. Wellisch, A. Stanton, N. Elsenberger, M. Irwin, and M. Lieberman. 2008. Craving love? Enduring grief activates brain's reward center. *NeuroImage, 42* (2): 969–72.

80. Ibid.

81. Georgiades, I. and I. Grieger. 2003. Counseling women for grief and loss. In M. Kopala and M. Keitel, *Handbook of counseling women,* pp. 220–240 Thousand Oaks, CA: Sage.

82. Ibid., p. 229.

83. Ibid., p. 230.

84. National Sudden and Unexpected Infant/Child Death and Pregnancy Loss Resource Center. 2005.

85. Ibid., (p. 2).

86. Schwab, R. 1996. Gender differences in parental grief. *Death Studies 20* (2): 103–13.

87. Wojnar, D. and K. Swanson. 2006. Why shouldn't lesbian women who miscarry receive special consideration? A viewpoint. *Journal of GLBT Family Studies 2* (1): 1–11.

88. Ibid.

89. Swanson, K. 2000. Predicting depressive symptoms after miscarriage: A path analysis based on the Lazarus Paradigm. *Journal of Women's Health and Gender-Based Medicine 9* (2): 191–206.

90. Swanson, K., D. Wojnar, A. Petras, and H. Chen. 2005. Gender differences in grief, depression, and satisfaction with support after miscarriage. Unpublished paper presented at Meeting Challenges of Pregnancy: 16th International Nursing Research Congress, July 15, Big Island, Hawaii.

91. Georgiades, I. and I. Grieger, Counseling women for grief and loss, p. 231.

92. Ibid. p. 231.

93. *Infertility.* 2003. www.medicinenet.com (retrieved March 16, 2009).

94. Georgiades, I. and I. Griger, Counseling women for grief and loss, p. 234.

95. Ibid., p. 233.

96. Ibid., p. 233.

97. APA, *Diagnostic and statistical manual of mental disorders.*

98. Korenstein, S. G., and B. A. Wojcik, 2002. Depression. In S. G. Kornstein and A. H. Clayton (eds.), *Women's mental health: A comprehensive textbook,* pp. 147–65. New York: Guilford.

99. Wells, M., C. J. Brack, and P. J. McMichen, 2003. Women and depressive disorders. In M. Kopala and M. Keitel (eds.), *Handbook of counseling women,* pp. 429–57. Thousand Oaks, CA: Sage.

100. Gotlib, I. H., and C. L. Hammen, eds. 2002. *Handbook of depression.* New York: Guilford.

101. APA, *Diagnostic and statistical manual of mental disorders.*

102. *APA Diagnostic and Statistical Manual of Mental Disorders.*

103. Nolen-Hoeksema, S. 1990. *Sex differences in depression.* Stanford, CA: Stanford University Press.

104. Canli, T., J. Desmond, Z. Zhao, and J. Gabrieli. 2002. Sex differences in the neural basis of emotional memories. *Proceedings of the National Academy of Sciences.* www.pnas.org/content/99/16/10789.abstract (retrieved March 16, 2009).

105. Furnham, A., and N. Greaves. 1994. Gender and locus of control correlates of body image dissatisfaction. *European Journal of Personality 8* (3): 183–200.

106. Downey, G. and J. C. Coyne. 1990. Children of depressed parents: An investigative review. *Psychological Bulletin,* 108: 50–76.

107. Brown, G. W., and P. M. Moran. 1997. Single mothers, poverty, and depression. *Psychological Medicine,* 27: 21–33.

108. Goodman, S. H. 2002. Depression and early adverse experiences. In I. H. Gotlib and C. L. Hammen (eds.), *Handbook of depression,* pp. 245–67. New York: Guilford.

109. Kendler, K. S., R. C. Kessler, M. C. Neale, A. C. Heath, et al. 1993. The prediction of major depression in women: Toward an integrated etiologic model. *American Journal of Psychiatry* 150: 1139–48.

110. Mazure, C. M., M. L. Bruce, P. K. Maciejewski, and S. C. Jacobs. 2000. Adverse life events and cognitive-personality characteristics in the prediction of major depression and antidepressant response. *American Journal of Psychiatry* 157: 896–903.

111. Maciejewski, P. K., H. G. Prigerson, and C. M. Mazure. 2001. Sex differences in event-related risk for major depression. *Psychological Medicine* 31: 593–604.

112. Brown, G., T. Harris, and C. Hepworth. 1995. Loss, humiliation and entrapment among women developing depression: A patient and non-patient comparison. *Psychological Medicine* 25 (1): 7–21.

113. Golding, J. M. 1999. Intimate partner violence as risk factor for mental disorders: A meta-analysis. *Journal of Family Violence* 14: 99–132.

114. Nolen-Hoeksema, S. 2000. The role of rumination in depressive disorders and mixed anxiety/depressive symptoms. *Journal of Abnormal Psychology* 109: 504–11.

115. Weiss, E. L., J. G. Longhurst, and C. M. Mazure. 1999. Childhood sexual abuse as a risk factor for depression in women: Psychosocial and neurobiological correlates. *American Journal of Psychiatry* 156: 816–28.

116. Fox, K., and B. Gilbert. 1994. The interpersonal and psychological functioning of women who experienced childhood physical abuse, incest, and parental alcoholism. *Child Abuse and Neglect* 18 (10): 849–58.

117. Andrews, B. 1995. Bodily shame as a mediator between abusive experiences and depression. *Journal of Abnormal Psychology* 104 (2): 277–85.

118. Silvern, L., J. Karyl, L. Waelde, and W. Hodges. 1995. Retrospective reports of parental partner abuse: Relationships to depression, trauma symptoms and self-esteem among college students. *Journal of Family Violence* 10 (2): 177–202.

119. McGrath, E., G. P. Keita, B. R. Strickland, and N. F. Russo, eds. 1993. *Women and depression: Risk factors and treatment issues.* Washington, DC: American Psychological Association.

120. Parry, B. L. 2000. Hormonal basis of mood disorders in women. In E. Frank (ed.), *Gender and its effects on psychopathology,* pp. 61–84. Washington, DC: American Psychiatric Press.

121. Young, E. A., A. Korszun, and M. Altemus. 2002. Sex differences in neuroendocrine and neurotransmitter systems. In S. G. Kornstein and A. H. Clayton (eds.), *Women's mental health: A comprehensive textbook,* pp. 3–30. New York: Guilford.

122. Nolen-Hoeksema, S. 2002. Gender differences in depression. In I. H. Gotlib and C. L. Hammen (eds.), *Handbook of depression,* 492–509. New York: Guilford.

123. Burt, V. K., and K. Stein, 2002. Epidemiology of depression throughout the female life cycle. *Journal of Clinical Psychiatry* 63, 9–15.

124. Misri, S. 2002. Is there an Andrea Yates in your practice? *The Journal of Family Practice, 1* (5). http://www.jfponline.com/Pages.asp?AID=508.

125. Ibid.

126. Misri, S. 2002. Is there an Andrea Yates in your practice? *The Journal of Family Practice, 1* (5). http://www.jfponline.com/Pages.asp?AID=508.

127. McGrath et al., *Women and depression.*

128. Carlson et al., *The women's concise guide to emotional well-being.*

129. Ibid.

130. APA, *Diagnostic and statistical manual of mental disorders.*

131. Misri. S. Is there an Andrea Yates in your practice? p. 2–3.

132. Ibid. p. 3.

133. McGrath et al., *Women and depression.*

134. Hobfoll, M., C. Ritter, J. Lavin, M. Hulsizer, et al. 1995. Depression prevalence and incidence among inner-city pregnant and postpartum women. *Journal of Consulting and Clinical Psychology* 63 (3): 445–53.

135. High, R., and P. Marcellino. 1994. Menopausal women and the work environment. *Social Behavior and Personality* 22 (4): 347–53.

136. McGrath et al., *Women and depression.*

137. Ibid.

138. Kendler, K., R. Kessler, E. Walters, and C. MacLean. 1995. Stressful life events, genetic liability, and onset of an episode of major depression in women. *American Journal of Psychiatry* 152 (6): 833–42.

139. Nolen-Hoeksema, S. 1994. An interactive model for the emergence of gender differences in depression in adolescence. *Journal of Research on Adolescence* 4 (4): 519–34.

140. APA, *Diagnostic and statistical manual of mental disorders.*

141. Nolen-Hoeksema, An interactive model for the emergence of gender differences in depression in adolescence.

142. Carlson et al., *The women's concise guide to emotional well-being.*

143. Wells, Brack, and McMichen. *Women and depressive disorders.*

144. McWilliams, N. 1994. *Psychoanalytic diagnosis: Understanding personality structure in the clinical process.* New York: Guilford.

145. Wells, Brack, and McMichen, *Women and depressive disorders,* pp. 433–34.

146. McGrath et al., *Women and depression.*

147. Ibid.

148. Ibid.

149. Centers for Disease Control and Prevention. August 26, 2011. *National vital statistics reports, volume 59, number 8.* www.cdc.gov/nchs/data/nvsr/nvsr59/nvsr59_08.pdf.

150. McGrath et al., *Women and depression.*

151. Gibson, P. 1989. Gay male and lesbian youth suicide. In *Prevention and intervention in youth suicide* (Report to the Secretary's Task Force on Youth Suicide), M. Feinleib, (ed.), vol. 3, pp. 110–42. Washington, DC: U.S. Department of Health and Human Services.

152. Centers for Disease Control and Prevention, National Center for Health Statistics. August 26, 2011. *National vital statistics report, volume 59, number 8.* http://www.cdc.gov/nchs/data/nvsr/nvsr59/nvsr59_08.pdf.

153. Pratt, L., Brody, D., Gu, Q. October, 2011. Antidepressant use in persons aged 12 and over: United States, 2005–2008. *NCHS Data Brief, Number 76.* U.S. Department of Health and Human Services, Centers for Disease Control and Prevention, National Center for Health Statistics.

154. Grohol, J. 2010. Top 25 psychiatric prescriptions for 2009. *Psych Central.* http://psychcentral.com/lib/2010/top-25-psychiatric-prescriptions-for-2009/.

155. APA, *The diagnostic and statistical manual of mental disorders.*

156. Ibid.

157. Grohol, J. Top 25 psychiatric prescriptions for 2009.

158. Centers for Disease Control and Prevention. July 1, 2011. Burden of mental illness. http://www.cdc.gov/mentalhealth/basics/burden.htm.

159. APA, *The diagnostic and statistical manual of mental disorders.*

160. Ibid.

161. Grohol, J. Top 25 psychiatric prescriptions for 2009.

162. Thorson, J., and F. Powell. 1994. Depression and sense of humor. *Psychological Reports* 73 (3): 1473–74.

163. Drebing, C., W. Gooden, S. Drebing, and H. Van de Kemp. 1995. The dream in mid-life women: Its impact on mental health. *International Journal of Aging and Human Development* 40 (1): 73–87.

164. Andrews, B., and G. Brown. 1995. Stability and change in low self-esteem: The role of psychosocial factors. *Psychological Medicine* 25 (1): 23–31.

165. Mayo Clinic Staff. 2007. *Seasonal affective disorder (SAD).* http://mayoclinic.com/health/seasonal-affective-disorder/DS00195/DSECTION=cause (retrieved March 17, 2009).

166. APA, *Diagnostic and statistical manual of mental disorders.*

167. Mayo Clinic Staff, Seasonal affective disorder (SAD), p. 2–3.

168. Ibid, p. 5.

169. Cornell Research Program on Self-Injurious Behavior in Adolescents and Young Adults. *What do we know about self-injury?* 2009 Cornell University Family Life Development Center. www.crpsib.com/whatissi.asp (retrieved March 16, 2009).

170. Ibid, p. 3.

171. Ibid, p. 3.

172. Pennebaker, J. 1990. *Opening up: The healing power of confiding in others.* New York: William Morrow.

Chapter Five

Managing the Stress of Life

CHAPTER OBJECTIVES

When you complete this chapter, you will be able to do the following:

◇ Describe the anatomy and physiology of stress

◇ Identify the warning signs of too much stress

◇ Summarize the different types of life stressors

◇ Describe the impact of stress on women

◇ Demonstrate effective coping strategies for stress management

CONCEPTS OF STRESS

You, like most people, have a lifestyle that, in one way or another, and at some time or another, can create stress in your life. **Stress** is the body's response to demands. A **stressor** is the demand itself. Such demands can include everyday life events such as getting up, going to work or school, being at work or school, rushing home to fix dinner, dashing off to play a quick game of tennis, spending time with the family in the evening, and catching up on work at home before going to bed at night. Stress is not something you can ever completely get away from; however, it is something you can learn to understand and to manage. Figure 5.1 identifies the types of stressors we encounter.

Stress and Perception

The way in which you might respond to an event depends greatly on how you may perceive that event. Perceptions can vary greatly from person to person. Perceptions can be impacted by immediate potential consequences and by an accumulation of life experiences. For example, students who must take a final exam may each have different stress responses to the event depending on their own expectations of self and/or the value of the event.

Where do the expectations you place on yourself and on others come from? Many psychologists believe that expectations come from your social environment—the messages you receive from your family, friends, and society that you integrate into your own belief and value system. These expectations can be less than, equal to, or exceed the demand of a particular situation. If your expectations of yourself are at a certain criterion for performance and you do not meet that criterion, then you will probably be greatly bothered by this failure. The level at which you set the criteria for success is going to affect how much stress you experience in trying to meet or surpass that goal. Having realistic expectations of yourself is important in managing your stress level.

Look outside of yourself and beyond family members by examining the goals and ambitions of your peers and healthy role models. This will help you determine what is realistic and what is not. This is not meant to imply that you should not strive toward excellence; instead,

FIGURE 5.1 Types of stressors.[1]

Stressors can be grouped into five categories

- Social stressors—noise, crowding, etc.
- Psychological stressors—anxiety, worry, etc.
- Psychosocial stressors—loss of a job, death of a family member, spouse, or friend, etc.
- Biochemical stressors—heat, cold, injury, pollutants, poor nutrition, etc.
- Philosophical stressors—value system conflict, lack of purpose, lack of direction, etc.

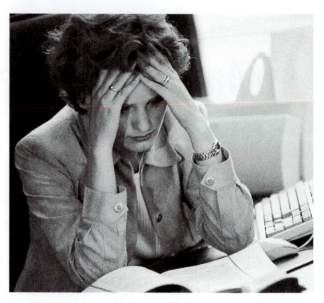

Too much to do and too little time to do it.

you should choose specific areas to excel in. Trying to excel in every area of life is too stressful and exhausting.

In some situations, some amount of stress is necessary to motivate you to perform and strive to do your best. Too little stress, as well as too much stress, can impede performance. A moderate amount of stress can drive you to try harder and to improve your current abilities. If you want to win the sports tournament or a grand prize at the state fair, then you have to work hard. Hard work involves stress.

The same kind of sensitivity to being realistic and self-aware may direct you to adjust the demands of a situation to your preferred stress level. Imagine that you were asked to perform the following tasks within the next week: write a professional paper, prepare a major presentation, have ten appointments, attend a wedding, and play in an all-weekend tennis tournament. How are you going to accomplish all of these tasks and still find time to do daily home chores, exercise, eat nutritionally, and find time to relax, much less sleep? It would be difficult to maintain this kind of schedule and expect to stay healthy for very long. In addition, you may not enjoy this high of a demand level; it may create much more stress in your life than you prefer. You might need to prioritize events and exercise assertiveness by saying "no" to some demands or by renegotiating completion dates. In addition, you might recruit some assistance for those tasks that you cannot complete alone within a realistic time span. We examine stress and time management strategies later in the chapter.

Positive versus Negative Stress

Not all stress is bad. There is constructive stress and destructive stress. Whereas debilitating or excessive stress is often referred to as **distress,** constructive stress is called **eustress** (prefix *eu* from Greek meaning "good").[2] Stress arousal can be a positive motivating force that improves the quality of life. Initially, as stress increases, so do health, performance, and general well-being. However, as stress continues to increase, an *optimal stress* level is

Journal
Activity

How Do You Handle Stress?

Think of some times in your life when you experienced stress from events in each of the five categories of stressors (see Figure 5.1). Write about each experience and suggest ways to alter or manage those stressors. Altering a stressor is finding a way to change the event to be less stressful by extending deadlines, getting assistance, and so on. Managing the stressor is finding a way to experience less stress during the stressor by practicing relaxation exercises, eating healthy foods, and so on.

obtained, and if stress continues beyond this point to *maximum stress,* performance quickly declines and health begins to erode. Complete *Journal Activity:* "How Do You Handle Stress?" to determine how you handle stress.

THE STRESS RESPONSE

Fight-or-Flight Response

The **fight-or-flight-or-freeze response** is your body's natural response to a perceived danger.[3] The body goes on alert, and various physiological changes occur that will allow you to survive the threat. For instance, imagine that you are walking through a beautiful mountain forest with luscious pine trees, and a fresh breeze is blowing your hair. You are relaxed and allowing your mind to wander and enjoy the experience. You hear the sound of thunder overhead. You look up and suddenly you realize that the thunder is actually the sound of a large boulder falling down from the cliff above and heading for your path. Instantly your body begins to respond to the threat. Blood vessels constrict, forcing more blood toward your heart and lungs. Your heart begins to pound, sending blood to vital organs. Your lungs open up and your breathing gets faster. Your pupils dilate so that you can see better. Adrenalin is sent into your system to give you a burst of strength. With all of this added metabolic help you are able to leap away from the boulder as it explodes past you. In this particular instance, you chose the "flight" response—and a wise choice it was because you would not have been able to defeat the large boulder in a fight and to "freeze" would have meant certain disaster. When the perceived threat is past, your body will begin to return to its prearousal condition. It takes longer for your body's systems to return to a state of relaxation than it does to become aroused. So you may be a little shaky for several minutes or so, depending on how often you replay the experience in your mind.

The stress response created by a life-threatening event is easy to recognize. However, your body has the ability to respond to stressors in varying degrees according to how important an event is perceived or imagined to be by you. Just getting out of bed and rushing to work or school can elevate the stress response, although to a degree much less noticeable than when running from an avalanche of rock. The stress response helps you to maximize your performance and to survive danger. However, if your stress response is not turned off periodically, it can create wear and tear on your body's systems. (See General Adaptation Syndrome, described below.) Your body will begin to break down and illness can set in. New research suggests that women and men respond differently to stress at the hormonal level (see *Women Making a Difference:* "Female Researchers Discover That Women Respond Differently to Stress Than Men Do," and *FYI:* "Stress Hormone Receptors Are Less Adaptive in the Female Brain").

General Adaptation Syndrome

The **general adaptation syndrome (GAS)** is a specific pattern of responses that your body experiences as a reaction to continuous life demands or threats.[4] The GAS has three stages: (1) alarm reaction (which is the same as the fight-or-flight response just described), (2) stress resistance, and (3) stress exhaustion. In the alarm reaction stage, hormones are released that create the arousal response in your body necessary to respond to the demand being placed upon it from the environment. The stress resistance stage is when your body tries to return to a state of internal balance that existed before the onset of the stress; this state is referred to as **homeostasis.** The persistent presentation of stressors throughout the day results in cumulative stress. As stressors continue to be presented and the stress response occurs followed by the body working to return to balance, your body eventually becomes exhausted. This is the stress exhaustion stage when parts of your body begin to break down.

You can learn to voluntarily control the stress response. Then you can give yourself the added burst when you need it, but also monitor the use of the stress response and turn it way down or even totally off frequently. You can conserve your stress response in the same way that you conserve electricity in your home: the less you use, the less you have to pay for later. To control your stress levels, learn to use some of the relaxation exercises described later in the chapter.

Anatomy and Physiology of Stress

An event in your life begins the journey to becoming a perceived stressor as a message to your cerebral cortex, the higher centers of the brain. (See Figure 5.2.) The thalamus, the part of the brain that serves as the main relay center for sensory impulses to the cerebral cortex, sorts the information, makes a decision that the event is indeed of a stressful nature and, thus, a stressor is perceived. Next, another part of the brain, the **hypothalamus,** is stimulated. Once the hypothalamus is stimulated, two major response pathways are activated in the body: the endocrine system and the autonomic nervous system.

Endocrine System

The **endocrine system** is activated by the anterior section of your hypothalamus. The anterior portion of the hypothalamus gland releases a hormone called the corticotropin-releasing factor (CRF). CRF stimulates the **pituitary gland** of the brain, and it releases **adrenocorticotropic hormone (ACTH).** ACTH is continuously released into the body via the bloodstream in small amounts during the day. However, a mental or physical demand can cause up to twenty times this amount to be secreted within seconds. ACTH stimulates the adrenal cortex of the **adrenal glands,** located on top of the kidney, which secrete **corticoids.** The adrenal glands secrete mostly glucocorticoids, primarily cortisol, and mineralocorticoids, primarily aldosterone.

Aldosterone, transported by the blood, acts on the kidney to increase sodium absorption. This creates an increase in osmotic pressure that forces extracellular fluid into the blood, causing an increase in blood volume and

Women Making a Difference

Female Researchers Discover That Women Respond Differently to Stress Than Men Do

Shelley Taylor of the University of California at Los Angeles (UCLA) and her colleague Laura Cousino Klein are researchers in the area of stress. One day they were discussing how men and women seem to respond differently to life stress. Men tend to respond to stress by aggressing toward the stressor in either an overt (open) or covert (secretive) fashion. Overt aggression might be to complain, to argue, or to quit their job; or, covertly, men may use drugs or alcohol to numb the effects of the stressor or exercise vigorously to release the stressor.[5] In contrast, women respond to stress much differently than men do.[6] When women are stressed they tend to seek support from other women (to befriend) and talk about their stress. Professional women and especially working professional mothers deal with their stress by redirecting energy to care for their homes and children (to tend). After discussing it at length, Taylor and Klein set out to discover the possible physiological source for the behavior difference between women and men in responding to stress.

Taylor and Klein discovered that the hormone oxytocin is released as part of the stress response in women. This hormone buffers the fight-or-flight responses and encourages women to tend to their children and to gather with other women. When women actually engage in this tending and befriending behavior, more oxytocin is released, which further counters stress and produces a calming effect. This finding may explain why men and women respond differently to stress and why women live longer than men. Men produce high levels of testosterone when under stress, which reduces the calming effects of oxytocin.

This tendency for men to aggress in response to a stressor (either overtly—"fight," or covertly—"flight"), and for women to tend and befriend in response to a stressor is a part of human primal survival instinct. According to Taylor, survival of the species meant that females had to learn to protect their young from danger, and, as there is strength in numbers, gathering with other females was an effective strategy for protecting the young and each other from predators and for finding support for coping with a variety of other types of stressors as well.[7] Thus, using Taylor's speculations as a basis for argument it seems reasonable and long overdue to reconsider the generally accepted concept of the fight-or-flight response. The traditional survival response to stress referred to in the stress literature for many years as the fight-or-flight response should be differentiated, one for men—the fight-or-flight response—and one for women—the tend-and-befriend response. This differentiation could explain why women tend to seek out professional counseling services at a significantly higher rate than do men: Under stress women seek out someone to talk to, whereas men tend to isolate. These different primal tendencies in response to stress may also explain some gender differences in relationship communication patterns—women like to talk about a stressor at length, whereas most men do not.

FYI

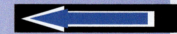

Stress Hormone Receptors Are Less Adaptive in the Female Brain

An understanding of why women experience more stress-related mental disorders like depression and post-traumatic stress disorder (PTSD) eluded science until new research with rats discovered that stress hormone receptors are less adaptive in the female brain. A team of researchers led by Dr. Rita Valentino and Dr. Debra Bangasser reported on their discovery online June 15, 2010 in the journal of *Molecular Psychiatry*.[8] Corticotropin releasing factor (CRF), which acts as both a hormone and a neurotransmitter, is a key player. In response to a stressor, CRF binds to receptors on cells in an alarm center deep in the brainstem, called the locus ceruleus. This telegraphs heightened emotional arousal throughout the brain via the chemical messenger norepinephrine. Such hyper-arousal can be adaptive for brief periods, but not if it becomes chronic. Runaway CRF is a core feature of depression. Previous studies suggested that this alarm system is more sensitive to CRF and stress in the female brain but scientist did not know why until now. Valentino's team used an electron microscope to see how the CRF receptor responds in male versus female rats—both unstressed and after exposure to a stressful swim. What they discovered was, "in response to a stressor, receptors for the stress hormone CRF remained exposed on the neuronal membrane in the female rat—taking the full hit. This increased CRF binding heightened the brain's stress reactivity. By contrast, in the stressed male rat, CRF receptors danced with internal proteins called arrestins, which enabled some to retreat into the cell's interior, where they could not bind with CRF. This adaptation—unique to the male brain—toned-down the neuron's stress sensitivity. Lack of such receptor internalization in the female brain could translate into impaired ability to cope with high levels of CRF—as occurs in depression and PTSD."[9]

an increase in blood pressure. Cortisol creates metabolic alterations in the body, increasing the **metabolic rate** in response to stress and decreasing the metabolic rate when stress is no longer perceived. The body attempts to get as much glucose into circulation as possible. Glucose is the body's most basic source of energy. If the stress response is maintained, glucose may become depleted and the body will then begin to draw off of the remaining energy reserves, fat deposits, and muscle tissue. As the body meets the demands and relief begins to occur, excess cortisol levels will act to shut down the production of CRF in the hypothalamus and the physiological stress response will begin to stop.

Autonomic Nervous System

The **autonomic nervous system (ANS)** is activated by the posterior section of your hypothalamus. The autonomic nervous system excites and inhibits various bodily functions. It stimulates motor functions, blood sugar production, and inhibitory functions. The ANS stimulates the adrenal medulla of the adrenal glands, which then secretes the catecholamines **epinephrine** (adrenalin) and **norepinephrine** (adrenalin-like substances). Norepinephrine increases blood pressure and the strength and frequency of the heartbeat. Epinephrine increases oxygen consumption, relaxes smooth muscles of the digestive system, increases carbohydrate metabolism, dilates arterials in the heart and skeletal muscles, accelerates heart rate, increases the volume of the blood, and decreases blood clotting time.

The shutdown of the digestive system during stress reduces the production of saliva, a fluid that contains digestive enzymes, and may result in a dry mouth. Also, decreased digestive activity can contribute to indigestion and stomachaches from poorly digested food.

DISTRESS AND THE BODY

Stress and "Dis-ease"

Prolonged stress can put your body at "dis-ease." The longer the body is under a strain, the more likely this disease will lead to uncomfortable and sometimes disabling symptoms or disorders. Your body is not capable of maintaining high levels of stress or arousal for prolonged periods of time without its systems beginning to break down. The stress response in humans is better designed for short bursts of energy and strength to survive immediate and short-lived challenges or dangers. Your body can maintain greater health status if there are sufficient periods of nonarousal between the heightened arousal episodes. The stress-adaptation theory suggests that stress depletes your reserve capacity, thereby increasing your vulnerability to health problems.[10] This relates to the general adaptation syndrome mentioned earlier.

Prolonged stress can lead to the development of a broad range of stress-related disorders, from the somewhat painful and annoying to life-threatening diseases. These stress-related disorders are called **psychosomatic disorders.** Just a few examples of these types of symptoms and disorders include tension and migraine headaches; muscle pain specific to the neck, back, or shoulders; insomnia; and anxiety. Chronic stress may contribute to serious conditions such as depression, digestive disorders (ulcers, colitis, and irritable bowel syndrome), cardiovascular disorders (high blood pressure, heart arrhythmias), and pancreatic disorders (diabetes). Your immune system is most vulnerable to the effects of prolonged stress. Hormones released during the stress response, specifically adrenal hormones, can have a destructive effect on important immune system cells. Under prolonged periods of stress, your immune system will become less capable of fighting off illness and disease, thus making you more prone to colds, flu, or bacterial infections.

Research has demonstrated on three different stress measures that participants reporting high stress were more likely than those reporting low stress to develop upper respiratory infections.[11] Conversely, persons with more social support networks have been shown to have greater resistance to upper respiratory illness.[12] It is likely that the social support diminished the effects of stress. The National Institutes of Health (NIH) report that stress slows the body's healing and recovery process by lowering levels of key immune system chemicals; thus wounds take longer to heal. This was demonstrated by significant differences in healing capacity of wounds created in a

FIGURE 5.2 The stress response: physiological reactions to a stressor.

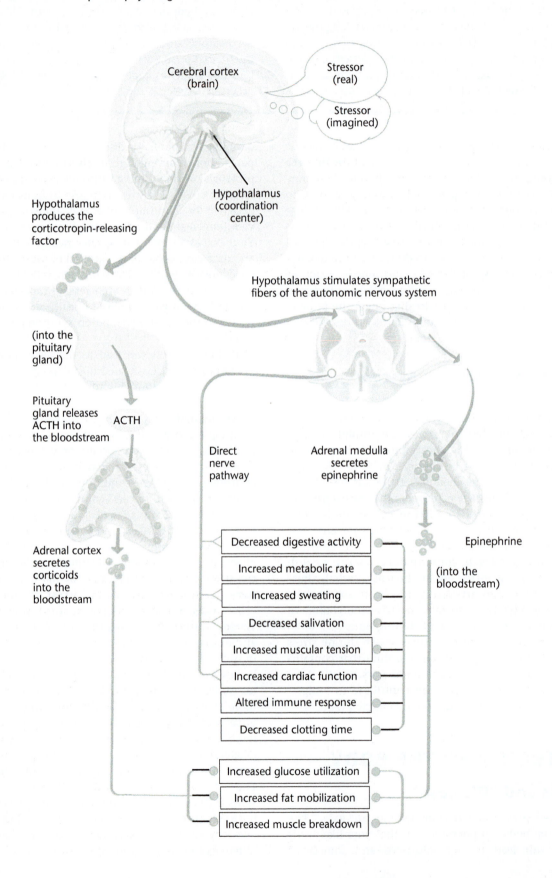

small-blister-causing chamber by persons who were in a stress stimuli group versus a non–stress stimuli group. A different study with mice demonstrated that increased levels of glucocorticoids as a result of a stress response was directly related to a suppressed immune system.[13] Such evidence supports the role of the stress response in negatively impacting the body's immune system.

Stressful major life events have been associated with a higher frequency of cutaneous symptoms (skin sensations such as burning, crawling, tingling, pricking, pins and needles, pain, tenderness, numbness, itching, and easy bruising).[14] The most frequently reported body region affected was the scalp (59.9 percent) and the most frequently reported symptom was itching (69.3 percent).

A landmark study determined that stress kills off telomeres, part of the cellular structure (the caps at the end of chromosomes).[15] This destructive process leads to premature aging. This research is the first evidence-based link between stress and aging. In this study, researchers examined thirty-nine women aged 20–50 who had been caring for a child with a serious chronic illness. They found that every time the cell structure divided in these women, the telomeres got shorter until they stopped functioning and the cell died. A key factor was the perception of stress. The more stresses a woman perceived in her life, the worse she scored on the level of stress. And the higher the level of stress, the greater damage was found to the telomeres.[16]

Investigating a possible link between stress and depression, researchers found that depressed women had significantly higher levels of perceived stress than depressed men.[17] They also found a connection between depression and day-to-day hassles in that not just major life events may cause depression but that everyday stressors may cause depressive symptoms as well.

Stress has been linked to eating disorders. After completing a baseline measure of restraint, forty-six binge-eating college women kept daily diaries assessing depressed affect, stress, coping, and binge eating for 30 days.[18] Regardless of depressed mood, higher stress was associated with increased risk of same-day binge eating; distraction coping was associated with increased risk of future binge eating; and social support was associated with decreased risk of same-day binge eating. In addition, vulnerability to binge eating in women who differ in terms of dietary restraint level was related to their coping responses to stress.

Stress has been related to problems with sleeping. A study investigated workplace characteristics and nocturnal sleep in 709 men and women employees.[19] Gender-stratified analyses revealed that high overcommitment was associated with poor sleep in men, while in women poor sleep was related to the amount of overcommitment in combination with perceived job reward. Thus, for men the amount of work effort is a significant determinant of disturbed sleep, and for women, the amount of work effort–reward balance is a significant determinant of disturbed sleep.

The NIH reports that stress hormones can contribute to osteoporosis in women by interfering with calcium absorption. The hormones secreted into your system during stressful events help you to survive in an emergency situation, but these hormones can contribute to brittle bones.

Stress, Obesity and Diabetes Does stress contribute to obesity? The relationship between stress and obesity has been elusive. In response to stress, some people lose weight and some people gain weight. Research has connected higher secretions of the stress hormone cortisol, resulting from environmental stress, with increases in abdominal fat.[20,21] Additional research has attempted to clarify the stress-obesity connection. Researchers have determined that it is not just the level of cortisol secretion that contributes to obesity but the pattern of secretion controlled by the hypothalamic-pituitary-adrenal axis and that available information suggest this may be programmed before birth.[22] A landmark study demonstrated that stress does exaggerate diet induced obesity through a peripheral mechanism in abdominal white adipose tissue (belly fat) that is mediated by neuropeptide Y (NPY).[23] In simple terms, the stress response causes the release of more NPY that in turn stimulates fat growth. Furthermore, these same researchers claim to be able to control weight gain and loss by manipulating NPY and the neuropeptide Y2 receptor (YR2). This mechanism based on neurotransmitters may explain why chronically stressed people put on more weight than would be expected from the calories they consume.

Does stress contribute to risk of diabetes? The NIH report an established physiological link between stress and diabetes in that stress levels in diabetes have been shown to have a relationship to diabetic complications due to destabilized glucose levels; but research has not yet established stress as a direct cause of diabetes. Stress hormones do impact a primary organ whose malfunction is directly related to diabetes. Chronic stress and the resulting release of hormones associated with the stress response may damage the pancreas over time and contribute to its eventual malfunction. When the pancreas can no longer manufacture insulin, the result is diabetes. The Centers for Disease Control and Prevention (CDC) explains that **diabetes mellitus** arises when insufficient insulin is produced, or when the available insulin does not function correctly. Without insulin, the amount of glucose in the bloodstream is abnormally high, causing unquenchable thirst and frequent urination. The body's inability to store or use glucose causes hunger and weight loss. Insulin-dependent diabetes—type 1 diabetes—is caused by the destruction of most or all of the beta cells in the islets of Langerhans in the pancreas. Type 1 diabetes usually appears before the age of 35, and most often between the ages of 10 and 16. Non–insulin-dependent diabetes—type 2 diabetes—occurs when the body does not produce enough insulin, and the insulin that is produced becomes less effective. Regular insulin injections are required to survive. Type 2 diabetes usually appears in people over the age of 40, and tends to have a more gradual onset. In most cases, glucose levels in the blood can be controlled by diet, or diet and insulin tablets, although sometimes insulin injections may be needed. About 90 percent of diabetics are non–insulin dependent.

The CDC reported in 2008 that 24 million people in the United States have diabetes, an increase of more than 3 million in 2 years. This means that nearly 8 percent of the U.S. population has diabetes. Among adults, diabetes increased in both men and women and in all age groups, but still disproportionately affects the elderly; 25 percent of those 60 years and older had diabetes in 2007. Diabetes disproportionately affects American Indians, African Americans, and Hispanics. After adjusting for population age differences, NIH 2004–2006 national survey data for people aged 20 years or older indicated that 6.6 percent of non-Hispanic whites, 7.5 percent of Asian Americans, 10.4 percent of Hispanics, 11.8 percent of non-Hispanic blacks, and 14.2 percent of American Indians/Alaska Natives had diagnosed diabetes. Among Hispanics, rates were 8.2 percent for Cubans, 11.9 percent for Mexican Americans, and 12.6 percent for Puerto Ricans.

Research suggests a link between stress and risk of diabetes for obese African American women.[24] Women with high epinephrine levels and more belly fat also had bigger increases in blood sugar levels during a stress test. While the nature of this association is not fully understood, it strongly suggests that women with abdominal obesity may be more vulnerable to the impact of stress, causing the body to increase blood sugar production and elevating their risk for diabetes. Further research is needed to determine exactly how epinephrine production affects blood sugar levels in black women. According to the American Diabetes Association, nearly one in four black women in the United States has type 2 diabetes.

Stress and Heart Disease

Does stress contribute to risk of heart disease? According to the American Heart Association, evidence suggests a relationship between the risk of cardiovascular disease and environmental and psychosocial factors, including job strain, social isolation, and personality traits. But more research is needed to determine how stress contributes to heart disease risk. Stress may affect other heart disease risk factors and behaviors, such as high blood pressure, cholesterol levels, smoking, physical inactivity, and overeating. Research has found a link between marital stress and heart disease among women. Scientists found that being in a strained relationship not only affected the mental health of women but increased levels of high blood pressure, obesity, and cholesterol—all symptoms that add up to "metabolic syndrome" (this result was not found in the husbands).[25] One of the largest studies on heart disease, with 5115 participants aged 18–30 years from four different states, showed a relationship between increased job strain and increased high blood pressure; job strain was defined as "a demanding and stressful work environment with little latitude, flexibility or option for coping with these demands."[26]

Stress and Cancer

Does stress contribute to the development and growth of cancer? According to the American Cancer Institute, studies done over the past 30 years that examined the relationship between stress and cancer have produced conflicting results. Although some studies have indicated an increased risk of developing cancer, a direct cause-and-effect relationship has not been proved.[27,28] Scientists have suggested that the effects of stress on the immune system may in turn effect the growth of some tumors.[29] Research with animal models suggests that the body's neuroendocrine response (release of hormones into the blood in response to stimulation of the nervous system) can directly alter important processes in cells that help protect against the formation of cancer, such as DNA repair and the regulation of cell growth.[30] Other research using animal models indicates that the body's release of stress hormones can directly affect cancer cell functions.[31] The stress hormone norepinephrine has been determined to stimulate growth of human cancer cells, thus linking the stress response to cancer growth, but not necessarily to the actual development of cancer.[32] Furthermore, this same research determined that beta-blockers (drugs that reduce the impact of stress hormones) slowed the growth of cancer cells; thus, this research shows promise in the treatment of cancer.

Stress Amenorrhea

Stress amenorrhea is specific to women. Stress amenorrhea is when menstruation stops because of physical or mental stress.[33] Stress can also cause irregularity in the menstrual cycle; that is, time between periods can vary significantly and so can flow rates. Fasting, irregular eating habits, or too much exercise can also place enough stress on the body to cause menstrual irregularity or cessation. If you experience menstrual cessation or irregularity, consult with your health care provider as you would with any other conditions of concern.

Migraine

The National Institute of Neurological Disorders and Stroke (NINDS) reports that migraine headaches affect 28 million Americans, of whom 75 percent are women. The migraine prevalence in the United States is 17.6 percent for females and 6 percent for males. The International Headache Society reports that a similar high prevalence is found in Europe and most parts of the world. In the United States, white women report more migraines (20.4 percent) than do African Americans (16.2 percent), and Asian Americans have the lowest levels of migraine (9.2 percent). This may indicate a genetic or cultural component. About 70 percent of migraine sufferers relate a positive family history for migraine. Migraine symptoms peak during productive years of life, between the ages of 25 and 55. In children, both males and females have a fairly equal prevalence before the age of puberty, and some studies suggest that the prevalence of migraine may be increasing in the United States.

Migraine symptoms occur in various combinations and include pain, extreme sensitivity to light and sound, nausea, and vomiting. Migraine is often described as an intense pulsing or throbbing pain in one area of the head. Some individuals can predict the onset of a migraine due to visual disturbances called the migraine aura.

Female sufferers often report that migraine has affected their ability to be in control of their life. It can affect confidence or ability to cope. Many describe feeling frustrated, angry, resentful of their condition, guilty for having the condition, or embarrassed by the condition. Many women do not realize how common this condition is and instead feel ashamed or weak because of it. (See *FYI:* "Migraine Sufferers.")

Health Tips

Migraine Triggers[35]

Experts know that people with migraines react to a variety of factors and events called triggers. These triggers can vary from person to person and do not always lead to a migraine. A combination of triggers—not a single thing or event—is more likely to set off an attack. A person's triggers also can vary from migraine to migraine. Many women with migraine tend to have attacks triggered by:

- Lack of or too much sleep
- Skipped meals
- Bright lights, loud noises, or strong odors
- Hormone changes during the menstrual cycle
- Stress and anxiety, or relaxation after prolonged or intense stress
- Weather changes
- Alcohol (often red wine)
- Caffeine (too much or withdrawal)
- Foods that contain nitrates, such as hot dogs and lunch meats
- Foods that contain MSG (monosodium glutamate), a flavor enhancer found in fast foods, broths, seasonings, and spices
- Foods that contain tyramine, such as aged cheeses, soy products, fava beans, hard sausages, smoked fish, and Chianti wine
- Aspartame (artificial sweetener)

To pinpoint your migraine triggers, keep a headache diary. Each day you have a migraine headache, put that in your diary. Also write down (1) the time of day your headache started, (2) where you were and what you were doing when the migraine started, (3) what you ate or drank 24 hours before the attack, and (4) each day you have your menstrual period, not just the first day. Talk with your doctor about what sets off your headaches to help find the right treatment for you.

FYI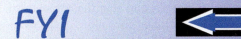

Migraine Sufferers

Women need to understand that migraine is a legitimate biological condition that can be quite disabling. Far too many women feel embarrassed by this condition. A telephone survey of 284 female migraine sufferers revealed that one-third felt that migraines have affected their ability to be in control of their life.[34] Twenty-one percent responded that it has affected their confidence or their ability to cope with life. These women reported feeling frustrated (80 percent), angry (52 percent), resentful (41 percent), guilty (33 percent), and embarrassed (20 percent). Some 14 percent reported that their self-esteem has been negatively affected by others' perception of migraine. The impact of migraine on family life is higher in women because of their child care and other family and general household responsibilities. Of all the women surveyed, 32 percent reported that migraine has had a negative impact on their relationship with their children, with the majority of these mothers reporting that they cannot engage in activities with their children during a migraine attack.

The cause of the migraine is not precisely known, but a strong genetic connection has been identified and specific abnormal genes may play a role in some forms of migraine. Traditional explanations of the cause of migraine headaches focused on the external environment or internal hormones that caused the blood vessels of the head to constrict and then dilate from built-up pressure, causing inflammation. The NINDS reports that new research is beginning to challenge the simplicity of this explanation. The onset of migraine is much more complex than simple constriction and dilation of the blood vessels in the head.

Investigators now believe that migraine is caused by inherited abnormalities in certain cell populations in the brain. Using new imaging technologies, scientists can see changes in the brain during migraine attacks. Scientists believe that there is a migraine pain center located in the brainstem, a region at the base of the brain. As neurons fire, surrounding blood vessels dilate and become inflamed, causing the characteristic pain of a migraine.

Various factors can trigger a migraine and, usually, it takes one or more of these together to cause an attack. Common migraine triggers include stress, the letdown after a period of stress, glare and eyestrain, changes in weather, sleep irregularities, certain medicines, tobacco or tobacco smoke, grinding or clenching your teeth, allergies, eating irregularly, fasting, and dietary factors (see *Health Tips*: "Migraine Triggers").

Both the frequency and the intensity of migraine headaches worsen at those times in a woman's life that are associated with hormonal fluctuation such as around menstrual periods and menopause. Researchers say that female sex hormones are related to migraine attacks. There are no consistent abnormalities found in patients who suffer from migraine, either chemical or hormonal, but it is suspected that changing levels of progesterone and estrogen, the main female hormones, are the trigger for menstrual migraine, and that it is mainly the withdrawal of estrogen which triggers the attack.[36] Menstrual migraine can be treated with the same protocol as nonmenstrual migraine. However, preventive therapy can be considered with nonsteroidal drugs or estrogen supplements.[37,38] Oral contraceptives may increase the frequency and severity of attacks in some women. A very small subgroup of women with migraine have an increased risk of stroke: those who suffer from migraine with aura (visual disturbances preceding the headache), who smoke, and who are taking combined oral contraception.[39]

A research study was conducted with 81 menstruating women with clinically diagnosed migraine in which the women kept a 98-day diary.[40] The results showed that an excess risk of headache occurred perimenstrually (around the menstrual period) and was highest on days 0 and 1 of the cycle (day 0 being the first day of menses). A significantly elevated risk on days 0 and 1 was observed for migraine without aura (visual disturbances that precede the headache) and for tension-type headache. Elevated risks were also observed in the 2 days before the onset of menses for migraine without aura. A significantly lower risk was observed around the time of ovulation for all kinds of headaches. Pain intensity was slightly greater for migraine headaches during the first 2 days of menses.

Another study was conducted with 1943 female students randomly selected from a university school of medicine and pharmacy who completed a questionnaire about headaches and the menstrual cycle.[41] Both migraine and nonmigraine headaches were found to be worse during menstruation, and the women with migraine headaches experienced more frequent, more severe, and more complex headaches than those with nonmigraine headaches. The researchers also found that both menstrually related migraine and menstrually related nonmigraine began on approximately the first day of menstruation. This shows that menstrual migraine occurs during peak fluctuation in estrogen levels. Women with nonmigraine headache can also experience fluctuation of these hormones, although to a lesser degree than in women with migraine.[42]

Migraine significantly decreases during pregnancy, disappearing in 70 percent of women migraine sufferers.[43] About 40 percent of women suffer from headaches the first week after giving birth. Migraine at this time is more frequent in women who had migraine headaches prior to becoming pregnant.

In strict medical terms, the menopause is actually the last menstrual period.[44] However, the term is often used for all the hormone fluctuations and resulting symptoms that women get both before and after the last menstrual period. Menopause is actually the failure of the ovaries to produce estrogen. The years leading up to menopause and shortly after are called the climacteric, or perimenopause. It is during perimenopause that many women find that migraine gets worse and those who previously had not noticed much of an association with their periods start having monthly migraine attacks. Hormone replacement therapy can help perimenopausal migraine.[45] You can read more about hormone replacement therapy in later chapters.

If you suffer from migraine headaches, it is a good idea to consult with your health care provider to get an accurate diagnosis. There are three basic ways to approach migraine treatment: prevention through health practices, prevention through medication, and reducing discomfort and restoring functioning with medication during an attack. Health prevention practices include taking care of your sinuses and watching what you eat and drink because some substances can trigger a migraine attack. Hormone therapy may help some women, and stress management strategies, such as exercise, relaxation, biofeedback and other therapies, may be helpful. In addition, medications to prevent a migraine may be taken on a daily basis. Some medications developed for epilepsy and depression may prove to be effective treatment options as well. Consult your health care professional to determine the treatment that is best for you.

A family of prescription medications designed to reduce discomfort and restore functioning during a migraine are triptans, which target specific groups of serotonin receptors that are known to play a role in migraine headaches.[46] Triptans have some negative side effects and are not suitable for all persons. Triptans currently available in the United States include sumatriptan (Imitrex), naratriptan (Amerge), zolmitriptan (Zomig), rizatriptan (Maxalt), eletriptan (Relpax), frovatriptan (Frova), and almotriptan (Axert). Imitrex is currently the most frequently prescribed medication for migraine.

To reduce discomfort and restore functioning during a migraine attack, the prescription drugs called *ergots* can be helpful.[47] However, ergots are known to have more side effects than triptans (discussed in the preceding paragraph). Ergots are a family of migraine medications that originally derived from a fungus that grows on rye. They interact with receptors for the brain chemical serotonin, which regulates mood, pain awareness, and blood vessel tone. Ergot drugs reduce inflammation and have a powerful effect on blood vessels, causing them to constrict. This vasoconstrictive property helps relieve the throbbing pain of migraine, but these drugs are not recommended for people with high blood pressure, heart disease, or peripheral vascular disease. Ergotamine tartrate is available in several different brands. Combinations containing caffeine in addition to ergotamine are available in tablets (Wigraine) and suppository (Ercf). Ergomar is a tablet that dissolves under the tongue, giving somewhat quicker results. Bellergal-S combines ergotamine with belladonna and phenobarbital. Ergotamine may produce nausea as a side effect; however, an antinausea drug taken beforehand can help with this. Dihydroergotamine is related to ergotamine but has a less powerful effect on blood vessel constriction, making it somewhat safer to use; it is also available in a fast-acting nasal spray (Migranal) or self-injection (DHE-45). Isometheptene (Midrin) is a migraine medication that contains acetaminophen and dichloralphenazone (a mild sedative) and is often chosen for migraine sufferers who cannot tolerate ergot drugs.

Simple over-the-counter analgesics can sometimes be helpful in reducing milder migraine pain.[48] Simple pain relievers include aspirin (Bufferin, Bayer), acetaminophen (Tylenol), ibuprofen (Advil, Motrin, Nuprin), ketoprofen (Orudis), and naproxen (Naprosyn, Aleve). These last three are nonsteroidal anti-inflammatory drugs (NSAIDs). Some NSAIDs are available in prescription strength or through injection at an emergency room, such as ketorolac (Toradol). Some over-the-counter pain relievers have drug combinations that contain caffeine; caffeine can constrict the blood vessels to reduce the inflammatory swelling (dilation) of the blood vessels. Extra Strength Excedrin and Excedrin for Migraine combine acetaminophen and aspirin with caffeine. Aspirin-Free Excedrin contains acetaminophen plus caffeine, and Anacin combines aspirin and caffeine. Over-the-counter analgesics can cause stomach irritation and are not recommended for people with ulcers. Frequent long-term use of some analgesics can cause liver damage.

STRESS AND PREGNANCY

Maternal stress, or stress during pregnancy, can be harmful for both expectant mothers and the babies they are carrying. The March of Dimes reported in 2007 that high levels of stress may increase the risk of preterm labor, infant low birth weight, labor and delivery complications, and miscarriage. Maternal stress hormones may influence fetal development directly or alter uteroplacental blood flow via maternal, placental, or fetal blood flow mechanisms. Catecholamines, produced by the adrenal glands during periods of stress, reduce uterine artery blood flow from 30 to 100 percent, resulting in fetal distress, low infant birth weight, and premature labor. Stress-induced blood vessel constriction (vasoconstriction) may reduce uteroplacental blood flow and exchange and contribute to intrauterine growth retardation. Finally, the immunosuppressive effects of hypothalamic-pituitary-adrenal axis activation that is typical with the stress response may result in maternal infection, which in turn is a risk factor for preterm labor.

Relaxation therapy including biofeedback can be very useful for pregnant women to learn to control and minimize the stress response. Biofeedback-assisted relaxation may also reduce labor and delivery time. Biofeedback therapy is discussed later in this chapter.

STRESS AND LIFESTYLE

Major Life Events

Major life events can create significant stress in your life. When you have a financial crisis, a death in the family, a break-off of a relationship, or so on, the pain of such an event and the adaptation required to adjust to the consequences generated by the event can present huge challenges for you. Several attempts to describe and measure the impact of such major life events have been made. However, the degree of stress experienced is dependent on how each individual perceives the event.

College Stress

It is difficult to specify the sources of stress for college students because they represent many diverse backgrounds located at many different institutions. It has been reported that up to 50 percent of the college students who seek counseling complain of difficulty studying or anxiety, tension, and depression due to poor grades, and fear of doing poorly in courses.[49]

Some of the more common factors related to college student stress include adapting to a new environment, expectations of parents, meeting demands of faculty members, pressure to achieve good grades, rising costs of higher education, and pressure to find employment before and after graduation. For the first time in their lives, many college students must find their own way in structuring and managing time for coursework, jobs, socializing, recreation, and daily chores.

Undergraduate college women are more likely than men to report an unacceptable stress level.[50] To reduce stress, college women are more likely to indicate

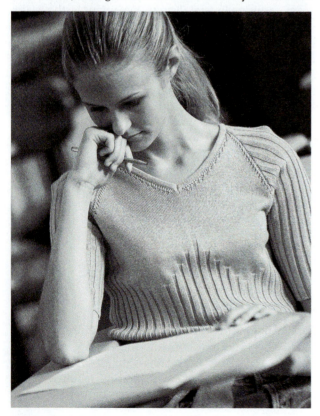

Many students suffer from test anxiety.

a need to limit commitments, exercise more, and worry less. Frequent reasons given by women in college for not reducing stress are lack of time and lack of self-discipline. Freshmen are probably the most vulnerable college group. The freshman class has the highest dropout rate, and 30 percent of first-year students frequently feel "overwhelmed by all I have to do." Nearly twice as many female students report feeling overwhelmed, 39 percent to only 20 percent of males. Why do women report higher levels of stress than men? In 2002, the Higher Education Research Institute at the University of California at Los Angeles conducted a study of attitudes and goals of first-year college students. The survey indicates women students spent more time working at goal-oriented tasks, and men students spent more time partying and playing. While women students' habits increased their stress, men students spent more time actively releasing stress. Women's high stress levels in college may be related to their plans while in college. For example, more women (44 percent) than men (33 percent) reported needing a job to pay for college, and women spent more time studying, volunteering, doing housework and child care, and joining student activities.

Most college students need assistance to adjust to the demands of college life. Among the most beneficial survival strategies are note-taking techniques, stress reduction tips, study skills tips, test-taking strategies, time management, writing skills tips, public speaking skills, financial management, and finding a supportive social group. Most college campuses have resources to help you in any of these areas.

College stress is very pronounced for the nontraditional student, one who is older, may be married with children, and perhaps commuting long distances to campus. The nontraditional student may also be holding down a part-time or full-time job. Also, difficult choices frequently have to be made, for instance, studying for a college exam versus taking a child to soccer practice. For these students, priorities are difficult to establish and maintain, and a great deal of help and support is needed from friends and family if they are to succeed in college.

Daily Life Hassles

It is not just major life events that can affect your stress level. Those little daily life hassles can eat away at your composure and elevate your stress level by a significant amount. Hassles are irritants that can range from minor annoyances to fairly major difficulties. Contrary to hassles, some daily events can uplift your life by creating good feelings. Uplifting events can serve as sources of peace, joy, or satisfaction. Some hassles and uplifting events occur often, whereas others are relatively rare.

It is often a combination of the presence or absence of hassles and uplifting events in your life that impacts your stress level and coping ability. Typical hassles are such things as misplacing or losing things, troublesome neighbors, the health problems of a family member, and having to wait in lines. Typical uplifting events are such things as being lucky, being rested, feeling healthy, and enjoying a hobby. Daily hassles prove to be a better predictor of the manifestations of stress symptoms than uplifting events, which are a deterrent to the manifestation of stress symptoms.[51] Thus, it seems that we may assign greater meaning to the hassles in life than we spend appreciating the uplifting events. Complete *Assess Yourself:* "Stress Checklist" to help determine your stress level.

IMPACT OF MULTIPLE ROLES

The demands on today's woman are extreme. They often involve any combination of the following: maintain a household, care for a family, and work in or outside of the home. A woman is expected to play multiple roles in her life, such as daughter, sibling, spouse, mother, boss, employee, pet owner, friend, neighbor, social volunteer, and hobbyist. Dedication to each of these various roles can create a major strain. It is often difficult for a woman to find time for herself, much less find time to relax, because of all the demands placed upon her. Society often views the woman as the "giver" of assistance rather than the "receiver" of assistance. Women may experience different levels and types of stress depending on the particular role they play. In addition, high demands in combination with a sense of low control over how tasks are done make a task more stressful.[52] Persons in nonprofessional positions, such as a secretary, have high demands placed on them, may find their jobs monotonous, and may experience boredom, frustration, and even a decline in self-esteem. Consequently, they have higher overall stress levels than do persons in professional positions, such as a teacher. Furthermore, women seem to cope better with stress than men; however, women seem to have more stress to handle.

Assess Yourself

Stress Checklist

Check the symptoms you have experienced in the past 3 months.
- _____ 1. Worrying
- _____ 2. Feeling anxious or uneasy
- _____ 3. Going over the same thing in your mind
- _____ 4. Feeling pushed
- _____ 5. Unable to concentrate
- _____ 6. Cold hands or feet occasionally
- _____ 7. Tiredness at the end of the day
- _____ 8. Sore or stiff neck
- _____ 9. Occasional headaches (one or two per month)
- _____ 10. Irritability
- _____ 11. Frequent headaches (more than two per month) or an occasional severe headache (at least one every 3 months)
- _____ 12. Indigestion or stomach problems
- _____ 13. Backaches
- _____ 14. Irregular sleeping pattern (either sleeping too much or not sleeping)
- _____ 15. Prolonged feelings of depression or anxiety (more than 1 week)

Interpretation: Items numbered 1–5 are typically associated with mild to moderate levels of stress. Items numbered 6–10 are typically associated with a moderate level of stress. Items numbered 11–15 are typically associated with a severe level of stress.

(*Note:* The Stress Checklist is not a thorough assessment instrument for stress. It is designed to be used for the purpose of a quick health screening. It is also important to consider additional possible causes for the symptoms listed other than stress. Stress symptoms can be evaluated for severity by trained professionals.)

- *Mild stress*—Changing your lifestyle or routine may help to reduce stress.
- *Moderate stress*—Although changing your lifestyle or routine may help to reduce stress, sometimes a more thorough assessment of the stress symptoms may be necessary. Direct intervention may be needed. This might include activities such as stress management instruction or biofeedback therapy to help prevent and/or alleviate symptoms.
- *Severe stress*—More thorough assessment and immediate intervention may be needed. The type of intervention will depend on the results of the more thorough assessment. Activities could include any or all of the following: a lifestyle modification to lessen the stress, stress management instruction, biofeedback therapy, physical and/or mental health counseling, or medication.

Stressors are different for employed women with children than they are for full-time homemakers with children. As a result, they require different kinds of support to enable them to cope effectively with their chosen roles.[53] One example is the cost of child care for employed women, which is a huge financial stressor on most families. Employed women identify work, children, and household duties as the most frequent stressors, whereas nonemployed women identify children, finances, and self-concerns as stressors.

There are advantages and disadvantages to being either a woman not employed outside of the home or a woman employed outside of the home.[54] Each experiences stress, but in different ways. Women employed outside of the home and women not employed outside of the home experience, on average, similar levels of depressive symptoms. Compared to women employed outside of the home, full-time homemakers benefit from having less responsibility for things outside of their control. Women employed outside of their home appear to benefit from having less routine work than full-time homemakers.

A national longitudinal survey of a representative sample of 1256 adults demonstrated that some of women's higher incidence of psychological distress than men's is associated with differences in men's and women's contributions to household labor.[55] Men performed on average 42.3 percent of the housework compared to 68.1 percent reported by women. Among married respondents, the gender differences in household labor were larger, with wives performing more than twice as many hours of household labor than husbands and doing over 70 percent of the housework as compared to 36.7 percent for men. The least distressed persons in the study were the ones who performed only about 50 percent of the housework. Those who did more than this or less than this had increasing levels of psychological distress. Thus, women are exceeding the amount of housework they should perform to receive maximum psychological benefits. And men, with an average of doing only 42.3 percent of housework, have room for increasing their contribution to housework without experiencing increased distress. This could benefit both genders.

Employment status moderates the effect of the division of household labor but not the effect of the amount of household labor. For those keeping house full-time, the least depressed perform almost 80 percent of housework, whereas for those employed full-time, the minimum level of depression occurs at performing 45.8 percent of housework.[56] Thus, persons with full-time employment and who performed more than or less than 45.8 percent of the housework had increasing levels of psychological distress.

The busy, stress-laden lifestyle of the modern woman has been described as "the hurried woman syndrome."[57] This is experienced primarily by women between the ages of 25 and 55 who have children living at home. The three major symptoms are fatigue or a low mood, weight gain, and low sex drive (libido). It is estimated that 50 million women suffer from these symptoms each year and reported that stress is probably the single most important factor that causes women to complain about hurried woman syndrome.

Women of middle age have a demanding multiple role position. As primary family caregivers, these women may be caring for their own children, their spouse, their grandchildren, and their elder parents. With the rising cost of child care, many young adults are turning to their parents to help take care of their kids. The middle-aged grandmother may be thrilled at the opportunity to spend time with her grandchildren, but it is a demanding task. In addition, the parents of the middle-aged woman may be experiencing a decline in health and require assistance with driving, cleaning house, preparing meals, and visits to a health care provider. These many roles that the middle-aged caregiver might fulfill can contribute to cumulative stress and have a negative impact on her emotional and physical health.

Researchers investigated autonomic and endocrine responses to acute stressors in twenty-seven women who were or are presently caring for a spouse with progressive dementia (high chronic stress group) and thirty-seven noncaregivers who were category matched for age and family income (low chronic stress group).[58] On measures prior to the presentation of the acute stressor, the caregivers reported greater stress, depression, and loneliness than the comparison group. The acute stressors were a math task and an evaluated speech task, each six minutes in length. Measures during and after the acute stressor reported that caregivers, compared to noncaregivers, exhibited a quicker response by stress hormones and higher blood pressure and heart rate. Progressive dementia is unpredictable, irreversible, and devastating to social relations. Many long-term caregivers for a spouse with progressive dementia live in strained relationships. Caregivers report more depressive symptoms than noncaregivers, and the impact of chronic psychological stress for caregivers carries physiological costs as well, making caregivers more vulnerable to the negative impact of acute stressors.

Researchers examined the relationship over time between women's paid work and their informal caregiving for aging or infirm relatives.[59] The sample was 293 white women who were wives and mothers born between 1905 and 1934. The results showed that women were equally likely to become caregivers regardless of whether they were employed. The investigation clarified the timing of women's caregiving and its association with their employment in several ways. First, caregiving was found to be an increasingly common role for U.S. women; over three-fifths of the women in this study were engaged in caregiving at some time in their lives and most typically in later midlife (ages 45–65). Second, the role of caregiver remains prominent as women age, even as they relinquish the role of paid worker. Third, while caregiving may be a major interruption in one's anticipated life experiences, researchers found that it does not necessarily interrupt women's labor force participation. Fourth, caregiving appears to be increasingly a role that is more, not less, characteristic of women's lives, as seen by the rising incidence of caregiving across succeeding birth cohorts. And fifth, position in social culture and level of education affect the likelihood of women working outside the home and caregiving at the same time. During the later years of adulthood, women with more education are more apt to be in the workforce than are women with less education, but the pattern is reversed for caregiving. It could be that women with only a high school education or less may not have the resources to pay for professional care or that women with a higher education tend to "invest" their time in paid work rather than in unpaid caregiving.

Women in middle adulthood are considered the **sandwich generation.** They are sandwiched between caring for their elderly parents while still providing for their children and sometimes even providing day care for their grandchildren. These multiple caregiver demands can put a severe financial and emotional strain on a woman.

In 2008, an estimated 65.7 million people in the United States served as unpaid family caregivers in the past 12 months to an adult or a child.[60] More than three in ten U.S. households (31.2 percent) report at least one person has served as an unpaid family caregiver within the past 12 months, leading to an estimate of 36.5 million households with a caregiver present. Caregivers are predominantly female (66 percent). They are 48 years of age, on average. One-third take care of two or more people (34 percent). A large majority of caregivers provide care for a relative (86 percent), with over one-third taking care of a parent (36 percent). One in seven care for their own child (14 percent). Caregivers have been in their role for an average of 4.6 years, with three in ten having given care to their loved one for 5 years or more (31 percent). The typical recipient of care is also female (62 percent) and averages 61 years of age. Seven in ten caregivers take care of someone 50 years of age or older, 14 percent take care of an adult age 18–49, while 14 percent take care of a child under the age of 18. When caregivers are asked what they perceive to be the main reason their recipient needs care, the top two problems they report are old age (12 percent) and Alzheimer's or dementia (10 percent). Other frequent mentions are mental/emotional illness (7 percent), cancer (7 percent), heart disease (5 percent), and stroke (5 percent). On average, caregivers spend 20.4 hours per week providing care. Caregiving is particularly time-intensive for those who live with their care recipient (39.3 hours per week), and those caring for a child under the age of 18 (29.7 hours per week). Female caregivers spend more time providing care than men do, on average (21.9 versus 17.4 hours per week). The longer a caregiver has been providing care, the more likely the caregiver is to report "fair" to "poor" health. In fact, 17 percent of caregivers feel their health has gotten worse as a result of caregiving. Those who have been providing care for five years or more are nearly twice as likely as shorter-term caregivers to report this decline (24 percent versus 14 percent). Three in ten caregivers consider their caregiving situation to be emotionally stressful (31 percent rating their stress as 4–5 on a 5-point scale). Women caregivers are more likely than men caregivers to feel high stress (35 percent versus 25 percent).[61]

Caregiver stress is the emotional and physical strain of caregiving. It can take many forms, for instance: feeling frustrated and angry with caregiver demands; feeling guilty because you think you should be able to provide better care; feeling lonely because of all the time you spend caregiving has hurt your social life; and exhausted when you go to bed at night.[62] Chronic caregiving can be very stressful. Common signs of caregiver stress include:

- Becoming easily irritated or angered.
- Feeling constantly worried.
- Often feeling sad.
- Frequent headaches, bodily pains, or other physical symptoms.
- Feeling tired most of the time.
- Feeling overwhelmed and irritable.
- Sleeping too much or too little.
- Gaining or losing a lot of weight.
- Losing interest in activities you used to enjoy.
- Abuse of alcohol or drugs, including prescription drugs.[63]

Talk to a counselor, psychologist, or other mental health professional right away if your stress leads you to physically or emotionally harm the person you are caring for. Too much stress, especially over a long time, can harm your health. As a caregiver, you are more likely to experience symptoms of depression or anxiety.[64] In addition, you may not get enough physical activity or eat a

Health Tips

Strategies for Dealing with Caregiver Stress[65]

The emotional and physical demands involved with caregiving can strain even the most resilient person. That is why it is so important to take advantage of available help and support. The strategies have helped others manage their caregiver stress:

Accept help. Be prepared with a list of ways that others can help you, and let the helper choose what he or she would like to do.

Focus on what you are able to provide. Do not give in to guilt. Feeling guilty is normal, but understand that no one is a "perfect" caregiver. You are doing the best you can at any given time.

Get connected. Organizations such as the Red Cross and the Alzheimer's Association offer classes on caregiving, and local hospitals may have classes specifically about the disease your loved one is facing.

Join a support group. A support group can be a great source for encouragement and advice from others in similar situations.

Seek social support. Make an effort to stay emotionally connected with family and friends. Set aside time each week for socializing, even if it is just a walk with a friend. Many have identified that maintaining a strong support system is the key to managing the stress associated with caregiving.

Set personal health goals. For example, set a goal to find time to be physically active on most days of the week, or set a goal for getting a good night's sleep and to eat a healthy diet.

See your doctor. Get recommended immunizations and screenings. Make sure to tell your doctor that you are a caregiver. Do not hesitate to mention any concerns or symptoms you have.

Two Internet resources for providing caregiver support are the websites for Today's Caregiver (www.caregiver.com) and Caregiver Stress (www.caregiverstress.com).

---

balanced diet, which only increases your risk of medical problems, such as heart disease and diabetes (see *Health Tips:* "Strategies for Dealing with Caregiver Stress").

A lack of knowledge and resources can significantly contribute to caregiver stress. These may include:

- Lack of knowledge of resources in a community.
- Lack of knowledge about alternative care facilities and their differences such as nursing homes, assisted living, and retirement homes.
- Lack of knowledge about Medicare/Medicaid.
- Lack of knowledge of home health aides or elder care services.
- Long-distance caregiving—caregiver living in a different city, state, or country than the person receiving care.
- Poorly coordinated community services for assisting the caregiver.
- Chronic care not receiving as much attention by the health community as acute care.

Many middle-aged women provide a significant portion of daily/weekly care for their grandchildren and/or have older children who still live at home. This trend is on the rise and seems to be related to:

- Higher divorce rates.
- Increases in the number of single-parent households.
- Cuts in federal funding for social services (especially child care).
- Increases in birthrates among teen-agers.

- Grandparents' being recruited by family and social services to care for a grandchild when a parent is no longer able to care for the child (because of substance abuse, emotional problems, unemployment, work-schedule conflicts, high cost of child care, incarceration, neglect, etc.).

Grandparents who provide significant care for grandchildren may feel out of control regarding the choices available; they may feel trapped by circumstances. They may feel uncertain about custodial rights and in their decision-making responsibility regarding the grandchild. While they have a responsibility to care for the child, they may not feel they have the legal right or power to exercise major decisions regarding him or her.

Stress is a common problem among women, especially among working mothers. From a sample of 1,000 British women who completed a survey, 79 percent indicated that they felt overly stressed.[66] The main manifestation was identified as increased irritability, this being most pronounced among working mothers with children under 16 years of age. Twenty-five percent of all women aged 15–24 turned to smoking, and 23 percent of subjects aged 25–34 turned to alcohol as a means of relieving stress.

Stress can lead to violence. Women who experienced violence in their relationship described stress as a significant predictor of marital aggression within one year following their wedding.[67] In other words, the greater the stress level that was present in the lives of each of the partners, the more violence was present in the relationship.

Stress, anxiety, and depression have been found to be among the most frequently reported health problems for women.[68] Significant factors contributing to these mental health problems include lower socioeconomic status, being an ethnic minority, being a member of a complex family structure, a lowered quality of family relationships, and intensity around participation in the labor market.

MULTICULTURAL ISSUES

Spiritual Beliefs

Cultural perspectives can impact health. Religious beliefs or, in the broader spectrum, spiritual beliefs can influence your frame of mind. Some beliefs emphasize a fatalistic philosophy—that one has no control over destiny. Other beliefs emphasize hope and a positive outlook on life—that one will reap positive rewards for efforts. Positive or hopeful attitudes seem to enhance health, whereas pessimistic or fearful attitudes can contribute to health deterioration.[69]

Ability to Acculturate

Degree of acculturation can impact health perspectives. Acculturation is how well an individual has adjusted to and become integrated into a community or country to which she or he has moved. Being a newcomer in a foreign environment can be stressful just because you do not know very many people, have not built up a good support system yet, and cannot utilize new resources. For example, Mexican American women who are more acculturated to the "Westernized" culture (one with a prevalent biomedical basis for health and well-being) have less belief in and reliance on traditional folk healing than do Mexican American women with less acculturation. Thus, the acculturated women experience less stress as a result of feeling more in control over medical outcomes.[70] The less acculturated women expressed having a somewhat lower sense of control over their own health.

Racial Issues

Ethnicity can impact the degree of stressors or support an individual experiences. Race, for example, is a significant predictor of both levels of social support and occupational stress for women. African American women report lower levels of coworker support than do Caucasian women.[71] Women in Japan are suffering significant stress from that culture's current emphasis on overwork.[72] Putting in long hours to beat the competition can take its toll on the body and the emotions. Being a member of an ethnic minority group can be stressful as a result of the amount of bigotry and discrimination that still exists in the world today.

Age Factors

Research has identified differences in numbers and types of stressors and resulting health problems for women by age groups.[73] The presence of healthy personality traits that may help cope with stress was also examined. Young women (18–29 years) reported high stressors (second to middle-aged women), less-healthy personality traits, and significantly more physical and emotional symptoms of health problems than middle-aged or older women. Middle-aged women (30–45 years) had significantly more stressors than the other women, but their healthy personality traits may have contributed to their having fewer health problems than younger women. Older women (46–66 years) had the fewest stressors, highest healthy personality traits, and fewest symptoms of health problems compared to the other age groups. According to this research, "In their roles and relationships as wives, mothers and employees, women experienced multiple stressors such as inadequate physical and emotional support from their spouse/partner, along with parenting and employee difficulties that contributed to their health problems. Young and middle-aged women were more stressed, juggling the multiple responsibilities and demands of their spouse, children, ageing parents, and their occupation, while trying to maintain their own 'inner balance.'"

Stressors can be more specific to certain age groups. Women in their twenties suffer from the syndrome referred to as the "type E woman"—being everything to everybody.[74] These women are divided among three competing goals in life: they want a career, a relationship, and a family. Retired women workers experience significant financial stress even in the early years after retirement.[75] This is even more significant for unmarried retired women workers. Women not only enter old age poorer than men but become poorer with age as a consequence of widowhood, higher health care expenditures, and pay and pension inequities.[76]

FINANCIAL STRESS

The ever-rising costs of living and unhealthy economic trends have placed a burden of financial stress on women. Many women are required to seek employment, and often work at more than one job, in order to pay all of the bills. The mobility of our society almost requires that women own their own mode of transportation or pay for public transportation. Paying rent or mortgage payments takes a huge bite out of women's income. The rising cost of food impacts pocketbooks daily. Clothes get more expensive all of the time, and women are expected to wear a variety of colors and designs. They are not supposed to wear just one or two types of suits or outfits to work whereas this is acceptable for men. Also, it is easy to accrue high-interest debts from using credit cards when cash is not available to purchase an attractive temptation such as clothing or to put food on the dinner table. Also, women are more likely to shop as a means to relax than are men.[77] Accruing finance charges can stretch the limits of a paycheck and create additional stress in the lives of women.

The Impact of Technology

The advancement of technology has made it difficult to remain an active and informed participant in the community without a financial investment. If you are unavailable, people expect to be able to leave a message on an answering machine or with an answering service, send you a letter via e-mail or fax, or get a more immediate response from a cell phone of text message. Access to television or radio programming is a vital link to staying informed about recent events so that you can understand what in the world everyone else is talking about. Employers or college professors may expect you to meet shorter deadlines because of the availability of desktop computers and the accessibility to computerized information networks and sophisticated software. Staying involved with a high-tech world is very expensive and very stressful.

The Workforce, Women, and Stress

A review of literature on working women and stress revealed that "occupational stress is a growing problem in U.S. workplaces and may be a problem of particular magnitude for working women, in part because of gender-specific job stressors (sex discrimination and difficulties combining work and family)."[78] This review included two national surveys showing that more employed women than men have reported high levels of stress and stress-related illnesses, and another survey where 60 percent of the women respondents reported that job stress was their number one problem.

> Job stressors commonly include job/task demands (work overload, lack of task control), organizational factors (poor interpersonal relations, unfair management practices, discriminatory hiring practices), and physical conditions. Additional sources of stress include financial and economic factors, conflict between work and family roles, sex-specific stressors (sexual harassment), training and career development issues, and poor organizational climate (values, communications styles, etc.).[79]

A frequently used model for studying the effects of job stress on worker health is the job strain model. "It characterizes jobs with low levels of job control (or decision latitude) and high workload demands as high strain and predicts that these types of jobs will be most likely to produce symptoms and illness."[80] Studies have examined the job strain model in populations of women and found health effects associated with high-strain jobs: "High-strain jobs have been linked with psychological distress, pain, and reduced physical functioning among nurses; increased sickness, absenteeism, and depressive symptoms among female workers in a wide variety of occupations; significant increases in blood pressure among more highly educated female white-collar workers; an increased risk of myocardial infarction; and more than twice the risk for short (24 days or less) menstrual cycles."[81]

Some women are not paid enough to make ends meet at the end of each month. Though some progress has been made over the years, the average wage earned by women is still significantly below that of men and this is an economic disadvantage that may affect health.[82]

Women are more than twice as likely as men to work in part-time jobs. These types of positions are even more segregated than full-time work and offer less training, fewer promotional opportunities, and fewer employment benefits. Women executives are significantly outnumbered by men, and more than 90 percent report that a glass ceiling prevents women from reaching the top in any great numbers. More than half say they have been sexually harassed on the job, but their most likely response was to ignore the harassment. Women executives are likely to be married and have children and are likely to report feeling stressed and burned out, the result of juggling work and a disproportionate load of family obligations.[83]

Many women are expected to be primary caregivers to their children and have a difficult time earning a wage while caring for their dependents. Women who receive financial assistance through social service programs often are not able to provide for themselves and their dependents and find the resources to invest in an education, training, or employment opportunity. Thus, these women are often not able to break from the cycle that keeps them dependent on social services and limits their opportunities to engage in self-development or careers.

It is quite common that women in a relationship are likely to have a spouse or partner who is also working. However, this is often still not enough to eliminate or significantly reduce financial worries. When both partners are working, an added stress is placed on the relationship. It becomes difficult to find time to spend with family members, and the time that is spent often is not of high quality, such as during family crises or hurried activities.

EMPLOYMENT AND HEALTH

Many women work outside of their home because they want to. A career is often a way to discover additional personal significance and self-worth. Employed women are physically healthier than nonemployed women, and participation in the labor force improves health over time.[84] Accumulating evidence suggests that, when compared with not working for pay, employment improves health. Thus, we can expect that women's lower likelihood for employment will negatively affect their health.[85]

Working against Stereotypes

Due to current social trends and to antidiscrimination legislation that has opened opportunities in the workplace to women, more women are exercising their right to pursue careers. Some are even in fields that were once, and may still be, dominated by men. The pressure to perform and not fail is constant for many women in the workplace. The entrance into fields once dominated by men is still relatively new. Thus, women are heavily scrutinized by men and by other women to determine if they are truly capable of performing their duties on the job. The nature of this scrutiny is often unfair for women in that they must far exceed the expectations placed on men in the same job in order to demonstrate that they are capable.

The "equal pay for equal work" principle led to the passage of legislation that makes it illegal to pay any worker (usually a female or a minority group member) lower rates of pay than that paid to others (usually white males). Some employers still use evasion to avoid compliance by using a different title for positions held by women and ethnic minorities, despite only minor differences in assigned duties, to justify a lower rate of pay.[86]

Women who are competing with negative social stereotypes are often forced to become superachievers. High and persistent achievement-oriented individuals are often referred to as "Type A" persons. Type A persons find it difficult to slow down and relax, often equating relaxation with laziness. Type A persons are more prone to developing and maintaining stress symptoms. Type A women have greater frequency of illness and higher blood pressure than do non–Type A women.[87] This could be a direct link to the rising numbers of cardiovascular illnesses reported among women.

ENVIRONMENTAL STRESS

Many elements in the environment can produce stress. Overcrowding in the home, in the neighborhood, or at work is a common cause of irritability and tension.

Chemical toxins and pollutants can create stress on the body that affects physical and psychological well-being.[88] Even everyday items can be toxic to most people. Toxins that we come into contact with on a daily basis include insecticides, household cleansers, and personal toiletries including shampoos and cosmetics. Just the odor from any of these chemicals can cause severe negative reactions in the body. The "closed-building syndrome" refers to the escalation of airborne infectious illnesses and allergic reactions to pollutants because of recycled air. Closed-loop ventilation systems provide minimal access to fresh air and little opportunity for contaminated air to escape. Spending time in a high-rise office building, shopping mall, or commercial airplane could be risky because many of these facilities do not have sufficient circulation of fresh air. (See *Viewpoint:* "Tired or Toxic?")

Noise pollution is a common and frequent stressor. Women have been found to be more sensitive to high-pitched noises, like the continuous machine noise from a computer. This noise generates high levels of irritability and stress for women, whereas it does not seem to bother men.[89] (See *FYI:* "Ergonomics.")

Just as some noise can create stress, other sounds have a relaxing effect. Music with a soft, slow, flowing movement created by the piano, cello, harp, or violin can soothe and calm the body and mind. Soothing sounds also occur naturally in the environment: rustling leaves on a tree; distant sounds of crickets, frogs, or birds; and water moving in a stream or from a waterfall, or ocean waves rolling onto the shore.

The concept of "safe neighborhood" is vital to consider in relation to stress levels. It is very difficult to relax when your life is endangered. There are numerous instances for which a woman or her family and friends

Viewpoint

Tired or Toxic?

Research suggests that the environment has become so toxic that it is giving rise to new illnesses such as atypical immune system dysfunction and chronic fatigue syndrome. The medical community is slow to accept this proposition despite existing evidence. Many women with these disorders are considered hypochondriacs because of the hesitancy by some health providers to diagnose the toxic effects of pollution on the body. What do you think about pollutants in the environment possibly having toxic effects on the body?

are at risk: from gunshots, bullets striking your home, or being hit by a stray bullet; the car breaking down on the side of the road; walking in an isolated area; and having to remember to lock yourself in at night and even during the day. The high incidence of rape and other violence against women is evidence that women are not safe in this world.

STRESS AND ANXIETY

There are a number of clinical anxiety disorders related to stress. (See *FYI:* "Clinical Anxiety Disorders" and *FYI:* "Prevalence Rates of Anxiety Disorders.") Specific phobia is the most common anxiety disorder and the second most common of all psychiatric disorders occurring in about 14 percent of women (and 7 percent of men) in the United States.[90] The only two anxiety disorders for which women are not at significant increased risk (over men) are social phobia and obsessive-compulsive disorder. The most effective mental health treatment for anxiety disorders is cognitive behavioral therapy.[91]

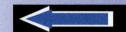

Ergonomics

Ergonomics is the science that seeks to adapt working conditions to suit the worker. A working environment that does not suit the worker can place stress and strain on the mind and the body. Let's look at the example of the computer station. Many people develop back or neck aches due to the strain of sitting in front of a computer for extended hours of work. Thus, through the study of postural positioning, new chairs were devised to help alleviate the strain on the body. These new "ergonomically correct" chairs range in design from an S-shaped chair that provides a padded knee rest to a giant rubber ball chair that provides complete leg and knee support; each of these designs straightens the back and pulls the shoulders back, thus preventing back and neck strain. Typing at the computer keyboard for long periods of time can lead to the development of a very sore wrist, hand, or arm and can be serious enough to be diagnosed as carpal tunnel syndrome. This condition was alleviated with the design of ergonomically correct keyboards, which do not require such a wide reach to each key. Carpal tunnel syndrome can be treated via physical therapy or biofeedback therapy. Some people even have surgery for this condition, which is recommended only as a last resort.

Now, let's examine the computer screen. The brightness of this screen can cause eyestrain and severe headaches. To alleviate this problem some computers now have the ability to adjust the color and brightness of the screen. Initially, computers were very noisy, which resulted in irritability and headaches for the user. Thus, computers are now designed to produce only minimal amounts of noise from the hard drive and the printer, so a quieter working atmosphere is created.

Take a look at your own working environment. Is there anything you can change that will make your work easier and more comfortable, and result in a happier and healthier place to work? How about your living environment? Can you make some adjustments in your home to create a safer and more pleasant place to live?

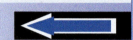

Clinical Anxiety Disorders[92]

- Panic attack—sudden onset of intense apprehension, fearfulness, or terror often associated with the feeling of impending doom. Symptoms include shortness of breath, palpitations, chest pain or discomfort, choking or smothering sensations, and fear of "going crazy" or losing control.
- Agoraphobia—anxiety about, or avoidance of, places or situations from which escape might be difficult; the anxiety typically leads to an avoidance of a variety of situations such as being alone outside of the home, being in a crowd of people, traveling, and being in an elevator.
- Specific phobia—anxiety provoked by exposure to a specific object or situation.
- Social phobia—anxiety provoked by exposure to certain types of social or performance situations.
- Obsessive-compulsive disorder—characterized by obsessions that cause marked anxiety and/or by compulsions that serve to neutralize anxiety.
- Posttraumatic stress disorder (PTSD)—persons who are victims of assault frequently experience PTSD. An individual suffering from PTSD will re-experience the traumatic event through dreams, recurrent images, or flashbacks. The person may try to avoid anything or anyone that reminds her of the event and will have persistent symptoms of increased arousal, such as difficulty sleeping, difficulty concentrating, irritability or outbursts of anger, an exaggerated startle response, and hypervigilance (being overly alert).
- Acute stress disorder—symptoms similar to those of PSTD but these occur within the first month after the trauma and are short lived.
- Generalized anxiety disorder (GAD)—persistent and excessive anxiety and worry for at least 6 months; individuals with GAD often worry about routine life circumstances such as job, finances, family, and daily chores and schedules.

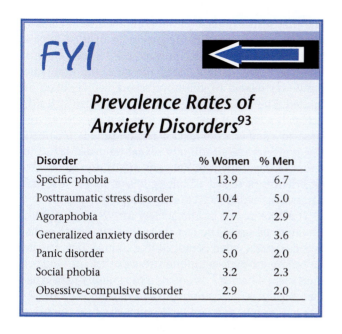

FYI

Prevalence Rates of Anxiety Disorders[93]

Disorder	% Women	% Men
Specific phobia	13.9	6.7
Posttraumatic stress disorder	10.4	5.0
Agoraphobia	7.7	2.9
Generalized anxiety disorder	6.6	3.6
Panic disorder	5.0	2.0
Social phobia	3.2	2.3
Obsessive-compulsive disorder	2.9	2.0

Cognitive-behavioral therapy recognizes the role that thoughts and emotions play in shaping behavior and assists an individual in recognizing and changing irrational thoughts and exaggerated feelings that result in dysfunctional behavior. Hypnotherapy is often used as an adjunct with cognitive-behavioral therapy for some anxiety disorders. Hypnosis creates a state of focused attention in which people can experience changes in perception, cognition, and emotion. Eye movement desensitization and reprocessing (EMDR) is also sometimes used in treating anxiety disorders. EMDR combines cognitive-behavioral and physiological interventions to reduce symptoms associated with posttraumatic stress disorder and other anxiety disorders. Relaxation training is incorporated into most treatment regimens for anxiety disorders, and biofeedback-assisted relaxation training is the most effective applied relaxation therapy. The most common medications for treating anxiety in 2009 were (listed by dispensed rank and number of U.S. prescriptions in 2009): Xanax (alprazolam), 44,029,000 prescriptions; Lexapro (escitalopram), 27,698,000 prescriptions; Ativan (lorazepam), 25,868,000 prescriptions; Zoloft (sertraline), 19 500,000; Prozac (fluoxetine), 19,499,000 prescriptions; Desyrel (trazodone), 18,873,000 prescriptions; Cymbalta (duloxetine), 16,626,000 prescriptions; Effexor XR (venlafaxine), 14,992,000 prescriptions; Valium (diazepam), 14,009,000 prescriptions; Vistaril (hydroxyzine), 9,770,000 prescriptions; Celexa (citalopram), 7,215,000 prescriptions; and Buspar (buspirone), 5,455,000 prescriptions.[94] Very often a combination of mental health treatment and drug therapy can get the best results in the early stages of treatment. As mental health treatment progresses, one goal is to move the client to the point of no longer needing drug therapy.

STRESS AND TRAUMA

Individuals who become victims frequently experience severe stress. The stress reaction can be immediate or delayed. It can be brief, or it may last for years. The stress reaction from trauma experiences can take on a variety of manifestations, including heightened startle and fear responses, anxiety and panic attacks, distancing from friends and family, and avoidance of strangers or crowded places. Mental health counseling can be effective in facilitating the healing process for trauma victims. (See *Her Story:* "Linda: Posttraumatic Stress Disorder.")

September 11, 2001, marked the single most disastrous terrorist event in U.S. history. Nineteen Islamic extremists hijacked four commercial airliners, crashing two into the World Trade Center towers in New York City, one into the Pentagon in Washington, D.C., and one in an open field in Pennsylvania. The victims of this tragedy included people of many different nationalities, along with rescue personnel who were caught in the rubble when the twin towers collapsed. Many of the bodies from the disaster were never found. The trauma experienced after this act was global. Almost every country in the world sent condolences and many declared "national days of mourning." Reports of insomnia, anxiety, generalized fears, and depression were common. Fear of flying left passenger airliners empty, and the aftermath of the attacks created great financial turmoil around the world. Many survivors of the September 11 terrorist event suffered posttraumatic stress symptoms, and most U.S. citizens experienced a heightened level of anxiety.

Women in New York City were two times more likely than men to have PTSD 5–8 weeks after the September 11, 2001, terrorist attacks.[95] Data from a telephone survey of randomly selected residents in Manhattan assessed demographic information, lifetime experience of traumatic events, life stressors, social support, event exposure variables, postevent concerns, perievent panic attacks (having a panic attack within the first few hours after the terrorist attacks occurred), and probable PTSD related to the attacks. The researchers concluded that specific behavioral and biographic factors explained most of the excess burden of probable PTSD among women after the terrorist attacks. The data suggested that the higher prevalence of PTSD in women after the attacks was largely explained by the effect of previous experience of unwanted sexual contact, the burden of acting as the primary caretaker for children in a household, concern for the community at large, a recent history of mental/emotional problems, and experience of a perievent panic attack. This research is significant because isolating the factors that increase the likelihood that women will develop PTSD may allow early identification and

Her Story

Linda: Posttraumatic Stress Disorder

Linda was assaulted by a stranger with a knife. She survived the attack. Along with some deep cuts on her hands, she experienced significant emotional trauma. She exhibited all of the symptoms relevant to PTSD. She was afraid to be alone, found crowds to be extremely anxiety provoking, and was startled by the smallest events, such as someone walking too close to her. After mental health counseling to help Linda recover from PTSD, which also incorporated many relaxation techniques, Linda's symptoms were all either significantly reduced or eliminated.

- Do you know anyone who has ever had anxiety from experiencing a traumatic event?
- Were they able to overcome it completely?
- Did they seek assistance from a mental health provider?

treatment of those at risk, reducing both the emotional and economic burden of PTSD after disasters.

Women in Combat

Officially, U.S. women serving in the military do not serve in combat; however, in the war in the Middle East, especially in Iraq and Afghanistan, traditional front lines did not exist and women were tasked to fill lethal combat roles more routinely than in any conflicts in U.S. history. The effects of Iraq and Afghanistan military service by women were described in a 2008 report by the Society for Women's Health Research (co-sponsored by the National Institute of Mental Health) titled, *PTSD in Women Returning from Combat: Future Directions in Research and Service Delivery*.[96] The report described an informal survey of health care providers at Walter Reed Army Medical Hospital and Bethesda Naval Hospital, where it was found that approximately 13 percent of active duty patients with PTSD were women. Of the responding clinicians to the survey, 35 percent stated their female patients reported more depressive symptoms than did their male patients. Male patients reported more irritability and anger, nightmares, and flashbacks. The responding clinicians also reported female patients are more receptive to psychotherapy while men expressed a stronger preference for medication. An important gender difference in PTSD in combat troops is that almost 65 percent of the clinicians responding to the survey

said that sexual trauma (either childhood or in combat theater) was an issue in the treatment of their female patients with PTSD. No clinicians cited sexual trauma as an issue for male patients. For men, the traumatic event was related to killing or seeing people killed or injured. The report by the Society for Women's Health Research addressed that, aside from trauma directly related to combat experiences, female service members face a greater risk of military sexual trauma (MST), the term the Department of Veterans Affairs uses to refer to experiences of sexual assault or severe, repeated sexual harassment experienced during military service.

The 2008 report by the Society for Women's Health Research discussed the fact that while all service members face stress when deployed to a combat area, female service members face unique stressors that may impact their mental health.[97] Women in the military may experience feelings of isolation and lack of support from colleagues, friends, and family. Women also bear the stress of often being the primary caregiver for family members. The stress of extended deployments for these women is compounded by the demands of caring for their families back home. In addition, the lack of safe hygiene facilities for women in combat can lead to both physical and mental health issues. For example, a lack of adequate facilities for urination can lead to an increase in bladder infection. Many latrines are isolated, so women face a real or perceived threat to their personal safety when using the facilities. These types of stressors can contribute to, compound, and/or complicate the diagnosis and treatment of PTSD for military service women serving in combat areas.

According to the U.S. Department of Veterans Affairs, trauma is common in women; five of ten women experience a traumatic event. Women tend to experience different traumas than men. While both men and women report the same symptoms of PTSD (hyperarousal, re-experiencing, avoidance, and numbing), some symptoms are more common for women than men. Women are more likely to be jumpy, to have more trouble feeling emotions, and to avoid things that remind them of the trauma. Men are more likely to feel angry and to have trouble controlling their anger than are women. Women may take longer to recover from PTSD and are four times more likely than men to have long-lasting PTSD. Women with PTSD also are more likely to feel depressed and anxious, while men with PTSD are more likely to have problems with alcohol or drugs. Both women and men who experience PTSD may develop physical health problems. After a trauma, some women may feel depressed, start drinking or using drugs, or develop PTSD. Women are more than twice as likely as men to develop PTSD (10 percent for women and 4 percent for men). There are a few reasons women might get PTSD more than men: Women are more likely to experience sexual assault; sexual assault is more likely to cause PTSD than many other events; and women may be more likely to blame themselves for trauma experiences than men. Not all women who experience a traumatic event develop PTSD. Women are more likely to develop PTSD if they: have a past mental health problem (e.g., depression or anxiety); experienced a very severe or life-threatening trauma; were sexually assaulted; were injured during the event; had a severe reaction at the time of the event; experienced other stressful events afterwards; do not have a good social support.[98]

COPING SKILLS FOR STRESS: PREVENTION, MANAGEMENT, AND TREATMENT

Social Support

One of the best buffers against stress is a satisfactory support system. Friends and family members who offer positive support can greatly diminish the impact of stress. In fact, research with undergraduate college women has shown that the presence of another woman who is perceived to offer nonevaluative, positive support to the research subject during an acutely stressful performance situation resulted in a significant reduction in the subject's cardiovascular responses to the stressor.[99] Women without a support person present had significantly greater cardiovascular responses (meaning a greater stress response). The perceived quality of the support modulated the impact of the stressor in that the more supportive the subject perceived the support person to be the less was the subject's stress response.

You Are What You Think

When an event occurs, you may make a judgment about that event that may impact how much stress you will or will not experience as a result of that event. If you take time to examine this process, you can understand it better and use it to your advantage; this is known as the technique of cognitive appraisal. **Cognitive appraisal** is the process of categorizing an encounter with respect to its significance for well-being.[100] The two main evaluative issues of cognitive appraisal are "Am I in trouble or being benefited, now or in the future and in what way?" and "What, if anything, can be done about it?"

Because the amount of stress experienced is so dependent on how a stress-eliciting event is perceived, one obvious technique for managing stress is to learn to alter your destructive thought patterns. There are numerous methods for altering negative patterns of thinking.[101] One important technique is **thought stopping.** Each

time a negative thought comes to mind, you immediately say to yourself "stop." The command "stop" acts as a distractor and interrupts the flow of self-defeating thinking. Thought stopping can be followed by substitutions of positively reassuring or self-accepting statements. Positive affirmations are self-statements that accentuate positive feelings or actions. Affirmations can be applied to any area of life. Example affirmations might be "I am confident and strong," "I feel good about myself," "I am calm and relaxed," "I am a beautiful and worthwhile person," and so on. You may not believe the statements at first, but with continued daily practice you will eventually begin to act as if you believe the statements. Before long, you will begin to, consciously or unconsciously, create the feeling or behavior you desire. Self-suggestion, whether it be positive or negative, has a powerful influence on the state of your mind and body. Complete *Journal Activity:* "Stop the Negative, Accentuate the Positive" to help accomplish this behavior.

Stress and Nutrition

Maintaining a well-balanced and nutritious eating pattern is vital for maintaining health and well-being and for countering the ill effects of stress. Although comprehensive coverage of nutrition is provided in a later chapter, it is important to note here that certain food substances can contribute to stress by stimulating the sympathetic stress response. Certain substances act as **vasoconstrictors,** in that they constrict the blood vessels of the body, causing an elevation in blood pressure and heart rate.[102] They also create a temporary

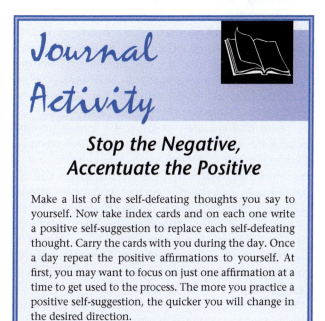

Journal Activity

Stop the Negative, Accentuate the Positive

Make a list of the self-defeating thoughts you say to yourself. Now take index cards and on each one write a positive self-suggestion to replace each self-defeating thought. Carry the cards with you during the day. Once a day repeat the positive affirmations to yourself. At first, you may want to focus on just one affirmation at a time to get used to the process. The more you practice a positive self-suggestion, the quicker you will change in the desired direction.

elevation in mood or energy level. Some of these stimulants are commonly present in our everyday life such as caffeine, found in coffee, tea, sodas, and some diet pills; chocolate or cocoa; processed sugar; and nicotine. These substances tend to interfere with the ability to reduce stress and anxiety levels. When the effects of these stimulants wear off, the individual often experiences a crash period. The body is exhausted from the pressure placed on it during the period of physiological elevation. These substances create elevations in stress or anxiety levels, and they also lead to greater fatigue and exhaustion. There is sometimes a temptation to take more of these substances in order to re-elevate the energy or mood level. Thus, these substances not only increase the stress and anxiety level, but for many people, they can be a part of an extremely detrimental addictive cycle. Reductions in types and amounts of these substances from one's diet should be gradual. These substances can produce such a strong physiological response in the body that some withdrawal symptoms may be present. If withdrawal symptoms become too uncomfortable, then an individual should consult with a health care provider for assistance in reducing and eliminating these substances from her diet. Women under stress may crave foods high in fat and sugar. These foods can cause a person to feel lethargic. Stress can also lead to bouts of overeating or undereating. Special attention should be paid to one's eating patterns during stressful times.

Emotional eating is the practice of consuming large quantities of food—usually "comfort" or junk foods—in response to feelings instead of hunger. Experts estimate that 75 percent of overeating is caused by emotions.[103] Depression, boredom, loneliness, chronic anger, anxiety, frustration, stress, problems with interpersonal relationships, and poor self-esteem can result in overeating and unwanted weight gain. By identifying what triggers you are eating, you can substitute more appropriate techniques to manage your emotional problems and take food and weight gain out of the equation (see *Health Tips*: "Triggers for Emotional Eating").

Some vitamins are thought to be helpful for cushioning the blow of stress on the body. The vitamin B category may be effective in countering stress and depression. The B vitamins, often referred to as B complex vitamins, help the body to convert food (carbohydrates) into fuel (glucose), which is used to produce energy. B complex vitamins also help the body metabolize fats and protein. B complex vitamins are needed for healthy skin, hair, eyes, and liver. They also help the nervous system function properly, and are needed for good brain function. B complex vitamins are sometimes called "anti-stress" vitamins because they strengthen the immune system and improve the body's ability to withstand stressful conditions.[105] Ask your health care

---

Health Tips

Triggers for Emotional Eating[104]

Situations and emotions that may trigger you to eat fall into five main categories:

Social. Eating when around other people—eating to fit in, relationship conflict, or feelings of inadequacy around other people.

Emotional. Eating in response to boredom, stress, fatigue, tension, depression, anger, anxiety or loneliness as a way to "fill the void."

Situational. Eating because the opportunity is there—eating after seeing an advertisement for food, or passing by a bakery. Eating while watching television or when going to the movies or sporting events.

Thoughts. Eating as a result of negative self-worth or making excuses for eating—scolding oneself for looks or lack of will power.

Physiological. Eating in response to physical cues—increased hunger due to skipping meals or eating to cure headaches or other pain.

To identify what triggers excessive eating in you, keep a food diary that records what and when you eat as well as what stressors, thoughts, or emotions you identify as you eat. You should be able to identify patterns to your excessive eating fairly quickly. After identifying your patterns of overeating, the second step is to break the habit by providing alternatives to eating such as: reading a good book or magazine, going for a walk or other relaxing exercise, talking to a friend, playing fun games, doing housework, or any other pleasurable or necessary activity.

---

provider about incorporating a regimen of healthy vitamins into your daily routine.

The intake of appropriate amounts of water is necessary to maintain a healthy body. Studies have shown that being just a half a liter dehydrated can increase your cortisol levels.[106] Cortisol is one of those stress hormones. Staying in a good hydrated status can keep your stress levels down. Furthermore, during times of stress you are more likely to forget to drink and eat well. Thus, stress can cause dehydration and dehydration can cause stress. It is a cycle that can be broken by building healthy amounts of water consumption into your day. Also, when an individual is under stress, toxins seem to build up more in the body. And because water aids in the process of removing waste products from your body, an increase in water consumption during stressful periods may be advised.

Use of Herbs

An herb is a plant or plant part used for its scent, flavor, or therapeutic properties. Herbal medicine products are dietary supplements that people take to improve their health. Many herbs have been used for a long time for claimed health benefits. They are sold as tablets, capsules, powders, teas, extracts, and fresh or dried plants. Herbal remedies have been used for calming stress and anxiety, as well as for combating the effects of stress.[107] Native healers from many continents have used herbs for healing since ancient times. The World Health Organization also recognizes the potential benefits to using herbal medicines.[108,109] Medicinal plants and herbs are important to the health of many communities; between 35,000 and 70,000 species have at one time or another been used for medical purposes, and international use of herbal medicines and natural products is steadily increasing. Today, healing herbs can be found in many local health food stores. However, the use of herbal medicines can be dangerous. In fact, some herbal medicines that have been in use for some time have been shown through research to be dangerous. One such instance was Aristolochia, which has been used in herbal remedies for centuries in Taiwan and China. Aristolochia was linked to cancer and kidney failure in 83 percent of the patients participating in a research study published online on April 9, 2012, in the journal *Proceedings of the National Academy of Sciences*.[110] To use an herbal product as safely as possible, the National Center for Complementary and Alternative Medicine recommends the following:

- Consult your doctor first.
- Do not take a bigger dose than the label recommends.
- Take it under the guidance of a trained medical professional.
- Be especially cautious if you are pregnant or nursing.[111]

It is important to consult a trained herbalist or herbal guide before utilizing these herbal remedies. Also, if you have allergies, exercise caution in using these substances.

Aromatherapy is the use of the scent or aroma from essential oils produced from certain herbs that benefit the individual. The use of essential oils can enhance recovery from particular mental and physical ailments. Essential oils can be used in baths, massage, as room fragrances, or as inhalants. Essential oils affect the body through the olfactory system. The olfactory system, used in the sense of smell, has a direct link to the limbic system, the part of the brain that deals with emotions.

Herbalists claim that the scent from certain oils can directly impact the brain, stimulating certain systems in the body that may facilitate healing.

Essential oils are very potent. It takes only a few drops of an essential oil in several ounces of a base oil for a massage, or a few drops of essential oil in bath water, to get the desired effect. Several essential oils can be helpful in countering stress and anxiety disorders, including jasmine, eucalyptus, rosemary, lavender, chamomile, clary sage, rose, and ylang ylang.[112] An individual who wishes to use aromatherapy should consult an aromatherapist or aromatherapy guide.

Massage and Reflexology

Massage involves systematically stroking, kneading, and pressing the soft tissues of the body to induce a state of total relaxation.[113] Massage works mainly on the muscles, ligaments, and tendons and affects particularly the body's balance of blood and fluids. A most effective massage can be obtained by visiting a certified massage therapist. However, individuals can learn some simple techniques to share with one another at home using a massage guide.

Reflexology is the use of compression massage on designated areas on the hands and feet. Reflexology is based on the principle that there are areas, or reflex points, on the feet and hands that correspond to each organ, gland, and structure in the body.[114] Reflexology is a means of helping the body attain balance in all its functions. It influences areas where weakened circulation has allowed waste matter to interfere with

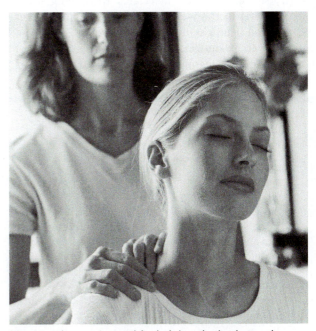

Massage therapy is good for helping the body to relax.

functioning. Through reflexology, the body is encouraged to renew itself so that all its processes are working in harmony. A basic understanding of human anatomy is vital for doing proper reflexology. Improper use of reflexology can be harmful, so it is recommended that you receive treatment from a trained reflexologist.

Acupressure and Acupuncture

Acupressure is a relaxing natural therapy that teaches the body to identify and release patterns of holding tension.[115] Acupressure has been used by Chinese healers for several centuries and is now in common practice in many cultures, including the United States. Acupressure treatments consist of slow, gradual finger pressure applied to designated sites on the body. These sites correspond with neural receptor sites. Acupressure is sometimes used to support conventional medical treatment. It can be used to recover from shock or trauma. Acupressure is frequently used for relaxation, improved circulation, tension release, and pain control.

Acupuncture, a therapy related to acupressure, is an ancient art that has been practiced for centuries in Asia. It utilizes fine needles inserted into acupressure points to stimulate relaxation and healing.[116] Consumers around the world utilize acupuncture; for instance, 77 percent of the pain clinics in Germany use acupuncture.[117] A national health survey conducted in 2002 in all 50 U.S. states and the District of Colombia revealed that 4.1 percent of respondents reported lifetime use of acupuncture, and 1.1 percent (representing 2.13 million Americans) reported recent use of acupuncture.[118] Results from the U.S. national health survey showed recent use was positively associated with being Asian female, living in the west or northeast, having poorer self-reported health status, a higher level of education, and being an ex-smoker. Among recent users, the most typical treatment regimen was two to four treatments (34.5 percent), with musculoskeletal complaints being the most frequently reported conditions, led by back pain (34.0 percent). Reports of perceived benefit were generally high. Many reported being referred to acupuncture by a conventional medical professional (25.3 percent).

Exercise

A regular exercise routine is a very effective approach to stress management. Exercise allows us to release pent-up anxiety and to stimulate and flush out the body's systems through movement. Exercise techniques are covered in a later chapter of this book. It is important to remember that simply taking the time to go for a walk can be an effective stress reducer.

Tai Chi is an exercise system specifically designed to calm the mind and emotions.[119] It is a low-impact exercise appropriate for any age group and is especially popular among older adults. Tai Chi is very effective at stretching muscles and enhancing flexibility of joints. It is also a form of meditation.

Time Management

Managing one's time effectively can reduce stress. This often requires some planning, prioritizing, and structuring.[120] High-achievement–oriented persons may not have trouble with the planning and structuring part, but they often have difficulty with prioritizing. They feel the obligation to get everything done. It takes some discipline to accept the idea that sometimes not everything will get done. Weighing the most important tasks (such as time with family versus time at work, or time for self versus time with the family), putting them in the order of most importance, and then just doing the best you can and not worrying about the rest is a healthy and realistic attitude. (See *Journal Activity:* "Time Management.")

Journal Activity

Time Management

Record how you use your time for 1 week. Study your record, and try to reduce those activities that take too much time or are less important than other activities. Now make a schedule by dividing your time into blocks so that similar activities can be scheduled together. (Purchasing a date book might be helpful here.) Classify activities into a few major areas of responsibility, such as chores, course work, job, recreation, and socializing. Schedule activities within each block of time. Schedule related activities in the same time block if possible. Complex activities need to be broken down into small steps or tasks so that you have a better chance of completing them. Be sure to schedule time for short breaks during long blocks of concentrated effort to minimize stress and fatigue. Reassess your time management activities occasionally and make adjustments when necessary.

Mind–Body Medicine: An Overview

The National Institutes of Health's National Center for Complementary and Alternative Medicine (NCCAM) advocates for the potential health benefits of mind–body medicine. As described by the NCCAM, mind–body medicine focuses on the interaction among the brain, mind, body, and behavior, and the powerful ways in which emotional, mental, social, spiritual, and behavioral factors can directly affect health.[121] It regards as fundamental an approach that respects and enhances a person's capacity for self-knowledge and self-care, and it emphasizes techniques that are grounded in this approach.

Mind–body medicine typically focuses on intervention strategies that are thought to promote health, such as relaxation, hypnosis, visual imagery, meditation, yoga, biofeedback, Tai Chi, cognitive-behavioral therapies, group support, calming self-talk, and spirituality. The field views illness as an opportunity for personal growth and transformation, and health care providers as catalysts and guides in this process. Certain mind–body intervention strategies, such as group support for cancer survivors, are well integrated into conventional care (and thus are mainstream approaches) and, while still considered mind–body interventions, are not considered to be complementary and alternative medicine (CAM).

Mind–body interventions constitute a major portion of the overall use of CAM by the public. In 2002 more than 30 percent of the adult U.S. population used at least one form of mind–body intervention, including relaxation techniques and imagery, biofeedback, and hypnosis. Prayer was used by more than 50 percent of the population.[122] The following is a presentation of selected research reviewed by the NCCAM that demonstrates some of the benefits of mind–body medicine.

Mind–Body Influence on Immunity

There is considerable evidence that emotional traits, both negative and positive, influence people's susceptibility to infection. Following systematic exposure to a respiratory virus in the laboratory, individuals who report higher levels of stress or negative moods have been shown to develop more severe illness than those who report less stress or more positive moods.[123] Recent studies suggest that the tendency to report positive, as opposed to negative, emotions may be associated with greater resistance to colds. These laboratory studies are supported by longitudinal studies pointing to associations between psychological or emotional traits and the incidence of respiratory infections.[124]

Mind–Body Interventions and Disease

Research on mind–body medicine stretching across 20 years has provided considerable evidence that psychological factors contribute to the development and progression of coronary artery disease.[125] There is evidence that mind–body interventions can be effective in the treatment of coronary artery disease, enhancing the effect of standard recurrences of cardiac rehabilitation in reducing mortality and recurrences of cardiac events for up to 2 years.[126] Multiple studies with patients who have various types of cancer suggest that mind–body interventions can improve mood, quality of life, and coping, as well as lessen disease and treatment-related symptoms, such as chemotherapy-induced nausea, vomiting, and pain.[127] Some studies have suggested that mind–body interventions can improve the function of the immune system; but it is unclear whether the improvement is large enough to have an impact on disease progression or prognosis.[128,129] Mind–body interventions have been applied to various types of pain associated with disease. Research demonstrates that these interventions may be particularly effective as complementary treatment in the management of arthritis, with reductions in pain maintained for up to four years and reductions in the number of physician visits.[130] Mind–body interventions have also been shown to be effective with more general acute and chronic pain management, headache, and low-back pain.[131]

Mind–Body Interventions for Surgical Preparation

Research has demonstrated that mind–body interventions can better prepare patients for the stress associated with surgery. Randomized controlled trials—in which some patients received audiotapes with mind–body techniques (guided imagery, music, and instructions for improved outcomes) and some patients received audio tapes without such techniques—found that subjects receiving the mind–body intervention recovered more quickly and spent fewer days in the hospital.[132] Mind–body interventions have been shown to reduce discomfort and adverse effects during vascular and renal procedures. Pain increased linearly with procedure time in a control group and in a group practicing structured attention, but remained flat in a group practicing a self-hypnosis technique. The self-administration of analgesic drugs was significantly higher in the control group than in the attention and hypnosis groups.[133]

The preceding body of research was reviewed by the NCCAM to demonstrate both preventive and recovery health benefits of mind–body medicine. The ultimate capacity for humans to consciously utilize the mind–body connection for healing and wellness has not yet been determined. It is clear that humans can use thoughts and emotions to affect health, yet relative to other areas, science has barely begun to explore this avenue of medicine. Much more research is required to help us understand the full potential for preventing illness and facilitating recovery with mind–body techniques.

Body Awareness

Your body talks to you. It tells you when it is getting too stressed. When you do not listen to it or choose to ignore what it is telling you, then it will start "screaming" at you with various aches, pains, and disorders. A body scream can take many forms. Many of these are listed in earlier sections of this chapter as stress symptoms and disorders. The longer it takes the body to get your attention, the more severe the manifestation of the body's scream.

You can refine your listening skills and respond to the body's needs before it gets to the screaming stage. Focus on your forehead. Stay aware of when you create lines or wrinkles due to tightening the forehead (frontalis) muscles. You do not need to "scrunch" the forehead while concentrating or focusing and certainly not while worrying. Keep the forehead as smooth and relaxed as possible at all times.

Be aware of your jaw. When you are truly relaxed, there should be a slight space between your upper and lower teeth while your mouth is closed. Tension in the jaw (masseter) muscles will prevent this. If you have carried high levels of tension in your jaw for a long time, it may take a while, sometimes several days, for it to completely relax.

Be aware of your neck and shoulders. As tension builds during the day, many people tend to start moving their shoulders gradually up toward their ears without even realizing it. Keep your shoulders down and relaxed. This will minimize the tension in those neck and shoulder (trapezius) muscles.

The few suggestions given regarding awareness refer directly to the body. However, a more relaxed body can also lead to a more relaxed mind and vice versa. The state of the body affects the mind and the state of the mind affects the body. They are interconnected. Attention to both the mind and the body will promote more holistic health.

Mindful Awareness

Mindfulness-based stress reduction is an approach to stress management and wellness that is growing in wide popularity in the United States. Mindful awareness is effective at helping you to live in the present moment in order to permanently change the way you handle stress. This approach involves techniques to become more aware and responsive to mind-body signals. It is effective at helping you live with less stress, fear, and anxiety and to cultivate more ease, connection, and well-being in your life.[134] Techniques that can assist one to enhance mindful awareness include relaxation exercises, meditation, yoga, spending time in nature, and so forth.

Since 2002, significant research has shown mindful awareness to address health issues such as lower blood pressure and boost the immune system; increase attention and focus; help with depression and anxiety; and enhance decision making, emotional flexibility, and empathy.[135] There are several books available on the subject including, *A Mindfulness-based Stress Reduction Workbook,* by Bob Stahl and co-authors. For more information, see the Mindful Awareness Research Center at the University of California, Los Angeles (website: www.marc.ucla.edu/).

Relaxation Exercises

Relaxation exercises are designed to calm the body, mind, and emotions. Practiced daily, they can be most effective in managing stress. Most relaxation exercises take only about fifteen minutes or less, so it is possible to incorporate at least one into your daily routine. **Progressive relaxation** is one of the most commonly used relaxation techniques.[136] This technique involves alternately tensing and releasing the muscles, beginning with the feet and slowly working through each section of the body. This technique enhances awareness of tension and facilitates relaxation in each part of the body. Many people are not aware that they are tense until they engage in a relaxation exercise.

Autogenic phrases is another commonly used relaxation exercise.[137] These are self-statements designed to calm the body and mind. (See *Journal Activity:* "Relaxation Exercise.")

It is possible to set aside only a minute or so and receive substantial benefits using certain brief techniques. The **relaxation response** is a technique through which one learns to quiet the body and mind by using long, easy exhalations, allowing the body to relax while sitting in a comfortable position.[138] Upon perceiving a stressful event, the "quieting reflex" is a set of specific responses, such as striving for a positive mental state, an "inner smile," and a deep exhalation with the tongue relaxed and the shoulders relaxed, which should be used immediately.[139] (See the example in *Journal Activity:* "Quieting Reflex.")

Biofeedback

Biofeedback is the use of electronic equipment to monitor the physiological state of the body while the individual learns techniques to voluntarily regulate the body's systems and reduce unwanted symptoms. Biofeedback for stress reduction is used with relaxation exercises. It enhances the learning of techniques for reducing mental, emotional, and physical tension. With biofeedback equipment, an individual can immediately see the negative effects of stressful thoughts and feelings and the

Journal Activity

Relaxation Exercise

Find a partner. Try this version of an autogenic training exercise. Sit in a comfortable position and close your eyes. Now have your partner read to you the phrases listed below. Be sure and have her read very slowly, pausing 5 seconds between each phrase, and read in a relaxed and mellow tone of voice. You can also record the script onto a tape and listen to it.

I feel quite quiet . . . I am beginning to feel quite relaxed . . . My feet feel heavy, heavy and relaxed . . . My ankles, my knees, and my hips feel relaxed and comfortable . . . The whole central part of my body feels relaxed and quiet . . . My hands, my arms, and my shoulders feel heavy, relaxed, and comfortable . . . My neck, my jaws, and my forehead feel relaxed . . . My whole body feels quiet, comfortable, and relaxed . . . My arms and hands are heavy and warm . . . I feel quite quiet . . . My arms and hands are relaxed, relaxed and warm . . . Warmth is flowing into my hands, they are warm, warm . . . I feel quite quiet . . . My mind is quiet . . . I withdraw my thoughts from my surroundings . . . I feel serene and still . . . I am awake but in an easy, quiet, inward-turned way . . . My mind is calm and quiet . . . I feel an inward quietness . . .

Maintain the inward quietness for about another minute or so and ask yourself the following questions: (1) What were your physical sensations during today's practice? (2) What were your feelings? and (3) What were your thoughts? Were they in words, images, or both? Reactivate by taking five slow, full breaths. Stretch and feel energy flowing through your body. Open your eyes. Write your experience in your journal.

Journal Activity

Quieting Reflex

Think of using four S's to help you remember to relax: smile, slack, sag, and smooth. As you take a deep breath in, put a smile on your face. Now, as you exhale slowly, let your jaw go slack and loose, sag your shoulders, and relax and smooth the muscles in your forehead. When you are confronted with a stressful event, try doing this slowly, three or four times in a row. Note any differences in the way you felt before the exercise and after. Write your experience in your journal.

positive effects of relaxation techniques on the body. Immediate and accurate feedback about the effects of stress and relaxation on the body facilitates the learning of voluntary control over the autonomic nervous system. Biofeedback is a noninvasive and painless therapy. Disorders or conditions that are effectively treated with biofeedback therapy include migraine and tension headaches, high blood pressure, neck and back pain, irritable bowel syndrome, Raynaud's disease (chronic cold fingers, toes, ears, nose, etc.), phobias, panic and anxiety, jaw pain, teeth grinding, and other stress-related disorders.

There are many types of biofeedback. The modality used depends on the nature of the presenting problem. Biofeedback is used to teach a person to voluntarily warm the hands and feet, which lowers blood pressure; to relax muscle tension, which reduces and eliminates pain; to facilitate healthy breathing for relaxation; and to alter brain wave patterns thereby allowing the individual to achieve and maintain a state of alert relaxation that is ideal for learning and performance.[140] Brain wave biofeedback, or **neurotherapy** (neurofeedback), is frequently used to treat learning disabilities, attention deficit disorder, and addiction disorders. Biofeedback therapy is available from mental or physical health therapists who have received specific education and training in biofeedback techniques.

Meditation

Meditation, one of the most common mind–body interventions, is a conscious mental process that induces a set of integrated physiological changes termed the relaxation response. It is a common technique utilized to foster health and well-being. It can facilitate feelings of personal balance and harmony, relaxation, and increased awareness of oneself and one's environment. It can assist with the development of intuition, self-insight, and greater self-trust. An expansion of consciousness often occurs from meditation that replaces feelings of isolation, provides greater personal security, and creates a sensation of being in communion with the universe. (See *Journal Activity:* "Meditation Exercise.")

Meditation can be a guided exercise or can take the form of completely blanking one's mind to allow for spontaneous imagery or insight. Meditations designed for healing purposes may involve a focus on the body and its healing mechanisms. A healing meditation may also be more abstract such as to visualize a swim in healing waters or to be

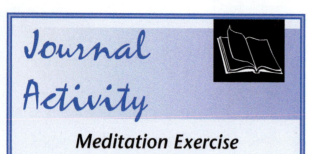

Journal Activity

Meditation Exercise

Try this beginning-level meditation exercise using the following steps: (1) lie in a comfortable position with eyes closed and breathe deeply, relaxing your mind and body; (2) imagine a very powerful presence within you and all around you that is totally loving, strong, and wise and that is nurturing, protecting, and guiding you; (3) relax and enjoy the feeling that you are being totally taken care of by the universe; (4) conclude the meditation with the following affirmation— "I feel and trust the presence of the universe in my life."[141]

This type of meditation encourages individuals to turn within for intuitive insight and creative ideas. What experiences did you have during this exercise?

---

emotional states. Moreover, in this same study, meditation was associated with increases in antibodies to influenza vaccine, suggesting potential linkages among meditation, positive emotional states, localized brain responses, and improved immune function.[144]

Yoga

Yoga involves the practice of body postures and poses to improve health by bringing the body into balance and reducing stress and tension. Hatha Yoga was developed in ancient India as a simple system of eight to ten poses that have evolved into the elaborate technique of today.[145] Yoga techniques range from very simple stretches to more complex twists and headstands. Yoga is an activity that can be used by persons of varying mobility and age.

Proper Breathing

Breath is life. Breathing is a variable rhythm that is linked to all metabolic functions.[146] Although breathing is automatic, it is affected by emotional and physiological

---

showered by a colorful rainbow that symbolically represents the chakras, hypothetically the main energy centers in the body. Tai Chi is used as a meditation of movement that simultaneously aligns the body with mind and spirit. A variety of schools or types of meditation exist.

Numerous benefits have been claimed from the practice of meditation: (1) meditations can bring about an increase in ego strength; (2) meditations can be applied to special problem areas and can be used to help explore a specific area and help loosen defenses (resistance to insight or change); (3) meditations assist with centering, the quality of feeling at ease with oneself and with one's environment; (4) meditations facilitate growth by teaching the individual to regard his or her being as something of real value and to give serious attention to the totality of being; and (5) meditations assist with growing beyond the ability to function in everyday life while being relatively pain-free.[142]

Functional magnetic resonance imaging (fMRI) has been used to identify and characterize the brain regions that are active during meditation. This research suggests that various parts of the brain known to be involved in attention and in the control of the autonomic nervous system are activated, providing a neurochemical and anatomical basis for the effects of meditation on various physiological activities.[143] Studies involving imaging are advancing the understanding of mind–body mechanisms. For example, meditation has been shown in one study to produce significant increases in left-sided anterior brain activity, which is associated with positive

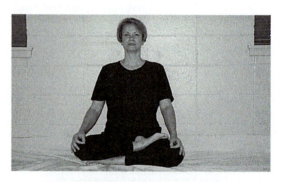

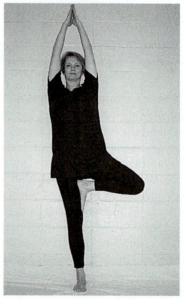

Yoga is good for relaxation and is a great fitness activity, too.

demands on the body. Short, quick, and shallow breathing that originates mostly from the chest area is the least effective pattern for full oxygenation of red blood cells. In chest breathing, known as thoracic breathing, the rib cage spreads and the chest goes up. Despite its appearance, this breathing mode results in very little air entering the lungs. This type of breathing is most common under stress.

Abdominal breathing, referred to as **diaphragmatic breathing,** is a healthy type of breathing. This is accomplished by alternately contracting the diaphragm and abdominal muscles that increase the space in the chest into which the lungs can expand to accept air.

Sometimes the individual is unaware of her breathing pattern. Training for proper breathing should begin with heightened awareness of current breathing patterns and then practice to create longer, deeper, and fuller breaths. For fuller benefits, breathing should be initiated from the abdomen (diaphragm), filling up the bottom of the lungs in the upper diaphragm with air and completing the task by filling up the top of the lungs in the chest. Exhaling reverses this pattern. Healthy, relaxing breaths should be easy and unlabored.

MAKE STRESS MANAGEMENT A PRIORITY

Many people claim they have no time for stress management. This simply implies that they have no understanding of what stress management is. Stress management makes life easier, not harder. It does not entail more work. Instead, it is fun and relaxing. Think of it as a form of entertainment and recreation. If you claim to have no time for stress reduction or management, then you should consider the reasons you are hesitant to relax. Now, go out and try some stress management for yourself. Remember, you are worth it.

Chapter Summary

- Stress is the physical, mental, and emotional response to the presence of a perceived stressor.
- The primary anatomical areas that are involved in the stress response are the cerebral cortex, the hypothalamus, the adrenal glands, the hormone ACTH, corticoids, and adrenalin.
- Life stressors fall into five major categories: social, psychological, psychosocial, biochemical, and philosophical.
- The immediate stress response is the mobilization of the body for confrontation or avoidance of challenge; this is referred to as the fight-or-flight response.
- The general adaptation syndrome is the long-term response to stress and consists of three stages: alarm, resistance, and exhaustion.

- There is good stress and bad stress. Eustress is considered good stress because it is motivational stress, whereas distress is debilitating stress. When stress is too great, it can become distress.
- The effects of stress are cumulative; symptoms may begin as relatively minor body aches and pains and gradually progress to more severe disorders and diseases. Major life events as well as daily hassles can produce stress.
- A variety of coping techniques can be easily learned and may prove to be beneficial in reducing stress.
- A positive attitude and taking time to play may protect some people from the potentially damaging effects of stressors.

Review Questions

1. What is stress and why do people perceive stressors differently?
2. What is optimal stress and what is the impact of going beyond this?
3. How does the stress response impact the endocrine system and the autonomic nervous system?
4. What are the three stages of the general adaptation syndrome?
5. What are some of the disorders or conditions that may result from prolonged stress?
6. Which stress-related disorders are more common in women than men?
7. What types of stressors exist for women in various roles?
8. What types of stressors are more specific to multicultural issues?
9. What are some effective strategies for coping with stress?

Resources

American Council for Headache Education
www.achenet.org
American Headache Society
www.americanheadachesociety.org
American Institute of Stress
www.stress.org

Association for Applied Psychophysiology and Biofeedback
www.aapb.org
Biofeedback Certification International Alliance
www.bcia.org
International Headache Society
www.i-h-s.org

The National Migraine Association
www.migraines.org
National Headache Foundation
www.headaches.org

National Institute of Neurological Disorders and Stroke (NINDS)
www.ninds.nih.gov
World Headache Alliance
www.w-h-a.org

References

1. Curtis, J. D., and R. A. Detert. 1981. *How to relax: A holistic approach to stress management.* Mountain View, CA: Mayfield.
2. Selye, H. 1975. *Stress without distress.* New York: New American Library.
3. Cannon, W. 1932. *The wisdom of the body.* New York: Norton.
4. Selye, *Stress without distress.*
5. Torkelson, E., and T. Muhonen. 2004. The role of gender and job level in coping with occupational stress *Work & Stress* 18 (3): 267–74.
6. Taylor, S., L. Klein, B. Lewis, T. Gruenewald, R. Gurung, and J. Updegraff. 2000. Biobehavioral responses to stress in females: Tend and befriend, not fight-or-flight. *Psychological Review* 107 (3): 411–29.
7. Taylor, S. E. 2002. *The tending instinct.* New York: Henry Holt.
8. Bangasser, D., A. Curtis, B. Reyes, T. Bethea, I. Parastatidis, H. Ischiropoulos, E. Van Bockstaele, and R. Valentino. June 15, 2010. Sex differences in corticotropin-releasing factor receptor signaling and trafficking: potential role in female vulnerability to stress-related psychopathaology. *Molecular Journal of Psychiatry, 15,* 877, 896–904.
9. Valentino, R. August 9, 2010. Stress hormone receptors less adaptive in female brain. National Institute of Mental Health, Science Update. http://www.nimh.nih.gov/science-news/2010/stress-hormone-receptors-less-adaptive-in-female-brain.shtml, pp. 1–2.
10. *Mosby's medical, nursing, and allied health dictionary.* 4th ed. 1994. St. Louis: Mosby-Year Book.
11. Cohen, S. 1996. Psychological stress, immunity, and upper respiratory infections. *Current Directions in Psychological Science,* 5: 86–90.
12. Cohen, S., W. Doyle, D. Skoner, B. Rabin, and J. Gwaltney, 1997. Social ties and susceptibility to the common cold. *Journal of the American Medical Association* 277 (24): 1940–44.
13. Curtin, N., N. Boyle, K. Mills, and T. Connor. 2009. Psychological stress suppresses innate IFN-y production via glucocorticoid receptor activation: Reversal by the anxiolytic chlordiazepoxide. *Brain, Behavior, and Immunity* 23 (3): 371–79.
14. Gupta, M. A., and A. K. Gupta 2004. Stressful major life events are associated with a higher frequency of cutaneous sensory symptoms: An empirical study of non-clinical subjects. *Journal of the European Academy of Dermatology and Venereology* 18: 560–565.
15. Epel, E. S., E. H. Blackburn, J. Lin, F. S. Dhabhar, N. E. Adler, J. D. Morrow, et al. 2004. Accelerated telomere shortening in response to life stress. *Proceedings of the National Academy of Sciences* 101 (49): 17312–15.
16. Ibid.
17. Farabaugh, A. H., M. Mischoulon, M. Fava, C. Green, W. Guyker, and J. Alpert. 2004. The potential relationship between levels of perceived stress and subtypes of major depressive disorder (MDD). *Acta Psychiatrica Scandinavica* 110: 465–70.
18. Freeman, L. M. Y., and K. M. Gil. 2004. Daily stress, coping, and dietary restraint in binge eating. *International Journal of Eating Disorders* 36: 204–12.
19. Kudielka, B. M., R. Von Kanel, M. L. Gander, and J. E. Fischer. 2004. *Work & Stress* 18 (2): 167–78.
20. Dallman, R., and P. Bjorntorp. 1998. Stress-related cortisol secretion in men: Relationships with abdominal obesity and endocrine, metabolic and hemodynamic abnormalities. *Journal of Clinical Endocrinology and Metabolism* 83 (6): 1853–59.
21. Bjorntorp, R., and R. Rosmond. 2000. Obesity and cortisol. *Nutrition* 16 (10), 924–36.
22. *Ibid.*
23. Kuo, L., J. Kitlinska, J. Tilan, L. LI, S. Baker, M. Johnson, E, Lee, M. Burnett, S. Fricke, R. Kvetnansky, H Herzog, and Z. Zukowska. 2007. Neuropeptide Y acts directly in the periphery on fat tissue and mediates stress-induced obesity and metabolic syndrome. *Nature Medicine* 13 (July): 803–11.
24. Georgiades, A. R. Williams, J. Lane, S. Boyle, B. Brummett, I. Siegler, J. Barefoot, C. Kuhn, and R. Surwit. 2009. Epinephrine levels interact with central adiposity in determining fasting glucose in African American women. *Psychosomatic Medicine* 71 (3). http://www.psychosomaticmedicine.org.
25. Henry, N., T. Smith, J. Butner, C. Berg, and B. Uchino. (2009). Marriage, depressive symptoms, and the metabolic syndrome: A couple's structural model. *Psychosomatic Medicine* 71 (3). www.psychosomaticmedicine.org.
26. Markovitz, J., K. Mathews, M. Whooley, C. Lewis, and K. Greenland. 2004. Increases in job strain are associated with incident hypertension in the CARDIA study. *Annals of Behavior Medicine* 28 (1): 4–9.
27. Garssen, B., 2004. Psychological factors and cancer development: Evidence after 30 years of research. *Clinical Psychology Review* 24 (3): 315–38.
28. Dalton, S. E. Boesen, and H. Morimoto. 2002. Mind and cancer: Do psychological factors cause cancer? *European Journal of Cancer* 38 (10): 1313–23.
29. Andersen, B., W. Farrar, and D. Golden-Kreutz. 1998. Stress and immune responses after surgical treatment for regional breast cancer. *Journal of the National Cancer Institute* 90 (1): 30–36.
30. Antoni, M., S. Lutgendorf, and S. Cole. 2006. The influence of bio-behavioural factors on tumour biology: Pathways and mechanisms. *Nature Reviews Cancer* 6 (3): 240–48.
31. Thaker, P., L. Han, and A. Kamat, 2006. Chronic stress promotes tumor growth and angiogenesis in a mouse model of ovarian carcinoma. *Nature Medicine* 12 (8): 939–44.
32. Yang, E., S. Kim, E. Donovan, M. Chen, A., Gross, J. Marketon, S. Barsky, and R. Glaser. 2009. Norepinephrine upregulates VEGF, IL-8, and IL-6, expression in human melanoma tumor cell lines: Implications for stress-related enhancement of tumor progression. *Brain, Behavior, and Immunity* 23 (2): 267–75.
33. *Mosby's medical, nursing, and allied health dictionary.*
34. Doctor's guide: Global edition. 1996. DG News: New study shows migraine hits women harder. www.docguide.com (retrieved September 22, 2006).
35. WomensHealth.gov. 2008. Migraine fact sheet. U.S. Department of Health and Human Services, Office on Women's

Health. http://www.womenshealth.gov/publications/our-publications/fact-sheet/migraine.cfm.

36. Eikermann, A. 2000. Headache, menstruation and oral contraceptives. *Headache World 2000—Headache and Hormones.* World Headache Alliance. http://w-h-a.org/wha2/Newsite/print.asp?idContentNews=26 (retrieved March 23, 2006).

37. Ibid.

38. MacGregor, E. A., et al. 2003. Estrogen supplements may help prevent menstrual migraine: Study results encouraging. World Headache Alliance. http://w-h-a.org/wha2/Newsite/print.asp?idContentNews=645 (retrieved March 23, 2006).

39. Eikermann, Headache, menstruation and oral contraceptives.

40. Stewart, W. F. R. B. Lipton, E. Chee, J. Sawyer, and S. D. Silberstein. 2000. Menstrual cycle and headache in a population sample of migraineurs. *Neurology* 55: 1517–23.

41. Dzoljic, E., et al. 2002. Prevalence of menstrually related migraine and nonmigraine primary headache in female students of Belgrade University. *Headache* 42: 185–93.

42. Ibid.

43. Massiou, H. 2000. Headache and pregnancy. *Headache World 2000—Headache and Hormones.* World Headache Alliance. http://w-h-a.org/wha2/Newsite/print.asp?idContentNews=26 (retrieved March 23, 2006).

44. MacGregor, A. 2000. Headache, the menopause and HRT. *Headache World 2000—Headache and Hormones.* World Headache Alliance. http://w-h-a.org/wha2/Newsite/print.asp?idContentNews=26 (retrieved March 23, 2006).

45. Ibid.

46. HealingWell.com. 2001. *Migraine medication.* www.healingwell.com/migraines (retrieved October 2001).

47. Ibid.

48. Ibid.

49. Whitman, N., D. Spendlove, and C. Clark. 1984. *Student stress: Effects and solutions.* Washington, DC: ERIC Clearinghouse on Higher Education.

50. Campbell, R., L. Svenson, and G. Jarvis. 1992. Perceived level of stress among university undergraduate students in Edmonton, Canada. *Perceptual and Motor Skills* 75 (2): 552–54.

51. Kanner, A., J. Coyne, C. Schaefer, and R. Lazarus. 1981. Comparison of two modes of stress management: Daily hassles and uplifts versus major life events. *Journal of Behavioral Medicine* 4 (1): 1–39.

52. Barko, N. 1983. Stress in professionals and nonprofessionals, men and women. *Innovation Abstracts* 5 (9).

53. Canam, C. 1986. Perceived stressors and coping responses of employed and non-employed career women with pre-school children. *Canadian Journal of Community Mental Health* 5 (2): 49–59.

54. Lennon, M. 1994. Women, work, and well-being: The importance of work conditions. *Journal of Health and Social Behavior* 35 (September): 235–47.

55. Bird, C. 1999. Gender, household labor, psychological distress: The impact of the amount and division of housework. *Journal of Health and Social Behavior* 40 (1): 32–45.

56. Ibid.

57. Bost, B. 2001. *The hurried woman syndrome: Healing for the 50 million women who suffer.* New York: Vantage.

58. Cacioppo, J. T., M. H. Burleson, K. M. Poehlmann, W. B. Malarkey, J. K. Kiecolt-Glaser, G. G. Bernstein, et al. 2000. Autonomic and neuroendocrine responses to mild psychological stressors: Effects of chronic stress on older women. *Annals of Behavioral Medicine* 22 (2): 140–48.

59. Moen, P., J. Robison, and V. Fields. 1994. Women's work and caregiving roles: A life course approach. *Journal of Gerontology* 49 (4): 176–87.

60. National Alliance for Caregiving and AARP. November 2009. Caregiving in the U.S. 2009. http://www.caregiving.org/data/Caregiving_in_the_US_2009_full_report.pdf.

61. Ibid.

62. Womenshealth.gov. May 2008. Caregiver stress fact sheet. Office on Women's Health, U.S. Department of Health and Human Services. http://www.womenshealth.gov/publications/our-publications/fact-sheet/caregivers-stress.cfm#c

63. Ibid.

64. Mayo Clinic staff. March 23, 2012. Caregiver stress: Tips for taking care of yourself. Mayo Clinic. http://www.mayoclinic.com/health/caregiver-stress/MY01231.

65. Ibid.

66. Wheatley, D. 1991. Stress in women. *Stress and Medicine* 7 (2): 73–74.

67. MacEwen, K., and J. Barling. 1988. Multiple stressors, violence in the family of origin and marital aggression: A longitudinal investigation. *Journal of Family Violence* 3 (1): 73–87.

68. Walters, V. 1993. Stress, anxiety and depression: Women's accounts of their health problems. *Social Science and Medicine* 36 (4): 393–402.

69. Siegel, B. 1986. *Love, medicine and miracles.* New York: Harper & Row; Borysenko, J. 1988. *Minding the body, mending the mind.* New York: Bantam.

70. Castro, F., P. Furth, and H. Karlow. 1984. The health beliefs of Mexican, Mexican American and Anglo American women. *Hispanic Journal of Behavioral Sciences* 6 (4): 365–83.

71. Snapp, M. 1992. Occupational stress, social support, and depression among black and white professional managerial women. *Women and Health* 18: 41–79.

72. "Koroshi"—Overwork—Taking its toll on women in Japan. *WIN News,* 1992. Winter, p. 61.

73. Kenney, J. W. 2000. Women's 'inner-balance': A comparison of stressors, personality traits and health problems by age groups. *Journal of Advanced Nursing* 31 (3): 639–50.

74. Francis, M., and C. Sacra. 1994. Stressed out? *Mademoiselle* (September): 190–93.

75. Logue, B. 1991. Women at risk: Predictors of financial stress for retired women workers. *Gerontologist* 31 (5): 657–65.

76. Minkler, M., and R. Stone. 1985. The feminization of poverty and older women. *Gerontologist* 25: 351–57.

77. Survey. 1994. *Orange County* (California) *Register,* October.

78. Swanson, N. 2000. Working women and stress. *Journal of the American Medical Women's Association* 55 (2): 76–79.

79. Ibid, p. 76.

80. Loc. Cit.

81. Loc. Cit.

82. Bird, C., and M. Fremont. 1991. Gender, time use, and health. *Journal of Health and Social Behavior* 32 (2): 114–29.

83. Presley, B. 1993. Women pay more for success. *New York Times,* July 4.

84. Marcus, A., T. Zeeman, and C. Telesky. 1983. Sex differences in reports of illness and disability: A further test of the fixed role hypothesis. *Social Science and Medicine* 17: 993–1002; Nathanson, C. 1980. Social roles and health status among women: The significance of employment. *Social Science and Medicine* 14a: 463–71; Verbrugge, L. 1983. Multiple roles and physical health of men and women. *Journal of Health and Social Behavior* 24: 16–30; Waldron, I., and J. Jacobs. 1988. Effects of labor force participation on women's health: New

evidence from a longitudinal study. *Journal of Occupational Medicine* 30: 977–83.

85. Ross, C., and C. Bird. 1994. Sex stratification and health lifestyle: Consequences for men's and women's perceived health. *Journal of Health and Social Behavior* 35 (June): 161–78.

86. Isaacson, L., and D. Brown. 1993. *Career information, career counseling, and career development.* 5th ed. Boston: Allyn & Bacon.

87. Lawler, K., and L. Schmied. 1992. A prospective study of women's health: The effects of stress, hardiness, locus of control, Type A behavior, and physiological reactivity. *Women and Health* 19 (1): 27–41.

88. Rogers, S. 1990. *Tired or toxic? A blueprint for health.* Syracuse, NY: Prestige.

89. Dow, C. 1988. Monitor tone generates stress in computer and VDT operators: A preliminary study. Presentation at the Annual Meeting of the Association for Education in Journalism and Mass Communications, Portland, OR.

90. McKee, D. B., and J. Dingee, 2003. Treatment of anxiety disorders. In M. Kopala and M. Keital (eds.), *Handbook of counseling women,* pp. 458–81. Thousand Oaks, CA: Sage.

91. Ibid.

92. American Psychiatric Association. 2000. *Diagnostic and statistical manual of mental disorders.* 4th ed., text revision (DSM-IV-TR). Washington, DC: APA.

93. McKee, D. B., and J. Dingee, 2003. Treatment of anxiety disorders. In M. Kopala and M. Keital (eds.), *Handbook of counseling women,* pp. 458–81. Thousand Oaks, CA: Sage.

94. Grohol. J. 2010. Top 25 psychiatric prescriptions for 2009. *Psych Central.* http://psychcentral.com/lib/2010/to-25-psychiatric-prescriptions-for-2009/.

95. Pulcino, T., S. Galea, J. Ahern, H. Resnick, M. Foley, and D. Vlahov. 2003. Posttraumatic stress in women after the September 11 terrorist attacks in New York City. *Journal of Women's Health* 12 (8): 809–20.

96. Society for Women's Health Research. 2008. PTSD in women returning from combat: Future directions in research and service delivery. http://www.womenshealthresearch.org/site/DocServer/PTSD_in_Women_Returning_From_Combat-reduced_file_size.pdf?docID=2661.

97. Ibid.

98. Vogt, D. 2009. *Women, trauma and PTSD.* National Center for PTSD Fact Sheet. United States Department of Veterans Affairs. www.ncptsd.gov (retrieved March 12, 2009).

99. Fontana, A. M., T. Diegnan, A. Villeneuve, and S. J. Lepore, 1998. Nonevaluative social support reduces cardiovascular reactivity in young women during acutely stressful performance situations. *Journal of Behavioral Medicine* 22 (1): 75–91.

100. Lazarus, R., and S. Folkman. 1984. *Stress, appraisal, and coping.* New York: Springer.

101. Chandler, C., and C. Kolander. 1988. Stop the negative, accentuate the positive. *Journal of School Health* 58 (7): 295–97; Peale, N. 1990. *The power of positive thinking.* New York: Doubleday.

102. Block, K., and M. Schwartz. 1995. Dietary considerations: Rationale, issues, substances, evaluation, and patient education. In Mark Schwartz (ed.), *Biofeedback: A practitioner's guide.* 2nd ed. New York: Guilford.

103. MedicineNet.com. 2012. Weight loss: Emotional eating. http://www.medicinenet.com/emotional_eating/article.htm.

104. Ibid.

105. University of Maryland Medical Center. June 26, 2011. Vitamin B1. http://www.umm.edu/altmed/articles/vitamin-b1-000333.htm.

106. Shaw, G. 2009. What's the link between water and stress reduction? WebMd. http://www.webmd.com/diet/features/water-stress-reduction

107. Balch, P. 2002. *Prescription for herbal healing: An easy-to-use A-Z reference to hundreds of common disorders and their herbal remedies.* Brea, CA: Avery Trade.

108. Zhang, X. 1996. Regulatory situation of herbal medicines: A worldwide review. World Health Organization (WHO). http://apps.who.int/medicinedocs/pdf/whozip57e/whozip57e.pdf

109. World Health Organization (WHO). 2002. WHO traditional medicine strategy 2002–2005. http://whqlibdoc.who.int/hq/2002/who_edm_trm_2002.1.pdf.

110. Preidt, R. April 12, 2012. Herbal remedy ingredient tied to cancer, kidney failure. MedlinePlus, U.S. National Library of Medicine, National Institutes of Health. http://www.nlm.nih.gov/medlineplus/news/fullstory_124028.html.

111. MedlinePlus. April 23, 2012. Herbal Medicine. U.S. National Library of Medicine, National Institutes of Health. http://www.nlm.nih.gov/medlineplus/herbalmedicine.html.

112. Keville, K., and M. Green. 2008. *Aromatherapy: A complete guide to the healing art, 2nd ed.* Berkeley, CA: Crossing Press.

113. Fritz, S. 2008. *Mosby's fundamentals of therapeutic massage.* 4th ed. St. Louis, MO: Mosby.

114. Faure-Alderson, M. 2008. *Total reflexology: The reflex points for physical, emotional, and psychological healing.* Rochester, VT: Healing Arts Press.

115. Reed Gach, M., and B. Henning Dipl. 2004. *Acupressure for emotional healing: A self-care guide for trauma, stress, and common emotional imbalances.* New York: Bantam.

116. Deadman, P. 2007. *A manual of acupuncture.* 2nd ed. San Diego, CA: Journal of Chinese Medicine Publications.

117. World Health Organization. May 16, 2002. WHO launches the first global strategy on traditional and alternative medicine. http://www.who.int/mediacentre/news/releases/releases38/en/.

118. Burke, A., D. Upchurch, C. Dye, and L. Chyu. September 2006. Acupuncture use in the U.S.: Findings from the National Health Interview Survey. *The Journal of Alternative and Complementary Medicine, 12* (7), 639–648. doi:10.1089/acm.2006.12.639.

119. Jwing-Ming, Y. 2010. *Tai Chi Chuan classical Yang style: The complete form Qigong.* Wolfeboro, NH: YMAA Publication Center.

120. Andrews, A. 2011. *Tell your time: How to manage your schedule so you can live free* [Kindle edition]. Amazon Digital Services. http://www.amazon.com.

121. National Center for Complementary and Alternative Medicine. 2005. Mind–body medicine: An overview. August. http://nccam.nih.gov/health/backgrounds/mindbody.htm (retrieved March 26, 2006).

122. Ibid.

123. Cohen, S., W. J. Doyle, R. B. Turner, et al. 2003. Emotional style and susceptibility to the common cold. *Psychosomatic Medicine* 65 (4): 652–57.

124. Smith, A., and K. Nicholson. 2001. Psychological factors, respiratory viruses and exacerbation of asthma. *Psychoneuroendocrinology* 26 (4): 411–20.

125. National Center for Complementary and Alternative Medicine, 2005.

126. Rutledge, J. C., D. A. Hyson, D. Garduno, et al. 1999. Lifestyle modification program in management of patients with coronary artery disease: The clinical experience in a tertiary care hospital. *Journal of Cardiopulmonary Rehabilitation* 19 (4): 226–34.

127. Mundy, E. A., K. N. DuHamel, and G. H. Montgomery. 2003. The efficacy of behavioral interventions for cancer treatment–related side effects. *Seminars in Clinical Neuropsychiatry* 8 (4): 253–75.

128. Irwin, M. R., J. L. Pike, J. C. Cole, et al. 2003. Effects of behavioral intervention, Tai Chi Chih, on varicella zoster virus specific immunity and health functioning in older adults. *Psychosomatic Medicine* 65 (5): 824–30.

129. Kiecolt-Glaser, J. K., P. T. Marucha, C. Atkinson, et al. 2001. Hypnosis as a modulator of cellular immune dysregulation during acute stress. *Journal of Consulting and Clinical Psychology* 69 (4): 674–82.

130. Luskin, F. M., K. A. Newell, M. Griffith, et al. 2000. A review of mind/body therapies in the treatment of musculoskeletal disorders with implications for the elderly. *Alternative Therapies in Health and Medicine* 6 (2): 46–56.

131. Astin, J. A., S. L. Shapiro, D. M. Eisenberg, et al. 2003. Mind–body medicine: State of science, implications for practice. *Journal of the American Board of Family Practice* 16 (2): 131–47.

132. Tusek, D. L., J. M. Church, S. A. Strong, et al. 1997. Guided imagery: A significant advance in the care of patients undergoing elective colorectal surgery. *Diseases of the Colon and Rectum* 40 (2): 172–78.

133. Lang, E. V., E. G. Benotsch, L. J. Fick, et al. 2000. Adjunctive nonpharmacological analgesia for invasive medical procedures: A randomized trial. *Lancet* 355 (9214): 1486–90.

134. Stahl, B., E. Goldstein, S. Santorelli, and J. Kabat-Zinn. 2010. *A mindfulness-based stress reduction workbook.* Oakland, CA: New Harbinger.

135. Mindful Awareness Research Center. 2012. About MARC. University of California, Los Angeles. http://www.marc.ucla.edu.

136. Davis, M., E. Eshelman, and M. McKay. 2008. *The relaxation and stress reduction workbook.* 6th ed. Oakland, CA: New Harbinger.

137. Ibid.

138. Benson, H. 1975. *The relaxation response.* New York: Avon.

139. Stroebel, C. 1978. *Quieting response training.* New York: BMA.

140. Schwartz, M. 2005. *Biofeedback: A practitioner's guide.* 3rd ed. New York: Guilford Press.

141. Gawain, S. 1986. *Living in the light.* Mill Valley, CA: Whatever Publishing.

142. LeShan, L. 1974. *How to meditate.* New York: Bantam.

143. Lazar, S. W., G. Bush, and R. L. Gollub. 2000. Functional brain mapping of the relaxation response and meditation. *Neuroreport* 11 (7): 1581–85.

144. Davidson, R. J., J. Kabat-Zinn, J. Schumacher, et al. 2003. Alterations in brain and immune function produced by mindfulness meditation. *Psychosomatic Medicine* 65 (4): 564–70.

145. Brown. C. 2003. *The Yoga bible.* Cincinnati, OH: Walking Stick Press.

146. Lewis, D. 2004. *Free your breath, free your life: How conscious breathing can relieve stress, increase vitality, and help you live more fully.* Boston, MA: Shambhala Publications.

Sexual and Relational Wellness

Part Three

Chapter Six

Building Healthy Relationships

CHAPTER OBJECTIVES

When you complete this chapter, you will be able to do the following:

◇ Explain the stages of dating

◇ Provide examples of different types of love based on Sternberg's triangular theory of love

◇ Describe the biochemistry of love

◇ Compare and contrast various types of relationships

◇ Describe relationship success and distress

◇ Explain how to resolve relationship conflicts

◇ Describe positive parenting relationships with children

FORMING RELATIONSHIPS

Healthy relationships evolve, they do not happen spontaneously. Young adolescents, as they begin to date, are learning how to connect and interact with someone else. The way adolescents interact is greatly influenced by the role models (parents, caregivers, media) they observed during childhood and, more accurately, by the adolescent's perceptions of how these role models interacted with each other. Most adults have never received training in appropriate methods and techniques for building, maintaining, and nurturing a relationship. This lack of skill development limits their ability to serve as healthy role models. As a result, adolescents have the difficult task of figuring out how to build healthy relationships without the benefit of previous modeling.

A lesbian adolescent may find it difficult to explore her attraction for other women during a time when it is most natural for her to do so. Lesbians often do not feel safe enough to begin the dating process with other women until they leave home and high school and migrate to a community that is more supportive of this type of relationship or where it is at least easier to be inconspicuous.

It is difficult for a lesbian to find role models for dating because much of this culture remains hidden. Thus, the lesbian is frequently forced to not only hide her desires and delay acting on her attractions, but she has little opportunity to learn from others about how to establish and maintain a healthy lesbian relationship.

Stages of Dating

The stages of dating include attraction, ritual, information sharing, activities, emotional intimacy, and, possibly, commitment.[1] These stages take time to evolve, and if women move too quickly through them, they may find themselves repeating destructive relationship patterns over and over.

Attraction The first stage of dating is attraction, sometimes called "chemistry." Physical attraction draws us to another person. You see him standing there, on the other side of the room. You think he's attractive. You see her at a bookstore and want to begin a conversation. She looks incredible. You make eye contact. Why did he catch your eye? Why did you want to talk to her? The physical appearance that appeals to one person may or may not appeal to another. Physical attraction doesn't suggest that this person will have the attributes or personality that you like, but it is a first step. Physically attractive people often benefit from their good looks. Studies suggest that they are perceived as being more intelligent, more socially skilled, happier, more successful, and better adjusted than are less attractive persons.[2] This perception occurs through the conscious or unconscious meaning we attach to the attraction; it isn't reality. It takes time to develop a complete picture of a person, and true reality can occur only with mutual self-disclosure and an unbiased observation of another person's behaviors.

Ritual   Rituals are the practices that help us create familiarity. These are the mannerisms, experiences, and behaviors that occur to deepen the bond between two people. Rituals are the shared experiences that lead to calling something "special" or "our favorite." It may be a song, a place to go for a walk, a special nickname, or anything that makes one person think fondly about the other. Rituals create meaning; meaning comes from doing; and doing takes time!

Information Sharing   Information sharing is the stage of getting to know each other better. It begins with impersonal dialog that allows two people to get to know each other: likes and dislikes, hobbies, career aspirations, worldview and politics, and other external issues. At this stage, she is attuned to how the other person communicates and interacts with her and others, what he says about others (either positively or negatively), and what draws her to this person. If she feels a sense of immediacy or desire to hurry through this stage, she should stop and evaluate why she is feeling this need. Is she feeling a need to be rescued, to rescue, to attach before he leaves or gets bored? Why isn't she willing to continue moving slowly? The information-sharing stage is only the beginning level of emotional intimacy. Eventually, she chooses to disclose more personal information about herself, such as information about her background, her family, and her inner thoughts and feelings. This disclosure will occur at a reasonably slow pace. Physical contact, such as kissing, hand holding, and other such behaviors, may also begin at this time. If she moves too quickly with physical contact, she may mistakenly think that the physical intimacy is synonymous with emotional intimacy. She may overlook characteristics and behaviors that otherwise could alert her to possible future problems (so-called red flags).

Activities   Activities play an important role in the dating process and keep the process moving slowly. These activities occur concurrently with the information-sharing stage, and now is the time to figure out if her interests are similar to the other person's interests. Does she like the same events, movies, or restaurants? Does she equally choose activities or is she always doing the activity planning? She should feel comfortable stating whether she prefers to do what he wants or if she prefers to do something else. She should feel comfortable saying that she wants to go out with friends or has made plans to do something without him. If conflicts arise, she and her partner have an opportunity to practice compromise and negotiation. If either person begins to sacrifice interests on a regular basis and goes along with the other's suggestions, inequity soon begins to infiltrate the relationship. (Complete *Assess Yourself:* "Are You Compatible as a Couple?" to reflect on the balance between alone time, time with your partner, and time with other friends.) Spending time alone and with other friends will help her move slowly. Throughout this dating process, she can decide whether to move forward toward a greater level of intimacy and more exclusivity, to keep the relationship at a more superficial level, to terminate the relationship, or to compromise on an acceptable level of interaction.

Emotional Intimacy   As two people spend more time together, their level of **emotional intimacy** continues to grow. Emotional intimacy is the feeling of knowing and being known. A key component of intimacy is good communication. It is knowing who you are and being willing to reveal yourself to someone else. It involves openly sharing important information about yourself while keeping your boundaries intact. Intimacy requires the same from your partner. Your partner must be willing to reveal herself and you must be willing to listen effectively. It is knowing where you begin and end and where she begins and ends. Emotional intimacy occurs when you disclose information in an open, honest, and authentic manner.[3]

Sometimes, as you become more intimate with a partner, you may encounter barriers that keep you from experiencing a meaningful intimate relationship. Such barriers may occur from being traumatized as a child, feeling fragmented, or having poor role models. Some children experience trauma (physical, emotional, or spiritual) and, in response, develop a psychological wall to protect themselves. This wall was useful for them as children, but as adults, it prevents them from being vulnerable and open with others. As they gain an understanding of their barriers, they begin to work toward overcoming the walls so that emotional intimacy can be attained.

As you share the parts of yourself that make you feel vulnerable, the psychological wounds you experienced as a child can begin to heal. Embracing those parts of yourself that you prefer to hide or disown and being truthful with a partner can provide a deeper level of emotional maturity. In an open, honest relationship, you can freely share those aspects while still accepting responsibility for your actions. Even small lies (whether through omission

Assess Yourself

Are You Compatible as a Couple?

Compatibility is an important component of relationships. You have probably heard that opposites attract; however, those differences can create problems if communication breaks downs. Rate the following twenty statements based on your feelings about your partner. The higher your score, the higher is the level of compatibility.

Always true   Frequently true   Sometimes true   Never true
    4   3   2   1

_____ 1. We communicate our inner thoughts and feelings effectively.

_____ 2. We trust each other.

_____ 3. We agree on whose needs come first.

_____ 4. We have realistic expectations of each other and ourselves.

_____ 5. Personal growth is important within our relationship.

_____ 6. We are committed to this relationship even if the other person doesn't change.

_____ 7. We discuss our personal problems with each other first.

_____ 8. We both do our best to compromise.

_____ 9. We usually practice fair fighting.

_____ 10. We try not to be rigid or unyielding.

_____ 11. We keep any needs to be "perfect" in proper perspective.

_____ 12. We agree on the amount of time spent together with time to be alone.

_____ 13. We both make friends and keep them.

_____ 14. Neither of us stays down or up for long periods.

_____ 15. We can tolerate the other's mood without being affected by it.

_____ 16. We can deal with disappointment and disillusionment.

_____ 17. Both of us can tolerate failure.

_____ 18. We can both express anger appropriately.

_____ 19. We are both assertive when necessary.

_____ 20. We agree on how our personal surroundings are kept.

or commission) impact a relationship. Truth and honesty permit you to openly experience your vulnerability, admit your mistakes, acknowledge your fears, express anger and sadness, and ask for what you need. These inner thoughts and feelings are easier to share if your partner demonstrates empathy (compassion), praise, and encouragement, and if you moved slowly through the initial stages of dating. Strong communication skills are a major asset to intimacy and a healthy relationship.

Commitment Commitment represents feelings of attachment and the desire to be in a more intimate relationship with the other person. People commit to a relationship for a variety of reasons, some more healthy than others. Three factors found to increase the potential of a person to remain committed to a relationship are a partner's satisfaction with the relationship, a partner's perceived lack of alternatives to the current partner, and the investment of important or numerous resources in the relationship.[4] Ultimately, staying or leaving depends on the willingness of the partners to commit to the relationship.

Gender-Role Attributes

Psychological factors such as masculinity and femininity have a profound influence on the development of relationships. Early studies of gender-role attitudes viewed masculinity and femininity as a unidimensional, bipolar concept. Traits designated for males and females were dichotomous and precluded each other. Masculinity was viewed as an absence of femininity; femininity was viewed as an absence of masculinity. This view was based on the belief that males and females differed in instinctive and emotional behavior—factors that shape personality. The female was characterized as sympathetic, nurturing, timid, jealous, suspicious, submissive, and nonaggressive. The male was described as aggressive, dominating, a leader, less religious, and strong.

In later studies, researchers suggested that masculinity and femininity were separate principles that coexisted to some degree in all individuals, irrespective of gender. They used a multidimensional model that was independent of gender. Individuals who scored high in attributes defined as masculine and low in those defined as feminine were classified as **masculine.** Individuals who scored high in feminine attributes and low in masculine attributes were classified as **feminine.** Those who possessed a high number of masculine and feminine traits were labeled **androgynous.** Androgynous individuals were believed to possess the traits that allowed them to function more equally in a relationship and to fare better psychologically.

A study of gender-role attitudes and dating behaviors in college students found differences in self-disclosure, power, and cohabitation among traditional and androgynous individuals. Traditional masculine males tended toward less self-disclosure and exerted more power in the dating relationship. Traditional masculine males and feminine females were also less likely to choose to be sexually active or cohabitate. In a follow-up of these couples 15 years later, traditional feminine women were more likely than androgynous women to have married their college sweetheart and to remain married.[5] However, this study ignored one apparent paradox of gender attributes: traditionally masculine males and feminine females have far from optimal relationships. In fact, another study suggested that marital happiness appeared to be related to high feminine traits in both males and females.[6]

More recently, the terms "instrumental" or "agentic" have been used to define masculine traits and "expressive" or "communal" to define feminine traits. These terms remove gender stereotyping and deemphasize gender differences. Instrumental or agentic traits include assertiveness, independence, and competence, whereas expressive traits include compassionate, affectionate, and interpersonal concern. An androgynous person exhibits a balance of instrumental and expressive traits and can appropriately display the necessary traits for the circumstances.

Sociological Factors

Sociological factors also impact the development of relationships. Socialization can contribute to the respective differences in attitudes and behaviors between males and females in interpersonal interactions. Some scholars suggest that women are more relational, whereas men are more autonomous. Women are more likely to define themselves in the context of relationships because of their socialization to be more dependent or interdependent. Men, on the other hand, define themselves as more independent, thus focusing on individual rights, self-centeredness, and self-interest.

Females and males tend to be socialized differently according to the values and beliefs of their culture. Individualistic societies focus on "the subordination of the goals of the collectives to individual goals." Men in these societies tend to pursue their self-interests and give the immediate family primary importance. Collectivistic societies, on the other hand, emphasize interdependence and the goals of the collective over an individual's goals.[7]

The United States is viewed as a more individualist than collective society. Some researchers have proposed that belonging to an individualistic society profoundly affects love and intimacy. They postulate that romantic love is more important to committed relationships in individualistic societies and that psychological intimacy (an important component in committed relationships) is difficult to develop.[8] Here, men tend to embrace the cultural and psychological aspects of an individualistic society, whereas most women tend to embrace the messages of a collective society. Men find it easier to

---

Journal Activity

Attractive and Unattractive Qualities

Create a list of ten qualities you find most attractive and least attractive in another person. Look at the qualities that you listed as most attractive in another person. Now, answer the following questions: To what degree do you possess these qualities? Would you like to develop these qualities more fully in yourself? Look at the qualities that you find least attractive in another person. To what degree do you possess these qualities? Do you try hard to avoid these qualities in yourself? Have you accepted your potential to possess these qualities? Do you accept these qualities as part of every human being's potential? Why or why not? Oftentimes, the qualities that we react to most strongly in another person are related to issues that we need to address within ourselves.

---

integrate societal messages and expectations for their role in relationships because these messages and expectations are congruent with an individualistic society. Women, on the other hand, grow up with the messages of interdependence (collective values) and can experience dissonance when trying to live by the rules of an individualistic society. This dissonance may lead to confusion if a woman seeks congruity between personal and societal values. Now complete *Journal Activity:* "Attractive and Unattractive Qualities."

THEORIES OF LOVE

Love is something that everyone seeks, yet when someone is asked how they know when they're in love or what to expect from love, the answers are varied. How do researchers describe love and its various forms? What ingredients do they feel are necessary for a couple to maintain a long-term love relationship?

Abraham Maslow divided love into two primary categories: D love and B love.[9] D love is based on deficiency, a desire to have another person meet one's unmet needs. As long as her needs are met, she is in love. D love has elements of possessiveness, jealousy, and dependence. B love is based on being. B love includes autonomy, interdependence, and mutual satisfaction. The relationship is secure and partners experience freedom to be themselves. Two other recognized theories of love are Sternberg's triangular model and Lee's six lovestyles.

Sternberg's Triangular Theory

Robert Sternberg's triangular theory of love focuses on three components: commitment, intimacy, and passion.[10] These components explain nine different combinations of love, but not why love occurs. One side of the triangle focuses on the emotional aspect of love (intimacy); the second side focuses on the motivational aspect of love (passion); and, the third side focuses on the cognitive side of love (commitment). The combinations of these three aspects explain different types of love, and changes in the components are illustrated by changes to the size and shape of the triangles. (See Figure 6.1.)

Liking occurs when only the emotional side of love (intimacy) is present. Two friends who trust each other, share similar values and beliefs, and communicate well form an intimate bond. They know the vulnerabilities and strengths of each other and form a close friendship. *Empty love* occurs when commitment alone is present. For example, when Julie states emphatically, "You know, I really don't like Ted anymore but I took a marriage vow. I said 'in sickness and in health, for better or for worse, until death do us part' and that's what I intend to honor. When I want to talk about intimate matters, I talk to my best friend. Besides, the children need a father and I can't find a job now." Julie's religious beliefs, the values

instilled during childhood, and limited financial earning potential keep her from leaving to seek a more fulfilling relationship. She may not like Ted as a person, but she married him and intends to stay with him. *Infatuation* occurs when passion is the sole dimension in the relationship. This concept can be summarized as "a crush." Kenitra isn't worried about Andre's values, beliefs, background, job, or anything else; she doesn't care. Andre is awesome, she's never seen anyone more attractive, and she thinks about him all the time. *Romantic love* involves the dimensions of intimacy and passion. Two people who like and are physically attracted to each other but do not have a commitment to form a romantic liaison. In one study, when men and women were asked, "What constitutes a romantic act?" both genders cited "taking walks together" most often. The women's list included taking walks together, sending or receiving flowers, kissing, candle-lit dinners, cuddling, declaring "I love you," love letters, slow dancing, hugging, and giving surprise gifts. The list for men looked similar and included taking walks together, kissing, candle-lit dinners, cuddling, hugging, flowers, holding hands, making love, love letters, and sitting by the fireplace.[11]

When passion and commitment result in a committed relationship without taking time to get to know each other, *fatuous love* results. Jill met Jackie at a softball game. It was the first game between their teams and the two players were immediately attracted to each other. After the game, they hugged and agreed to meet later at the bar. They ended the night at Jill's place and the sex

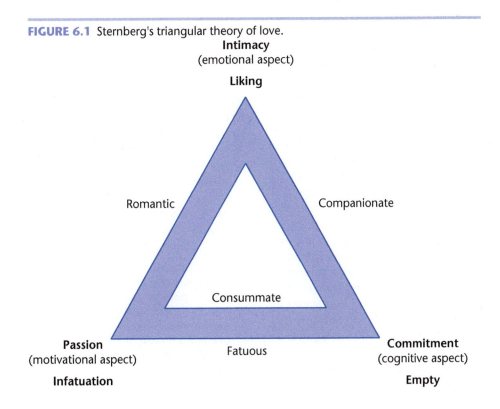

FIGURE 6.1 Sternberg's triangular theory of love.

was great. The next week, Jill asked Jackie to move into her apartment. They were "in love" and ready to commit to a lifetime together. Six months later they shook their heads, wondering how they could have possibly been attracted to each other. They ran out of things to talk about and had very little in common. *Companionate love* involves intimacy and commitment without passion. In some long-term relationships, the physical attraction may die but the intimacy and commitment provide the ingredients for a long-term friendship. The partners are best friends. When all three components are present in the relationship, *consummate love* or complete love occurs. This love is what partners strive to create and to maintain. It requires nurturing, physical attraction, vulnerability, and a commitment to growing together. When all three components are absent in the relationship, Sternberg calls this *nonlove*. These are just casual interactions that occur without any form of relationship evolving.

Lee's Six Lovestyles

I love him, but I'm not in love with him. I like him, but I'm not sure I love him. What do we mean by such words? Psychologist John Alan Lee, in *The Colors of Love*, identifies six different lovestyles.[12] He identifies three primary lovestyles (*eros, storge,* and *ludus*) and three secondary lovestyles (*mania, pragma,* and *agape*). **Erotic love** occurs when lovers get involved quickly and base their attraction on physical attributes and sexual passion. This love is based on "chemistry" and "love at first sight." Eros is a major ingredient in relationship success.

Ludic love is an uncommitted alliance with more than one partner. The partners may be very different from one another because love is based on game playing rather than romance. A partner is "kept guessing" and distancing occurs when dependency develops. Ludus tends to be negatively related to satisfaction with relationships.

Pragmatic love draws two people together for practical reasons such as financial security or parental potential. It is "pragmatic" and fills certain specifications for a partner such as similar background, good job, or good parent. It is often present in long-term relationships.

Manic love is often portrayed in the "heart throb" of Hollywood, the perfect match. The emotional highs and lows remind one of a roller-coaster ride, and possessiveness, dependency, and jealousy abound. Mania leads to total focus on and fear of losing one's partner.

Altruistic love places the needs of the partner above one's own needs. It is selfless and nondemanding, and one chooses self-sacrifice rather than hurting a partner. This love is sometimes referred to as **agape**, a more spiritual relationship.

Storgic love is more like friendship, without the passion. It provides a secure, trusting relationship that evolves from a deep, abiding friendship and leads to long-term relationships.

BIOCHEMISTRY OF LOVE

Helen Fisher is a leading researcher in the biochemistry of love. Functional magnetic resonance imaging (fMRI) brain scans performed by her research team confirmed her hypothesis that the neurotransmitter dopamine is a major player in romantic love. The brain scans were taken while each subject stared at a picture of his or her beloved. The researchers discovered that while many brain parts became active in each subject who was experiencing love, two regions appeared to be central to the experience: the caudate nucleus and the ventral tegmental area (VTA).[13] The caudate nucleus is a large C-shaped region that lies deep near the center of the brain and is considered part of the limbic system, known as the primitive emotional brain. The brain scans showed that parts of the body and the tail of the caudate nucleus became very active as a lover gazed at the photo of a sweetheart. The caudate nucleus, according to Fisher, "is part of the brain's 'reward system,' the mind's network for general arousal, sensations of pleasure, and the motivation to acquire rewards. The caudate helps us to detect and perceive a reward, discriminate between rewards, *prefer* a particular reward, anticipate a reward, and expect a reward. It produces motivation to acquire a reward and plans specific movements to obtain a reward. The caudate is also associated with the acts of paying attention and learning." Not only did the subjects exhibit activity in the caudate, but the more passionate they were, the more active their caudate was: those who scored higher on a self-report measure taken as part of the study, the Passionate Love Scale, also showed more activity in a specific region of the caudate when they looked at the picture of their sweetheart. The researchers "also found activity in other regions of the reward system, including the septum and a brain region that becomes active when people eat chocolate. Chocolate can be addictive." Fisher maintains that romantic love is addictive, too. The other area where activity was discovered on the fMRI brain scans by Fisher's research team was the VTA, a central part of the reward circuitry of the brain.

> The VTA is a mother lode for dopamine-making cells. With their tentacle-like axons, these nerve cells distribute dopamine to many brain regions, including the caudate nucleus. And as this sprinkler system sends dopamine to many brain parts, it produces focused attention, as well as fierce energy, concentrated motivation to attain a reward, and feelings of elation, even mania—the core feelings of romantic love. . . . No wonder lovers talk all night or walk till dawn. . . . Drenched in chemicals that bestow focus, stamina, and vigor, and driven

by the motivating engine of the brain, lovers succumb to a Herculean courting urge.[14]

While Fisher and her colleagues were in the middle of their project, a London research team, headed by Andreas Bartels and Semir Zeki, announced in 2000 the completion of a study that was coincidentally similar to what Fisher was working on.[15] Similar to what Fisher's team was finding, Bartels and Zeki also found activity in the same brain structure for those persons in love, the caudate nucleus. In addition, the London team discovered that their subjects, who reported being in love for an average of 2.3 years, had activity in two more regions—the anterior cingulate cortex and the insular cortex (the Fisher study had involved subjects who reported being in love for only an average of 7 months). This prompted Fisher to go back and look at subjects varying in how long they reported being in love. Fisher discovered that those who were in relatively longer relationships showed activity in the anterior cingulate cortex and the insular cortex, just like the London study.

> We don't actually know what this means. The anterior cingulate gyrus is a region where emotion, attention, and working memory interact. Some parts are associated with happy states; others involve awareness of one's own emotional state and the ability to assess other people's feelings during social interactions; and some are associated with split-second emotional reactions to a win or a loss, thereby judging a reward's value. The insular cortex collects data from the body regarding external touch and temperature, as well as internal pain and activities of the stomach, gut, and other viscera. . . . Parts of the insular cortex also process emotions. . . . So we established that as a relationship lengthens, brain regions associated with emotions, memory, and attention begin to respond in new ways. Exactly what these brain parts are doing, no one knows.[16]

The brain physiology research on love and relationships is relatively new and the full ramifications of this information are yet to be discovered. Based on the research findings, it seems that one part of the brain's pleasure center, one associated with the hunt (seek) and reward system, is most active during the first 2 years of a relationship, being bombarded with very high levels of the neurotransmitter dopamine. These early courtship months manifest euphoric feelings accompanied by obsession with and passion for one's dating partner. When the relationship is about 2 years old, it seems that a different part of the brain's pleasure center becomes more active, a part associated with pleasurable memories (instead of seek and reward). This shift in brain physiology corresponds with the couple settling into a comfortable, mutual familiarity, and while some passion and thoughtfulness remain, the levels of obsession and passion (associated with the first 2 years) are much lower because less dopamine is being generated in this second

area of the brain's pleasure center. The couple has moved into the phase of a long-term relationship. It is interesting to consider if this physiological brain shift after 2 years of courtship may explain why some couples fear that the "love" has gone out of their relationship after about 2 years because they experience less passion and obsession than they had the first 2 years of the relationship. In fact, it is likely that it is just that the brain physiology has shifted—a probable necessity to enable the couple to become established and settled and perhaps, raise a family. This shift would likely be necessary for species survival. Many couples miss the feelings of euphoria associated with the first 2 years of dating. Counselors who work with couples encourage them to find new and different things to try together to renew and sustain the passion in the relationship, such as hobbies, sports, a special date night, and variations of emotional and physical intimacy. Fun, new, and exciting activities can initiate temporary surges in neurotransmitter secretion (especially dopamine), providing stimulation of the pleasure center in the brain.

It is interesting to further speculate if the shift in brain physiology after 2 years of dating could at least partially explain why people have extramarital or extrarelationship affairs, in that one partner may miss the euphoria of the early dating phase and seek it outside of a more established relationship. At the same time, they may not want to let go of the comfort and security of an established, long-term relationship. So they remain in the long-term relationship, but secretly have an affair outside of the relationship. Some people might even get addicted to the euphoria stage of dating, which may result in a series of extrarelationship affairs.

The body's hormone of sexual desire is testosterone (and, to a lesser degree, other male sex hormones). "Men and women who have higher circulating levels of testosterone tend to engage in more sexual activity."[17]

> When it comes to sexual desire, people vary, in part because levels of testosterone are inherited. Levels also fluctuate according to the day, the week, the year, and the life cycle. Moreover, the balance of testosterone, estrogen, and other bodily ingredients, as well as social circumstances and a host of other factors, all play a role in when, where, and how often we feel lust. Nevertheless, testosterone is central to this appetite.[18]

Just as the presence of testosterone stimulates sexual desire, declining levels in testosterone can lead to lessened sexual desire. Testosterone levels naturally decline with age. "Both sexes have fewer sexual fantasies, masturbate less regularly, and engage in less intercourse as they age. . . . Some two-thirds of middle-aged women do not experience any decline in libido, however. . . . As the estrogens decline with menopause, levels of testosterone and the other androgens become unmasked: these potent hormones can finally express themselves more fully."[19]

Researchers have recently focused on understanding which brain chemicals produce a feeling of attachment or emotional bonding with a long-term mate. "Most now believe that vasopressin and oxytocin, closely related hormones made largely in the hypothalamus and the gonads, produce many of the behaviors associated with attachment."[20] Research with male prairie voles discovered that as "the male prairie vole ejaculates, levels of vasopressin increase in the brain, triggering his spousal and parenting zeal." Injections of vasopressin into the brains of virgin male prairie voles resulted in instant behaviors of territorial protection (an aspect of pair formation), and when introduced to a female the males became immediately possessive of her. Blockage of vasopressin production in the brain of the virgin male prairie voles resulted in actions of copulation, abandonment, and moving on to another female for another mating opportunity. Like vasopressin, oxytocin is made in the hypothalamus as well as the ovaries and testes.[21] Oxytocin has been most recognized for its role in birthing: contracting the uterus and stimulating mammary glands to produce milk. "But scientists have now established that oxytocin also stimulates bonding between a mother and her infant . . . [and] many now believe that oxytocin is also involved in the feelings of adult male–female attachment." Vasopressin and oxytocin (referred to as the satisfaction hormones) are secreted during stimulation of the genitals and/or nipples and during orgasm. "At orgasm, levels of vasopressin dramatically increase in men and levels of oxytocin rise in women. These 'cuddle chemicals' undoubtedly contribute to that sense of fusion, closeness, and attachment you can feel after sweet sex with a beloved."[22] (*Note:* Sexual function and dysfunction are covered in a later chapter.)

TRAITS OF A SUCCESSFUL RELATIONSHIP

What attributes or characteristics are needed to create a healthy relationship in which both partners indicate happiness? Researchers have identified a number of attributes that contribute to a happy, successful relationship. Researcher Judith Wallerstein's study of fifty happily married couples indicated that nine psychological tasks had to occur for marital satisfaction to be achieved.[23] The nine tasks couples had to achieve are

1. Separating emotionally from the families of origin and creating a new family. The lines of connection to the original families had to be redefined.
2. Maintaining autonomy and balancing it with togetherness. Mutual identification and shared intimacy are essential for overall satisfaction.
3. Establishing a vital sexual relationship that remains free from the distractions of work and family

obligations. Setting aside quality time for each other is important.
4. Recognizing the changes that occur with parenthood and keeping communication open while time demands and responsibilities shift. Privacy is important and should be protected.
5. Confronting crises (they will happen in every relationship) and facing adversity together.
6. Determining safe ways to express differences, conflict, and anger, and seeking resolution when differences occur.
7. Creating humor that keeps the little things in perspective and maintains the dynamic stimulation to avoid boredom and isolation.
8. Nurturing and comforting each other, allowing dependency and vulnerability to feel safe.
9. Remembering the early romantic, idealized images of love for the partner while facing the reality of shifts in the relationship.

These tasks are important in any committed relationship regardless of whether the couple is married, cohabitating, heterosexual, homosexual, bisexual, or transgendered. Happiness within the relationship requires both partners to keep the relationship a high priority. Now complete *Journal Activity:* "Attributes That Contribute to Relationship Success."

Journal Activity

Attributes That Contribute to Relationship Success

Many components are important for creating and maintaining a successful relationship. Write one or two feeling statements regarding the importance and meaning of each attribute.

ability to nurture	competence	touch
commitment	empathy	authenticity
devotion	(compassion)	confidence
honesty	ability to	generosity
sacrifice	apologize	openness
responsibility	remember own	respect
support	needs	self-disclosure
acceptance	sacrifice	trust

What other attributes are necessary for relationship success? Can any of the above attributes be removed from the list?

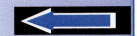

FYI

Mutually Supportive Relationship[24]

In a mutually supportive, creative relationship each person realizes that

To bring one's thoughts and to hear the other's,
To express one's enthusiasm and to delight in the other's,
To reveal one's self and to reflect the other,
To value one's self and to esteem the other,
To enjoy one's creations and to treasure the other's,
To pursue one's growth and to nurture the other's,
To cherish one's solitude and to honor the other's,
To follow one's interests and to encourage the other,
To act on one's pace and to accept the other's,
To indulge one's self and to give to the other,
To involve one's self and to assist the other,
To protect one's self and to comfort the other,
To see one's self and to behold the other,
To be one's self and to let the other be,
Is to love one's self and to love the other.

Health Tips

Basic Rights in a Relationship[25]

The right to goodwill from the other.
The right to emotional support.
The right to be heard by the other and to be responded to with courtesy.
The right to have your own view, even if your mate has a different view.
The right to have your feelings and experience acknowledged as real.
The right to receive a sincere apology for any jokes you find offensive.
The right to clear and informative answers to questions that concern what is legitimately your business.
The right to live free from accusation and blame.
The right to live free from criticism and judgment.
The right to have your work and your interests spoken of with respect.
The right to encouragement.
The right to live free from emotional and physical threat.
The right to live free from angry outbursts and rage.
The right to be called by no name that devalues you.
The right to be respectfully asked rather than ordered.

Equity in a relationship is key to a healthy, satisfying, and thriving relationship. When one partner has power over the other partner, then the relationship is not equal and the partner with less personal power is in a position not to have personal needs met. Also, the partner with less personal power is more susceptible to exploitation and verbal, emotional, or physical abuse. In a healthy relationship, mutuality and co-creation sustain personal power for each partner. "Both parties bring themselves to the relationship as whole and separate people. They are secure in their relationship to themselves. Because of this security, neither has a need to exert power over the other."[26] (See *FYI:* "Mutually Supportive Relationship.")

Each person in a relationship needs to feel safe and respected. When respect and goodwill are present, then individual and relationship issues can be more easily addressed. For instance, when "there is *no* verbal abuse there *is* openness and a willingness to discuss the hopes, fears, desires, needs, and expectations of both parties."[27] (See *Health Tips:* "Basic Rights in a Relationship.")

TYPES OF RELATIONSHIPS

Marriage and Other Committed Relationships

Over the past 50 years in the United States, there has been a decline in marriage and rise of new families. The preeminent family unit of the mid-twentieth century—mom, dad, and the kids—no longer has the stage to itself. In 1960, 72 percent of American adults were married; by 2008 it had fallen to 52 percent. Public attitudes toward marriage reflect these dramatic changes. When asked in the Pew Research Center survey if marriage is becoming obsolete, about four in ten Americans (39 percent) said that it is.[28] The National Center for Health Statistics reported the number of marriages in the United States in 2010 as 2,077,000.[29] The overall rate of marriage for 2010 was 6.8 per 1000 population, which was a decline from 7.8 per 1000 population in 2004. The six states with the highest marriage rates for 2010 were Nevada (38.3), Hawaii (17.6), Arkansas (10.8), Vermont (9.3), Tennessee (8.8), and Idaho (8.8). In most states, the marriage rate has decreased from 2004 to 2010, with the exceptions of the District of Columbia (5.2 to 7.6), New Mexico (6.6 to 7.7), and Vermont (8.9 to 9.3). In 2009, 48 percent of Americans reported to be married, and 73 percent of women reported to have been married at some stage during their lifetime.[30,31] The patterns of marriage and cohabitation have changed across time, with the proportion of married (husband-wife) couples with children continuing to decline: 1970, 40.3; 1980, 30.9; 1990, 26.3; 2000, 23.5; and 2010, 20.2 percent.[32] In addition, the median age at first marriage has shown a steady increase across time: 1970—men 23.2, women

20.8; 1980—men 24.7, women 22.0; 1990—men 26.1, women 23.9; 2000—men 26.8, women 25.1; and 2010—men 28.2, women 26.1.[33] So it seems that individuals in the United States are waiting longer to get married and fewer are choosing to have children.

David Olson and his colleagues have studied the marital relationships of more than 8000 couples and found seven basic types of marriage.[34] They established profiles based on ten scales including personality issues, communication, conflict resolution, financial management, leisure activities, sexual relationship, children and parenting, family and friends, egalitarian roles, and religious orientation. These ten issues are most frequently cited as areas of conflict for couples. Seven distinguishable marriage typologies were derived from these scales: devitalized, financially focused, conflicted, traditional, balanced, harmonious, and vitalized marriages. *Devitalized* marriages (40 percent) were characterized by dissatisfaction in all areas. These couples were extremely unhappy and both partners had considered divorce at some point in the relationship. They tended to be young, married a short period of time, and not financially secure. They stayed together because of limited alternatives and often came from families with divorced parents. In contrast, *vitalized* marriages (9 percent) were characterized by satisfaction with all dimensions of the relationship and reciprocal liking. Partners had well-integrated personalities and agreed on most external issues. They tended to be older, Protestant, in their first marriage, and from intact families. Couples in *financially focused* marriages (11 percent) were unhappy in their communication but stayed together for money and financial rewards. Careers were more important than the relationship, and financial management was their only relationship strength. Couples in *conflicted* marriages (14 percent) had unresolved conflicts between them but gained satisfaction from outside sources such as leisure, children, or friends. Couples in *traditional* marriages (10 percent) were moderately satisfied with their relatively stable relationship. These couples tended to be older, married longer, white, and Protestant. Their major sources of distress were sexual and communication conflicts. Couples in *balanced* marriages (8 percent) were moderately satisfied with their relationship, particularly in areas of communication and problem solving. Their source of distress was financial stability, whereas agreement occurred in areas such as leisure and child rearing. Couples in *harmonious* marriages (8 percent) were extremely satisfied with each other, including sexual and affectional dimensions. They tended to be self-centered and preferred to have no children. In all seven types, women were less satisfied than men in the relationships and were more likely to have considered divorce. Although generalizing to all types of relationships (heterosexual or homosexual)

has some inherent reliability and validity problems, this research has implications for all types of committed relationships.

Predicting Marital Success Olson and his colleagues also consolidated their typologies and attempted to predict marital success in premarital couples. Couples categorized as vitalized had a high degree of overall relationship satisfaction. They preferred egalitarian roles, viewed religion as important, resolved conflicts appropriately, and liked each other. Harmonious couples had a moderate level of relationship satisfaction. They liked their partner's personality and habits and enjoyed family and friends, and resolved conflicts appropriately. They did not view religion as important and had somewhat unrealistic expectations of relationships. Their strengths were in the areas of interpersonal communication and sexual relationships. Traditional couples had a moderate level of relationship dissatisfaction. They were realistic about the relationship, were least likely to have cohabitated before marriage, and placed a higher value on religion. Their strengths were in the area of children, family, and developing well-defined plans. Conflicted relationships reported dissatisfaction with the relationship. They disliked their partner's personality and habits and had problems with the sexual relationship and relating to their partner's family and friends. Results of Olson's longitudinal study showed that conflicted couples were more likely to cancel wedding plans or divorce if they got married, traditional couples were least likely to divorce or separate, and vitalized couples demonstrated more marital satisfaction after 3 years.[35]

Attitudes regarding keys to a successful marriage seem to have shifted over time in that the percentage of adults that consider children very important to a successful marriage is now much lower, while the sharing of household chores is considered as pivotal. A 2007 Pew Research Center survey of 2,020 adults on the topic of marriage and parenting found that "children had fallen to eighth out of nine on a list of factors that people associate with successful marriages—well behind 'sharing household chores,' 'good housing,' 'adequate income,' 'a happy sexual relationship,' and 'faithfulness.' In a 1990 World Values Survey, children ranked third in importance among the same items, with 65 percent saying children were very important to a good marriage. Just 41 percent said so in the 2007 Pew survey. Chore-sharing was cited as very important by 62 percent of respondents, up from 47 percent in 1990." The 2007 survey also found "that, by a margin of nearly 3-to-1, Americans say the main purpose of marriage is the 'mutual happiness and fulfillment' of adults rather than the bearing and raising of children."[36]

Peer Marriages Pepper Schwartz, coauthor of *American Couples,* coined the phrase **peer marriages** to describe egalitarian partnerships between two people. In a large research study of American couples, she found that true companionship came in the form of equity and equality with both partners sharing talents, resources, and decision-making skills. In these couples, both partners had equal say in major decisions and equal sharing of money decisions and discretionary funds, and they supported and valued each other's work. Peer couples enjoyed their mutual friendship and greater emotional intimacy and exhibited a stronger commitment and interdependence. The major difficulties faced by peer couples were the lack of role models, lack of support by others, and loss of passion. Near peers emulated these couples but differed in several key areas: when arguing, the male usually dominated; in child rearing, the male did not participate equally; and in money matters, the male still assumed a provider role.[37]

Coupled Households

The U.S. Census reported there were 64.3 million coupled households in 2010.[38] This number includes the total number of married (opposite-sex) couples (56.5 million) and unmarried-partner households (7.7 million), with unmarried-partner households including both unmarried opposite-sex couples (6.8 million) and unmarried same-sex couples (.9 million). At the time of the 2010 U.S. Census, the idea of "legally" married same-sex partners was a relatively new and widely rejected construct in the United States and, for the most part, still is with legal recognition in only a few states (see the latest on same-sex marriage laws at the Human Rights Campaign web site: www.hrc.org). The 2000 U.S. Census was the first in the history of the country to include unmarried same-sex partner households as a demographic variable. Even so, this number is still likely to be underreported given the fear by lesbians and gay men of discrimination or retaliation in a country that has a large number of persons who are homophobic or heterosexist.

Cohabitation, that is, unmarried-partner households, has greatly increased across time, and with this increase has come a need to study its impact on marital stability, family formations, race and ethnic differences, and single-parent or stepparent families. The U.S. Census Bureau recognizes that the current number of cohabiting couples, whether heterosexual or homosexual, continues to be underestimated (up to 10 percent of all households). In addition, many households with children are reported as "single parent" when they may actually be cohabiting couples. The increase in cohabitation is evidenced by the increased reporting of this arrangement in Census reports. Fewer than 500,000 people were unmarried and living together in

1970 compared to 5.4 million in 2000. There were a little over 6.5 million unmarried-partner households reported for 2009.[39] These households were reported with the following configurations: female householder and male partner—2.8 million; female householder and female partner—0.30 million; male householder and female partner—3.0 million; and male householder and male partner—0.28 million.

The U.S. Department of Health and Human Resources reported the percentage of women who were currently cohabiting (living with a man in a sexual relationship) rose from 3.0 percent in 1982 to 11 percent in 2006 to 2010 (the 4 years over which the National Survey of Family Growth was conducted).[40] This number was even higher in some groups, including Hispanic groups and the less educated. In 2006–2010, women and men married for the first time at older ages than in previous years. The median age at first marriage was 25.8 years for women and 28.3 for men. Premarital cohabitation contributed to the delay in first marriage for both women and men. Only half of cohabiting relationships end in marriage after 5 years.

The increase in cohabitation is one of the most significant shifts in family demographics of the past century.[41] Cohabitation has become much more common, with an estimated 50 to 60 percent of couples living together before marriage in the United States.[42] Yet, various research studies published from 2002 to 2004 showed cohabitation prior to marriage in the United States has been consistently associated with poorer marital communication quality, lower marital satisfaction, higher levels of domestic violence, and greater probability of divorce.[43] Though premarital cohabitation is now considered "the norm" the associated risks are not abating; the association between premarital cohabitation and poorer marital outcomes is known as the "cohabitation effect." Common characteristics of the "cohabitation effect" include more negative commitment in marriage, lower levels of marital satisfaction, erosion over time of the value and view of marriage and childrearing, and greater likelihood of divorce.[44]

The impact of the cohabitation effect is most pronounced for those who seem to "slide into marriage"; that is, they decide to go ahead and get married after they have already been cohabitating—referred to as the "cohabitation inertia effect."[45] A 2004 study found those who began cohabitating prior to marital engagement had more negative interactions, lower levels of interpersonal commitment to their partners, lower relationship quality, and lower levels of confidence in their relationship than those who cohabitated only after marital engagement or not at all before marriage.[46] A 2009 study published results of a random telephone survey of men and women (1050) married within the past 10 years that showed those who cohabitated before marital engagement (43.1 percent) reported lower marital satisfaction, dedication, and confidence as well as more negative communication and greater potential for divorce than those who cohabited only after marital engagement (16.4 percent) or not at all until marriage (40.5 percent).[47] There were no significant differences between those who cohabitated only after marital engagement and those who did not cohabitate before marriage. Thus, not cohabitating before marriage or only cohabitating after a formal commitment to marriage (engagement) seems to dampen the "cohabitation effect."

Researchers used data from the National Institute of Child Health and Human Development Study of Early Child Care and Youth Development to assess how cohabitation of unmarried two-biological-parent families is associated with characteristics of young children's family environment.[48] After controlling for demographic differences, researchers found that stably cohabitating mothers reported more depressive symptoms and were less sensitive with their children than were married mothers. They also found that cohabitating couple relationships were characterized by more ambivalence and conflict. Thus, family environment can be negatively affected by a cohabitation parental status.

For both women and men, there was a significant increase in the percentage of first births that occurred within a cohabitating union between 2002 and 2006–2010 (the 4 years over which was conducted the National Survey of Family Growth).[49] Among the 46 percent of first births that were premarital in 2006–2010, nearly one-half were to women in cohabitating unions. Nearly four of ten (39 percent) first births to Hispanic men and three of ten (30 percent) first births to Hispanic women were within cohabitating unions, the highest of any race and Hispanic origin group. The percentage of mothers who had a birth within a cohabitating relationship nearly doubled from 17 percent in 2002 to 30 percent in 2006–2010. The increase in births within a cohabitating relationship for men was more modest, rising from 25 percent to 33 percent.

Interracial and Mixed-Race Couples

In 1967 the U.S. Supreme Court overturned a Virginia antimiscegenation law, paving the way for interracial marriages in all geographic regions. Although many interracial marriages experience some discrimination, our society tends to exhibit more hostility toward unions between African Americans and other races than for unions between any other races. Non-Hispanic white unions with Asian Americans, Hispanics, or Native Americans are more tolerated than African American unions with non-Hispanic whites, Asian Americans, Hispanics, or Native Americans.[50]

The degree of discrimination, prejudice, and animosity these couples (and their children) will face depends, to some extent, on their socioeconomic status, the diversity within their community, and their educational status. Their relationship, particularly if they are an African American and white couple, faces demands not experienced by other couples, including other intermarriage groups. These demands create opportunities for extraordinary growth and maturity within the couple, as well as potential downfalls that can contribute to a higher than normal divorce rate. Couples who find themselves in interracial relationships need support and encouragement, not only from each other, but from friends and family. (See *Her Story:* "Michelle: An Interracial Relationship Encounters Family Bigotry.")

Children's identities are changing as the blurring of color lines is accelerating. Under pressure from mixed-race Americans, the U.S. Census Bureau changed its rules in 2000 to allow for selection of a new race/ethnicity category, that of biracial or multiracial. The increase in the number of biracial and multiracial children has presented a need to additionally consider cultural identity development from biracial and multiracial perspectives.[51]

The Pew Research Center's analysis of data from the U.S. Census Bureau's American Community Survey in 2008 to 2010 and findings from three of the center's own nationwide telephone surveys that explore attitudes toward intermarriage lead to the following conclusions.[52] About 15 percent of all new marriages in the United States in 2010 were between spouses of a different race or ethnicity from one another, more than double the share in 1980 (6.7 percent). Among all newlyweds in 2010, 9 percent of whites, 17 percent of blacks, 26 percent of Hispanics, and 28 percent of Asians married outside of their race or ethnicity. Looking at all married couples in 2010, regardless of when they married, the share of intermarriages reached an all-time high of 8.4 percent; in 1980, that share was just 3.2 percent. Regarding gender patterns, about 24 percent of all black male newlyweds in 2010 married outside their race, compared with just 9 percent of black female newlyweds. Among Asians, the gender pattern runs the other way. About 36 percent of Asian female newlyweds married outside their race in 2010, compared with just 17 percent of Asian male newlyweds. Intermarriage rates among white and Hispanic newlyweds do not vary by gender. When viewed as two large groups, recent newlyweds who married outside their race and those who married inside their race have similar characteristics regarding income and education. In 2008 to 2010, the median combined annual earnings of both groups are similar: $56,711 for newlyweds who "married out" versus $55,000 for those who "married in." In about one in five marriages of each group, both the husband and wife are college graduates. Spouses in the two groups marry at similar ages (with a 2- to 3-year age gap between husband and wife), and an equal share are marrying for the first time. When examining the data further by race/ethnicity subgroups some sharp differences do emerge. For example, white/Asian newlyweds of 2008 through 2010 have significantly higher median combined annual earnings ($70,952) than do any other pairing, including both white/white ($60,000) and Asian/Asian ($62,000). Regarding educational characteristics, more than half of white newlyweds who marry Asians have a college degree, compared with roughly a third of white newlyweds who married whites. Among Hispanics and blacks, newlyweds who married whites tend to have higher educational attainment than do those who married within their own racial or ethnic group. There are regional differences regarding intermarriage that tends to tilt west. About one in five (22 percent) of all newlyweds in Western states married someone of a different race or ethnicity between 2008 and 2010, compared with 14 percent in the South, 13 percent in the Northeast, and 11 percent in the Midwest.

Is more intermarriage viewed as good for society? In 2008–2010, more than four in ten Americans (43 percent) said that more people of different races marrying each other has been a change for the better in our society, while 11 percent said it has been a change for the worse, and 44 percent said it has made no difference.[53] Minorities, younger adults, the college-educated, and those who describe themselves as liberal and those who live in the Northeast or the West are more disposed than others to see intermarriage in a positive light. More than one-third of Americans (35 percent) said that a member of their immediate family or a close relative is currently married to someone of a different race. Also, nearly two-thirds of Americans (63 percent) said it "would be fine" with them if a member of their own family were to marry someone outside their own racial or ethnic group. In 1986, nearly three in ten Americans (28 percent) said people of different races marrying each other was not acceptable for anyone, 37 percent said this may be acceptable for others, but not for themselves, and only one-third of the public (33 percent) viewed intermarriage as acceptable for everyone.

Lesbian Couples

The U.S. Census Bureau estimates from the 2010 Census, there were 131,729 same-sex married couple households and 514,735 same-sex unmarried partner households in the United States.[54] Lesbian couples have a unique opportunity to experience the best and also the most challenging aspects of what it means to be "female" in a relationship.[55] For lesbians,—both partners are relationship-focused. This focus encourages equality and equity, regardless of whether they are in a committed, long-term relationship or an intimate friendship.

Her Story

Michelle: An Interracial Relationship Encounters Family Bigotry

Michelle, a 24-year-old senior, met Tony at a nightclub. She found him physically attractive, but more important, she enjoyed talking with him. When she discussed her work, he showed genuine interest. When he asked her out on a date, she wondered what her parents would think. They never told Michelle that she could not date a black man. But she could recall a time when she was 9 or 10 years old and her father commented negatively about an interracial couple at a restaurant. However, she decided to go ahead with the date.

Michelle told her mother about Tony immediately but waited nearly 6 months before telling her dad. Her mother was pretty open-minded about it, but her father could not accept it. She had always been "Daddy's little girl," had followed the path that made him happy, and now, she just couldn't understand his feelings. Maybe with some time, he would accept it. Why didn't he trust her to make the right decisions for herself?

They had been dating for 2.5 years when Michelle became pregnant. It wasn't planned, but they were excited about having a baby. Michelle would be graduating soon, and Tony had an excellent job as a business consultant. Her mother handled the news pretty well; she didn't like the idea that they weren't married. Her dad, however, went through the roof . . . he said he hadn't accepted the relationship so he most certainly wasn't going to accept this! He didn't even want her in the house anymore; he didn't want to see her. Michelle was devastated; how could he treat his own daughter this way? Would her baby ever know her grandfather? What should she tell her little girl as she grew up and wanted to know about her grandparents?

- How would your parents respond to an interracial grandchild?
- What would you do if you were in Michelle's situation?

However, lesbians, by virtue of being same-sex couples, encounter additional challenges in their relationships. One potential difficulty is maintaining personal boundaries, which easily can become blurred when both partners focus on emotional intimacy and exclude personal autonomy. Maintaining balance between autonomy and intimacy is an important consideration. Another potential difficulty for lesbian couples is the lack of adequate role models for "peer relationships." Within the lesbian community, long-term relationships are often "closeted," particularly among older lesbians who grew up during more discriminatory times. Many lesbian couples form committed relationships but do not receive the same benefits as married couples, for example, health insurance, help in finding a job for one partner when the other is relocated, tax benefits, and family support.

In the past, lesbian couples didn't have the option of raising children unless one or both partners had children from a previous heterosexual relationship. Today, the number of lesbian couples choosing to have children is rising steadily, and their options include adoption, artificial insemination, or other arrangements. Children provide the same parental bond for lesbian couples as they do for heterosexual couples but may create some additional parenting issues.[56] Difficulty can arise when others, particularly those opposed to lesbian lifestyles, question the ability or right of lesbians to raise children. They suggest that children raised in a same-sex household may differ from other children emotionally or that the children may be raised to be lesbians or gay. A study comparing men and women raised by heterosexual single mothers and lesbian mothers found that these young adults exhibited similar behavioral patterns regardless of the sexual orientation of the parent. Almost all (including twenty-three of twenty-five lesbian-raised adults) described themselves as heterosexual and indicated a desire for marriage and children.[57]

Support for equal rights for same-sex couples seems to be on the rise in the United States, while opposition to same-sex marriage is on the decline. The Pew Research Center for the People and the Press conducted a poll in 2012 of individuals in the United States regarding public opinion regarding same-sex marriage.[58] Results showed 47 percent favor allowing gays and lesbians to marry legally, while 43 percent are opposed. The public has gradually become more supportive of granting legal recognition to same-sex marriages over the past 15 years, with support increasing more steeply in recent years—39 percent were in favor in 2008, while 31 percent were in favor in 2004. Religious groups show the greatest opposition toward legal same-sex marriage, but a Pew Research Center poll in 2011 showed there to be some differences in opinion between the various religions.[59] White, evangelical Protestants express the greatest opposition to same-sex marriage, with 74 percent saying they oppose allowing gay and lesbian couples to marry legally. A large majority of black Protestants also oppose same-sex marriage (62 percent). The views of these two groups have not changed since 2010. Compared with evangelicals and black Protestants, white mainline Protestants are more supportive of same-sex marriage, with 54 percent saying they favor allowing gay and lesbian couples to get legally married; this is an increase from 49 percent in favor in 2010. Among Catholics as a whole, supporters of same-sex marriage now outnumber opponents (53 percent versus 37 percent). This is a change from 2010 where Catholics were more evenly divided on the issue, with 46 percent favoring same-sex marriage and 42 percent expressing opposition.

The Human Rights Campaign lists 10 top reasons for same-sex marriage equality:

1. There are at least 1049 protections, benefits, and responsibilities extended to married couples under federal law, according to a 1997 study by the General Accounting Office.
2. No religious institution would be required to perform a ceremony.
3. The Constitution promises liberty and justice for all Americans, not just the majority.
4. There are hundreds of ways in which state laws take marital status into account, including some of the most basic of human rights.
5. Marriage provides families stability and security.
6. Gay, lesbian, bisexual, and transgender (GLBT) people deserve equal access to the American dream.
7. Public support is growing.
8. Separate is not equal.
9. Marriage protects couples nationwide (recognized across state lines).
10. Marriage equality would build on America's tradition of moving civil rights forward and erasing the inequities of the past.[60]

The Human Rights Campaign reports the cost of marriage inequality for same-sex couples is compounded for seniors.[61] The loss of Social Security benefits for surviving partners amounts to an average loss of $5,528 each year. Surviving partners are routinely forced to pay tens of thousands of dollars in taxes when they inherit a retirement plan from an unmarried partner, while married spouses in the same situation are charged no taxes at all. A surviving gay, lesbian, or bisexual partner is charged an estate tax on the couple's home, even if the house had been jointly owned. In conclusion, the report stated, "Equality in access to marriage, and the many benefits and protections that go with it, would bring equity to the taxation of and benefits provided to all seniors, regardless of sexual orientation. Specifically, granting same-sex couples the right to marry would guarantee that the 'widows' and 'widowers' of same-sex couples would not be hit with undue estate tax and income tax burdens—nor deprived of Social Security survivor benefits—upon the death of a partner. Marriage equality also would decrease the risk of losing their homes that gay, lesbian, and bisexual seniors now face when a partner enters a nursing home or dies."[62]

Bisexual Couples

An estimated 3.5 percent of adults in the United States identify as lesbian, gay, or bisexual and an estimated 0.3 percent identify as transgender.[63] This implies that there are approximately 9 million LGBT Americans. Among adults who identify as LGB, bisexuals comprise a slight majority (1.8 percent compared to 1.7 percent who identify as lesbian or gay). Women are substantially more likely than men to identify as bisexual. Bisexuals comprise more than half of the lesbian and bisexual population among women. Conversely, gay men comprise substantially more than half of gay and bisexual men. Estimates of those who report any lifetime same-sex sexual behavior and any same-sex sexual attraction are substantially higher than estimates of those who identify as LGB. An estimated 19 million Americans (8.3 percent) report that they have engaged in same-sex sexual behavior and nearly 25.6 million Americans (11 percent) acknowledge at least some same-sex attraction.

Bisexuals have no preference of attraction for one gender over the other. They form a relationship based on love, attraction, and compatibility, regardless of the gender of their partner. Bisexuals have had relationships with both genders. Bisexuals are an often misunderstood minority, relative to couple formations. When a bisexual woman is partnered with a man, she is viewed by many in society as heterosexual; and when she is partnered with a woman, she is viewed by many as homosexual. When and if she should, through the course of dating, move from one spectrum, say an opposite-sex partner, to the other spectrum, a same-sex partner (or vice versa), she risks losing the friendships and associates from the prior relationship. This is because our current social structure does not tolerate ambiguity very well and there is pressure to belong to a well-defined group. A bisexual woman rarely receives, but from the most open-minded associates, recognition and acceptance for her true relationship identity, that of a bisexual. Because, today, society does not readily accept the idea of bisexuality, bisexuals often do not receive the type and amount of support and encouragement that heterosexual or homosexual coupled relationships receive from their own cohort. Because of a lack of positive recognition and support, bisexuals may feel as if they do not belong to any group and may struggle with a sexual identity. It is helpful for a bisexual woman to focus on developing a sound self-concept as a bisexual woman and, if necessary, invest in strengthening her own self-esteem and self-confidence in relationships.[64] To do this, she may need to surround herself with friends and associates who accept and understand her. She may even want to seek assistance from a mental health counselor to help her on her journey of self-acceptance. Another potential concern is that a bisexual's current relationship partner may feel threatened by the bisexual's lack of gender preference and thus the partner may experience anxiety that he or she may not be able to fulfill the bisexual's desires. This lingering fear may degrade the quality of the relationship if it is not addressed by both partners, and couples counseling may be a viable option in this case. A further demonstration of a bisexual's potential frustration with society's views on relationships is that when in a relationship with a partner of the opposite sex, the bisexual has the option of legal marriage, but when in a relationship with a partner of the same sex, the bisexual does not have the option of legal marriage, except in just a few states in the United States.

Transgender Couples

Transgendered persons have a sexual identity different from their sexual physiology. A transgendered woman feels trapped inside a body that is physiologically male. She feels more comfortable dressing, acting, and living as a woman; this can be complicated, since her sexual physiology does not match her lifestyle. A transgendered man feels trapped inside a body that is physiologically female and he feels more comfortable living the lifestyle of a male. A transgender couple can have one or both partners who are transgendered. Transgender couples face unique legal issues with regard to marriage. The way many U.S. state laws are worded, a transgender person can enter into a legal marriage with either a same-sex partner or an opposite sex partner.

Some people are aware that transgender individuals are often able to enter into a heterosexual marriage after undergoing sex-reassignment. What may be less well-known, however, is that a transgender person may also be married to a person of the same sex. The situation arises, for example, when one of the spouses in a heterosexual marriage comes out as transsexual and transitions within the marriage. If the couple chooses to stay together, as many do, the result is a legal marriage in which both spouses are male or female. Alternatively, in states that do not allow a transgender person to change his or her legal sex, some transgender people have been able to marry a person of the same sex. To all outward appearances and to the couple themselves, the marriage is a same-sex union. In the eyes of the law, however, it is a different-sex marriage because technically speaking, the law continues to view the transgender spouse as a legal member of his or her birth sex even after sex-reassignment. In short, marriage is a very real option for a variety of transgender people in a variety of circumstances.[65]

Transgender people often experience a lack of societal understanding and support. By some unenlightened individuals, a transgendered person is viewed as abnormal and ostracized. For this reason, many transgender people may keep their situation a secret from those who they feel may not understand or accept them. Being transgendered can be very stressful, most especially if one does not have a supportive environment.[66] A study of transgender youth aged 15 to 21 reported 45 percent had thought seriously of killing themselves, and half of these said their thoughts were related to their transgender status. Those who had attempted suicide, compared with those who had not, had experienced more physical and verbal abuse from their parents.[67] Another study of transgender persons of all ages found that 83 percent of transgender people had thought about suicide and 54 percent had attempted it.[68] The greatest risk factors for attempted suicide for transgender individuals were found to be: younger (under age 25), depression or history of substance abuse, forced sex, and gender-based victimization and discrimination[69] (see *Her Story*: "Janet Mock, a Transgender Woman").

It is fortunate that today's medicine can offer transgendered persons the option to change their sexual physiology to more closely match their sexual identity, if they choose. But available sex-change procedures, some hormonal and some surgical, can be very uncomfortable and expensive. This is the reason why many transgendered persons choose not to undergo actual physiological transformation. It is highly recommended, and required by most physicians, that transgendered persons receive mental health counseling prior to making the decision to undergo physiological sex change procedures.

TROUBLED RELATIONSHIPS

When a relationship gets into trouble, a variety of patterns can ensue that exacerbate existing problems and prevent resolution. As conflict and distress increase, the familiar pattern occurs more quickly, and partners become more entrenched in their role of perpetuating the pattern. Couples continue to cycle through these patterns until the relationship ends or they seek help.

Terminating a Relationship

The National Center for Health Statistics estimated rates for divorces and annulments in the United States shows the trend has slowed somewhat since the year 2000 (rates per 1000 population): 2010, 3.6; 2009, 3.5; 2008,

Her Story

Janet Mock, A Transgender Woman[70]

Janet Mock, a People.com editor and popular blogger, came out as a transgender woman in 2011. Mock was born with a male body, but she identified as female from a young age and was lucky to have friends and a mother who supported her. She began taking estrogen in high school and saved enough money for gender reassignment surgery by winter break of her freshman year at college. Thus, many of the people in her adult life, including coworkers, did not know about her past. In addition to coming out publicly, Mock has created an It Gets Better video and is working on a memoir about her journey—she says that telling her story has helped her celebrate her history, "I have a thriving career as a Web editor for a very popular magazine. My coworkers don't know about my past, mostly because I never wanted to be the poster child for transsexuals—pre-op, post-op, or no-op. But the recent stories about kids who have killed themselves because of the secrets they were forced to keep has shifted something in me. That's why I decided to come out in the pages of *Marie Claire*, why I'm writing a memoir about my journey. It used to pain me to hear my birth name, a heartbreaking insult classroom bullies would shout to get a rise out of me. But talking and writing about my experiences have helped me finally accept the past and celebrate the fact that I was once a big dreamer who happened to be born a boy named Charles. I hope my story resonates with other big dreamers, lets them know that no matter how huge, how insane, how unreasonable or unreachable your goals may seem, nothing—not even your own body—can hold you back if you are certain and fearless and, yes a little ballsy in your quest."

3.5; 2007, 3.6; 2006, 3.7; 2005, 3.6; 2004, 3.7; 2003, 3.8; 2002, 3.9; 2001, 4.0; 2000, 4.0.[71] It is believed this slower trend is at least partially a result of the decline in marriage rates over this same period: 2010, 6.8; 2009, 6.8; 2008, 7.1; 2007, 7.3; 2006, 7.5; 2005, 7.6; 2004, 7.8; 2003, 7.7; 2002, 8.0; 2001, 8.2; 2000, 8.2. According to the U.S. Census Bureau, men and women in the South had higher rates of divorce in 2009 than in other regions of the country (10.2 and 11.1); in contrast men and women in the Northeast had the lowest rates of divorce (7.2 and 7.5).[72] Divorce rates tend to be higher in the South because marriage rates are also higher in the South; in contrast, in the Northeast, first marriages tend to be delayed and the marriage rates are lower, meaning there are also fewer divorces. The U.S. Census Bureau reported the rate of first divorce in the United States was 17.6 per 1000 women 18 years and older in a first marriage.[73] Research from the National Center for Family and Marriage Research shows there is substantial variation in the first-time divorce rate when it is broken down by race and education.[74] Regarding first-divorce rates and race or ethnicity, the study found that Asian women have the lowest rate, 10.0 divorces per 1000, in a first marriage. The first-divorce rates of white and Hispanic women are somewhat similar at 16.3 and 18.1, respectively. African American women have substantially higher rates of first divorce compared to all other racial and ethnic groups, at 30.4 divorces per 1000 women in a first marriage. The association between education and first-divorce is curvilinear with the least (no high school diploma or GED) and the highest (college degree) educated women sharing the lowest rate of divorce, with 14.4 and 14.2 per 1000, respectively. With the exception of Asians, the highest rate of first divorce was among women with some college, regardless of race or ethnicity.

Divorce is one of the most stressful things a person can go through in life. The emotional and financial effects of divorce are generally greater for women than for men. A research study found divorced middle-aged women are 60 percent more likely to get cardiovascular disease—even when they remarry—than women who remain married; divorce, however, does not increase the odds of heart disease among middle-aged men.[75] Emotional distress and a decline in financial status were the main factors linking divorce to heart disease in women. The effects of divorce did not go away with time, showing divorce's effects on women's cardiovascular health appear to linger long after the divorce. Researchers of the study "found that divorced women have the lowest household income and wealth, compared to married women, widows and women who remarry. Divorce clearly leads to a drop in financial resources. Add that to the emotional distress that can stem from a change in residence, loss of social support or the potential of single parenting, and divorced middle-aged women are facing incredible stress that puts them at a distinct disadvantage when it comes to their cardiovascular health."[76]

Women are especially vulnerable to the effects of divorce if they are older women, ending a long-term relationship, have limited work experience, or have relied on the husband as the wage earner. Information about the financial and emotional effects of breakups on cohabiting women supports a similar trend. Cohabiting women have the added burden of limited or no legal remedies. These women may experience more difficulty in gaining emotional support than divorcing women because their relationships are less acceptable or recognized by the general population. A breakup of a relationship (lesbian, cohabiting, or divorcing) can cause a number of disruptive consequences in women's lives, including depression, lower self-esteem, anxiety, feelings of betrayal or abandonment, as well as changes in child rearing, career decisions, finances, and housing.

Love Addiction

The idea that love might be connected to "addiction" seems contradictory; however, loving relationships built on healthy emotional and physical intimacy differ significantly from "addictive," incomplete relationships built on faulty thinking and feeling. This addictive pattern has been described as love/avoidance addiction.[77] It occurs when one partner, the **love addict,** feels the need to be rescued and the other partner, the **avoidance addict,** attempts to avoid involvement with the partner. The primary fear of the love addict is abandonment; the primary fear of the avoidance addict is intimacy. The secondary fear of each is reversed, thus both have the same two fears: abandonment and intimacy. Unless both partners make a concerted effort to break these cycles (usually through making conscious decisions to understand and change behaviors that contribute to these patterns), the relationship will deteriorate further until one partner leaves.

Potential Sources of Conflict

Conflict is a ubiquitous aspect of any close relationship—it is common, and to be expected. There are many common areas of what couples fight about. One researcher studied, over a 1-year period, both partners from 75 gay, 51 lesbian, and 108 heterosexual couples who did not reside with children and discovered the couple types were very similar in (a) how often and about what they would commonly argue about and (b) how this related to current relationship satisfaction, and overall relationship satisfaction across the 1-year period.[78] Couple scores fell into six clusters that represented areas of conflict regarding power, social issues, personal flaws, distrust, intimacy, and personal distance. Each partner's current relationship satisfaction was strongly negatively related to the frequency of arguing in areas reflecting power and intimacy. And a decrease in each partner's relationship satisfaction over a 1-year period was linked to frequent arguing in the area of power.

Imbalance of Power An imbalance of power in a relationship can cause distress and distrust that results in relationship conflict. Imbalance of power results when one of the partners is seeking "power over" rather than both partners promoting "personal power" for each other.[79] Implementing power over someone in a relationship can take many forms and may include self-absorption, excessive ambition, feelings of inferiority or superiority, criticism, contempt, or defensiveness. Self-absorbed partners always put their own needs ahead of their partner's needs. They are unable or unwilling to meet their partner's needs if those needs interfere with their own. A partner with excessive ambition will make getting ahead in the material world a higher priority than the relationship. Most women prefer intimacy and relationship, not goals connected to ambition. Whether a partner has feelings of inferiority or superiority, she is masking the usnderlying malady, low self-esteem. The behaviors and interaction with a partner will manifest differently, but the root cause is the same. A partner with feelings of inferiority will defer to her partner because she believes he has more rights, is more knowledgeable, or is more deserving. A partner with feelings of superiority will believe she has more rights, knows more, and "is more" than her partner. A critical partner attacks his partner for who she is rather than her behaviors. This type of attack can certainly be construed as emotional abuse of a partner and creates few opportunities for changing the pattern. A partner who feels contempt for his partner can intentionally hurt her with words or actions. A partner exhibiting defensiveness may deny responsibility or make excuses for his actions. If she complains, his complaint will be louder, stronger, worse, one better. He may "dig in" on his position and not see any alternatives. The distancer will put up a wall and shut the other person out with silence. This position inhibits emotional intimacy and keeps the other person "guessing."

A number of warning signs may signal a troubled relationship, including an increase in physical symptoms by a partner, an increase in alcohol or drug consumption, silence or emotional withdrawal by a partner, more frequent arguments, more fantasies of separation, or more divergent lives. These signs may manifest in actual behaviors such as a partner's affair, lying or other deceit, inattentiveness, lack of sexual interest, outside influences, and illegal activity. Several of these behaviors and issues are described in the following sections.

External Affair Sexual infidelity may occur for different reasons. Some affairs result because expectations were not met; others are viewed as a payback or punishment; whereas others involve emotional intimacy and closeness. The four words, "I'm having an affair" can be a wake-up call or a death knell to relationships. These words and the act itself certainly signal problems in a relationship. Affairs exacerbate the problems that currently exist, and the person isn't necessarily running to something as much as running away from something. A common reason why a woman has an affair is "I wanted more warmth and intimacy." According to biological anthropologist Helen Fisher, and author of *Why*

We Love, women tend to have an emotional connection with their lover and are more likely to have an affair because of loneliness; in contrast, men are more likely to cite sexual motivations for infidelity and are less likely to fall in love with an extramarital partner.[80] Women who have an extramarital affair tend to be more unhappy with the relationship they are in, while men can be a lot happier in their primary relationship and also cheat. Women are more interested in supplementing their marriage or jumping ship than men are—for men, it is a secondary strategy as opposed to an alternate. In one of her studies, Fisher found only 34 percent of women who had affairs were happy or very happy in their marriage, while a much greater percentage of men who had affairs, 56 percent, were happy in their marriage.

In one study of dating, cohabiting, and married women, the researchers found that the length of a relationship and number of previous partners were positively related to the potential for a secondary sex partner.[81] Women who had four or more sex partners before the current relationship were nearly ten times more likely to have another sex partner. Married women with multiple previous partners were twenty times more likely than their counterparts with no previous partners to have a secondary sex partner. And, as the length of the relationship increased, the potential for a secondary sex partner also increased. The researchers found that cohabiting women were less committed than married women to monogamy. Four percent of married women compared to 20 percent of cohabiting women had a secondary sex partner.

Nonmonogamy within the relationship, whether heterosexual or lesbian, increases the likelihood of a breakup. Although an affair has the potential to destroy a relationship, it doesn't have to end the relationship. The end of an affair can be the new beginning to an existing relationship. The outcome depends on the willingness of both individuals to work through broken expectations.

Money Research has shown that the most frequently reported issue that couples argue about in first marriages was money (in re-marriages it was conflict about children).[82] Money issues are often a major consideration because the amount of money earned determines power within the relationship. And power equates with freedom to make important decisions.

The key to resolving money issues in a relationship is understanding one's own habits and communicating with a partner regarding the management of money and power within the relationship. A couple must set joint priorities and appreciate the differences that exist in philosophy and patterns of handling money. (See *Viewpoint:* "Spending Differences Can Impact Relationships.")

Viewpoint

Spending Differences Can Impact Relationships

Money conflicts within relationships are common, particularly if expectations differ when it comes to the management and control of money. Money harmony is difficult to maintain and requires flexibility and communication. Olivia Mellan, author of *Money Harmony: Resolving Money Conflicts in Your Life and Relationships*, calls money harmony "a balanced state in which both partners feel free to spend, save, or invest money in ways that support their deeper desires, values, and sense of themselves."[83] Money harmony can occur only if partners are willing to discuss and explore their beliefs and behaviors related to money. Mellan identified seven common money personality types: spenders, hoarders, avoiders, amassers, money monks, worriers, and bingers. Spenders use the slogans "shop till you drop" or "power shopping." This person enjoys spending and has a hard time saving money. Hoarders are the misers, the stingy money savers who put money away for a rainy day. The miser has a strict budget and will not part with her money unless absolutely

necessary. Managing money is a difficult, overwhelming task for avoiders. This person waits until the last minute to pay her bills and often is late with her payments. She is overwhelmed by the concept of budgeting and saving, thus seldom budgets or saves. Amassers base their self-worth on net worth. An amasser will accumulate money to feel good about herself, and workaholism is common. Money monks view the love of money as the "root of all evil," therefore they tend to give money to socially worthwhile projects or religious endeavors. They seldom accumulate money so as to avoid the temptation of valuing it too highly. Worriers, on the other hand, see money as a scarcity and are extremely cautious. They review the budget and expenditures over and over, looking for corners to cut or making sure to account for every dime. Bingers use money to fill an emotional need, and the "rush" that comes from spending money dissipates with the empty feelings that follow the binge.

How proactive is your money management style?

Household Labor Gender is the major criterion used by heterosexual couples for the distribution of household tasks and child rearing. Women do the majority of household tasks and child rearing, estimated at two to three times that of men. Even for couples who appear to divide household labor more equally, men do not assume more responsibility; instead, women, in effect, choose to do less. This condition of inequity exists irrespective of education, income, and presence of children. The assigning of tasks based on gender may be efficient, but it often relegates women to subordinate roles in the relationship, leading to depression and a sense of powerlessness. Women who feel relegated to this role and powerless to change it are more likely to experience psychological distress. This sense of inequality can lead to marital distress, and in a larger sense, gender inequalities within the relationship (unpaid household labor and child care) may produce gender inequalities outside the relationship.[84] Research has found that lesbian couples are more careful to divide household labor equally (maybe because few women enjoy doing these tasks) than married or male gay couples.[85] This equal sharing of responsibility for menial tasks and sense of personal power in choosing to share the tasks acts as a protective factor in preventing emotional distress.

Resolving Conflicts—Fighting Fair

How couples fight or handle fundamental disagreements has been shown to be a major predictor of whether the relationship will last. John Gottman, founder of the Gottman Relationship Institute, studied 73 couples at two time points, 4 years apart, and discovered a typology of five groups of couples who differed by marital interactions.[86] There were two groups of unstable couples: hostile and hostile/detached, who could be distinguished from each other on problem-solving behavior and on specific negative and positive emotions. There were three groups of stable couples: validators, volatiles, and avoiders, who could be distinguished from each other on problem-solving behavior, specific emotions, and persuasion attempts.

Validators would discuss their differences, attempting to understand the other's viewpoint, and strive to reach a compromise. Volatile reactors shouted at each other and attempted to outmaneuver their partner to a position of submission. Conflict avoiders, the least successful of the three types, did everything possible to avoid conflict. When disagreements occurred, these couples just agreed to disagree, not looking for compromise or a change in stance of the other partner. John Gottman and Robert Levenson designed a model that accurately predicted divorce over a 14-year period with

93 percent accuracy.[87] Couples who were negative during conflict early in their marriages were more likely to divorce early in their marriages. Couples who were disengaged or had a lack of emotions in events-of-the-day and conflict discussions predicted later divorcing, rather than earlier divorcing in the marriage.

Gottman and Levenson conducted a 12-year longitudinal research study of twenty-one gay couples and twenty-one lesbian couples.[88] They found that satisfaction and stability in gay and lesbian relationships are related to similar emotional qualities as in heterosexual relationships. Their research did uncover some differences, however. Gay and lesbian couples are more upbeat in the face of conflict. Compared to heterosexual couples, gay and lesbian couples use more affection and humor when they bring up a disagreement, and partners are more positive in how they receive it. Gay and lesbian couples are also more likely to remain positive after a disagreement. Gay and lesbian couples use fewer controlling, hostile emotional tactics than heterosexual couples. Gottman and Levenson also discovered that gay and lesbian partners display less belligerence, domineering and fear with each other than heterosexual couples do. The researchers suggest that fairness and power-sharing between the partners is more important and more common in gay and lesbian relationships than in heterosexual relationships. In a fight, gay and lesbian couples take it less personally. In heterosexual couples, it is easier to hurt a partner with a negative comment than to make one's partner feel good with a positive comment. This appears to be reversed in gay and lesbian couples. Gay and lesbian partner's positive comments have more impact on feeling good, while their negative comments are less likely to produce hurt feelings. Unhappy gay and lesbian couples tend to show low levels of physiological arousal. This is just the reverse for heterosexual couples whose physiological arousal signifies ongoing aggravation. For gay and lesbian couples this lower level of arousal shows they are able to soothe one another. Gottman and Levenson found differences in how gay versus lesbian couples express themselves in conflict; these differences were mostly attributed to gender differences. In a fight, lesbians show more anger, humor, excitement and interest than conflicting gay men. This suggests that lesbians are more emotionally expressive, both positively and negatively, than gay men. Gay men need to be especially careful to avoid negativity in conflict. If the initiator of conflict in a gay relationship becomes too negative, his partner is not able to repair as effectively as lesbian or heterosexual partners.

In *The Dance of Anger*, psychologist Harriet Lerner discussed some ineffective techniques women may use to handle anger.[89] These techniques (silent submission, ineffective fighting and blaming, and emotional distancing) are used by women to keep a relationship harmonious, but often at the expense of authenticity. These patterns happen during times of stress or overload and may change depending on the individual with whom the woman is arguing. The patterns of expressing anger are classified as pursuers, distancers, underfunctioners, and overfunctioners. Pursuers value talking through an issue and want a partner to do the same. They seek closeness when disagreements occur and feel hurt when the other person seeks distance. Distancers want to be left alone, emotionally and physically, when disagreements occur. They attempt to figure things out away from the pressure of the moment. They address the issue again when they are ready. Underfunctioners appear weak and submissive, fragile, or irresponsible. They fall apart under stress and become disorganized or nonfunctional. They have difficulty appearing competent to those close to them. Overfunctioners are the "fixers" who give advice and move in quickly to resolve a dispute.

The first step in fair fighting requires that both partners agree to engage in the discussion. When they are willing to engage in the discussion, the partner with the complaint should state it clearly and ask for what is needed or wanted. When the other person has heard and restated the complaint, several options are available: agree to the request, ask for clarification, offer an alternative, or agree to disagree (say no). Successful negotiation occurs when both parties have heard each other and have committed to change the pattern, found an acceptable compromise, or have reached an agreement to disagree.[90] Difficulties arise in all relationships; the difference between successful and unsuccessful resolution is the willingness of both partners to openly share their concerns and negotiate for change.

Marshall Rosenberg's *Nonviolent Communication: A Language of Life* describes an approach to communication that enhances both personal and other awareness of needs and desires that may contaminate our communication. Rosenberg's "NVC process" assists to transform conflict into mutually satisfying outcomes by defusing anger and frustration peacefully and teaching how to create personal and professional relationships grounded in mutual respect, compassion, and emotional safety.[91] NVC involves an exploration of four components:

- The concrete actions we *observe* that affect our well-being
- How we *feel* in relation to what we observe
- The *needs*, values, desires, etc. that create our feelings
- The concrete actions we *request* in order to enrich our lives

The two major parts of NVC focus on teaching a person to (1) express honestly through the four components and (2) receive empathically through the four components.[92]

Couples in conflict may benefit from attending psycho-educational groups designed to enhance effective relationship communication and conflict resolution. In addition, a mental health counselor who specializes in couples counseling can be very beneficial in assisting a couple to resolve conflicts and obtain greater relationship satisfaction. Couples in the early stages of their relationship may be able to avoid many conflicts by participating in couples counseling to learn how to communicate effectively before major conflicts arise.

CELEBRATING MOTHERHOOD

On Sunday, May 11, 2008, the Mother's Day celebration reached its 100th anniversary. The woman credited for the idea of having a "Mother's Day" was Anna Jarvis, who got the idea after her mother said it would be nice if someone created a memorial to mothers.[93] "Three years after her mother died in 1905, she organized the first official mother's day service at a church where her mother had spent more than 20 years teaching Sunday school," the Andrews Methodist Episcopal Church located in Grafton, Taylor County, West Virginia—this is considered the "mother church" of

Mother's Day and it was incorporated as the International Mother's Day Shrine on May 15, 1962, as a tribute to all mothers. West Virginia became the first state to recognize Mother's Day in 1910. President Woodrow Wilson approved a resolution in 1914 marking the second Sunday in May a nationwide observance. Now Mother's Day is celebrated on the second Sunday in May in 52 countries.

In 2008, there were 85.4 million mothers of all ages in the United States.[95] The average number of children that women in the United States aged 40 to 44 had given birth to as of 2008 was 2.3; this was down from 3.4 children in 1976, the year the Census Bureau began collecting such data. The percentage of women aged 40 to 44 who had given birth as of 2008 was 82 percent; this was down from 90 percent in 1976.[96] There were 5 million stay-at-home mothers nationwide in 2010; this was down from 5.1 million in 2009, and 5.3 million in 2008.[97] Stay-at-home mothers were more likely to be

- Younger (44 percent were under 35 compared with 38 percent of mothers in the labor force).
- Hispanic (27 percent compared with 16 percent of mothers in the labor force).
- Foreign-born (34 percent compared with 19 percent of mothers in the labor force).

Women Making a Difference

Working Mother of the Year

WorkingMother.com has announced its Working Mother of the Year awards for 2008. One recipient is Beth Hope, age 47. She is the founder of Hope House and vice president of sales for Autoland in Woodland Hills, California. She is the mother of Erin, 19, Sean, 14, Brittany, 11, and Connor, 6. Beth started Hope House because of her concern for homeless women on the streets. "She'd not only stop and offer a sandwich and some money, sometimes she offered her sofa". Friends suggested that Beth formalize her good deeds, so in 1989 she took out a personal loan and rented a suburban house for homeless women that was soon filled with extraordinary stories. Tormented by everything from drug addiction to domestic abuse, the women at Hope House have for 17 years benefited from food, shelter, medical care and links to public programs that can help them turn their lives around. Beth's empathy comes from a personal place. She was born and raised in Monterey, CA, by a single mother who worked three jobs. Beth attended an excellent school on full scholarship and then moved to Los Angeles, where she earned a bachelor's degree from UCLA. After that, she waited tables to save money for law school. But a serendipitous

encounter with a customer changed all of that: The owner of Autoland, the nation's largest credit-union auto-buying service, was so impressed with Beth (her ability to push the dessert tray was notorious) that he hired her. 'The rest is history,' says Beth, who 21 years later is vice president of sales ($270 million yearly!)." Beth's daughter, Brittany, who nominated her mom for this award, said that even with her many work and home demands her mom gives some special time to each of her children. Brittany wrote in her nomination that, "Beth sees it this way: 'I want my children to know that not everyone has it as good as they do, and those of us who have it pretty good have an obligation to give back. If they understand this, then I've done my job.'"[94]

This is a good example of a successful career woman who can put her family first while excelling in her career and contributing to her community. Do you think that working mothers must deny their family's basic needs to create and maintain a professional career or to get or keep a job? What factors may allow some working mothers to dedicate more time to their family? What factors keep some working mothers from dedicating more time to their family?

- Living with a preschool-age child (57 percent compared with 43 percent of mothers in the labor force).
- Without a high school diploma (19 percent versus 8 percent of mothers in the labor force).[98]

The number of single mothers living with children younger than 18 in 2010 was 9.9 million; this was up from 3.4 million in 1970.[99]

Nonmarital Childbearing

According to the National Survey of Family Growth, 2006–2010, there is a growing trend to have children outside of marriage. Over the past several decades nonmarital childbearing has increased among women in all ages and Hispanic origin and race groups.[100] In 1970, only 11 percent of all live births were to unmarried women, compared with 42 percent in 2002. Among men and women who have ever had a biological child, nearly one-half had a child outside of marriage. Of those same men and women who have ever had a biological child, about one in three had that child in a cohabiting union.

There continues to be an increase in the percentages of women and men who have had a nonmarital birth.[101] Among women who ever had a live birth, the percentage with a nonmarital birth increased from 42 percent in 2002 to 49 percent in 2006–2010, and among men, the percentage of nonmarital births rose from 40 percent to 47 percent. Among those who had a biological child, black men (79 percent) and black women (82 percent) were most likely to have had a nonmarital birth, followed by Hispanic men (61 percent) and Hispanic women (57 percent).

The Pew Research Center for the People and the Press reported in 2010, that less traditional family arrangements get mixed reviews from the public, but fall far short of getting an endorsement.[102] More than four in ten (43 percent) say that the trend toward more unmarried couples raising children is bad for society, and an equal percentage say it does not make much difference. Only 10 percent say that it is good for society. Similarly, 43 percent say more gay and lesbian couples raising children is bad for society, 41 percent say it does not make much difference and 21 percent say it is good for society.

The increasing trend to have children outside of marriage may significantly impact parenting styles and strategies. Mothers (or fathers) not in a relationship may require extended family support and community resources to help care for their children. Community health services must be able to address the needs of single mothers (and fathers) that may not be able to afford health insurance or health care for their children. Furthermore, as discussed earlier in the chapter, cohabitating mothers tend to have more depressive symptoms

and less sensitivity toward their children than married mothers, thus parenting may be more challenging for cohabitating mothers than for mothers who are married. Education, mental health, and other community services need to provide training, services, and support for single parents or cohabitating parents who are challenged in their parenting styles or provision of child care.

Positive Parenting Relationships

The responsibility of every parent is to protect and nurture a child and also to prepare that child for success and happiness in family relations, school achievement, work satisfaction, and other life challenges. (See *Women Making a Difference:* "Working Mother of the Year.") The style of parenting used to attempt to fulfill parental responsibilities is vital to the success or failure of that goal. There are three common types of parenting, two of which are dysfunctional and one that is recommended.[103] One dysfunctional parenting style is referred to as "Giving Orders"—to be too controlling by giving orders, setting unreasonable limits, and giving children little or no freedom. Another dysfunctional parenting style is referred to as "Giving In"—to be too permissive by giving children lots of freedom but no limits. The most functional parenting style is referred to as "Giving Choices"—to help children learn a balance between freedom and limits by offering them choices and allowing them to experience the natural and logical consequences of those choices. "Giving Choices" is a **democratic parenting style** and will help parents raise a responsible child by (1) setting limits for children and (2) giving children choices within those limits. For example, "You have math and science homework. Which would you like to do first?" or "You may choose to remove your muddy shoes, or you can choose to clean the muddy tracks from the floor. You decide."

All children need to feel accepted, to have a sense of belonging in a family, and to be acknowledged as a significant member of that family.[104] Children need guidance, encouragement, and support to develop and thrive and to feel as if they belong. A child who chooses negative behavior as a way of feeling she or he belongs is a **discouraged child.** A discouraged child often misbehaves to accomplish one of the following goals: (1) to gain attention, (2) to achieve power, (3) to seek revenge, or (4) to display inadequacy. (See *FYI:* "Identifying the Four Goals of Children's Misbehavior.") Understanding and recognizing which one of the four goals of misbehavior the child is seeking will help a parent to respond adequately to the child's needs, thereby moving the child from a state of discouragement to one of encouragement. A key to successful parenting is to remember that if what you are doing is not working, then change your response to the child's behavior.

Therapists recommend four ingredients for forming strong relationships with children: (1) showing respect, (2) having fun, (3) giving encouragement, and (4) showing love. Giving encouragement means believing in children. "We must believe in our children if they are to believe in themselves:

- To feel capable and loved, children need lots of encouragement.
- To be ready to truly cooperate, children need to feel good about themselves."[105]

The democratic parenting style is successful because it provides opportunities for a child to succeed. Children who experience success will begin to believe in themselves again and be willing to cooperate.

Mothers and Teen Daughters

Roni Cohen-Sandler, a clinical psychologist and author who specializes in mother–daughter relationships, provides tips for parenting teen daughters.[107] She says that girls report being more stressed out than boys. One reason is that in today's fast-paced world, mothers are often girls' role-models and appear to be superwoman, juggling jobs, families, the home, volunteer work, and more. This busy lifestyle sets up the expectation that girls need to be living their lives as they see their mothers'. According to Cohen-Sandler, what girls do not realize is that stress in not normal, and is not necessary for successful, healthy lives. One powerful thing parents can do to help their daughters is to model a stress-reduced lifestyle. It is also very useful for parents occasionally to model failure for their children. Children that are only allowed to see their parents succeed at everything may set self-expectations very high and this may create a drive for perfectionism. But when a parent tells about a failure, it shows children that failure is a fact of life and something we all can learn from. Some things a parent can do to help reduce stress on children, specifically daughters, are:

- Help children to set realistic goals so they are not set up for failure and feelings of guilt when they don't meet (unrealistic) expectations. Instead, nurture your daughter's dreams and encourage her to go for it.
- Don't use social pressure as punishment. For example, do not take time away from friends for a bad grade in school. Teens need social acceptance and limiting social contacts may create additional anxiety and stress.
- Don't bombard girls with questions as soon as they walk in the door. Give them time to decompress.
- Don't overschedule kids. Let your daughter choose one or two activities to focus her gifts and talents.[108]

Cohen-Sandler feels that because mothers are their safest and most available targets, daughters usually take their anger out on them.[109] Girls know that if they take their anger out on their friends they will be shunned, but their mothers, who love them unconditionally, will not shun them. Mothers need to help daughters learn how to channel their anger constructively. Mothers want their daughters to speak up, to protect themselves in relationships, and to be able to express anger constructively so that they are not inciting violence. An important thing

---

FYI

Identifying the Four Goals of Children's Misbehavior[106]

HOW A PARENT FEELS	WHAT A PARENT USUALLY DOES	HOW THE CHILD USUALLY RESPONDS	MISBEHAVIOR GOAL OF THE CHILD
Bothered, annoyed	Remind, nag, scold	Stops temporarily; later, misbehaves again	Attention
Angry, threatened	Punish, fight back, or give in	Continues to misbehave, defies, or does what is asked slowly or sloppily	Power
Angry, extremely hurt	Get back at child, punish	Misbehaves even more, keeps trying to get even	Revenge
Hopeless, like giving up	Give up, agree that the child is helpless	Does not respond or improve	Display inadequacy

for mothers to teach their daughters is that anger is a perfectly normal human emotion. And if you are in a close relationship with someone, anger and conflict is probably inevitable. But a girl needs to know how to handle the anger so she can stay connected in the relationship and not harm the relationship or the people in it.

Cohen-Sandler explains that girls are experiencing puberty earlier and earlier. So many of their emotional issues that used to start at 11 or 12 are now starting at 9 or 10—the over-sensitivity, the self-consciousness, irritability, moodiness, and anger. Speculation around why girls are maturing earlier includes better nutrition and the possibility that girls' bodies are impacted by the hormones found in food and water. Also, with mothers in the work force and less available, kids are left alone more to manage on their own. In addition, the media plays a role in influencing young girls to act more adult-like. This early puberty onset means that girls are now in social situations sooner than they are emotionally and cognitively equipped to handle them. So while a young girl may feel she is ready for seductive dress, adult activity, and little supervision, mothers must take responsibility for reining daughters in and having them participate in activities that are more age appropriate.[110]

Chapter Summary

- Statistics suggest that relationships are more difficult to maintain in today's society. Over one-half of all first marriages end in divorce.
- Relationships have undergone a number of changes as gender roles and attitudes have converged.
- Sternberg's triangular theory of love suggests that relationships can be envisioned as the sides of a triangle. The sides include commitment, intimacy, and passion.
- Healthy relationships are characterized by attributes such as trust, respect, honesty, and authenticity.
- Unhealthy relationships are characterized by traits such as self-absorption, jealousy, feelings of inferiority or superiority, and distancing.

- Marriage, cohabitation, same-sex unions, and remarriages are different types of relationships.
- People spend money according to different personality profiles.
- Resolving conflicts by fair fighting is important to the happiness of partners in a relationship.
- The four ingredients for forming strong relationships with children are show respect, have fun, give encouragement, and show love.

Review Questions

1. What gender-role attributes seem best suited to relationships?
2. What are the differences between individualistic and collectivistic societies?
3. What are the key components of each stage of dating?
4. What is the difference between physical and emotional intimacy?
5. What is consummate love based on Sternberg's theory?
6. Which two areas of the brain are most active during the early stages of romantic love, and what two additional areas of the brain are most active with longer romantic involvement?
7. Which neurotransmitter has been identified by Fisher to be actively involved in the experience of romantic love?
8. Which hormone stimulates sexual desire?
9. Name the male hormone and the female hormone that produce behaviors associated with emotional attachment.
10. What are the lovestyles described by John Alan Lee?
11. What are the differences between vitalized and devitalized marriages?
12. What is a peer marriage?
13. What characteristics do cohabitators share with married couples? with singles?
14. What are some challenges to interracial and mixed-race couples?
15. What are some challenges to lesbian, bisexual, and transgender couples?
16. What characteristics are exhibited by love addicts? by avoidance addicts?
17. What are the major issues in troubled relationships?
18. What is the most effective parenting style?
19. What are the four goals of misbehavior for children?
20. What are the four ingredients for forming a strong relationship with children?

Resources

American Association for Marriage and Family Therapy
http://www.aamft.org

References

1. Presented by Michel Ann Fultz, Louisville Center for Adult Children, Louisville, Kentucky, 1996.

2. Adams, G. R. 1982. The physical attractiveness stereotype. In A. G. Miller (ed.), *In the eye of the beholder: Contemporary issues in stereotyping*. New York: Praeger; Berscheid, E. 1985. Interpersonal attraction. In G. Lindzey and E. Aronson (eds.), *Handbook of social psychology*. New York: Random House.

3. Lerner, H. G. 1990. *The dance of intimacy: A woman's guide to courageous acts of change in key relationships*. New York: Harper & Row.

4. Sacher, J. A., and M. A. Fine. 1996. Predicting relationship status and satisfaction after six months among dating couples. *Journal of Marriage and the Family* 58: 21–32.

5. Peplau, L. A., C. T. Hill, and Z. Rubin. 1993. Sex role attitudes in dating and marriage: A 15-year follow-up of the Boston couples study. *Journal of Social Issues* 49 (3): 31–52.

6. Antill, J. K. 1983. Sex role complementarity versus similarity in married couples. *Journal of Personality and Social Psychology* 45: 145–55.

7. Hui, C. H., and H. C. Triandis. 1986. Individualism-collectivism: A study of cross-cultural researchers. *Journal of Cross-Cultural Psychology* 17: 225–48.

8. Dion, K. K., and K. L. Dion. 1993. Individualistic and collectivistic perspectives of gender and the cultural context of love and intimacy. *Journal of Social Issues* 49 (3): 53–69.

9. Eysenck, M. 2004. Maslow's hierarchical theory. *In Psychology: An international perspective*, pp. 65–67. New York: Psychology Press.

10. Nevid, J. S., and S. A. Rathus. 2005. *Psychology and the challenges of life: Adjustment in the new millennium*. 9th ed. Hoboken, NJ: John Wiley & Sons.

11. Livermore, B. 1993. The lessons of love. *Psychology Today* 27: 30–39.

12. Lee, J. A. 1976. *The colors of love*. New York: Prentice-Hall.

13. Fisher, H. 2004. *Why we love: The nature and chemistry of romantic love*. New York: Henry Holt, pp. 68–72.

14. Ibid., pp. 68–72.

15. Ibid., pp. 72–73.

16. Ibid., pp. 72–73.

17. Ibid., pp. 81–82.

18. Ibid., pp. 81–82.

19. Ibid., p. 82.

20. Ibid., p. 88.

21. Ibid., p. 89.

22. Ibid., p. 89.

23. Wallerstein, J. S., and S. Blakeslee. 1995. *The good marriage: How and why love lasts*. Boston: Houghton Mifflin.

24. Evans, P. 1996. *The verbally abusive relationship*. Holbrook, MA: Adams Media, p. 37.

25. Ibid., p. 122.

26. Ibid., pp. 36–37.

27. Ibid., p. 123.

28. Pew Research Center. November 18, 2010. The decline of marriage and rise of new families. Pew Social & Demographic Trends. http://www.pewsocialtrends.org/2010/11/18/the-decline/of-marriage/and-rise-of-new-families/2/.

29. National Center for Health Statistics. 2010. Marriage and divorce. Centers for Disease Control and Prevention. http://www.cdc.gov/nchs/fastats/divorce.htm

30. U.S. Census Bureau. 2010. American community survey data on marriage and divorce. http://www.census.gov/hhes/socdemo/marriage/data/acs/index.html.

31. The Heritage Foundation. 2012. FamilyFacts.org. http://www.familyfacts.org/charts/marriage-and-family.

32. U.S. Census Bureau. April 2012. Households and families: 2010. http://www.census.gov/prod/cen2010/briefs/c2010br-14.pdf.

33. U.S. Census Bureau. 2010. Estimated median age at first marriage, by Sex: 1890 to the Present. http://www.census.gov/population/socdemo/hh-fam/ms2.xls.

34. Lavee, Y., and D. H. Olson. 1993. Seven types of marriage: Empirical typology based on ENRICH. *Journal of Marital and Family Therapy* 19: 325–40; Olson, D. H., D. Fournier, and J. Druckman. 1986. *PREPARE/ENRICH Counselor Manual*. 2nd ed. Minneapolis, MN: PREPARE/ENRICH, Inc.

35. Fowers, B. J., K. H. Montel, and D. H. Olson. 1996. Predicting marital success for premarital couple types based on PREPARE. *Journal of Marital and Family Therapy* 22: 103–19.

36. Crary, D. 2007. *Study: Shared chores key in marriage* www.aolsvc.timeforkids.kol.aol.com (retrieved July 5, 2007).

37. Schwartz, P. 1994. Modernizing marriage. *Psychology Today* 27: 54–59.

38. U.S. Census Bureau. April 2012. Households and families: 2010.

39. U.S. Census Bureau. 2009. American Community Survey, B11009, "Unmarried-Partner Households and Household Type by Sex of Partner." http://factfinder.census.gov/.

40. U.S. Department of Health and Human Services. March 22, 2012. First marriages in the United States: Data from the 2006–2010 National Survey of Family Growth. http://www.cdc.gov/nchs/data/nhsr/nhsr049.pdf.

41. Smock, P. 2000. Cohabitation in the United States: An appraisal of research themes, findings, and implications. *Annual Review of Sociology* 26 (1): 1–20.

42. Stanley, S., S. Whitton, and H. Markman. 2004. Maybe I do: Interpersonal commitment levels and premarital or nonmarital cohabitation. *Journal of Family Issues* 25: 496–519.

43. Stanley, S., G. Rhoades, and H. Markman. October 2006. Sliding versus deciding: Inertia and the premarital cohabitation effect. *Family Relations* 499–509.

44. Ibid.

45. Ibid.

46. Kline, G., S. Stanley, H. Markman, P. Olmos-Gallo, M. St. Peters, S. Whitton, and L. Prado. 2004. Pre-engagement cohabitation and increased risk for poor marital outcomes. *Journal of Family Psychology* 18: 311–318.

47. Rhoades, G., S. Stanley, and H. Markman. 2009. The pre-engagement cohabitation effect: A replication and extension of previous findings. *Journal of Family Psychology* 23 (1): 107–111.

48. Klausli, J., and M. Owen. 2009. Stable maternal cohabitation, couple relationship quality, and characteristics of the home environment in the child's first two years. *Journal of Family Psychology* 23 (1): 103–106.

49. U.S. Department of Health and Human Services. April 12, 2012. Fertility of men and women aged 15–44 years in the United States: National Survey of Family Growth, 2006–2010. http://www.cdc.gov/nchs/data/nhsr/nhsr051.pdf.

50. Besherov, D. J., and T. S. Sullivan. 1996. One flesh: America is experiencing an unprecedented increase in black–white intermarriage. *New Democrat* 8 (4): 19–21.

51. Hud-Aleem, R., and J. Countryman. 2008. Biracial identity development and recommendations in therapy. *Psychiatry* 5 (11): 37–44.

52. Wang, W. February 16, 2012. The rise of intermarriage: Rates, characteristics vary by race and gender. Pew Research Center. http://www.pewsocialtrends.org/2012/02/16/the-rise-of-intermarriage/.

53. Ibid.

54. U.S. Census Bureau. September 27, 2011. U.S. Census Bureau News: Census Bureau releases estimates of same-sex married couples. http://2010.census.gov/news/releases/operations/cb11-cn191html.

55. Clunis, D., and G. Green. 2004. *Lesbian couples: A guide to creating healthy relationships.* Berkeley, CA: Seal Press.

56. Istar Lev, A. 2004. *The complete lesbian and gay parenting guide.* New York: Berkley Trade.

57. Tacker, F., and S. Golombok. 1995. Adults raised as children in lesbian families. *American Journal of Orthopsychiatry* 65: 203–15.

58. Pew Research Center for the People & the Press. April 25, 2012. More support for gun rights, gay marriage than in 2008 or 2004. http://www.people-press.org/2012/04/25/more-support-for-gun-rights-gay-marriage-than-in-2008-or-2004/.

59. Pew Research Center for the People & the Press. February 7, 2012. Religion and attitudes toward same-sex marriage. http://www.pewforum.org/Gay-Marriage-and-Homosexuality/Relgion-and-Attitudes-Toward-Same-Sex-Marriages.aspx.

60. Human Rights Campaign. 2009. *Top 10 reasons for marriage equality*, pp. 1–2. www.hrc.org/issues/5491.htm (retrieved January 16, 2009).

61. Bennett, L. 2004. *The cost of marriage inequality to gay, lesbian and bisexual seniors.* A Human Rights Campaign Foundation Report, Washington, D.C., pp. 2, 4, 5, 6. www.hrc.org (retrieved January 16, 2009).

62. Ibid, p. 7.

63. Gates, G. April 2011. How many people are lesbian, gay, bisexual, and transgender? The Williams Institute, University of California, Los Angeles. http://www.williamsinstitute.law.ucla.edu/wp-content/uploads/Gates-How-Many-People-LGBT-Apri-2011.pdf.

64. Bieschke, K., R. Perez, and K. DeBord. 2006. *Handbook of counseling and psychotherapy with lesbian, gay, bisexual, and transgender clients.* Washington, D.C.: American Psychological Association.

65. Ibid.

66. Kriger, I. 2011. *Helping your transgender teen: A guide for parents.* New Haven, CT: Genderwise Press.

67. Grossman, A. & A. D'Augelli. 2007. Transgender youth and life-threatening behaviors. *Suicide and Life-Threatening Behavior* 37 (5): 527–537.

68. Dean, L., I. Meyer, K. Robinson, R. Sell, R. Sember, V. Silenzio, et al. 2000. Lesbian, gay, bisexual, and transgender health: Findings and concerns. *Journal of the Gay and Lesbian Medical Association* 4 (3): 102–151.

69. Clements-Nolle, K., R. Marx, and M. Katz. 2006. Attempted suicide among transgender persons: The influence of gender-based discrimination and victimization. *Journal of Homosexuality* 51 (3): 53–69.

70. Mock, J., and K. Mayo. May 18, 2011. I was born a boy. *Marie Claire.* http://www.marieclaire.com/born-male, pp. 1–4.

71. National Center for Health Statistics. January 10, 2012. National marriage and divorce rate trends. Centers for Disease Control and Prevention. http://www.cdc.gov/nchs/nvss/marriage_divorce_tables.htm.

72. U.S. Census Bureau. August 25, 2011. Divorce rates highest in the South, lowest in the Northeast, Census Bureau Reports. http://www.census.gov/newsroom/releases/archives/marital_status_living_arrangements/cb11-144.html.

73. Ibid.

74. National Center for Family and Marriage Research. November 3, 2011. First-time divorce rate tied to education, race. Bowling Green State University, Bowling Green, Ohio. http://www.bgsu.edu/offices/mc/news/2011/news103463.html.

75. Zhang, Z., and M. Hayward. 2006. Gender, the marital life course, and cardiovascular disease in late midlife. *Journal of Marriage and Family* 68: 639–657.

76. Hayward, M. August 22, 2006. Divorced middle-aged women more prone to heart disease than those who remain married, study shows. The University of Texas. http://www.utexas.edu/news/2006/08/22/sociology/, p. 1.

77. Mellody, P., A. W. Miller, and J. K. Miller. 1992. *Facing love addiction: Giving yourself the power to change the way you love.* San Francisco: HarperCollins.

78. Kurdek, L. 1994. Areas of conflict for gay, lesbian, and heterosexual couples: What couples argue about influences relationship satisfaction. *Journal of Marriage and Family* 56: 923–934.

79. Evans, P. 1996. *The verbally abusive relationship.*

80. Worth, T. 2010. Why women cheat: Insights into common reasons why women have affairs. WebMD. http://women.webmd.com/features/why-do-women-cheat.

81. Forste, R., and K. Tanfer. 1996. Sexual exclusivity among dating, cohabitating, and married women. *Journal of Marriage and the Family* 58: 33–47.

82. Stanley, S., H. Markman, and S. Whitton. 2002. Communication, conflict, and commitment: Insights on the foundations of relationship success from a national survey. *Family Process* 41: 659–675.

83. Mellan, O. 1994. *Money harmony: Resolving money conflicts in your life and your relationships.* New York: Walker.

84. Major, B. 1993. Gender, entitlement, and the distribution of family labor. *Journal of Social Issues* 49: 141–59.

85. Kurdek, L. A. 1993. The allocation of household labor in gay, lesbian, and heterosexual married couples. *Journal of Social Issues* 49: 127–39.

86. Gottman, J. 1993. The roles of conflict engagement, escalation, and avoidance in marital interaction: A longitudinal view of five types of couples. *Journal of Consulting and Clinical Psychology* 61 (1): 6–15.

87. Gottman, J., and R. Levenson. 2000. The timing of divorce: Predicting when a couple will divorce over a 14-year period. *Journal of Marriage and the Family* 62: 737–745.

88. Gottman, J., R. Levenson, J. Gross, B. Fredrickson, K. McCoy, L. Rosenthal, A. Ruef, and D. Yoshimoto. 2003. *Journal of Homosexuality* 45 (1): 65–91.

89. Lerner, H. 2005. *The dance of anger: A woman's guide to changing the patterns of intimate relationships.* New York: Perennial Currents/HarperCollins.

90. Lerner, H. 2002. *The dance of connection: How to talk to someone when you're mad, hurt, scared, frustrated, insulted, betrayed, or desperate.* New York: William Morrow/HarperCollins.

91. Rosenberg, M. B. 2003. *Nonviolent communication: A language of life.* Encinitas, CA: Puddle Dancer Press.

92. Ibid.

93. Vitello, A. 2008 (May 11). Mother's day celebration reaches 100th anniversary. Associated Press, *Denton Record-Chronicle,* p. 11A.

94. Roberts, M. 2008. *2007 Working mothers of the year. Working Mother.* www.workingmother.com (retrieved January 17, 2009).

95. U.S. Census Bureau. February 22, 2012. Newsroom: Facts for features & special editions. http://www.census.gov/news room/releases/archives/facts_for_features_special_editions/cb12-ff05.html.

96. U.S. Census Bureau. March 17, 2011. Newsroom: Facts for features & special editions. http://www.census.gov/newsroom/releases/archives/facts_for_features_special_editions/cb11-ff07.html.

97. U.S. Census Bureau. 2010. Families and living arrangements: 2010. http://www.census.gov/population/www/socdemo/hh-fam/cps2010.html.

98. U.S. Census Bureau. 2007. Families and living arrangements: 2007. http://www.census.gov/newsroom/releases/archives/families_households/cb09-132.html.

99. U.S. Census Bureau. 2010. Families and living arrangements: 2010.

100. U.S. Department of Health and Human Services. April 12, 2012. Fertility of men and women aged 15–44 years in the United States: National Survey of Family Growth, 2006–2010.

101. Ibid.

102. Pew Research Center. November 18, 2010. The decline of marriage and rise of new families.

103. Dinkmeyer Sr., D., G. McKay, and D. Dinkmeyer Jr. 1997. *The parent's handbook.* Circle Pines, MN: American Guidance Service, pp. 3, 6.

104. Dinkmeyer, McKay, and Dinkmeyer, *The parent's handbook,* pp. 10–11.

105. Ibid., p. 19.

106. Ibid., pp. 14–15.

107. Rutson, D. 2009. Westonite Roni Cohen-Sandler. *Girls are more stressed out than boys.* www.acorn-online.com (retrieved January 18, 2009).

108. Ibid.

109. Cohen-Sandler, R. 2000. *I'm not mad, i just hate you! A new understanding of mother–daughter conflict.* New York: Penguin.

110. Ibid.

Chapter Seven

Preventing Abuse against Women

CHAPTER OBJECTIVES

When you complete this chapter, you will be able to do the following:

◇ Identify the extent of violence and abuse against women in the United States

◇ Categorize the various types of abuse committed against women

◇ Develop protective plans to avoid the possibilities of rape

◇ Summarize the characteristics of women who are abused

◇ Explain common elements present in all types of abuse

◇ Identify the types of consequences abused women experience

◇ Develop strategies for leaving an abusive relationship

◇ Utilize information and methods necessary to heal from the wounds of an abusive relationship

◇ Determine methods by which violence and abuse against women can be reduced and prevented

◇ Identify the various sources of assistance available to abused women and children

THE REALITY OF VIOLENCE AGAINST WOMEN

Maria gently pressed the cold towel against her cheek and ear. Painfully she removed the numbing cold compress and looked at her inflamed, swollen face in the mirror. Why? . . . she asked herself . . . why does this happen to me? She hated it. She hated him, yet, here she was, and remained, an abused wife. As she looked once again at her physical wounds, she knew that her most profound wounds were hidden within.

Violence against women is a major public health concern and a violation of human rights. The concept and treatment of women as the lesser sex is documented throughout history. For example, during the Stone Age, duties essential to survival—working the land, finding shelter, preparing food—were, for a time, shared by men and women. As metals were discovered and agriculture using heavy tools increased, man used the strength and labor of other men, reducing some men to slaves and diminishing the role of women to the position of servitude. Thomas Aquinas, the thirteenth-century Christian theologian, stated that woman was created to be man's helpmate, but her unique role is in conception . . . since for other purposes men would be better assisted by other men.[1] The attitude of a woman "belonging" to and serving the needs of man too often has led to men "controlling" or "disciplining" women by punishment in whatever manner was deemed necessary or appropriate. According to an old English common law doctrine, a husband could punish his wife for any behavior he considered inappropriate. This law, called the "Rule of Thumb," permitted a husband to beat his wife with a stick no larger than the circumference of his thumb.

In the early history of the United States, violence, especially domestic violence, was met with varying degrees of concern. Scholars who have studied domestic violence believe there is a direct relationship between the degree of male dominance in a society and the extent of violence toward women.[2] Female servants in the South in the eighteenth and nineteenth centuries often fell victim to rape by their "owners"; prostitutes often are beaten by a man who "owns" them for the brief period of time for which he paid.

Abuse of women encompasses a wide spectrum of behaviors, from derogatory remarks to rape and from battering to murder. Tragically, in the United States, nearly one in five women and one in 71 men have been raped at some time in their lives, with more than 51 percent of female victims reported being raped by an intimate partner and almost 41 percent by an acquaintance. Additionally, nearly one in four women have experienced severe physical violence by an intimate partner.[3]

Prevalence of violence against women varies little among all cultures, among unmarried and married couples, and among socioeconomic groups. The wife of a Fortune 500 company president is just as likely to be abused as is the wife or partner of a blue-collar laborer. Abused women of all races and cultures seek refuge in safe shelters, utilize community agencies, and seek the support of the legal system.

Violence and abuse against women is a perplexing phenomenon. The perpetrator is usually someone the victim knows—and often loves: the husband, boyfriend, father, or other relative. Nearly 4.7 million incidents of intimate partner violence (IPV) occur each year against U.S. women aged 18 and older.[4] As former U.S. Attorney General Richard Carmona stated in an address to the Symposium on Family Violence: "At a fundamental level it is a violation, a betrayal of the trust and love that should occur within our families and intimate relationships. Family violence is beneath us as individuals; it is beneath us as a nation."[5] An adult female today is more likely to be raped, beaten, and/or stalked by her current or former husband, her boyfriend, or her date than by any other person.[6] Incidents, such as the following, are recounted in state and federal government reports and illustrate the extent of violence and abuse inflicted against females. A 9-year-old girl in Texas reports that she was raped by her father; a 15-year-old Connecticut girl was stabbed by her boyfriend; an Idaho woman was raped by her boss; a 46-year-old woman in New Mexico was thrown out of a moving car by her husband; a 31-year-old Baltimore woman was beaten, choked, and raped by a former friend who was helping her move; and an Arizona woman, 8 months pregnant, fled her home after her husband beat her with a broomstick and threatened to kill her. The wide diversity of these incidents reveals that no one is immune; violence happens to women from all walks of life, old and young, rich and poor, homemakers and homeless, and it is usually inflicted by someone they know. These incidences are called **acquaintance violence,** meaning violence and abuse committed by a parent, relative, coworker, neighbor, or friend.

Women may be victimized more by individuals they know due to the fact that society and/or the legal system has not, in the past, disapproved of acquaintance violence. Abuse committed in the home, called **domestic abuse,** is often perpetrated by an individual whose belief system is grounded in extremes—it can only be right or wrong: the dinner was prepared or it was not, performance of some duty was carried out or it was not. Family violence, according to Dobash and Dobash,[7] has existed for centuries and has been accepted as being a part of a "patriarchal terrorist" system. By virtue of observation and/or experience, children often perpetuate family traditions by engaging in and/or accepting those behaviors that they have seen or experienced in their own family environment. Children from abusive families are more likely to grow up to be abusive parents.[8] In addition to witnessing family violence, children witness more than 100,000 acts of violence on TV by the time they complete elementary school and 200,000 acts of violence on TV by the time they graduate from high school.[9]

THE EXTENT OF THE PROBLEM

Statistics regarding IPV may vary due to different data sources and how IPV is defined and the data are collected. However, IPV, sexual violence, and stalking are major public health problems in the United States and throughout the world. It is an epidemic that too often results in physical injury and mental health consequences, such as depression, anxiety, low self-esteem, and/or suicide attempts. As children observe or experience violence in their homes, these behaviors time and again spiral into the next generations, and the victim becomes the victimizer. The Centers for Disease Control and Prevention launched a nationwide survey, entitled *the National Intimate Partner and Sexual Violence Survey*[10] in 2010 to determine (1) the prevalence and characteristics of sexual violence, stalking, and IPV, (2) who is most likely to experience these forms of violence, (3) the patterns and impact of the violence experienced by specific perpetrators, and (4) the health consequences of these forms of violence. Selected results of this survey were as follows:

Violence by an intimate partner

- One in three women (35.6%) have experienced rape, physical violence, and/or stalking by an intimate partner in their lifetime.

- One in three women experienced multiple forms of rape, stalking, or physical violence.
- One in four women (24.3%) have experienced severe physical violence by an intimate partner (slapped, hit with fist, beaten, slammed against something).
- One-half of all women in the United States have experienced psychological aggression by an intimate partner.

Sexual violence by any perpetrator or intimate partner

- One in five women (18.3%) in the United States have been raped at some time in their lives.
- Nearly one in ten women has been raped by an intimate partner in her lifetime.
- Most female victims of completed rape (79%) experienced first rape by age 25.
- 1.3 million women reported being raped by any perpetrator in the twelve months prior to taking the survey.

Stalking victimization by any perpetrator or intimate partner

- One in six women (16%) have experienced stalking victimization at some point during their lifetime.
- An estimated 10.7% of women have been stalked by an intimate partner during their lifetime.

Violence experienced by race/ethnicity

- Approximately one in five black (22%) and white (18.8%) non-Hispanic women and one in seven Hispanic women (14.6%) have experienced rape at some point during their livetime.
- Approximately one in three multiracial non-Hispanic women (30.6%) and one in four American Indian or Alaska Native women (22.7%) reported being stalked during their lifetime.
- Approximately four of every ten women of non-Hispanic Black or American Indian or Alaska Native race/ethnicity and one in two multiracial non-Hispanic women have experienced rape, physical violence, and/or stalking by an intimate partner in their lifetime.

Crandall et al.[11] found that 44 percent of women murdered by their intimate partner had visited an emergency room within two years of the homicide and, of these women, 93 percent had at least one injury visit. See *FYI:* "The Violence Against Women and Department of Justice Reauthorization Act of 2005" to learn about the current federal legislation to reduce and prevent violence against women.

Why Women Stay in Abusive Relationships

Virginia, married for 23 years to an abusive executive, remained in the relationship because she was, for many years, economically dependent on her husband. Forgoing her education to assist him through college, she maintained the house and raised the children. Over the years, Virginia developed few job skills, had no training outside the home, and had no other place to live. When Virginia talked about leaving, her husband threatened her with more abuse and the possible loss of the children. Feeling trapped and fearing physical, legal, and financial retaliation, Virginia felt she had no choice but to remain in the relationship.

Situational factors such as financial dependency, lack of education, lack of job skills, or job inexperience are all too real for women involved in abusive relationships. Statistically, a woman with children who leaves the home has a 50 percent probability that her standard of living will drop below the poverty level. Moreover, a woman is often in greater physical danger

---

FYI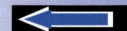

The Violence Against Women and Department of Justice Reauthorization Act 2005[12]

The Violence Against Women Act was reauthorized in the fall of 2005 and signed into law by President Bush in January 2006. This act

- enhances core programs and policies in the criminal justice and legal systems and reaffirms the commitment to reform systems that affect adult and youth victims of domestic violence, dating violence, sexual assault, and stalking;
- makes new strides to end domestic and sexual violence and stalking by addressing currently unmet needs;
- provides practical solutions to improve response of the criminal justice and legal systems for local groups, to enhance collaboration between victim service organizations and civil legal assistance providers, and to enforce protective orders;
- includes the reauthorization of critical programs and the development of new services that respond to evolving community needs; and
- works to provide transitional housing options, protect the safety and confidentiality of homeless victims, and ensure that victims can access the criminal justice system.

when she attempts to leave the relationship. She fears for her safety, her children's safety, and sometimes the safety of anyone who attempts to help her. Fear is the major reason that women stay in an abusive relationship. A victim's chances of being killed or injured increase by 75% when she leaves the abusive relationship.[13]

Emotional factors such as fear of social isolation and lack of emotional and financial support from family and friends may contribute to women staying in unhealthy and abusive relationships. Abused women frequently lose touch with supportive friends and family due to the isolative nature of abuse. Cultural constraints (for example, men are the dominant sex) and religious beliefs (for example, divorce is a sin) may also keep women from leaving these relationships. Women generally accept the responsibility for success or failure of the relationship; to leave is to feel like a failure.

Love for the abuser is one reason for not reporting abuse inflicted by a partner. Laura, a woman who had been abused by her husband for a number of years, cried as she said, "I love him; I don't want him arrested; I don't want to hurt him, but I don't want him to hurt me either. I don't know what to do." The partner may be the father of her children; they love him, therefore, she is reluctant to eliminate his presence from the home.

Curiously, abused women often are concerned about their husbands' inability to survive on their own. They might ask themselves, "If I should die, would he be able to survive?" The answer is, of course, "Yes!" Concerns about survival if she remains in the abusive relationship and the fears associated with having independence and major life changes if she leaves create much ambivalence about the situation. And she can live with the false hope that he will change. Feeling trapped in the relationship, women may determine that some place to live, even if abusive, is better than no place to live, especially if children are involved. (See *Her Story:* "Pat: Choosing to Leave an Abusive Marriage.") Society's view of domestic violence is often a barrier to a woman's willingness to admit that she has been abused.

People may not understand why abused women do not leave the relationship, or think they may deserve the abuse or even enjoy it. The fact is that many barriers exist that discourage this abuse from being reported. Even the legal system may create a barrier to gaining a proper perspective concerning the actual incidences of violence and abuse. Slow to respond to the needs of violated women, the legal system in some states doesn't even consider spousal violence and abuse a felony until after the second conviction of the abuser.

Her Story

Pat: Choosing to Leave an Abusive Marriage

It wasn't easy for me to leave my spouse because, first of all, I still loved him. We had invested 24 years in our marriage, and I had never been totally on my own. Finally after several breakups, numerous arguments, and fights with some of them being near fatal on both our parts, I realized it was time for "Me" to do something different, and healthy. So I moved out for the last time. Since that time I have grown more spiritually and mentally. I've learned how to become an optimistic person, which means for me: Things will be and are bad at times, but things won't be and aren't bad all the time. Marriage is a good example of that statement because so many years of my marriage were bad, but out of all of that, he and I have a daughter and son we love. Through our children we were blessed with two precious and loving grandsons.

I thank God and every person who helped and encouraged me: the residential shelter, my adult children, the counseling center. Even with all of that help, it would not have worked had I not made the decision to help MYSELF, even though it took time and extreme courage. I thought I would never reach a serene point or fulfill my life goals, but I did and I have. I started college in the spring, I have a job, a car, an apartment, but most of all, I have peace of mind! Thank you God, thank you everybody.

- What type of feelings do you have as a result of reading this story?
- What do you think was the impetus for Pat leaving the relationship?
- What do you think of Pat's explanation of being an optimistic person?

Once violence becomes part of a relationship, it usually escalates in severity and frequency. An innocent remark, a push, or a criticism often initiates a response that ranges from a slap, kick, or punch to permanent damage (physically and/or psychologically) or even death. The resulting consequences negatively affect the victim/survivor, her children, and perhaps the perpetrator.

TYPES OF ABUSE

Abuse against women takes many forms, each with varied and far-reaching consequences. Perhaps an awareness and understanding of the major types of violence and abuse inflicted upon women and the resultant consequences may be helpful in the prevention of abuse. Perhaps a clearer understanding of the destructive effects will motivate women to take action and resolve the abuse or dissolve the relationship, either through family counseling or by leaving. Following is a brief description of the major types of violence that women may experience during various stages in their lives.

Childhood Abuse

One of the most serious problems in our society is abuse inflicted on children. It is often the root of abusive adult relationships. **Childhood abuse** consists of maltreatment of a child before age 18 through physical or mental injury, sexual abuse or exploitation, and/or negligent treatment by the individual(s) who are responsible for the child's welfare. There are four different types of childhood abuse: physical abuse, neglect, emotional abuse, and sexual abuse.

- *Childhood physical abuse* can result in cuts, burns, contusions, frequent pain without obvious injury, bites, or any other intentional pain that results in injury. Slapping, hair pulling, even tickling—especially to the point of hysteria—are also forms of childhood abuse. Physical abuse may begin as physical punishment and escalate into injurious, painful acts. Implements such as belts, switches, or paddles may be used to hit the child anywhere on the body. Frequent use of enemas or laxatives, unnecessary medical probing, and other intrusive procedures physically intrude on a child's right to privacy and respect.

- *Childhood abuse by neglect,* which is a less obvious form of physical abuse, is described as not providing a child with basic necessities (for example, shelter, food, clothing, medical needs, or a hygienic environment). Obvious malnourishment, fatigue and listlessness, lack of personal cleanliness, or habitually dressing in torn and/or dirty clothes are noticeable signs of neglect. Less obvious types of neglect are being unattended for long periods of time; needing glasses, dental care, or other medical attention; and not receiving emotional support or attention.

- *Childhood emotional abuse* is the most perplexing type of child abuse. Although there may be no physical evidence of emotional abuse, there are telltale indications that this type of abuse is occurring. Parents can inflict emotional abuse on a child by depriving her or him of an essential sense of self-worth. Emotional abuse includes continually criticizing or belittling the child, talking perpetually to the child in negative terms, threatening severe punishment or abandonment, and ignoring the child. Demanding perfection (for example, a perfect appearance or performance), excessive control by denying spontaneity and creativity, and disallowing social peer interactions are further types of emotional abuse. Learning problems, behavioral extremes such as isolation or aggressiveness, expressions of depression, and apathy are often consequences of emotional abuse.

- *Childhood sexual abuse* refers to oral, anal, or vaginal intercourse, fondling, unwanted touching, and/or using instruments on a child's genitalia. Forcing a child to view adult genitalia, to watch a pornographic scene or movie, or to undress or expose herself or himself to an adult are also forms of child sexual abuse. Eighty-five percent of childhood sexual abuse is done by an individual the child knows (for example, a parent, relative, or neighbor). Harmful and serious physical, emotional, behavioral, and social consequences often are the result of childhood sexual abuse. High-risk behaviors, depression, anxiety, alcohol or illicit drug abuse, eating disorders, which can lead to long-term physical health problems such as STIs, cancer, or heart disease, often result from childhood abuse.[14]

- Children who experience sexual abuse often have a poor sense of self-worth. They withdraw, isolate, and may be suicidal. One common result of childhood sexual and physical abuse is **posttraumatic stress disorder (PTSD).** PTSD develops over a period of time as a result of some traumatic event, such as war, a violent act, or abuse. Symptoms such as irritability, edginess, and insomnia among others do not arise at the time of the trauma but occur at a later time in life. These are similar to the PTSD symptoms people experience as a result of being at war as well as going through other traumatic life events. As adults, women can begin to experience these symptoms and may not understand why the symptoms are developing. Children who experienced childhood sexual abuse may, as adults, develop PTSD and have involuntary memories, flashbacks, nightmares, and physical reactions when exposed to reminders of the events.[15]

More than 3.6 million referrals concerning the welfare of children were reported to the U.S. Children Protective Services in 2006.[16] Of the 905,000 children who were found to be victims of maltreatment, 64 percent experienced neglect, 16 percent were physically abused, 8.8 percent were sexually abused, 6.6 percent were psychologically maltreated, and 2.2 percent were medically neglected. In addition, 15 percent experienced "other" types of maltreatment, such as abandonment or threats to harm a child. Forty-eight percent of the victimized children were boys and 52 percent were girls, ranging in age from infant to 16; the younger the child, the more likely to be neglected, while children in the 12–15 age range were more likely to be physically and sexually abused. These children were from all ethnic groups: One-half of all victims were white (44.8 percent); almost one-quarter (21.9 percent) were African American; and 21.4 percent were Hispanic. For all racial categories except Native Hawaiian and Pacific Islander, the largest percentage of victims suffered from neglect. Nearly 81 percent of victims were abused by a parent acting alone or with another person. Approximately 37 percent of child victims were maltreated by the mother acting alone; another 19 percent were maltreated by their father acting alone, and 18 percent were abused by both parents.[17] More than 1,537 children died as a result of abuse or neglect in 2010, with more than 29 percent of the children killed under the age of 3. This is a sad commentary on our society, and it is a problem that has far-reaching consequences because children, both males and females, who are abused very often become child and/or spousal abusers as adults.

Abuse and Adult Women

Females who are abused during childhood often expect to be abused or feel they deserve abuse during their adult relationships. Prevention and treatment programs often address the worthiness and respect of self as a way to overcome this misconception. Abuse inflicted on adult women often takes forms similar to child abuse.

Physical Abuse Physical abuse, or battery, is the most overt type of domestic violence adult women encounter. Being kicked, hit, bitten, choked, pushed, having hair pulled, being thrown across the room or down on the floor, and/or being assaulted with some type of weapon are examples of battery. Perpetrators may target certain areas of the body for abusing, such as the breast, face, hairy areas of the body where bruises or abrasions are difficult to detect, or even the abdomen of a pregnant woman.

Abuse, especially physical abuse, tends to be cyclic in nature and typically involves three stages: increased tension building, the acute battering incident, and finally, the "honeymoon" phase, a loving, calmer, less tense period of time. The cyclic nature of this tragedy predicts that it will be repeated over time. Further explanation of these phases is found in *FYI*: "The Cycle of Abuse."

Psychological Abuse **Psychological abuse,** unlike physical abuse, is clandestine and insidious. It is traumatic, often long-lasting, more difficult to assess, and less likely to lead to intervention and/or prosecution of the perpetrator.

Psychological abuse comes in many forms and can include some or all of the following conditions:

- *Financial disadvantages.* This is characterized by the perpetrator having control over household finances. The woman may not be allowed to work, and therefore she becomes financially dependent on her partner. If she is working, she may have to account for all the money she earns, thus reducing her sense of freedom or independence outside the relationship.
- *Young children at home.* This includes threatening to take children from their mother, abusing the children, or using the children to degrade or belittle their mother. Statements such as "You're stupid, just like your mother," or "How can you ever amount to anything, just look at who your mother is" produce a psychological environment that hinders the development of worthiness and positive self-concept, degrading both the mother and the children.
- *Fear for herself and her children.* A woman may be frightened by her partner's looks, gestures, voice, destruction of property, or harming of children or pets. The worry that he may explode and express verbal degradation, curse, and call her or the children names can further contribute to her humiliation and fear. The home as a safe environment no longer exists.
- *Threatening harm.* The perpetrator inflicts harm on the children or threatens to take them away. He may even allude to committing suicide. The perpetrator may also threaten to kill her, the immediate family, other relatives, or close friends. His threats are designed to create anxiety, fear, & control in his partner and the children.
- *Ultimate control of behavior.* The perpetrator may limit his partner's activities by controlling her freedom to join organizations, limiting contact with companions, and not allowing her to go on errands or to travel. He fears the loss of control and influence over her life if she is absent too often or too long from the home. His extreme possessiveness or jealousy creates the need to know with whom and where his partner is at all times.
- *Isolation.* The perpetrator controls all social contacts and movements of a woman. Severe jealousy and frequent accusations serve to isolate the woman, keep her psychologically off balance, and contribute to the abusive environment. The systematic destruction of a woman's self-esteem results from continual psychological abuse. This type of abuse is often present when physical and/or sexual violence are also present.

Sexual Assault **Sexual assault** is a term used to describe numerous forms of sexual improprieties and sexual violence toward another individual. It can result from manipulation or coercion as well as through

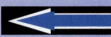

FYI

The Cycle of Abuse

Phase I –Tension/Buildup

Phase characterized by increased arguments, minor forms of verbal/physical abuse. Perpetrator wants to control, victim is aware of consequences if she doesn't "obey" his demands.

Perpetrator– isolates her, withdraws affection, put downs, yelling, destroys property, sullen, isolates her.

Victim – nurtures him, agrees, keeps kids quiet, cooks favorite meals, tries to reason, calms him, walking on egg shells. She may be willing to seek help and assistance.

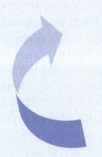

Phase III – Calm or "Honeymoon" Phase

Couple has feelings of reconciliation, calmness, and reminders of earlier, loving times. Usually shorter than tension phase and usually disappears over time as battering becomes more frequent and severe. He attempts to justify his behavior by blaming others, alcohol, the victim. Intervention for batterer may be possible in this phase.

Perpetrator – Begs forgiveness, promises to seek help, sends flowers/gifts, brings presents, goes to AA, promised to never to it again, says he loves her/children, cries, tries to get family to help.

Victim – attempts to stop legal process, sets of counseling appointments, agrees to stay, takes him back, feels happy and hopeful. As she stays, cycle starts to repeat.

Phase II – Abusive Incidents

For perpetrator, situations cause tension/anger and exceed his ability to cope, results in angry/violent responses; attempts to change "her" behavior through acts of violence toward her and/or the children.

Perpetrator – slapping, beating, choking, rape, use of knife or other weapon, humiliates, locks her up, throwing her down.

Victim – Attempts to protect self and children, calls for help (police, neighbor), tries to reason with him, calm him, leaves, fights back.

After acute abuse, both may be amenable to intervention: he feels shame/guilt; she feels hurt, angry, frightened.

physical force. Rape, a type of sexual assault, is sexual intercourse that is forced on women and is considered an act of violence, aggression, power, and control rather than an act of sexual desire.

The prevalence of rape is astounding. Sexual violence is a serious problem that affects millions of people every year. One in five women (18 percent) and one in 71 men (1.4 percent) reported experiencing forced rape at some time in their lives.[18] Three out of four who reported being raped and/or physically assaulted since age 18 stated that a current or former husband, cohabiting partner, or date was responsible.[19] Women who were raped by a stranger were more likely to report the rape to police.

The United States is the most rape-prone contemporary society in the world. These tragic numbers reflect a dark and shameful side of human nature. Each statistic is reflective of a woman whose life is forever changed as a result of a violation inflicted on her by another human being. The number of reported and unreported sexual assaults is staggering. But even *one* sexual assault is one too many.

A woman may be raped by a male who she knows or by a male who is a stranger to her. Each type of rape presents its own set of circumstances and consequences. **Acquaintance rape** is the sexual assault of a woman by a man whom she knows, such as a man who is in her class or lives in her residence hall. **Date rape,** a form of acquaintance rape, refers to the rape of a woman by a man who she has agreed to see socially. Some rapists prefer to know their victims because they are able to get closer to them or trap them in a vulnerable position without creating alarm. Acquaintances are also able to gain more information about the routine, friends, and living conditions of the intended victim, and perhaps believe that a woman will be less willing to report the rape if she knows the rapist.

Date and acquaintance rape are characterized by physical attacks on the woman's breasts or genitals, sexual sadism, and forced sexual activity. Acquaintance rape occurs more frequently among college students, especially freshman women, than among any other age group. According to research conducted on a number of campuses, approximately 18 to 20 percent of college women experience rape or some sort of sexual assault during their college years.[20] One study revealed that one in two college women said they had experienced some type of sexual aggression, and one in four or five reported being the victim of rape or attempted rape. Nine out of ten victims of rape knew their attackers as dating partners or acquaintances at the time of the assault,24 with the majority taking place in living quarters. Yet only 5 percent of completed or attempted rapes of college women were reported to law enforcement.[21]

Characteristics of a Rapist
Acquaintance rape can often be prevented by being aware of certain male behaviors. A man who demonstrates a disrespectful attitude toward other individuals, especially women, may indicate that he sees women as second-class citizens. Furthermore, the potential acquaintance rapist often lacks concern for a woman's feelings, may express extreme jealousy, or may attempt to be domineering. He often is highly competitive and may use physical violence as a means of coping with stress-filled situations. He may also speak negatively about women's rights or tell jokes that are demeaning to women.

Women should avoid individuals who exhibit these behaviors and seek out companions who display behaviors that are conducive to developing a healthy and enjoyable relationship. *Health Tips:* "Avoiding Date Rape" offers guidelines to use to avoid being placed in a position of possible danger. Four main factors increase the risk of being sexually assaulted:

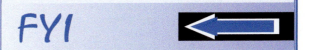

Sex Trafficking

Sex trafficking is a modern-day form of slavery where women, men, girls or boys under the age of 18 are forced into various forms of commercial sexual prostitution, pornography, stripping, live-sex shows, and/or being mail-order brides. It is estimated that over 50,000 women become victims of sex trafficking in the United States each year. Victims, usually women and girls, are lured into sex trafficking with a promise of a good job in another country or a false marriage proposal, then being sold into the sex trade by parents, husbands, or boyfriends or being kidnapped by traffickers. The perpetrators of sex trafficking may hold the victim in debt-bondage, stating that the victim must "work" until they pay back the costs of bringing them to another country and supplying them with essentials for survival: food, clothing, shelter.

Physical and psychological health risks for the victim occur as a result of their involvement in various sex acts. Drug/alcohol addiction, physical abuse, rape, gang rape, sexually transmitted infections, and other diseases are too often experienced by the victim. Psychological harm includes fear, distrust, shame, grief, hatred of self or men, suicide, posttraumatic stress disorder, depression, and other issues for victims. Victims of sex trafficking may be placed as street prostitutes, in brothels, or at massage parlors, spas, strip clubs, and other fronts for prostitution.

The Trafficking Victims Protection Act of 2000 (TVPA) made sex trafficking a federal law violation. The U.S. government can assist victims, if identified, by adjusting their immigration status and obtaining support to help rebuild their lives. The National Human Trafficking Resource Center (1-888-3737.888) can be contacted for any type of assistance related to sex trafficking.

Health Tips

Avoiding Date Rape: Guidelines for Men and Women[22]

Men

- *Know your sexual desires and limits.* Communicate them clearly. Be aware of social pressures and realize it's okay not to score.
- *Being turned down when you ask for sex is not a rejection of you personally.* Women can express their desire not to participate in a single act of sex. You may think your desires are beyond control. However, your actions are certainly within your control.
- *Accept a woman's decision.* "No" means "no." Don't read other meanings into the answer. Don't continue after you are told "No!"
- *Don't assume that just because a woman dresses in a sexy manner and flirts that she wants to have sexual intercourse.*
- *Don't assume that previous permission for sexual contact applies to the current situation.*
- *Avoid excessive use of alcohol and other drugs.* Alcohol and other drugs interfere with clear thinking and effective communication.

Women

- *Know your sexual desires and limits.* Believe in your right to set those limits. If you are not aware, stop and talk about it with your date.

- *Communicate your limits clearly.* If someone starts to offend you, tell him so firmly and immediately. Polite approaches may be misunderstood or ignored. Say "no" when you mean "no."
- *Be assertive.* Often men interpret passivity as permission. Be direct and firm with someone who is sexually pressuring you.
- *Be aware that your nonverbal actions send a message.* If you dress in a sexy manner and flirt, some men assume you want to have sex. This does not make your dress or behavior wrong, but it is important to be aware of a possible misunderstanding.
- *Pay attention to what is happening around you.* Watch the nonverbal clues. Do not put yourself into a vulnerable situation.
- *Trust your intuition.* If you feel you are being pressured into unwanted sex, you probably are.
- *Avoid excessive use of alcohol and other drugs.* Alcohol and other drugs interfere with clear thinking and effective communication.

- Frequently drinking enough to get drunk
- Being unmarried
- Previously being a victim of sexual assault
- Living on campus (for on-campus victimization only)

Marital rape appears to be mainly an act of violence and aggression, in which sex is the method used to humiliate, hurt, degrade, and dominate the spouse, usually the female partner. The violence and brutality in an abusive sexual relationship of a couple seems to escalate with time. The sexual violence is frequently accompanied by life-threatening acts or warnings.

Compassion, caring, and believing a woman are important responses supporters can provide when assisting someone following an act of rape. *Health Tips: "What to Do If You Are Raped"* provides suggestions for what to do if you find yourself or a friend to be the victim of a rape.

Relationship among Alcohol, Drugs, and Sexual Assault
Drugs can affect judgment and behavior and place a woman at risk for unwanted or risky sexual activity. Alcohol is the drug most commonly used when a sexual assault is committed. When a person drinks too

much alcohol, her or his judgment is impaired and can cause a distortion of thinking and reasoning abilities. Alcohol, as well as other drugs, can lessen the ability to recognize danger signals, such as changes in a man's behaviors, suggestions, and intentions. A woman may have lessened ability to communicate her feelings about what she does and does not want to do sexually. Words such as "no" or "maybe" may be interpreted to mean "yes" if the man and/or woman have been drinking. Men may urge women to drink more to increase the chances that she will be unable to resist pressure to have sex. Under the influence of alcohol, men are more likely to be more aggressive in regard to sex; women may have a diminished ability to recognize danger signs.

To compound the concerns related to alcohol and sexual assault, specific drugs, usually slipped into a woman's drink, can produce disinhibition and amnestic effects for the potential victim. Rohypnol ("roofies"), gammahydroxy butyrate (GHB), and ketamine hydrochloride (Special K), described in detail in Chapter 12, are used as an accessory to date or acquaintance rape on or near college campuses.[23] Easy to place in the potential victim's drink, these drugs are tasteless and odorless and difficult to detect. Effects include increased confusion,

Health Tips

What to Do If You Are Raped

- Contact a friend or someone for support. There is always someone who will help you.
- Seek medical attention at once. All injuries are not immediately present.
- Do not bathe, douche, change your clothes, or rinse your mouth. If there is any possibility that you will report the crime, you don't want to destroy any evidence. Take a clean change of clothes with you to the hospital. Ask for tests to detect any sexually transmitted infections.
- You have the option of reporting the crime to the police. There are trained personnel who can assist

you in making that decision. They will explain the legal process to you.
- Write down what happened, in your own words. This will be helpful to you if charges are filed, the case goes to trial, and you decide to testify.
- Even if you decide not to testify, provide information about the rapist to the police which could help solve other rape cases.
- Get follow-up help and support. Counseling centers, rape centers, and health centers may be of help.
- Do not blame yourself for the incident.

relaxation or a dreamy state, and eventual unconsciousness; the victim usually is unable to remember what happened, which makes prosecution difficult.

Murder Intimate partner homicides comprise 40 to 50 percent of all murders of women in the United States. In 70 to 80 percent of intimate partner murders, regardless of which partner was killed, the man physically abused the woman before the murder.[24] These women were the victims of the one person in their life who professed to love and honor them—their partner. Unfortunately "until death do us part" came all too soon for the female partner. Murder is frequently the ultimate end to long-term and escalating abuse—abuse that, for unknown reasons, had been tolerated over time and was neither punished nor treated.

Crisis centers across the United States report case after case of deadly outcomes of abusive relationships. For example, Christine in New Mexico was stabbed twenty times by her former husband; Louise was shot to death by her estranged husband as she picked up their children after a weekend with their father; Joycelyn's throat was slashed by a former boyfriend as she left a restaurant with a date. Although the manner in which each woman was killed differed, the underlying circumstances were quite similar: Each woman was killed by a past or present husband or lover. Murder may be the final statement men make to their partners. A violent end to a relationship is often marked by desperate and barbarous acts on the part of the male partner.

The highest profile criminal and civil murder case of all time may well be that of O. J. Simpson. Simpson, a well-recognized professional athlete, TV personality, and actor, was accused of murdering his former wife and her male friend. In the development of the murder

case against Simpson, prosecutors uncovered a history of harassment and verbal and physical abuse of his wife. Claus von Bulow was tried and convicted of attempting to murder his wealthy wife and then won a reversed decision on appeal; actor Robert Blake was eventually acquitted of murdering his wife, Bonny Lee Bakley; and Scott Peterson was convicted of murdering his wife and unborn son and is now on death row at San Quentin Prison. (The Unborn Victims of Violence Act, making it a crime to harm an unborn, viable fetus, was signed into law in April 2004.)

Same-Sex Domestic Violence Violence against gay individuals and gay partners has increased significantly in recent years according to a study by the National Gay and Lesbian Task Force. Incidents of victimization include verbal harassment and threats, physical assaults, murder, and abuse by police. In 2003, lesbians, gays, bisexuals, and transgender (LGBT) people experienced 6,523 incidents of domestic violence. Six of these incidents resulted in murder.[25]

Domestic violence is usually discussed as a concern of heterosexual partners, but domestic violence occurs at similar rates in LGBT relationships. Numerous barriers exist for LGBT partners who are dealing with domestic violence. Already experiencing condemnation, discrimination, and denial, revealing additional "dirty laundry" may place same-sex partners in an even more precarious position. LGBT relationships are often condemned and exist in secret, and partners are often denied the rights of married couples; to reveal that domestic violence occurs in these relationships provides more ammunition to people who already condemn same-sex partnerships. Therefore, the wall of silence grows stronger.

FYI

Cyberstalking

Cyberstalking is a method by which the perpetrator(s) uses technology, usually the Internet, to harass another individual, group, or organization. The behavior includes false accusations, monitoring, transmission of threats, identity theft, solicitation of minors for sexual purposes, and gathering information for harassment purposes.[26] Characteristics of true cyberstalking will include one or several of the following: malice, premeditation, repetition, distress, obsession, vendetta, disregard of warnings to stop, harassment and/or threats.[27] Perpetrators meet or target their victims via Internet search engines, chat rooms, bulletin boards, and online communities such as MySpace or Facebook, or the victim may be a personal acquaintance of the perpetrator. While some cyberstalking may involve physical stalking, usually the perpetrator will post negative or derogatory comments that will include false accusations, false information, and may claim false victimization. The perpetrator may attempt to find information about the victim, encourage others to harass the victim, may send viruses to the victim's computers or order products in the victim's name, such as ordering sex toys and having them sent to the victim's workplace.

The first cyberstalking law went into effect in California in 1999 and a number of other states have followed with anti-cyberstalking laws. The Violence Against Women Act, reauthorized in 2005, made cyberstalking a part of the federal interstate stalking act. While the federal government is making some strides in addressing cyberstalking, the majority of legislative action is occurring at the state level.

What can individuals do to prevent cyberstalking? Consider the following: Do not give out personal information anywhere online; do not use your real name or nickname in chat rooms or online communities; be extremely cautious about meeting online acquaintances in person; log off immediately if the online chat becomes hostile or hints at unwelcome sexual behaviors. If you are being cyberstalked, make it clear that you do not want contact with the stalker, save all communications, attempt to block or filter messages from the stalker, contact the stalker's Internet service provider (ISP) and ask the ISP to contact the stalker or to close his account. The local police should be called and the stalker reported; provide the information needed to support your claim. The National Domestic Violence Hotline, 1-800-799-SAFE, can be contacted for assistance when reporting cyberstalking.

Care and assistance for LGBT victims of domestic violence are limited, and few shelters around the country reach out to victims of same-sex violence. People who are not "out" may be reluctant to report violence at the hands of their partners, and laws may make it difficult to obtain protective orders. An excellent assistance program is the Los Angeles Gay & Lesbian Center's STOP Partner Abuse/Domestic Violence Program. This center provides intervention and prevention services that address the unique needs of youth and adults in the LGBT community. Services include survivors' groups, a court-approved batterers' intervention program, crisis intervention, individual counseling, specialized assessment, education and consultation, and a multifaceted prevention program.[28] Educating mental health service providers and medical and law enforcement personnel about the special issues related to violence in LGBT partners will ensure that services are sensitive, appropriate, and accessible.[29] More shelters, more resources, and better training for professionals who work with LGBT victims of violence are critical needs.

Sexual Harassment Although **sexual harassment** is not violent in nature, it is abusive. It represents abuse of power and position, and, furthermore, it is a criminal offense. Taking place most often in the workplace or educational setting, it can also be a type of domestic abuse, wherein the abuser dominates his partner so that she feels unable to refuse sexual requests.

Types of sexual harassment include unwanted and unwarranted comments with sexual overtones or sexual innuendos, unwanted and uninvited touching or staring, and requests for sexual favors. Jokes, comments, or personal questions with sexual overtones that are offensive to the listener are also considered sexual harassment. Sexual harassment includes working, being, or living in a hostile, offensive, or intimidating environment in which actions or talk of a sexual nature exists because of gender. Female college students may be asked to provide a sexual act in return for a favor or preferential treatment provided by a professor. Men as well as women may be victims of sexual harassment; however, more commonly women are harassed by men. (See *Viewpoint:* "Is This Sexual Harassment?")

Health Tips: "Strategies for Addressing Sexual Harassment" contains suggestions for resolving concerns of sexual harassment. Have you ever experienced sexual harassment? If so, do you think these suggestions are beneficial?

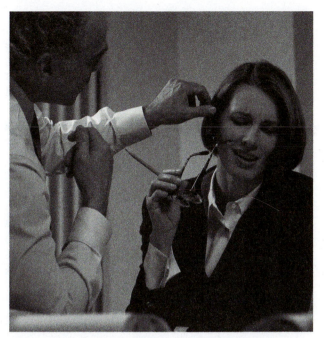

Unwanted touching is a type of sexual harassment.

Viewpoint

Is This Sexual Harassment?

Michelle worked in a department dominated by males. She brought to this job prior sales experience and qualities that made her effective in working with employees and customers. Her immediate supervisor developed a habit of telling his stories of sexual conquests to male employees when Michelle was near enough to hear. She politely asked him to wait until she was unable to hear the conversations before sharing the details of his sexual ventures. He refused, stating that he was not talking to her in the first place, and second, if she found the conversations so disturbing, to move far enough away so that she was unable to hear. If you were in Michelle's position, would you consider this a sexual harassment situation? If yes, what would you do about it? If you don't consider it sexual harassment, do you find it offensive?

ELDER ABUSE

As the population of the United States continues to age, the reality of **elder abuse** is more evident and more prevalent. Each year hundreds of thousands of older persons are abused, neglected, and exploited by family members and others. Many victims are people who are older, frail, vulnerable and cannot help themselves, and depend on others to meet their most basic needs. Most alleged perpetrators

Health Tips

Strategies for Addressing Sexual Harassment

- Do not ignore innuendos or degrading statements; otherwise, they will not stop. Clearly and firmly state your objections immediately. (Perhaps the harasser did not understand that the words or gestures were offensive.) You may need to share the incident(s) with a trusted individual in case you file charges later.
- Write down any incident(s) or written communication made by the harasser; date and file the information. Be sure to include the time, place, date, and witnesses, if any were present. Include what occurred and your response.
- Give the written information to another trusted individual as well as verbally share the incident with her or him. This person may be needed for verification if you elect to file charges either now or in the future.
- Confront the harassment by reporting it to authorities; you may be able to keep this from happening to others. If desired, talk to a professional counselor who can help you deal with any emotional distress related to the incident.
- Be truthful and accurate about the incident. Do not place the reputation of yourself and someone else in jeopardy if you are unsure about what happened. The fallout for you and the accused can have serious and embarrassing consequences.

are adult children (32.6 percent) or other family members (21.5 percent); and spouses/intimate partners accounted for 11.3 percent of the total.[30] Typically, elder abuse is defined as various types of abuse against someone age 60 or 65 and older. The types of abuse may include: physical, sexual, and emotional abuse; financial exploitation; neglect, self-neglect, and abandonment. The following describes the various types of abuse that are inflicted on the elderly:[31]

- **Physical abuse** is inflicting, or threatening to inflict, physical pain or injury on a vulnerable elder, or depriving them of a basic need.
- **Sexual abuse** is the infliction of nonconsensual sexual contact of any kind.
- **Emotional or psychological abuse** is the infliction of mental or emotional anguish or distress on an elder person through verbal or nonverbal acts.
- **Financial or material exploitation** is the illegal taking, misuse, or concealment of funds, property, or assets of a vulnerable elder.
- **Neglect** is the refusal or failure by those responsible to provide food, shelter, health care, or protection for a vulnerable elder.

Journal Activity

Incidents of Abuse

Having just read about abusive and violent acts against women, write down any incidents that you have experienced. Did you respond in any way to the perpetrator? If so, what did you say or do? Did you share the incident with anyone? Was the incident serious enough that you needed to involve the legal system? Was there a way to handle the situation better than you did? If so, what would that have been?

- **Self-neglect** is characterized as the behavior of an elderly person that threatens his/her own health or safety.
- **Abandonment** is the desertion of a vulnerable elder by anyone who has assumed the responsibility for care or custody of that person.

Reporting suspected abuse is extremely important; it is the moral and ethica l action to take. Contact the local police, and/or call the adult protective services in your state. If the abuse is occurring in a nursing home or other long-term care facility, along with contacting the police, contact the nursing home licensing agency in the state in which the abuse is occurring.

Having just read about the many types of violence and abuse against women, it is easy to see that incidents of abuse appear in many forms and range from minimal to very severe. A woman may quite easily experience several incidents, such as obscene telephone calls or being stalked, during her lifetime. No such experience should be considered inconsequential. Complete *Journal Activity:* "Incidents of Abuse" to evaluate how you would handle this situation. Unwanted touching is a type of sexual harassment.

COMMON ELEMENTS IN ALL TYPES OF ABUSE

All forms of abuse share four common elements and are linked with concerns regarding resolution of abusive situations. These elements reflect common thought that influences public opinion and often hinders effective legal and societal resolutions, delays the victims' efforts to seek help and counseling, and/or slows the process of healing. These common elements are discussed below.

Minimization

The public often thinks that violence and abuse are rare and that official statistics accurately represent prevalence. Violence against women can be likened to an iceberg: The tip of the iceberg represents the reported amount of violence; the larger portion of the iceberg, which remains unseen, is the actual occurrence and is estimated to be two to three times greater than abuse that is reported.

Directionality

Violence occurs largely in one direction: men victimize women. Incest is generally from father or stepfather to daughter or stepdaughter; generally men make obscene phone calls to women; date rape almost always involves men assaulting women.

Trivialization

Violence against women is often viewed in a joking way: "Incest is the game the whole family can play," "If you're going to be raped, just lie back and enjoy it." Remarks and jokes tend to negate the impact and seriousness of violence against women and promote a sporting aspect to men's violence.

Blaming the Victim

This occurs not only in violence but in such crimes as car theft or house burglaries. Worldwide, studies identify events that purportedly "trigger" violence. Examples of these includes not obeying her husband, talking back, not having food ready on time, not caring for children or home as instructed, questioning him about money or girlfriends, refusing sex, or going somewhere without permission. Little girls are accused of behaving "seductively," and women are held responsible for not stopping men sooner when kissing leads to an assault. An underlying assumption is that women are careless, men are not responsible for their actions, and self-control is much more difficult for men than for women.

CHARACTERISTICS OF BATTERED WOMEN

What are the traits of women who have been abused or violated? Why do they often remain in abusive relationships, either unable or unwilling to leave or seek assistance? Do these women develop these traits prior to experiencing abuse, or as a result of the abuse?

Personal Feelings and Beliefs

Battered women tend to feel degraded, worthless, isolated, and depressed, often leading to poor self-esteem.[32] Abused women often underestimate their abilities. A woman may assess her worthiness as it relates to success as wife or mother. If she is in a stormy, abusive relationship, even if she is successful in other areas of her life, feelings of inadequacy and negative self-concept can develop. Feelings of hopelessness may be a trait of the female both before and during an abusive relationship. She may feel that she cannot "do any better" than the partner she is currently with, or she may be so emotionally and financially dependent on her partner that she is afraid and/or unable to resolve the abusive situation. Feeling emotionally and psychologically helpless, a woman may become indecisive and unable to trust her ability to think or act outside of the relationship with her partner.

Mistaken personal beliefs such as "Battering is part of a loving relationship," or "If only I didn't make him mad, I wouldn't get hit" may originate in childhood and develop further in subsequent abusive relationships. These beliefs interfere with development of self-worth and prevent the woman from developing life-enhancing behaviors. Abused women may have watched their mothers or sisters being abused and can equate abuse with love and believe that this is how women are supposed to be treated by husbands, fathers, and other men. They come to believe that those who love you, abuse you.

Abused women may hold to the traditional belief that a man is the head of the household and a woman is subservient. Whatever her perception prior to the union, his violence eventually convinces her that yielding to him, maintaining the household, and taking care of the relationship and the children are safer behaviors than behaviors exemplified in "liberated partnerships." Abused women, often blaming themselves for causing the partner's violence, are socialized to believe they are responsible for maintaining the relationship. Consequently, if the relationship is unhappy, disturbed, or abusive, the abused woman feels the responsibility to "repair" it or soothe whatever is bothering the abuser. She may believe that if she were only a better lover, wife, mother, or worker, she would not be abused. As a result, the woman may believe she is deserving of the abuse and the abuser may camouflage abusive acts under the cloak of discipline. He teachers her a lesson, perhaps, as her or his father did to his wife during violent episodes that may have been witnessed during childhood.

Codependency

Women often have a codependent relationship with the abuser. **Codependency** means developing an emotional dependency with the abuser and the abuser's problem(s) to the point of self-neglect. Codependent women think and feel responsible for the needs of other people. These responsibilities may include their feelings, thoughts, actions, choices, wants, needs, well-being, lack of well-being, and ultimate destiny. Therefore, a codependent woman who is in an abusive relationship often feels responsible for the abuse and is willing to endure it so that she can be available to care for the abuser.

Perception of Partner

An abused woman's perception of her violent partner is often one of need; that is, the perpetrator needs her. She may believe that she is the only person who can help him overcome his problem; therefore, she feels compassion and pity. If her partner is a chemically dependent batterer, she may believe he will stop the abuse if he stops using alcohol and/or other drugs. She may believe that if she leaves him, he may abuse alcohol and drugs to the point of illness or death. Even in relationships having a history of long-term battering, women often love the batterer and are emotionally dependent upon the relationship.

CONSEQUENCES OF ABUSE

Consequences of abuse are varied and depend on the duration, type, and severity of the abuse. Over time, continual abuse will result in one or more of the following consequences.

Physical Consequences

Depending on the type of abuse inflicted, a woman can experience a plethora of physical consequences. Cuts, burns, punctures, bites, bruises, bleeding, dislocations, and bone fractures are physical manifestations of abusive encounters. Over time, physical abuse usually escalates in both severity and frequency. Abused women usually have a history of many visits to emergency rooms. Medical care providers are trained to screen injuries that may indicate various types of abuse. (See *FYI:* "Physical Abuse Scale.")

Physical wounds inflicted on women may eventually result in chronic, long-term disorders and disabilities. Conditions such as chronic arthritis, hypertension, gastrointestinal disorders, or asthma, which can develop because of stress, may be consequences of long-term physical abuse.

Emotional and Psychological Consequences

Women are likely to experience negative psychological effects as a result of abusive relationships. Continual abuse will cause women to feel depressed and worthless,

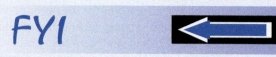

Physical Abuse Scale[33]

These acts of violence are listed in priority from less severe to most severe. The progression of physical abuse can be used in domestic abuse evaluations to determine the level of violence at which the perpetrator is operating and acts as a guide to determine the level of protection needed by the victim.

1. Throwing things; punching the wall
2. Pushing, shoving, grabbing, throwing things at the female
3. Slapping with an open hand
4. Kicking, biting
5. Hitting with a closed fist
6. Attempted strangulation
7. Beating up (pinning the victim to the wall or floor, repeatedly kicking or punching her)
8. Threatening with a weapon
9. Assault with a weapon

Her Story

Sue Anne: Surviving Incest

Sue Anne recounted the incestuous relationship with her father that always occurred in the mornings. After her mother left early for work, her father would come into the room as she was dressing for school. As the incest continued, it became broader in its scope, until Sue Anne had all but become her father's full-time lover. She escaped as much as possible by participating in as many school functions as possible. Sue Anne did not date until well into her college years, then married someone who was emotionally distant and withdrawn. She reported that as a married adult it was impossible to have sexual relations with her husband in the morning, and they continually argue about sexual issues. Sue Anne has difficulty with other intimate relationships, even to the point of feeling uncomfortable holding her own children, believing that she will "infect" her children if she is physically too close to them.

- What are some positive steps Sue Anne could take to begin healing from the abuse she experienced from her father?
- How can Sue Anne establish a support system that can assist her in this issue?
- Can Sue Anne's husband play a role in the process of her healing from her early experiences?

experience anxiety attacks, and feel they are going crazy. As a result of these feelings, women experience major emotional distress. The most devastating psychological effects appear as a result of being abused by a trusted person who was known to the victim (for example, a father, stepfather, or brothers).

As children, girls who have been sexually abused may develop feelings of anxiety, depression, anger, hostility, guilt, shame, and/or inferiority. These feelings can develop as an immediate response to the abuse, or they may develop in adulthood. As adults, these women often experience nightmares, relationship distress, and sexual dysfunction. Women who were sexually abused as children may have problems relating to their own parents as well as to both men and women; these women also experience difficulty in responding to their own children in a healthy manner. The severity of emotional and psychological consequences depends on the length of time since the abuse, the length of time the abuse lasted, the woman's age at the time of abuse, and her relationship to the perpetrator. (See *Her Story:* "Sue Anne: Surviving Incest.")

Another young woman, describing the emotional pain she experienced as a result of abuse, proclaimed her self-hatred by saying, "I had an oil slick oozing goo inside me. I knew I was filled with something evil, and that evil rubbed off on everyone I came in contact with. So I didn't let anybody really get near me."[34]

Women who have been victimized will experience an immediate postvictimization distress response that includes a pattern of fear and avoidance, disturbances of self-concept and self-esteem, and sexual dysfunction.

Spiritual Consequences

The very basic values of meaningful life and meaningful relationships are undermined as a result of early abuse, especially when the abuse is inflicted by individuals who are supposed to nurture and protect (for example, father, stepfather, grandfather, uncle). Females may find that core values such as trust, honesty, respect, and concern are impaired or lost as a result of abusive relationships, especially abuse inflicted by supposedly caring men. Abused women report an inability to trust and respect others, especially men. Perhaps of greater concern is the fact that these women may mistrust their *own* perceptions of other people's behaviors and motives. Abuse in the family destroys the very foundation on which healthy functioning relationships are built.

Social Consequences

Violence and abuse manifest themselves with a variety of societal consequences. For example, increased use of dwindling health care resources causes the costs of medical care to rise, overloads medical personnel, and may lead to hasty diagnoses and sometimes too-aggressive treatments for many disorders. Emergency care is the most costly and most frequently used form of medical care following incidents of abuse. Communities experience overburdening of police, judicial, and human resources systems that lead to increases in taxes and increases in social problems such as drug abuse, violence, and homelessness. Society as a whole suffers from abusive relationships—not just monetarily—but with the negative consequences of violence cycling into the next generation, violence of all types is continued. In general, abuse contributes to decreases in the quality of life for everyone, not just for those in abusive relationships.

Economic Impact of IPV

The physical, emotional, psychological, spiritual, and social consequences of IPV are staggering and undermining of the most essential component of our society—healthy human individuals and family. Additionally, this epidemic of personal violence has a significant economic impact for families, states, and the nation. The cost of intimate partner violence exceeded $8.3 BILLION annually, which included $460 million for rape, $6.2 BILLION for physical assault, $461 million for stalking, and $1.2 billion in the value of lost lives.[35] Victims of severe IPV lose nearly 8 million days of paid work—the equivalent of more than 32,000 full-time jobs—and almost 5.6 million days of household productivity each year.[36] For women who experience severe aggression by men, they often are not allowed to go to work or school, or they may have their or their children's lives threatened. These women cannot be productive in the workforce and may lack marketable skills if they elect to leave the abusive relationship.

LEAVING THE ABUSIVE RELATIONSHIP

Deciding to Leave

Some women stay in abusive relationships, but others leave. Abused women typically leave an abusive environment five to seven times before they feel safe enough and have accumulated the resources needed to leave for good. Women frequently return to perpetrators following a visit to a safe shelter or a relative's home. Following her return, methods for eliminating the abuse without terminating the relationship, if both partners desire, need to be developed. However, if the abuse continues following each return, then she should seek assistance to leave the relationship permanently.

During the course of abuse, women may have involved the legal system in a number of ways. Calling the police during bouts of abuse, gaining protection for children, and obtaining restraining orders to keep the abuser at a distance are all proper and probable ways to use the legal system. As a woman prepares to leave a relationship, she may need to again use the resources of the legal system. Occasionally a safe escort out of the home is required, as well as accompaniment to secret and safe housing for her and her children. Community resources can be invaluable to a woman who has decided to remove herself and her family from an abusive environment.

Developing a Safety Plan

Once a woman makes the decision to leave the relationship, perhaps her most critical concern is developing a safety plan and determining a means of survival. The safety plan needs to include a means of leaving, a list of people to call in case of emergency, and a suitcase containing clothing, personal items, money, Social Security cards, bankbooks, children's birth certificates and school records, and other important documents. Immediate survival needs consist of locating a safe place to live once she has left the relationship, being able to feed and clothe herself and the children, and determining a way to become financially self-sufficient. Long-term survival may include finding a job, completing some type of education, or developing necessary job skills. It may also include locating dependable quality child care.

Answering the following questions may assist women in determining the essential elements necessary for their survival and their children's survival: Are there family or friends where she can stay? If not, does she know how to access alternative means of shelter? Does she need to contact the police or obtain legal aid? Does she need counseling services? What other community agencies might assist her? Let's take a close look at some possible answers to these questions.

Locating Safe Shelter

This can be as simple as calling the police and asking for help. Currently there are several thousand safe shelters throughout the United States in which women can find safety, as well as advocacy, support, and other needed services. Check the phone book under "domestic violence," "women's shelter," "shelter for battered or abused women," and "crisis hotline" to locate the nearest safe shelter. In rural areas where safe housing may not be available, women can contact a local church or community center for assistance in locating temporary safe shelter.

Knowing what to expect is beneficial and may lessen the anxiety of leaving the abusive environment. Safe-shelter personnel will usually transport women and their children from an emergency room, the police station, or any other designated place to the shelter and away from the abusive partner.

Women and their children often arrive at the shelter with only the clothes they are wearing and return to their home to retrieve their belongings only when their partners are absent. They may need to utilize the shelter's resources for a time. Women and their children are usually allowed to remain in the safe shelter for 30 days with the option of increasing the time if the situation warrants it, unless other women are waiting to move in. During their stay, women help with the routine care and maintenance of the shelter, cook meals for themselves and their children, and wash and care for personal clothing.

Planning for the future without the abusive partner is also an important task during a woman's stay at the shelter. Depending on their individual needs, women may receive personal, group, and/or job-related counseling. Shelter personnel provide access to government assistance programs such as Women, Infant and Children (WIC), food stamps, and drug abuse counseling, if needed. Women may also receive help obtaining Medicaid and Social Security benefits. Other important tasks may include seeking employment, locating child care, filing protective orders, and starting divorce proceedings.

Locating Other Resources

Because safe shelters are temporary and serve only as a short-term bridge, finding other resources beyond the shelter is essential. Financial assistance may be temporarily obtained from Aid for Dependent Children (AFDC), the American Red Cross, the Social Security Administration, or local church charities. Phone numbers and addresses for these agencies can be found in local telephone directories. (See *Health Tips:* "Locating Local Resources.") A multitude of resources can be found on the Internet, and it is possible to "hide" Web site searches so no one can discover the search.

Housing can often be found through the local housing authority, Housing and Urban Development Office (HUD), or local property management offices, which often have apartments for rent at lower rates. Addresses and information for agencies that provide child care are usually provided to women during their stay at the safe shelter. Child care arrangements, sometimes at a reduced rate, are often made between the shelter and child care providers. Additionally, churches often have day care centers that are made available to local safe-shelter

---

Health Tips

Locating Local Resources

Locate addresses and phone numbers for the following list of helpful resources in your town that can be used by women who are in need of assistance. Add any additional agencies or individuals who can be beneficial. Attach a city map and highlight helping agencies.

Agency	Phone #	Address
Emergency		
Crisis hotline		
Police		
Ambulance		
Safe house		
Legal aid		
Child protective service		
Doctor		
Friend		
Other:		

---

children on a temporary basis. Women who are making the effort to move forward following an abusive relationship may elect to share child care responsibilities, caring for one another's children while each works at different times.

Job training is available through a variety of sources. Communities offer adult learning centers with computer classes, Graduate Equivalence Diploma (GED) classes, and literacy volunteers. Social services departments offer job counseling, skill testing, and contact persons for job location through state or county employment commissions. Many temporary personnel agencies provide on-the-job training programs, which can lead to employment opportunities for women who already possess job skills. Many towns and cities have community colleges at which job training or job-skill refresher courses are available for women who seek assistance. State, county, and local agencies provide emotional and financial counseling, often without charge.

HEALING FROM ABUSE

Healing from violence and abuse is possible. In fact, it is probable if a woman makes the choice to heal and then takes the steps, sometimes long and painful steps, to move forward and to thrive. Thriving means to flourish, bloom, to become whole, whole in one's own life and also in friendships, family relationships, and love relationships. Healing means

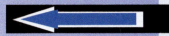

FYI

The Process of Healing

- Commit to heal, and begin to move toward self-change.
- Processing memories of the abusive incidents and the accompanying feelings is often painful and depressing; remember that it is transitional and will go away.
- Admit to yourself that the abuse did occur. Share this essential step with a trusted person who can help you with any feelings of shame associated with the incidents.
- Place the heavy blanket of guilt and shame on its rightful owner—the perpetrator. In no way was the abuse the fault of the victim.
- Develop realistic and appropriate feelings toward other people by getting in touch with the vulnerable child within—that child you may have lost in the process of coping with the agony that can accompany abuse.
- Listen to your instincts; listen to your own feelings, mind, and body. This promotes learning to trust oneself and builds a foundation from which to approach life situations.

- Recognize and feel all the losses related to an abusive relationship: loss of childhood, loss of trust, loss of idealized relationship, loss of respect, loss of joy, and so much more. This enables you to confront the pain, feel it, express it, and move forward.
- Use the freeing emotion of anger, considered the backbone of healing, and direct it to where it belongs: toward the perpetrator and the individuals who were not protective.
- Confront the perpetrator and disclose the abuse, if possible, because this can be an empowering and freeing activity for women who choose to do it.
- Forgiving the perpetrator is highly recommended, though it is not necessary for healing. But forgiving yourself is a must.
- Spiritual renewal through religion, nature's beauty, meditation, and/or contributing to society is important to the process of resolution and moving forward.

moving beyond repair of the damage to body, mind, and soul. It also means being able to feel at peace, to feel genuine love, and to gain satisfaction with one's life and contribute to one's immediate and expanding environment.

One survivor said that healing and recovery are beautiful parts of life. Her healing "family" not only consisted of her present, nonabusive husband, her children, and grandchildren, but also included her fellow travelers—other survivors she learned to love and trust. The gift she had given herself was to allow all of her healing family to express love, warmth, and kindness.

Survivors of abuse recount the stages and feelings they experienced as they progressed toward healing and moved forward with their lives. These women have come to realize that they survived the traumatic time of abuse and became adults. From this awareness, women can move forward through the necessary stages into a life of satisfying relationships and contributions.

In their book *The Courage to Heal,*[37] Bass and Davis identify fourteen stages that women experience as they progress toward healing and recovering from abuse. It should be noted that survivors may not experience every stage and may not go through them in any particular order. *FYI:* "The Process of Healing" is a paraphrased summary of these stages.

HOW TO HELP

Helping a woman who is leaving an abusive relationship and is attempting to move forward with her life may not always be the responsibility of the legal, judicial, or social systems. Women often turn to friends and family first for support and assistance. Family, friends, and professionals who are available and knowledgeable about how to help these women can go a long way in aiding their chance to develop a healthy and contributing lifestyle.

How can friends and family help? How can you help? Consider the following suggestions developed by the U.S. Center for Mental Health Services titled *Supporting the Survivor.*[38]

- *Listen.* Talking about the experience, when the survivor is ready, will help validate what happened to him or her and can reduce stress and feelings of isolation. Let the survivor take the lead in conversations and respond when appropriate.
- *Research.* If the victim/survivor wants more information, would like to report a crime, or has other concerns, help her find the answers and resources.
- *Reassure.* As strange as it may sound, survivors often question whether an incident was their fault or wonder what they could have done to prevent the crime against them. They may need to hear that it was not their fault and be assured that they are not alone.

- *Empower.* Following trauma, victims can feel as though much of their lives is beyond their control. Aiding them in maintaining routines can be helpful, as well as offering options or possible solutions.
- *Be patient.* Every journey through the healing process is unique. Try to understand that it will take time, and do what you can to be supportive. The healing process has no predetermined timeline.
- *Ask.* The survivor may need help with any number of things or have questions on many different topics. Even a favor as mundane as running a few errands or keeping the children temporarily can be helpful.
- *Encourage.* Suggest that the survivor seek professional support in addition to your support.

Time and space will be required for a woman to proceed through the stages of healing. As a friend or family member, express compassion for and validation of her feelings, such as feelings of fear, anger, guilt, and pain. Also, helping her through the stages of healing will produce changes in your relationship with her. Be prepared to make some changes in your attitude and behaviors toward her.

Equally important, children must be taught that the use of violence to resolve problems and exert control over others is unacceptable behavior. Children may need as much emotional support as their mother after leaving an abusive environment. Many of the same support systems that have been discussed for women also offer opportunities for healing and growth for children. Children need both healthy role models and structure and discipline without abuse.

MOVING FORWARD

I kept working on change . . . slowly, slowly I moved ahead. My body cells replace themselves. . . . I can replace and remove the damage, the pain. Yes, I have more work, but I have come a long way, baby! I now have the skills and the desire to move ahead; I will use them and I will find peace.

—A Survivor

Women can develop skills that enable them to heal from abusive relationships. Moreover, they can engage in activities that foster resolution of the abuse and promote progression toward a joyful and fulfilling life.

Building Resiliency

Resiliency is the ability to recover, to overcome adversity, to bend and bounce back like a willow tree in a wind-storm. Resiliency can be developed as a skill and utilized to recover from the adverse effects of an abusive relationship. Finding and developing support systems outside the abusive environment can assist women in recognizing characteristics of healthy relationships. Having contact with "healthy" individuals who believe in the woman will promote belief in herself. These supportive relationships also provide conditions that enable women to feel worthwhile and valued. Susan, leaving home as a young teen following years of incest, found support and acceptance in a church group. She told of how the church group assisted her in developing a sense of purpose and value. Spirituality, too, can promote the development of resiliency because it fosters a sense of worthiness and a purpose for living. As a result, women should seek to discover and fulfill that purpose. Abused women report recognizing potential personal power as a way to take control of their lives and develop resiliency. Becoming self-directed, making personal decisions, taking responsibility for oneself, and being self-sufficient are methods by which personal power can be discovered.

Even though the history of the abuse cannot be erased, moving through and acting on these stages allows a woman to discover stability, develop a positive perspective, experience peace, and move forward to a satisfying and contributing life.

Self-Caring

"Why would I care for myself when no one else cared for me? Besides, I was too busy taking care of everyone else. Caring for myself made me think I was 'selfish,'" stated one survivor of domestic abuse. **Self-caring** or self-nurturing means taking care of one's own physical, emotional, and spiritual needs. Having concern for others should not be neglected, but concern for others should not be at the expense of oneself. Self-caring is often a major change in behavior for women who have been in abusive relationships. Self-care enables women to recognize the value of self and to act accordingly by making healthy, nurturing choices. Engaging in fun and enjoyable activities is indicative of moving ahead with life and practicing the art of self-care.

What would you do if you were asked to demonstrate self-care activities? Answers to this question often reflect the stage of healing and growth that survivors are in at any given point. "Having a quiet meal or a complete night's sleep" may be indicative of initial stages of moving ahead with life. Women who, perhaps, have moved further through the healing and growth process may provide such answers as enjoying a hot tub, working in the garden, watching movies, reading books, exercising, cooking a favorite meal, buying flowers, or sharing loving embraces. Whatever the method, engaging in self-care activities is an important move away from former negative beliefs and toward a healthier life.

Assess Yourself

Recognizing and Meeting Personal Needs

Identify and briefly explain some of the things a woman can do to meet the various needs that are important to moving forward with her life.

Needs	Who	How	Where
Survival			
Security			
Love/acceptance			
Self-worth			
Self-actualization			

Meeting Needs

Except for the most basic survival needs, such as food, shelter, and clothing, a woman's higher level needs often go unmet in an abusive relationship. Moving forward certainly means moving beyond survival needs and toward needs that promote progression and growth. Abraham Maslow, whose hierarchy of needs model was introduced in Chapter 3, provides an excellent guide to determining human needs. The need for security, love and acceptance, self-worth, and self-actualization (the fulfillment of a woman's potential) are discussed by Maslow as necessary for basic well-being and continual growth. Adhering to the suggestions found in the section titled "Leaving the Abusive Relationship" and utilizing the resource information presented here can provide the means by which these needs can be recognized and met. Now complete *Assess Yourself:* "Recognizing and Meeting Personal Needs."

PREVENTING ABUSE

Preventing abuse against women must be addressed at all levels: personal, community, state, and federal. Support and advocacy can be addressed at each level, as can strategies that enable women to stop abusive episodes or, even better, prevent abusive patterns from ever occurring.

Personal Level

At the personal level, consider the following suggestions that provide empowerment for women, enabling them to recognize and partner in a nonabusive and whole relationship.

- Teaching women to be intolerant of any form of abuse inflicted upon them or their children is an essential component of prevention.
- Educating girls and boys from an early age about the characteristics of healthy and long-lasting relationships will set the foundation for preventing abuse in adulthood. These characteristics include respect, love, shared values, trust, honesty, commitment, mutual caring, and communication.
- Improving the self-worth of women may assist them to think well enough of themselves and to accept that they do not deserve and should not tolerate any abusive behaviors. Personal self-worth leads to the desire to live in a healthy and whole family environment.
- Creating awareness of the negative consequences for women and children, both short-term and long-term, that result from involvement with an abusive partner can assist in preventing relationship abuse.

Healthy relationship awareness not only is a means of empowerment for females but also is a way of changing patterns of socialization for the two sexes. From an early age, boys must be taught that relationships are a partnership in which both participants share in all areas of decision making, responsibilities, and promotion of the relationship's success.

In thinking back on boys and young men in your life, can you remember characteristics that created an uneasy or skeptical feeling in you about them? Do you remember any of the following traits or behaviors that have been identified as characteristics of potential abusers: very little tolerance for others who have different ideas, opinions, or beliefs; low self-esteem; feelings of inadequacy as a man; being quick to anger; rigid and controlling behaviors or demands; overuse of alcohol and use of other drugs; blaming others for anything that doesn't work out; criticizing others; or being from a family in which there was abusive treatment of the mother and/or children.

Community Level

A community effort to prevent violence and abuse against women is essential because abuse is a social problem, not a private or secret problem. These community actions have been initiated in some areas to address violence and abuse against women as a major social concern:

- Coordination of agencies and programs that can serve to reach families in the community has been accomplished in some areas of the country. The legal, medical, social, and educational agencies have developed formal and, in some instances, informal linkages to educate and provide services to families.
- Parenting classes, relationship-building skills, and stress management seminars are a few of the

components that communities offer that can promote healthy family relationships, family preservation, and support for families in need of these services. When the health and well-being of individuals and families are destroyed by family violence, the quality of community life deteriorates.

- Programs for men, especially abusive men, are being developed in which they learn to take responsibility for their actions, develop better partnering skills, and find support for change and growth among other participants.
- Extended-day programs for children and youth have been developed, either at school sites or at community centers. Providing recreational and educational activities and sometimes personal and social guidance, these centers offer a safe, fun, and caring environment for youth from all types of families.
- Increasing community awareness, speaking out about individual and victims' rights, and holding men accountable for their abusive actions is critical, not only in preventing violence and abuse against women but in stopping it as well.

State and Federal Levels

State and federal legislation, legislators, agencies, and other governing entities are making inroads into accepting the fact that women *are* abused and that not only the perpetrators but also the systems that allow this to go unchallenged must be stopped. State and federal governments are continuing to enact legislation to prevent violence and abuse against women as well as prosecuting individuals who dare to commit this crime against another human being, especially human beings whom they profess to love.

- Laws to protect the rights of women against violence and abuse are being passed at the state and federal government levels.
- Reporting any injury that medical personnel, during the time of treatment, perceive to be the result of violence or abuse is required by many states. A physician who fails to report suspected abusive wounds of any type (for example, cuts, burns, bruises, or bullet wounds) is subject to fines or even a possible jail sentence.
- The Violence Against Women Act is a landmark mandate that continues to strengthen law enforcement strategies and promote safeguards for victims of domestic and sexual assault. This law has provisions related to safe streets, safe homes for women, civil rights and equal justice for women in the court system, rights against stalking, and protection for battered immigrant

---

Autobiography in Five Short Chapters

I.

I walk down the street.
There is a deep hole in the sidewalk.
I fall in
I am lost . . . I am helpless
It isn't my fault
It takes forever to find a way out.

II.

I walk down the same street.
There is a deep hole in the sidewalk.
I pretend I don't see it.
I fall in again.
I can't believe I am in the same place
but, it isn't my fault.
It still takes a long time to get out.

III.

I walk down the same street.
There is a deep hole in the sidewalk.
I see it is there.
I still fall in . . . it's a habit
my eyes are open.
I know where I am.
It is my fault. I get out immediately.

IV.

I walk down the same street.
There is a deep hole in the sidewalk.
I walk around it.

V.

I walk down another street.

by Portia Nelson[39]

women and children. The Department of Justice coordinates efforts with other federal agencies as well as state, local, and tribal law enforcement agencies.

- The Trauma Act, passed in 2003, expands research on the psychological aftereffects of violence against women and enhances research on socioeconomic and sociocultural correlates of violence, research related to special populations, and violence screenings.[40]

It is clear that violence and abuse against women are raging crimes in this country. Varied and complex negative consequences result—not only for women, but for our children, who are possibly future victims or perpetrators. To rectify and to prevent this, actions at all levels—from the individual to the federal government—must continue. Until violence and abuse are absolutely condemned by everyone, abuse will continue and women will remain trapped in a potentially lethal cycle of violence.

Chapter Summary

- Abuse against women has been documented throughout history.
- Domestic abuse, sexual assault, child abuse, elder abuse, and other forms of abuse against women are an epidemic in this country and produce serious physical, mental, emotional, and social consequences for men, women, and their children.
- Financial concerns, self-blame, emotional issues, codependency, and perception of her partner are reasons women often remain in abusive relationships.
- Fear for their children's lives and safety as well as their own is sometimes the impetus for leaving an abusive relationship.
- Sex trafficking © cyberstalking are a serious concern for young woman, both in the United States and in other countries.

- Having a plan that includes safe facilities, a support system, and accessibility to a variety of resources is an important asset when leaving an abusive relationship.
- As women heal from abusive relationships, they generally experience the healing process in a number of stages.
- Family and friends can aid women who have left abusive relationships in moving forward with their lives. Survivors can develop skills that assist their efforts to improve the quality of life for themselves as well as their children.
- Developing a widespread and comprehensive approach to prevention of abuse and violence against women must be a personal priority as well as a priority at the local, state, and federal government levels.

Review Questions

1. Historically, why have women been considered the lesser or weaker sex?
2. Why is it that women often believe they deserve the abuse they receive in a relationship?
3. How and why is the perpetrator socialized into a belief system?
4. Why are women reluctant to report domestic abuse?
5. What barriers in society reduce the likelihood that domestic abuse will be reported to law enforcement authorities?
6. What is meant by psychological abuse, and what are a number of the resulting consequences?

7. What are the behaviors of a potential rapist, and how can women avoid being in a situation where a rape could occur?
8. What are some methods that can help resolve issues related to sexual harassment?
9. What characteristics are associated with women who are abused? How do they develop?
10. What are some of the physical, psychological, spiritual, and social consequences when experiencing abuse?
11. What are the types of resources available to enable a woman to leave an abusive relationship?
12. What are the indicators of healing that show that women are moving ahead with their lives after abuse?

Resources

Arming Women against Rape & Endangerment
  www.aware.org
Asian & Pacific Islander Institute on Domestic Violence 415-568-3315
  www.apiidv.org
Battered Women's Justice Project
National Clearinghouse for the Defense of Battered Women 800-903-0111 ext. 3
  www.ncdbw.org

Casa de Esperanza 651-646-5553
  www.casadeesperanza.org
Child Help National Child Abuse Hotline
  www.childhelpusa.org
Institute on Domestic Violence in the African American Community
  www.dvinstitute.org

Men Can Stop Rape
www.mencanstoprape.org
National Center for Lesbian Rights
nclrights.org/index.htm
National Center for Victims of Crime
www.ncvc.org/ncvc/Main.aspx
National Coalition against Domestic Violence
www.ncadv.org
National Domestic Violence Hotline 1-800-799-7233
1-800-787-3224 (TTY)
www.ndvh.org
National Health Resource Center on Domestic Violence
888-792-2873
www.futureswithoutviolence.org/health
National Indigenous Women's Resource Center 406-465-1638
www.niwrc.com

National Latino Alliance for the Elimination of Domestic
Violence/Alanzia Latino National para Erradicar La Violencia
Domèstica
www.dvalianza.org
National Resource Center on Domestic Violence 800-537-2238
www.nrcdv.org and www.vawnet.org
Rape, Abuse, and Incest National Network (RAINN)
www.rainn.org
Resource Center on Domestic Violence: Child Protection and
Custody 800-527-3223
www.ncjfcj.org/dept/fvd
Survivors of Incest Anonymous
www.siawso.org
Violence against Women Office (National)
www.usdoj.gov/ovw

References

1. *Women's history in America.* 1995. Retrieved July 9, 2012, from www.wic.org/misc/history.htm
2. Dobash, R. E., and R. P. Dobash. 1977–1978. Wives: The "appropriate" victim's of marital violence. *Victimology: An International Journal* 2: 429.
3. Black, M.C., K. C. Basile, et al. 2011. *The National Intimate Partner and Sexual Violence Survey (NISVS): 2010 Summary Report.* Atlanta, GA: National Center for Injury Prevent and Control, Centers for Disease Control and Prevention.
4. Ibid., p. 38.
5. U.S. Surgeon General. 2003. *Family violence as a public health issue.* Presented to the Symposium on Family Violence: The Impact of Child, Intimate Partner, & Elder Abuse. Retrieved July 9, 2012, from http://www.surgeongeneral.gov/news/speeches/violence08062003.htm
6. Tjaden, P., and N. Thonnes. 2002. *Extent, nature, and consequences of intimate partner violence.* Washington, DC: National Institute of Justice, and Atlanta, GA: Centers for Disease Control and Prevention.
7. Dobash, R. E., and R. P. Dobash. Wives: The "appropriate" victims of marital violence.
8. Tran, C. 2005. Monkey see, monkey abuse. *Science Now.* (June 27).
9. The Children's Partnership. 2002. *America's children: Challenges for the 21st century.* Retrieved July 9, 2012, from www.childrenspartnership.org
10. Black, M. C., K. C. Basile, et al. 2011. *The National Intimate Partner and Sexual Violence Survey (NISVS): 2010 Summary Report.*
11. Crandall, M., A. B. Nathens, M. A. Kernic, V. L. Holt, and E. P. Rivara. 2004. Predicting future injury among women in abusive relationships. *Journal of Trauma-Injury Infection and Critical Care* 56 (4): 906–83.
12. National Task Force to End Sexual and Domestic Violence Against Women. 2005. *The Violence Against Women Act: 10 Years of progress and moving forward.* Retrieved July 10, 2012, from http://www.ncadv.org/files/OverviewFormatted1.pdf
13. Arkansas Coalition Against Domestic Violence. (2009). *Why do the abused stay?* Retrieved July 10, 2012, from http://www.domesticpeace.com/ed_whystay.html
14. U.S. Department of Health and Human Services. National Clearinghouse on Child Abuse and Neglect. (2008). *Long-term consequences of child abuse and neglect.* Retrieved July 10, 2012, from http://www.childwelfare.gov/pubs/factsheets/long_term_consequences.cfm
15. Moelker, W. 2008. *Consequences of sexual abuse; Effects of child abuse; Symptoms of child molestation; Child sexual abuse signs.* Retrieved July 10, 2012, from http://web4health.info/en/answers/sex-abuse-effects.htm
16. U.S. Department of Health and Human Services. Administration on Children, Youth and Families. (2010). *Child Maltreatment 2010.* Retrieved July 10, 2012, from http://www.acf.hhs.gov/programs/cb/pubs/cm10/cm10.pdf#page=31
17. Ibid.
18. Black, M.C., K.C. Basile, et al. 2011. *The National Intimate Partner and Sexual Violence Survey (NISVS): 2010 Summary Report.*
19. Ibid.
20. National Institute of Justice. 2008. *Measuring Frequency.* Retrieved July 10, 2012, from http://www.nij.gov/nij/topics/crime/rape-sexual-violence/campus/measuring.htm
21. Fisher, B. S., F. T. Cullen, and M. G. Turner. 2000. *The sexual victimization of college women.* Washington, DC: U.S. Department of Justice, Office of Justice Programs.
22. Payne, W., D. Hahn, and E. Lucas. (2007). *Understanding our health.* 9th ed. New York: McGraw-Hill.
23. National Women's Health Information Center. 2004. *Date rape drugs fact sheet.* Retrieved on July 10, 2012, from http://womenshealth.gov/publications/our-publications/fact-sheet/date-rape-drugs.cfm
24. National Institute of Justice. 2007. *How Widespread Is Intimate Partner Violence?* Retrieved July 10, 2012, from http://www.nij.gov/nij/topics/crime/intimate-partner-violence/extent.htm
25. National Coalition of Anti-Violence Programs. 2004. *Lesbian, gay bisexual, and transgender domestic violence: 2003 supplement.* New York: National Coalition of Anti-Violent Programs. Retrieved July 10, 2012, from www.avp.org
26. Bocij. P. 2004. *Cyberstalking: Harassment in the internet age and how to protect your family.* p. 14. London: Praeger.
27. Ibid., pp. 9–10.
28. National Coalition of Anti-Violence Programs, *Lesbian, gay, bisexual, and transgender domestic violence: 2003 supplement.*

29. McClaughlyn, K. 2002. *Domestic violence: The hidden secret of LGBT community.* Archived newsletter from the Office of Minority Health. Washington, DC: U.S. Office of Public Health and Human Services, Office of Minority Health, pp. 10–11.

30. Administration on Aging. 2004. *Elder rights and resources.* http://www.aoa.gov/eldfam/Elder_Rights/Elder_Abuse/Elder_ Abuse.aspx

31. Ibid.

32. National Council on Child Abuse and Family Violence. 2012. *Spouse/partner abuse information.* Retrieved July 11, 2012, from http://nccafv.org/spouse.htm

33. Strauss, J., R. J. Gelles, and S. K. Seinmetz. 1988. *Behind closed doors: Violence in the American family.* Garden City, NY: Anchor.

34. Bass, E., and J. Davis. 1992. *The courage to heal: A guide for women survivors of child sexual abuse.* New York: Harper & Row, p. 181.

35. Max, W., D. P. Rice, E. Finkelstein, R. A. Bardwell, and S. Leadbetter. 2004. The economic toll of intimate partner violence against women in the United States. *Violence Vict.* 19(3): 259–72.

36. Centers for Disease Control and Prevention (CDC). 2003. *Costs of intimate partner violence against women in the United States.* Atlanta, GA: CDC, National Center for Injury Prevention and Control.

37. Bass, E., and J. Davis. 1992. *The courage to heal: A guide for women survivors of child sexual abuse.*

38. U.S. Department of Health and Human Services, Center for Mental Health Services. 2005. *Supporting the Survivor.* Retrieved July 12, 2012, from www.mentalhealth.samhsa.gov/ publications/allpubs/SMA05-4028/victimforprint.pdf

39. Nelson, P. 1993. *There's a hole in my sidewalk.* Hillsboro, OR: Beyond Words.

40. Office of Legislative Policy and Analysis, S 1811-. 2003. *Expanding Research for Women in Trauma Act of 2003.* Retrieved July 12, 2012, from http://olpa.od.nih.gov/tracking/ senate_bills/session1/

Chapter Eight

Exploring Women's Sexuality

CHAPTER OBJECTIVES

When you complete this chapter, you will be able to do the following:

◇ Describe the female reproductive anatomy

◇ Describe the phases of the menstrual cycle

◇ Recognize the signs and symptoms of uterine fibroids

◇ Contrast the stages of the female sexual response cycle

◇ Explain the advantages and disadvantages of menopausal hormone therapy

This chapter covers female sexuality, including female reproductive anatomy and physiology, breast health, the human sexual response cycle and sexual dysfunction. It looks at the changes you can expect to experience from menarche to menopause. This information is important in raising awareness about your body, how it functions, and the changes you can expect throughout your lifetime.

FEMALE REPRODUCTIVE ANATOMY AND PHYSIOLOGY

The chapter begins with a discussion of the female reproductive anatomy and physiology, particularly the external genitalis, the internal genitalis, and the breasts.

External Genitalia

The external genitalia, termed the pudendum or **vulva,** refers to those parts that are outwardly visible. The vulva includes the mons pubis, labia majora, labia minora, clitoris, urethral opening, vaginal opening, and perineum. Individual differences in size, coloration, and shape of the external genitalia are common.

Mons Pubis   The **mons pubis** is a triangular, mounding area of fatty tissue that covers the pubic bone. During adolescence, pubic hair begins to appear on the mons pubis as a result of increased sex hormones. This hair, varying in coarseness, curliness, amount, and thickness, covers the mons and may extend to the navel. The mons protects the pubic symphysis (the place where the pubic bones join) and cushions the woman's body during sexual intercourse.

Labia Majora   The **labia majora** are two longitudinal folds of adipose tissue covered with skin. They are sometimes referred to as the "large lips" and have darker pigmentation than the labia minora. The labia majora protect the vaginal and urethral openings and are covered with hair and sebaceous (oil) glands. The inner surfaces tend to be smooth, moist, and hairless. After childbirth, the labia majora may separate and no longer fully cover the vaginal area. The labia majora become more flaccid as a woman gets older.

Labia Minora   The **labia minora,** sometimes referred to as the "small lips," consist of erectile, connective tissue that darkens and swells during sexual arousal. The labia minora, located inside the labia majora, are more sensitive and responsive to touch than the labia majora. The labia minora enclose the clitoris. The upper folds form the prepuce, while the lower folds form the frenum of the clitoris. At the bottom, the folds blend together to form the fourchette, the anterior edge of the perineum.

Clitoris

The **clitoris** is a highly sensitive organ composed of nerves, blood vessels, and erectile tissue. It is covered with a thin epidermis. It can be found under the prepuce, clitoral foreskin, by separating the folds of the labia majora. The clitoris consists of a shaft and a glans that becomes engorged with blood during sexual stimulation. It is homologous to the penis in males, meaning that they develop from the same embryonic tissue. The clitoris is the key to sexual pleasure for most women, and consequently, some misogynist cultures practice female circumcision.

Urethral Opening

The urethral opening is located directly below the clitoris. It is the opening through which a woman urinates. The urethral opening, urethra, and bladder are unrelated to reproduction. Urinary tract and bladder infections can occur with transmission of bacteria from the vagina or rectum.

Urinary Tract Infections   The urinary tract includes the kidneys, ureters, bladder, and urethra. UTIs are caused when bacteria reaches the urinary tract, which can happen more easily in women than men. The most common UTIs are bladder and urethra infections. Signs and symptoms of UTIs may include a burning sensation when urinating, feeling a need or urge to urinate more frequently but little urine output, leaking of urine, or cloudy, smelly, or bloody urine. The reasons women are more likely to get UTIs include having a shorter urethra than men, the urethra is located near the rectum, and sexual activity can push bacteria into the urethra. If bacteria are present, an antibiotic may be prescribed. Symptoms should disappear in one to two days. Women who are prone to UTIs may want to drink plenty of water or cranberry juice, wipe from front to back after a bowel movement, urinate after sex to wash away bacteria, choose a birth control method other than the diaphragm or cervical cap, refrain from using douches or feminine sprays, and take showers rather than tub baths.[1]

Urinary Incontinence   Bladder control problems (leaking of urine) are two times more common in women than men, and more common in older women than younger women. Incontinence can result from medical conditions such as neurologic injury, birth defects, strokes, multiple sclerosis, or physical problems associated with aging. Episiotomies may cause temporary incontinence, as can pregnancy when the baby presses against the bladder. Incontinence also occurs in women after menopause.[2] The types of incontinence include:

- Stress incontinence—leakage happens with coughing, sneezing, exercising, laughing, lifting heavy things, and other movements that put pressure on the bladder. It is the most common type of incontinence. It can be treated and sometimes cured.
- Urge incontinence—this is sometimes called "overactive bladder." Leakage usually happens after a strong, sudden urge to urinate. The sudden urge may occur when you don't expect it, such as during sleep, after drinking water, or when you hear or touch running water.
- Functional incontinence—leaking because you cannot get to a toilet in time. People with this type of incontinence may have problems thinking, moving, or speaking that keep them from reaching a toilet. For example, a person with Alzheimer's disease may not plan a trip to the bathroom in time to urinate. A person in a wheelchair may be unable to get to a toilet in time.
- Overflow incontinence—leaking urine because the bladder does not empty completely. Overflow incontinence is less common in women.
- Mixed incontinence—two or more types of incontinence together, most often stress and urge incontinence.
- Transient incontinence—leaking urine for a short time due to an illness such as a bladder infection. Leaking stops when the illness is treated.

Kegel Exercises   A woman can practice **Kegel exercises** to prevent incontinence or reduce leakage. It may take several weeks before seeing results. The following steps are designed to strengthen the pelvic floor:

1. Initially, practice these exercises lying down.
2. Squeeze the muscles in your genital area as if you were trying to stop the flow of urine or trying to stop from passing gas. Try not to squeeze the muscles in your abdomen, legs or buttocks at the same time.
3. Relax. Squeeze the muscles again and hold for ten seconds. Then relax for ten seconds. Do this eight more times.
4. When your muscles get stronger, do your exercises sitting or standing. You can do these exercises any time, while sitting at your desk, riding the car, waiting in line, doing homework, etc.
5. Be patient. It may take six to eight weeks to notice improvement.[3]

Vaginal Opening

The vaginal opening may be covered by a thin sheath called the **hymen.** Hymens vary in size, shape, and thickness and usually have an opening in the center through which menstrual blood flows.

A common myth is that an intact hymen indicates virginity and that it breaks during a young woman's first sexual intercourse. Using the presence of an intact hymen for determining virginity is erroneous. The hymen can be perforated by many different events, such as the first menstrual blood, the use of a tampon, strenuous exercise, or some mishap. Some women are born without hymens, and some women retain intact hymens despite several experiences of sexual intercourse.

Perineum   The **perineum** is the part of the muscle and tissue located between the vaginal opening and the anal canal. It holds up and surrounds the lower parts of the urinary and digestive tracts. The perineum contains an abundance of nerve endings that make it sensitive to touch. A common practice in Western medicine was to perform an **episiotomy,** an incision of the perineum, for widening the vaginal opening to facilitate childbirth. However, the American College of Obstetricians and Gynecologists now urges restricting its use and no longer considers the procedure routine.[4] The number of episiotomy procedures in the United States has declined during the past decade. Women's advocates and medical researchers challenged the need for the practice as a routine procedure and suggested that the incision greatly increased the probability of tears into and through the anus.[5]

Internal Genitalia

The internal genitalia consist of the vagina, cervix, uterus, fallopian (uterine) tubes, and ovaries.

Vagina   The **vagina** connects the cervix to the outer body and lies between the bladder and the rectum. The vaginal canal serves three important functions. First, the menstrual flow and uterine secretions pass through the vagina to the vaginal opening. Second, the vagina serves as the birth canal during labor and can expand during childbirth to several inches in width. Third, the vagina is lubricated by two Bartholin's glands located on either side of the vaginal opening and is the female organ of copulation. During puberty, the vagina begins to produce a clear or white discharge. This self-cleaning process, called leukorrhea, gives the vulva its characteristic smell. Douching or hygiene products are unnecessary and may actually disturb the normal pH balance. Unpleasant odors may be a sign of infection, and if they continue, a health care provider should be visited.

A common myth is that the size of a penis contributes to sexual satisfaction. In reality, the vagina expands to accommodate the size of any penis. Another myth is that a penis may become trapped within the vagina. In fact, unlike animals with a bone in the penis, a male's penis becomes flaccid after ejaculation and cannot be trapped in the vagina.

Cervix   The **cervix** is the portion of the uterus that protrudes into the vaginal cavity. It has a smooth, glistening mucosal surface. The cervical opening to the vagina is small, thus preventing tampons and other objects from entering the uterus. During childbirth, the cervix dilates to accommodate the passage of the fetus. The dilation of the cervix is an early sign that labor has begun. The cervical opening is small and round in a nulliparous (never having given birth) woman but becomes wider after one or more deliveries. When a woman has a Pap smear, the cells are scraped from the cervix and examined under a microscope to detect cancer or precancerous conditions. A Pap smear is both a visual inspection and a cell culture. A negative result is normal.

Uterus   The **uterus** is often described as being pear shaped and about the size of a clenched fist. The powerful muscles of the uterus expand to accommodate a growing fetus and contract strongly to begin the birth process and push the fetus through the birth canal. The **endometrium,** the complex inner lining of cells, consists of blood-enriched tissue that sloughs off each month during the menstrual flow if fertilization does not occur. It is the organ in which the fertilized egg becomes implanted and the fetus matures. An endometrial biopsy can be used to detect diseases or infertility problems.

Women Making a Difference

Dr. Susan M. Love: A Pioneer in Women's Breast Health and Menopause Research

Susan M. Love is one of the founding mothers of the breast cancer advocacy movement and serves on the Boards of the Y-ME, the National Breast Cancer Coalition, and the Young Survivor's Coalition. She is a clinical professor of surgery at UCLA and the founder and director of the Dr. Susan Love Research Foundation, whose mission is to eradicate breast cancer.

Dr. Love is best known for her groundbreaking books: *Dr. Susan Love's Breast Book* and *Dr. Susan Love's Menopause and Hormone Book.* Her lectures are visionary and challenging to existing medical practices. Her continued work in the area of breast cancer research provides hope for the many women who live with breast cancer today.[6]

Uterine Cancer   There is no known cause for uterine cancer. Most uterine cancers begin in the endometrium, the inner lining of the uterus. Most endometrial cancer begins as adenocarcinomas (cancers that begin in cells that make and release mucus and other fluids). The American Cancer Society (ACS) estimates about 46,470 new cases of uterine cancers (endometrial and uterine sarcomas) will be diagnosed and 8120 women will die from cancers of the uterine body in 2011.[7] Uterine cancer usually occurs after menopause, or around the time menopause begins. Abnormal bleeding or discharge, difficult or painful urination, pain during intercourse, and pain in the pelvic areas are symptoms of uterine cancer. These symptoms also may occur in more benign conditions, such as uterine fibroids. Uterine cancer is discussed more fully in Chapter 16.

Uterine Fibroids   Uterine fibroids are common tumors of the uterus composed of muscle and fibrous tissue. Nearly 80 percent of all women have uterine fibroids, and 25 percent of them have severe enough symptoms to require treatment. Fibroids may cause heavy vaginal bleeding, pelvic discomfort, pain, constipation or pressure on other organs. There is no known cause or reason why some women have severe symptoms while others have no symptoms. Age, race/ethnicity, lifestyle, and genetics can play a role in who gets uterine fibroids, which often begins between the ages of 40 to 50 years. African American women are two to three times more likely to be at risk than white women. The first goal of treatment is to alleviate the symptoms. Surgical removal of the fibroid, shrinking the tumors, or a hysterectomy may be required to alleviate the symptoms.[8]

Fallopian (Uterine) Tubes   The fallopian tubes, or oviducts, serve as a pathway for the ovum (egg) to the uterus and as the site of fertilization, typically in the upper third of a fallopian tube. The sperm travel through the vagina, cervix, and uterus to fertilize the egg in one of the fallopian tubes. The fertilized egg takes approximately 6–10 days to travel through the fallopian tube to implant in the uterine lining.

Ovaries   The **ovaries** are the female gonads (sex glands) that develop and expel an ovum each month. A woman is born with approximately 1 million eggs that steadily die throughout the life cycle. At puberty a young women has about 300,000 immature eggs, called follicles. The majority of the follicles disappear before puberty. Usually none are found after menopause. Very few of these follicles reach full maturity; about 300–400 are developed and released for possible fertilization during a woman's reproductive years. The follicles in the ovaries produce the female sex hormones progesterone and estrogen, which are important in preparing the uterus for the implantation of a fertilized egg. The ovaries are homologous to the male's testes.

Polycystic Ovarian Syndrome (PCOS)   PCOS occurs when the ovaries produce excessive amounts of male hormones (androgens) and multiple small cysts develop. Among nonpregnant women, ovarian conditions (PCOS and ovarian failure) are the most common causes of amenorrhea. PCOS is diagnosed when women have two of the following: clinical or biochemical evidence of excessive amounts of androgens, menstrual irregularity due to too few or no ovulatory cycles, or polycystic-appearing ovaries on ultrasound. PCOS is suspected when menstrual irregularities begin following puberty and include signs of hyperandrogenism (excess body hair following a male pattern, male pattern balding, or acne). Health care providers also screen for glucose tolerance and type 2 diabetes because of the association of PCOS with insulin resistance. Treatment for PCOS depends on the symptoms.[9]

Breasts

The breasts function as organs of sexual arousal, contain the mammary glands that nourish a newborn baby, and consist of two main types of tissues, glandular and stromal (supporting). Glandular tissues house the milk-producing lobules and ducts, through which milk passes. Each breast contains fifteen to twenty-five clusters called lobes, which have smaller sections called lobules. Lobes and lobules are connected by main ducts opening into the nipple. The ducts join together to form ampulla, the collecting sacs located just behind the nipple. The nipples, composed of erectile tissue, become temporarily erect with cold temperature, sexual stimulation, or lactation. The pigmented portion around the nipple of each breast is called the areola, which usually darkens during pregnancy and in women who have had children. The core of the nipple is the opening of the fifteen to twenty-five ducts and contains sebaceous glands that keep the nipple lubricated during breast feeding. Figure 8.1 shows the structures of the breast. The supporting structure of the breasts is connective tissue, composed mainly of collagen, a material that also makes up bone and tendons. Stromal tissues include fatty and fibrous connective tissue.

Breast size is determined primarily by heredity and depends on the existing amount of fat and glandular tissue. Breasts may exhibit cyclical changes, including increased swelling and tenderness just before menstruation. Small changes in weight also can influence breast size. After menopause, the glandular tissue shrivels and the breasts are composed mainly of fat.[10]

Benign Breast Conditions   Benign breast conditions are often detected by clinical breast examination, routine mammography, or breast self-examination.

FIGURE 8.1 Structures of the breast.

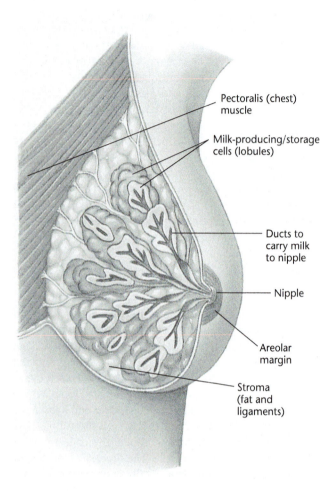

Pectoralis (chest) muscle

Milk-producing/storage cells (lobules)

Ducts to carry milk to nipple

Nipple

Areolar margin

Stroma (fat and ligaments)

FYI

Benign Breast Conditions

Lumps, breast pain, and nipple discharge are the most common breast complaints in women seeking medical attention. Benign breast conditions are common changes in breast tissue with no cancerous breast abnormality. Some of the more common changes are discussed.

Nipple discharge: Fluid coming from the nipple(s). Typically spontaneous milky, clear, yellow, or green discharge from both nipples. Persistent discharges should be evaluated by a health care provider, but in most cases the condition is benign, typically caused by hormonal imbalance or papillomas.

Lobular carcinoma in situ (LCIS): Not classified as a cancer but, rather, a precancerous condition. LCIS begins in the lobules and is typically monitored closely by a health care provider.

Fibrocystic breast condition: Describes a variety of changes in glandular and stromal tissues in the breast(s). Symptoms include cysts, fibrosis (excess fibrous connective tissue), lumpiness, areas of thickening, tenderness, and breast pain.

Cysts: Accumulations of fluid in the breast. Cysts are noncancerous and present as smooth, rounded lumps that are movable. They respond to the body's hormone levels and are most common in premenopausal women.

Fibroadenomas: Common benign breast tumors that are found more often in African American women than in other women. They are usually too small to feel by self-examination. Fibroadenomas tend to be round and have borders.

Intraductal papillomas: Noncancerous wartlike growths inside the breast. These often involve the large milk ducts near the nipple.

Mastitis: Most commonly affects women while they are breast-feeding. Bacteria enter the breast duct and attract inflammatory cells.[11]

The most common benign breast conditions include fibrocystic breast condition, benign breast tumors, and breast inflammation. (See *FYI:* "Benign Breast Conditions.")

Fibrocystic breast condition is a catchall phrase for any signs or symptoms not related to breast cancer. It is not a disease but, rather, a variety of changes in the glandular and stromal tissues of the breast. Women may have cycles of pain, tenderness, and swelling in the breast tissue, particularly during the 1–2 weeks before menstruation. (See *Health Tips:* "Treatment of Fibrocystic Breasts.") These symptoms may occur concurrently with lumps or masses of overgrown breast tissue. Benign (noncancerous) breast changes are most common in the upper-outer quadrant of the breasts, followed by the lower-outer quadrant of the breasts. Many women, nearly 70 percent, experience benign breast changes, that is, breast lumps, pain, tenderness, or nipple discharge during the menstrual cycle. The ACS suggests that nine out of every ten women have some type of abnormality when breast tissue is examined under a microscope. The diagnosis of whether a mass is benign (noncancerous) or malignant

(cancerous) is usually confirmed by observing the lump over time, imaging tests, or biopsy. Approximately 10 percent of the women who get mammograms will require a breast biopsy to determine whether the mass is benign or malignant. Just remember, 85–90 percent of lumps are benign and most do not require biopsy.

Lumps, breast pain, and nipple discharge are the three most common breast complaints of women seeking medical attention. Nipple discharge, fluid from the nipple(s), is typically caused by hormonal imbalances or papillomas. Nearly 20 percent of women may experience spontaneous fluid nipple discharge. Bloody or watery nipple discharge, especially if it is from one side or a single duct, is considered abnormal. Only around

Health Tips

Treatment of Fibrocystic Breasts

Women with fibrocystic breasts should consult a health care provider for recommendations. Suggestions may include:

- Wear extra support bras.
- Avoid caffeine.
- Use oral contraceptives.
- Use aspirin, acetaminophen, or Motrin.
- Maintain a low-fat diet.
- Apply heat.
- Reduce salt.
- Take vitamin E, vitamin B-6, niacin, or other vitamins.
- Take prescribed medications.[14]

10 percent of abnormal discharges are cancerous.[12] The following discharge may be of concern:

- Bloody or watery with a red, pink, or brown color
- Sticky or clear in color
- Brown to black in color (opalescent)
- Appears spontaneously without squeezing the nipple
- Persistent
- On one side only
- A fluid other than breast milk[13]

If a women experiences a change in the breasts (lumps, dimpling changes, skin irregularities, or nipple discharge), she should immediately contact her health care provider.

Breast Self-Examination (BSE) The American Cancer Society (ACS) no longer recommends BSE as a technique for detecting breast cancer. However, BSE can help a young woman in her twenties or thirties be proactive in knowing normal monthly breast changes from abnormal breast changes. A young woman can become familiar with the shape and feel of her breasts, and recognize changes such as lumps, dimpling changes, skin irregularities, and nipple discharge. Most of these breast conditions are normal (see *FYI:* "Benign Breast Conditions"), but when changes occur, a health care provider should be notified. BSE is optional, and can even be done irregularly. The best time to do BSE is when the breasts are not tender. Some women choose a particular day of the month such as a birthday or anniversary day.

Clinical Breast Examination (CBE) CBE should be part of every average-risk, asymptomatic woman's periodic health examination, about every 3 years for women in their twenties and thirties and annually for women 40 and older. As part of the periodic health examination, the health care provider can discuss BSE, normal changes in breasts, risk factors, and early detection testing. The health care provider should recommend annual mammography to women age 40 and older, and discuss its benefits and limitations. She will also discuss earlier detection testing and additional testing for women at increased risk for breast cancer.

Mammography Mammography is an X-ray of the breast that serves as the gold standard for early detection of breast cancer. Most mammography units are screen-film units, which means they produce the mammography picture on X-ray film. Full-field digital mammography units capture the picture on an electronic digital detector, and the image is then displayed on a video monitor. ACS recommends that all women get a screening mammogram every year beginning at 40 years of age as part of a periodic health examination for as long as they are healthy. Individual research studies and meta-analysis studies continue to show the benefits of mammography beginning at age 40, including significant mortality reduction. Women should be told about the limitations and risks of mammography. Mammography will miss some cancers, and may lead to follow-up screenings or biopsies that are not cancer. Women with a family history of breast cancer or known to be at increased risk for breast cancer may benefit from earlier initiation of early detection testing and/or the addition of breast ultrasound or MRI.[15]

The ACS recommends that women at high risk for breast cancer should get an MRI and a mammogram every year beginning at age 30. ACS defines high risk as about 20 percent or greater lifetime risk of developing breast cancer based on a profile completed by your health care provider.

Women at moderate increased risk, defined as 15–20 percent lifetime risk, should discuss the pros and cons of adding MRI to their early mammogram screening. Yearly MRI is not recommended for women whose lifetime risk profile is lower than 15 percent.

Women who have breast augmentation surgery are encouraged to have yearly clinical breast exams. They may also choose to conduct regular BSE so they can inform the health care provider of the edges of the saline (saltwater) implants. Mammography on women with implants involves special views to see both the breast tissue and the implant. Women who have breast reduction surgery should have yearly mammography after the age of 40.[16]

MENSTRUATION

Changes in the physiology of the body brought about as the result of hormonal influences signal the end of childhood and the beginning of puberty. Young adolescent females experience their bodies becoming much fuller in the breasts, hips, and thighs as they move from girlhood to womanhood with the initiation of monthly menstrual cycles. Biologically, all of these changes occur to prepare the female body for potential reproduction. The onset of menstruation, **menarche,** is a central focus of body politics. Menarche not only is a physiological happening, but it is experiential. In the 1930–1940s, the common wisdom was that menstruation was accompanied by fatigue and cold sensitivity, so young women were discouraged from physical activity, including anything athletic. In the 1950–1960s, these precautions were debunked as myths, yet many young women persisted in the belief that one should rest and be sedentary with menses. Female athletes were not believed to be able to reach peak performance if they menstruated. And today, young women are being told that they can avoid menstruation completely by taking synthetic hormones. In fact, using synthetic hormones to prevent menses is being marketed and extolled as a healthy lifestyle choice. However, little scientific evidence supports the claim that hormone-induced amenorrhea is "good for you." Like hormone replacement (HRT), marketing precedes science.[17]

Menarche sets the stage for how a young woman perceives her sexuality. How she views menstruation can affect how she feels about her body, her femininity, her relationships with men, and reproduction. The medicalization of menstruation may cause young women to see menstruation as an inconvenience, a pathology rather than a cleansing process. Most young girls anticipate their period with a range of emotions from fear, disgust, and embarrassment to joy and excitement. Indeed, researchers have suggested that a young woman's attitude toward menstruation is influenced and shaped by how the media, popular culture, and others portray it.[18]

Over the past century, a decrease of about 3–4 months in age of onset of menstruation has occurred every decade. Today, the average preadolescent's body begins to change around age 10 or 11, but for some young girls, it begins much earlier.[19] Nearly 48 percent of African American and 15 percent of non-Hispanic white girls show pubic hair and develop breast buds by the age of 8. Researchers found that the median age of menarche for U.S. girls is 12.43 years, with less than 10 percent starting to menstruate before 11 years, and 90 percent menstruating by age 13.75 years. African American girls begin menstruating significantly earlier than white girls, and Hispanic girls are significantly earlier than white girls. Since 1973, the age of onset of menarche has stabilized based on findings from the Third National Health and Nutrition Examination Survey.[20] The onset of menstruation can be affected by a variety of factors, including genetics, socioeconomic conditions, nutritional status, and in some cases, exercise regimens.

Overweight and obesity also are known factors for early puberty. The emotional, as well as physiological, changes can have an impact on young girls. They may feel "different" from their friends, and it can seem as if the world changed overnight. What are your personal recollections of menarche? Were your experiences the same as your friends'? How do the media influence your attitudes toward menstruation today? Record your responses in the *Journal Activity:* "Your Recollection of Menarche" and discuss them with friends.

Six primary hormones are involved in regulating the female reproductive system: gonadatropin releasing hormones (follicle stimulating hormone–releasing factor [FSH-RF] and luteinizing hormone–releasing factor [LH-RF]) from the hypothalamus, FSH and LH from the pituitary gland, and estrogen, progesterone, and the male hormone testosterone from the ovaries. Puberty begins when FSH and LH are released from the pituitary gland (the master gland), which stimulates the ovaries to produce more estrogen. Estrogen is responsible for developing the secondary sex characteristics of puberty. These changes may include an increase in body hair, the beginning of breast growth, distribution of body fat, size of larynx and its influence on the voice, and a widening of the hips or pelvic area.[21] A growth spurt of several inches may occur at this time. For many girls, the first menstrual cycles may not be associated with ovulation. However, once menstruation begins, a young woman must assume that ovulation and fertility can occur.

The menstrual cycle is generally subdivided into three phases: follicular (or proliferate), ovulatory, and luteal (or secretory). Day 1 of your menstrual cycle marks the beginning of the **follicular** phase. Menstrual blood flow occurs for several days of the follicular cycle, the uterus is at its thinnest and estrogen is at its lowest.

Journal Activity

Your Recollection of Menarche

The menstrual cycle is something that every young person, male or female, should understand. Sharing our stories about menarche can take away the secrecy that some of us experienced. Write a paragraph or two about your experience with menarche. If it was positive, write about the events that made it positive. If it was negative, write about how you would have liked the experience to have been.

The hypothalamus is activated to release gonatotropin releasing hormones to stimulate the release of FSH and small amounts of LH from the anterior pituitary gland. FSH causes follicles on the ovaries to begin maturing. The selected follicle, the graafian follicle, continues to mature on one of the ovaries and holds the ovum. Concurrently, the endometrium begins to build up and thicken and estrogen levels increase. When estrogen reaches a certain level, LH-RF causes the pituitary to release a large amount of LH (LH surge). LH causes the mature follicle to burst and release the mature egg. Many types of birth control prevent the surge in LH, thus inhibiting ovulation. Just before ovulation, an abundance of clear, stretchy mucus is secreted by the cervix. Women who use the cervical mucus method (or Billings method) of birth control will note the change in mucus color and texture. Women who use the basal body temperature (BBT) method of birth control will note a slight elevation in BBT by about 0.1° to 0.4° until menstruation occurs. The follicular phase is the most variable in length and determines the length of time until the next menstrual cycle. With a 28-day menstrual cycle, ovulation will occur on day 14. With a 35-day menstrual cycle, ovulation will occur on day 20. The **ovulatory** phase begins when the largest follicle bursts and the mature egg is released into one of the fallopian tubes. The cell and tissue changes following ovulation are quite constant through the next 14 days. Once the egg is released, menstruation will occur in about 14 days unless fertilization occurs. The corpus luteum (the temporary structure formed from the follicle following the release of the mature egg) accounts for the stable time between ovulation and day 1 of the next follicular phase. Again, the BBT will remain elevated throughout the ovulation phase. Progesterone, from the corpus luteum, is responsible for the rise in BBT. After ovulation, the mature egg remains viable for about 24–48 hours while travelling through the fallopian tube. Sperm can stay alive inside a woman's body for 3–4 days, but possibly as long as 6–7 days. Intercourse, before or after ovulation, can result in pregnancy. The fertile time frame is about 7–10 days during the middle of a menstrual cycle and depends upon the length of the follicular phase. The only safe time frame to avoid pregnancy is when the egg is no longer viable after ovulation. The empty follicle becomes the corpus luteum during the **luteal** phase. The corpus luteum secretes estrogen and large amounts of progesterone. These hormones are essential in maintaining a pregnancy by preparing the endometrium for a fertilized egg. If the egg is fertilized, the thickened blanket of blood vessels becomes the placenta. If the egg is not fertilized, the corpus luteum (yellow body) disintegrates and becomes the corpus albicans (white body). Estrogen and progesterone levels drop and the endometrium is sloughed off. The amount of menstrual bleeding varies from woman to woman, and the expulsion of blood clots (pooled blood in the vagina) is common. Blood can vary in color from bright red to dark brown. Normal periods can last from 4–8 days, and cycles can vary from 20–40 days. While some women experience no discomfort, others experience fluid retention, cramping, mood swings, weight gain, breast tenderness, diarrhea, or constipation.[22,23]

Pelvic Examination and Pap Test

Pelvic Examination   Regular screening with a pelvic examination and Pap test is important for any sexually active woman. A pelvic examination should be conducted annually for 3 consecutive years for all women who are or have been sexually active or are over age 21. If the results are negative (no abnormalities), less frequent Pap test can be conducted at your discretion in consultation with your health care provider, who may still recommend annual exams.

The pelvic examination includes a visual screening to ensure that the reproductive organs look normal in size, shape, and location, a Pap test to screen for cervical cancer, and a bimanual check of the ovaries, fallopian tubes, and uterus. The health care provider visually checks the vaginal area for signs of herpes, tumors, or genital warts. She then gently inserts a speculum into the vagina to view and check the internal organs for abnormalities. It is helpful if a woman can remain relaxed during the examination. Many women feel embarrassed or apprehensive about the pelvic examination, but relaxing the stomach and vaginal muscles makes the pelvic examination easier. A Pap test and then a bimanual examination follow the visual examination. The bimanual examination requires the health care provider to place two gloved fingers (with lubricating jelly) into the vagina to feel for abnormalities in the fallopian tubes, ovaries, and uterus, sometimes followed by a rectal examination. She checks for tumors, tenderness to the area, and the location of the organs.[24]

When a woman is making an appointment for her first pelvic examination, she should inform the nurse or health care provider that it is her first exam. The young woman should NOT use vaginal creams or douche, use tampons, or have sex, for 48 hours before the examination. At the exam, she will be weighed, her height will be measured, and her blood pressure will be taken; then she will be given a gown to put on and a sheet to put over her stomach and legs. The exam table has stirrups (holders for the feet) and with the woman's knees bent, the health care provider will conduct the examination. The exam may include the external (visual) exam, the speculum exam, and the bimanual exam.

Pap Test The Pap test is a standard part of any pelvic examination. The best time to have a Pap test is 10–14 days after the first day of the last menstrual period. The Pap test is conducted by taking a sample of cells from the cervical area, called the squamous epithelium. This area is the site where 90 percent of all cervical cancers begin. The speculum separates the vaginal walls and exposes the cervical opening. A brush or Thin-Prep is used to scrape some cells from the part of the cervix that protrudes into the vagina, and then the cells are smeared onto a slide. Another sample is taken from the endocervical canal and wiped onto another slide; then the speculum is removed. Sometimes a woman will spot blood after a pelvic examination; this is normal and does not require treatment unless the area remains tender.

The primary purpose of having a Pap test is to prevent invasive cancer from occurring. Precancerous cervical lesions (or dysplasia) can be detected when small and easily treated. If left untreated, the normal history of progression is from dysplasia to cancer. Cervical cancer develops slowly and is nearly 100 percent curable if detected when localized. A minute or two of discomfort (whether emotionally or physically) is well worth the benefit of early detection. A woman's failure to undergo an annual examination is more common than a failure by the physician to obtain an accurate smear or the lab technologist to misread a slide. The most important preventive measure is to comply with the guidelines for annual pelvic examinations. All women should begin having Pap tests at age 21 or prior to that age if sexually active. At age 30, women who have had three normal Pap results in a row may decided to get screened every 2 or 3 years. At age 70, women who have had three or more normal Pap tests in a row and normal test results for the past 10 years may decide to forego any future cervical cancer screenings. Any woman with a history of cervical cancer, DES exposure before birth, HIV infection, HPV infection or a weakened immune system, chemotherapy, or chronic steroid use should continue to have annual screenings. Women who have had a total hysterectomy may also choose to stop having cervical cancer screenings unless the hysterectomy was done to treat pre-cancerous growths or cervical cancer. If a woman had a partial hysterectomy without removal of the cervix, she should continue to follow ACS guidelines.[26]

Menstrual Disorders

Endometriosis **Endometriosis** occurs when the endometrium (the lining of the uterus) fragments and lodges in other parts of the body, most commonly in the pelvic cavity. It can lodge on the uterosacral ligaments, on the ovaries, fallopian tubes, and supporting broad ligaments. The fragments build up tissue each month and then break down and bleed, causing inflammation, scarring, and adhesions.[27] The cause of endometriosis remains unclear, but scientists are continuing to explore possible causes, including reverse flow of menstrual blood and tissue, immune system problems in destroying endometrial tissue, and blood and lymphatic transport of endometrial tissue outside the uterus. Nearly 5 million females in the United States have endometriosis. Treatment of endometriosis depends upon age, the severity of symptoms, severity of the disease, and whether a woman wants have children. Treatment includes hormonal therapy, laparoscopic surgery, pain medication, and major surgical management, depending upon the needs of the woman. Treatment may alleviate the symptoms, but removal of endometrial tissue does not mean a woman is cured. Chronic endometriosis can be frustrating and disabling for women and is a common cause of dysmenorrhea, dyspareunia (painful intercourse), chronic pelvic pain, and infertility.[28]

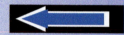

FYI

American Cancer Society Guidelines for Cervical Cancer Screening

All women should have Pap tests about 3 years after they begin having sexual intercourse, but no later than age 21. Screening should be done every year, with the regular Pap test or every 2 years using the newer liquid-based Pap test.

Beginning at age 30, women who have had three normal Pap test results in a row may get screened every 2 to 3 years. Another reasonable option for women over 30 is to get screened every 3 years (but not more frequently) with either the conventional or liquid-based Pap test, plus the HPV DNA test. Women who have certain risk factors such as diethylstilbestrol (DES) exposure before birth, HIV infection, or a weakened immune system due to organ transplant, chemotherapy, or chronic steroid use should continue to be screened annually.

Women 70 years of age or older who have had three or more normal Pap tests in a row and no abnormal Pap test results in the last 10 years may choose to stop having cervical cancer screening. Women with a history of cervical cancer, DES exposure before birth, HIV infection or a weakened immune system should continue to have screenings as long as they are in good health.

Women who have had a total hysterectomy (removal of the uterus and cervix) may also choose to stop having cervical cancer screening, unless the surgery was done as a treatment for cervical cancer or pre-cancer. Women who have had a hysterectomy without removal of the cervix should continue to follow the guidelines above.[25]

Dysmenorrhea Painful menstrual cramps, dysmenorrhea, is the most cited reason for missing school or lost workdays for young women. Although most women occasionally experience menstrual cramps, 5–10 percent of women will experience painful, incapacitating cramps for several hours to a couple of days. Primary **dysmenorrhea,** painful menses without evidence of a physical abnormality, is a normal body response to forceful, frequent uterine contractions that result from increased production of prostaglandins. A number of other symptoms may occur as well, including nausea, vomiting, gastrointestinal disturbances, and fainting. Some women alleviate painful cramps with OTC medications such as ibuprofen (Advil, Nuprin, Motrin IB), with drugs designed specifically for menstrual symptoms (Midol, Pamprin), or with prescription nonsteroidal anti-inflammatory drugs. If medications do not work, oral contraceptives that contain both estrogen and progesterone may be prescribed. Women who suffer from dysmenorrhea may try to increase their physical activity, cut down on salt to reduce possible fluid retention, or rest more because of feelings of fatigue. Secondary dysmenorrhea may be due to anatomic abnormalities such as a congenital abnormality of the uterus, presence of fibroids or endometrial polyps, an IUD, pelvic inflammatory disease, or endometriosis. Secondary dysmenorrhea is diagnosed during a pelvic exam, ultrasound, or laparoscopy, and treatment depends on the type of disease or disorder.[29]

Amenorrhea It is not unusual for women to miss some periods during their lifetime. Primary **amenorrhea** indicates a significant physical disorder characterized by delayed puberty, the failure to menstruate by age 15, or lack of menses by age 14 along with the absence of secondary characteristics such as breast development and increased body hair. The incidence of primary amenorrhea in the United States is less than 1 percent. Multiple causes for the disorder have been identified including a normal delay of onset (up to ages 14–15), drastic weight reduction or malnutrition, chronic illness, extreme obesity, and congenital defects and abnormalities such as Turner's syndrome and hermaphroditism. The treatment of amenorrhea depends on the cause but often includes hormonal supplementation, surgery, or both. Secondary amenorrhea is failure to menstruate for more than 6 months after prior establishment of menstruation. The incidence of secondary amenorrhea is approximately 5–7 percent of menstruating women with a length of 3 months. Some missed periods are quite normal, such as after childbirth or after discontinuing birth control pills. The most common cause of secondary amenorrhea in premenopausal women is pregnancy or the onset of menopause.[30,31]

The prevalence of amenorrhea in young female athletes, particularly dancers, gymnasts, and long-distance runners, has received considerable attention. The Female Athlete Triad is identified as low energy availability (with or without disordered eating), amenorrhea, and osteoporosis. Restrictive eating, excessive training, extreme stress, and low body-fat percentage all predispose a female athlete to amenorrhea. A young, elite athlete who participates in sports for which a slender appearance or low body fat is advantageous is at greatest risk. The endocrine profile of an athlete in "thin-body" sports may show an estrogen deficit similar to that in menopausal women. This profile has implications for infertility, premature osteoporosis, and poor psychological well-being. Studies show between 25 and 60 percent of young female athletes in "thin-body" sports have episodes of amenorrhea compared to 2–5 percent of the general female population.[32]

Premenstrual Syndrome

Premenstrual syndrome (PMS) is a politically charged and "culture-bound" issue. PMS can be perceived as another medicalization of a woman's normal cyclical pattern. Women who experience PMS tend to have a grouping of symptoms. For this reason, PMS symptoms may be categorized under four main headings:

- *Type A.* A stands for anxiety. This type of PMS is most notable for its emotional symptoms of anxiety, irritability, and mood swings. Type A accounts for 80 percent of all PMS sufferers.
- *Type C.* C stands for carbohydrate cravings. Along with the sugar cravings are exhaustion and headaches (all symptoms of low blood sugar).
- *Type D.* D stands for depression. Depression is accompanied by mental confusion, an inability to think clearly, and poor memory.
- *Type H.* H stands for hyperhydration, which is like waterlogging. You may suffer from Type H PMS if you have swelling of the abdomen, hands, or feet. Fluid retention will also cause your breasts to swell and become tender.[33]

PMS symptoms may fall into one or a combination of these categories. Most symptoms of PMS taper off with the onset of menstruation although some women may continue to experience symptoms throughout the period. Changes in symptoms of PMS may be attributed to factors such as childbearing, the approach of menopause, and aging. Now complete *Assess Yourself:* "Physical and Emotional Symptoms and PMS" to determine which symptoms you experience.

Nearly half of women with PMS have symptoms unrelated to a cycle-dependent pattern. Health care providers diagnose PMS by eliminating coexisting medical

Assess Yourself

Physical and Emotional Symptoms and PMS

Over 150 symptoms have been associated with PMS, a condition that women can experience 1–2 weeks before menstruation. Listed below are some common experiences associated with PMS. Keep a daily diary of the changes in your physical and emotional state for 1 month, using a severity index of 1–10, with 10 being the most severe. Divide experiences into physical and emotional and begin on day 1 of menstrual bleeding (follicular phase). Record any of the following experiences you have before menstruation: acne, anxiety, depression, dizziness, fatigue, headaches, irritability, panic, swelling, rashes, nausea, weight gain, hives, breast swelling, irregular heartbeats, joint pain, mood swings, muscle aches, paranoia, gastrointestinal symptoms, water retention, food cravings, moodiness, insomnia, withdrawal, sadness, crying, impatience, overreactivity, self-criticism, extreme sensitivity, distractibility, indecision, suicide ideation, violence.

- Did you experience any other symptoms during your menstrual cycle? Record them as well.
- Did you practice any nutritional or health behaviors to alleviate these symptoms? If so, what outcomes did you experience?
- What other suggestions to alleviate symptoms might you try?

Health Tips

Eating Healthy to Avoid PMS[35]

Poor nutrition and low-quality foods contribute directly to the incidence of PMS. Some foods are known to worsen your problems.

Foods to Avoid

- Refined carbohydrates such as white bread, cakes, cookies, refined breakfast cereals, crackers, candy, and chocolate
- Foods that are high in fats, including dairy products and red meat
- Synthetic foods that are highly processed and full of chemical additives
- Caffeinated drinks such as coffee, tea, and soda
- Alcohol
- Salt and heavily salted foods

Foods to Add to Your Diet

- Complex carbohydrates, such as whole-grain bread, brown rice, whole-grain pasta, and whole-grain cereals
- Plenty of fresh fruits and vegetables
- Low-fat protein sources, such as fish, chicken, and vegetarian proteins
- Vegetable oils rich in essential fatty acids. Poly and monounsaturated oils

---

disorders and charting symptoms through several consecutive menstrual cycles. Symptoms that consistently occur during the second half of the menstrual cycle may be caused by PMS, and these symptoms can worsen with age before tapering off after menopause.

The best approach to dealing with PMS symptoms is to alleviate them through noninvasive strategies such as relaxation techniques, biofeedback, nutritional changes, and exercise. (See *Health Tips*: "Eating Healthy to Avoid PMS.") Medications can help alleviate most premenstrual abdominal cramping, headaches, nausea, vomiting, and diarrhea. A health care provider can work closely with a woman experiencing PMS to alleviate discomforting symptoms.[34]

Premenstrual Dysphoric Disorder (PMDD)

Why is PMDD defined as a clinically pathological disorder while PMS is seen as normal? That's the question many women's health advocates have asked. While women are seeking relief from feeling "out of sorts,"

specialists choose to label it mental illness, which raises questions about the social construction of a disease. **Premenstrual dysphoric disorder (PMDD)** is defined as a severe form of PMS, including marked disruption of quality of life and bouts of significant premenstrual depressed mood, anxiety, sadness, or anger that occur one week before menses and impair a woman socially or occupationally.[36] The disorder, according to the *Diagnostic and Statistical Manual of Mental Disorders–IV,* must have five or more of eleven symptoms during the last week of the luteal phase in most menstrual cycles. The symptoms often resolve within a few days after menstruation begins. PMS may affect as many as 80 percent of all women, whereas PMDD affects 3–8 percent. The symptoms of PMDD include the following:

- Feelings of sadness or hopelessness, possible suicidal thoughts
- Feelings of tension or anxiety
- Mood swings marked by periods of teariness
- Persistent irritability or anger that affects other people
- Disinterest in daily activities and relationships
- Trouble concentrating

- Fatigue or low energy
- Food cravings or bingeing
- Sleep disturbances
- Feeling out of control
- Physical symptoms such as bloating, breast tenderness, headaches, and joint or muscle pain[37]

Many health care professionals have voiced concern that normal behavior in women may be labeled inappropriately or explained away as "that time of month." They believe that PMDD is a socially constructed condition that exists normally for most women and should not be labeled "clinically pathological" or lead to stigmatizing a woman. When PMDD is diagnosed, the recommended first line of drug therapy for PMDD is selective serotonin reuptake inhibitors (SSRIs). The main point: Whether PMDD exists or not, a woman who is experiencing hormonal symptoms should be validated for her experience of those symptoms.

Hysterectomy

Every minute, a hysterectomy is performed in the United States, and nine of twelve of them may not meet the guidelines of the American College of Obstetricians and Gynecologists. The good news is that the rates of hysterectomy have been decreasing steadily since 2000. The most recent statistics available from the National Hospital Discharge survey suggested that an estimated 3.1 million U.S. women had a hysterectomy in the time frame 2000–2004. In 2004, the hysterectomy rate decreased slightly from 5.4 per 1000 in 2000 to 5.1 per 1000. Rates remained highest for women aged 40–44 but decreased significantly in women aged 50–54 (from 8.9 per 1000 to 6.7 per 1000) and in the Northeast (from 4.9 per 1000 to 3.7 per 1000).[38,39] Hysterectomies are the second most common major surgery performed in the United States (the most common are cesarean sections). The most common reason for this surgery is uterine fibroids, followed by endometriosis and uterine prolapse. A **hysterectomy** is an operation to remove a woman's uterus and, sometimes, the fallopian tubes, ovaries, and cervix. A hysterectomy is performed through an incision in the abdomen (abdominal hysterectomy, or laparoscopic hysterectomy) or the vagina (vaginal hysterectomy). Vaginal hysterectomies are performed if possible because they require less hospital and recovery time. A woman can return more quickly to normal activities. Yet, abdominal hysterectomies remain the more commonly performed procedure.

The most common type of hysterectomy is a complete or total hysterectomy, which entails removal of the cervix as well as the body of the uterus. A subtotal hysterectomy removes the upper part of the uterus but not the cervix. When both ovaries and fallopian tubes are also removed, the surgery is known as a bilateral salpingo-oophorectomy. A radical hysterectomy removes the uterus, the cervix, the upper part of the vagina, and supporting tissues. This surgery is usually reserved for advanced cases of cancer. (See Figure 8.2 for visual representation of the different types of hysterectomy.) Whenever possible, the ovaries should be conserved. Ovarian conservation for benign conditions benefits long-term survival for women, whereas removal increases risk of death due to premature heart disease and hip fractures. However, estrogen replacement is used to counter these effects.

Women today are recognizing that many conditions that previously called for hysterectomies may be treated with alternative therapies. Hysterectomy may be the best choice for certain conditions, particularly cancer, but women should seek a second opinion, ask about alternative options to try first, and ask about possible complications of surgery. A woman should make an informed decision and choose her best option.

FIGURE 8.2 Types of hysterectomy.

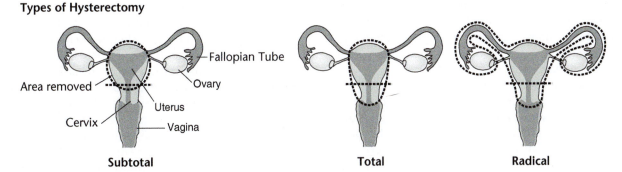

Types of Hysterectomy

Fallopian Tube — Area removed — Ovary — Cervix — Uterus — Vagina

Subtotal   **Total**   **Radical**

Note: Dotted lines show area removed.

MENOPAUSE

Natural Menopause

Menopause and hormone replacement therapy are the hottest women's health topics of the baby boomer generation. An unprecedented number of American women, about 1.25 million annually, are experiencing menopause. This generation of women has grown up believing that informed decisions are based on adequate information. They want answers to questions that previously were not asked. They want to know what to expect physiologically and psychologically as they enter this next life transition. This generation has removed the shroud of secrecy around a number of health topics, from breast cancer to menopause.

Menopause normally occurs between the ages of 40 and 58, with premature menopause occurring before 40 and delayed menopause occurring after 58. Nearly half of American women experience menopause by 50. Physiologically, menopause is the time when ovulation and menstruation cease, but in the social context menopause includes the entire time period from 3–7 years before the last menstrual period to a year after the last period. Physically, the four stages of menopause include premenopause, perimenopause, menopause, and postmenopause.

Perimenopause is the period of time (3–7 years) before and after the last menstrual period during which the menstrual cycle becomes erratic and hot flashes begin. During this phase, the ovaries begin to shrink and FSH is slightly elevated and LH stays within the normal range. A woman may skip one or two periods, she may experience lighter or heavier menstrual flow, and the length of the menstrual period may be shorter or longer than usual. **Hot flashes,** sudden bursts of intense heat, often accompany irregular bleeding. Nearly 85 percent of all perimenopausal women experience hot flashes. Hot flashes alter skin and core temperature and precede increases in LH and FSH. Symptoms may include feelings of warmth in the face or upper body, profuse sweating, and even tremors or shaking. Some women experience anxiety, tenseness, dizziness, heart palpitations, or nausea before the hot flash. The actual cause of hot flashes is unknown, but researchers believe that mixed signals from the hypothalamus cause skin temperatures to rise while internal body temperature drops. Other symptoms include night sweats, mood disturbances, vaginal dryness, and reduced skin elasticity.[40]

Menopause results from the normal aging of the ovaries, when estrogen levels fall and ovulation and menstruation have ceased for 12 months. A significant increase in both FSH and LH occurs due to the rapid depletion of ovarian follicles. Estrogen depletion contributes to other body changes, including varying degrees of atrophy of the internal and external genitalia. The uterus, uterine cavity, fallopian tubes, vagina, and clitoris all become smaller. The breasts may become less firm and full. Bone loss accelerates, and osteoporosis with accompanying risk of fractures becomes more likely. Other possible changes include vaginal dryness, less vasocongestion, and decreased vaginal expansion.[41] Any vaginal bleeding after this time is considered abnormal and should be reported to a health care provider.

Postmenopause begins when menstruation has ceased for one year. Once a woman is past menopause, she will be postmenopausal for the rest of her life. Regular exercise is especially important during this phase of a woman's life. Exercise prevents or delays osteoporosis and heart disease, enhances sleep, and contributes to overall well-being.[42]

Premature Menopause

Premature menopause is menopause that happens before the age of 40, whether it is natural or induced. The body immediately stops producing estrogen and progesterone, causing an array of physical and emotional symptoms similar to those of natural menopause, like hot flashes, night sweats, arrhythmias, irritability and mood swings, insomnia, vaginal dryness, and decreased sex drive. Women with premature menopause also tend to be at increased risk for osteoporosis. The reasons for premature menopause are numerous, including chromosome defects (e.g., Turner's syndrome, where ovaries do not form normally), genetics (family history), autoimmune diseases (e.g., thyroid disease or rheumatoid arthritis may cause the immune system to attack the reproductive system), surgical removal of the ovaries (often with hysterectomy), and chemotherapy or pelvic radiation treatments for cancer that damage the ovaries. If a woman has a hysterectomy without removal of the ovaries, she no longer has menstrual bleeding and will go through menopause naturally.[43]

Menopausal Hormone Therapy (MHT)

Menopausal hormone therapy was touted as the answer for maintaining health and well-being in postmenopausal women. The cessation of menstruation and the concurrent loss of estrogen were viewed as a health problem in women. Anecdotal evidence and some observational studies suggested that women who were on hormone replacement therapy (whether estrogen alone or estrogen plus progesterone) lived longer and had better mental health outcomes. Scientific evidence was sorely lacking. The Women's Health Initiative began in 1991 as a 15-year project sponsored by the National Institutes of Health, National Heart, Lung, and Blood Institute and involved 161,808 women aged 50–79 and was the most definitive set of clinical trials and an observational study ever conducted on women in the United States. The overall goal of WHI was to reduce coronary heart disease, breast and colorectal cancer, and osteoporotic fractures in women. Coronary heart disease is the leading cause of death in women, breast cancer is the second leading cause of cancer death in women, colorectal cancer is the third leading cause of cancer death in women, and one-sixth of all women has osteoporotic fractures during her lifetime.[44] The WHI had three components: a randomized clinical trial studying hormone therapy, diet modification, and calcium/vitamin D; an observational study of the relationship between lifestyle, health and risk factors, and disease outcomes; and a community prevention evaluation of eight university-based model health programs for women aged 40 and over. In the clinical trials studying hormone therapy, women who had not had a hysterectomy were enrolled in the estrogen-plus-progestin study and women who had a hysterectomy before joining were enrolled in the estrogen-alone study. In 2002, after 5.2 years of follow-up data, the estrogen-plus-progestin study was discontinued because there were more risks than benefits to women enrolled in the study. (See Figure 8.3).

The estrogen plus progestin study found that only 2.5% of women had the health events found in Figure 8.3. *For every 10,000 women* taking estrogen plus progestin in one year, the researchers expected:

- Seven more women with heart attacks. In other words, 37 women taking estrogen plus progestin would have heart attacks compared to 30 women taking placebo.
- Eight more women with strokes.
- Eight more women with breast cancer.
- Eighteen more women with blood clots.

The results also suggested that *for every 10,000 women* taking estrogen plus progestin, researchers expected:

- Six fewer colorectal cancers.
- Five fewer hip fractures.
- Fewer fractures in other bones.[45]

Viewpoint

What Should We Believe?

The Women's Health Initiative was the first definitive study of hormone replacement therapy. The findings were astounding and confusing. The clinical trial of women who were receiving CEE and progestin was discontinued because the researchers found a 41 percent increase in strokes, 29 percent increase in heart disease, 100 percent increase in blood clots, and 26 percent increase in breast cancer. The reductions in colorectal cancer and fractures were outweighed by the risks. The clinical trial of women who were receiving CEE only was discontinued two years later. The researchers found that the risks far outweighed the benefits.[46] Critics of the recommendation to discontinue MRT suggest that the results of the study do not adequately represent women aged 40–55. The average age of women who participated in the WHI was 63 years and many of them had underlying atherosclerosis. These researchers believe HRT has a role in treatment of the symptoms of menopause. Some have found decreases in heart disease, hip fractures and osteoporosis with use of HRT. The decision whether to use HRT should be made with the knowledge of the pros and cons of HRT and through discussions with one's health care provider.[47] What do you think? What choice would you make based on the research to date?

FIGURE 8.3 Disease rates for women on estrogen plus progestin or placebo.

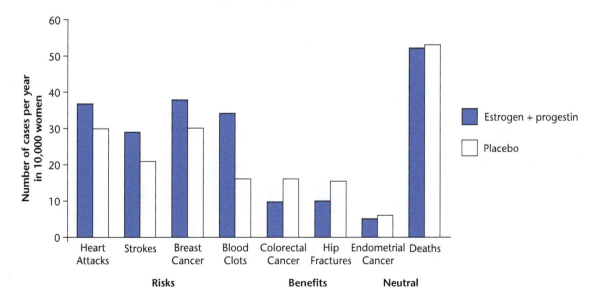

After the CEE-plus-progestin study was discontinued, WHI continued to follow up on the women involved in the study and found that women taking the combination were no longer at increased risk for cardiovascular disease, were at the same risk level for colorectal cancer, and were at the same risk level for osteoporotic fracture of the hip. The 3-year follow-up found women who were taking the combination hormone therapy had an increased risk of all cancers and mortality was somewhat higher.[47] The global index was 12 percent higher and suggested that health risks outweighed health benefits from the beginning of the study through the 3-year follow-up. Findings confirmed that HRT should not be used to prevent diseases in healthy, postmenopausal women.[48]

In 2004, after 6.8 years of follow-up data, the estrogen-alone study was discontinued because there were more risks than benefits to women enrolled in the study. Women taking CEE alone had more strokes but fewer hip fractures than women taking the placebo. The findings that CEE did not increase breast cancers or decrease colorectal cancers were different from the estrogen-plus-progestin study. The researchers concluded that CEE should not be used to prevent chronic diseases overall, and heart disease in particular[49] (see Figure 8.4). Secondary analyses of the data have supported the finding that hormone therapy (HT) should not be used at any age for heart disease prevention and that while risks may differ according to age or years since menopause, the decision to use HT should be carefully weighed in light of previous findings. Health care providers who support the benefits of HT for moderate or severe symptoms of hot flashes or vaginal dryness should shift to lower daily doses, suggest short-term use, and consider the age of the menopausal woman. They should evaluate the severity of the symptoms, the underlying risks for cardiovascular disease and breast cancer, discuss risks and benefits of HT with the woman, and discuss alternatives for addressing the prevailing symptoms.

Natural or Alternative Therapies

Women should consider alternatives to MHT whenever possible. Postmenopausal women are at greater risk for heart disease, stroke, and osteoporosis because of the decrease in estrogen production. Therefore, exercise and healthy eating become even more important in preventing chronic diseases.

Preventing Chronic Conditions

Exercise   Exercise is a key protection against chronic diseases. Exercise helps prevent osteoporosis, reduces the risk of cardiovascular diseases, helps with joint and muscle strength, and helps control weight. Experts agree that walking and some strength training are excellent forms of exercise for all women, but particularly important for post-menopausal women.

Nutrition   Pay attention to healthy eating plans. Be sure to eat adequate fruits and vegetables, whole grains, fat-free or low-fat dairy products (milk, cheese, yogurt, etc.), fish caught in low chemical pollutant environments, skinless poultry, dry beans and nuts, and polyunsaturated and monounsaturated fats. Saturated fats, trans fat, cholesterol, sodium, and added sugars should be used sparingly, if at all. Alcohol can be eliminated or if used, it should drunk in moderation (never more than one drink per day).

FIGURE 8.4 Effects of estrogen alone and placebo on disease rates.

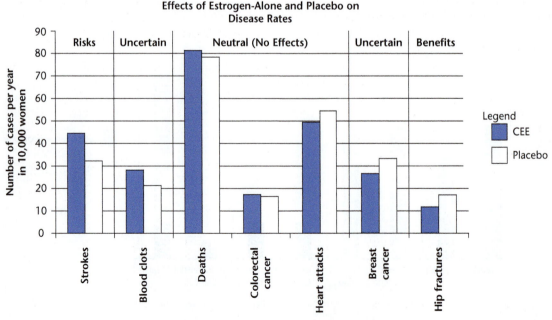

Preventing Menopausal Symptoms

Menopausal symptoms may also be alleviated or managed through natural or alternative therapies. Hot flashes may be addressed through lifestyle changes, phytoestrogens, or antidepressants. Foods to avoid may include spicy foods and caffeine. Wearing layered clothes to be able to adjust as necessary can also help with hot flashes. Phytoestrogens (estrogen-like products from plants) can be found in soy products. Soy may help with mild hot flashes but is contraindicated for women who are at risk for breast cancer, particularly estrogen-dependent breast cancer. A number of herbs act like estrogen produced in the body. These herbs include black cohash, wild yam, Dong quai, and Valerian root. These herbs are often included as the active ingredients in products marketed specifically for menopausal symptoms in women. Herbs and herbal remedies are not FDA-approved so the dose strength may vary from product to product and within product lot numbers. Mild cases of vaginal dryness can be countered with OTC vaginal lubricants and moisturizers. More severe cases may require products such as vaginal creams, Vagifem (vaginal suppositories), and Estring (plastic ring). Mood swings may be helped with adequate physical activity and sleep, relaxation strategies, or antidepressant and antianxiety drugs. Insomnia may be alleviated through OTC sleep aids, milk products drunk prior to bedtime, avoiding physical activity late in the evening, and taking a hot shower or bath immediately before bedtime. Memory problems may be helped through mental exercises such as crossword puzzles and Sudoku and adequate physical activity and sleep.[50]

Sexuality

Sexuality begins at birth and includes sexual knowledge, values, attitudes, and behaviors as well as the anatomy and physiology of reproduction. Sexuality is more than simple mechanics involving genitalis, intercourse, and orgasm. In almost all cultures, behavior, including sexual behavior, is divided into male and female; masculine and feminine; man and woman. As we grow, society rewards or punishes us for behaving in gender appropriate or inappropriate ways. These rewards and punishments impact our entire being. In the following section, we look at some of the influences of biology and psychosocial factors that influence our values, feelings, desires, and activities.

Biological Bases of Human Sexuality   At conception, the sex of a baby is determined by the genes from the mother and father. A fertilized ovum with XX sex chromosomes is biologically female and the fertilized ovum with XY sex chromosomes is biologically male. Genetics forms the most basic level of biological sexuality. The growing embryo develops male gonads around the seventh week and female gonads around the twelfth week. Male embryos develop male reproductive structures with the presence of androgens and mullerian inhibiting substance. Female embryos develop female reproductive structures with the absence of these male hormones. At puberty, maturation in the female includes the budding of breasts, growth of pubic and underarm hair, and the onset of menstruation. In males, maturation includes genital enlargement, growth of pubic and underarm hair, the lowering of the voice, facial hair, and nocturnal emissions.[51, 52]

Psychosocial Bases of Human Sexuality   As human beings, we have the ability to be more than just reproductive beings. By the eighteenth month of development, the infant has the language and ability to self identify as male or female. **Gender identity** is the ability to correctly identify their gender. By preschool, the child takes on the appearance and behaviors that are typically associated with gender. **Gender preference** refers to the emotional and intellectual understanding and acceptance of one's biological gender. It determines how women think, feel and act as feminine, masculine or androgynous. **Gender adoption** refers to the process of acquiring and personalizing gender preferences. As a woman develops and matures into an adult, she consciously makes decisions related to the roles and behaviors she adopts. At some point, she forms a **gender identification**. As an example, a child can correctly identify herself as female. She takes on traits and characteristics that align with traditional or nontraditional feminine choices as part of her gender preference. As she ages, she adopts and personalizes feminine preferences. Her gender identity is woman. In another example, a child can correctly identify herself as female. She prefers the traits and characteristics that align with traditional male and masculine choices such as being physically active, playing sports, and being independent and autonomous. She adopts and personalizes masculine preferences and prefers an androgynous gender adoption. Her gender identification is woman. There are multiple variations of patterns from gender identity to gender identification that evolve through thinking, feeling, and acting as a male or female. These patterns can be heavily impacted by cultural and social variables.[53]

Human Sexual Response Cycle   The human sexual response cycle was first described by Havelock Ellis and elaborated on by Alfred Kinsey and colleagues. Kinsey and his colleagues' research provided some of the first empirical findings related to the physiological response of women to orgasm. It was their work that lead to further study by Masters and Johnson who reported their seminal findings in *Human Sexual Response*.[54] They found that the human sexual response cycle followed a pattern through four stages with individual variability in duration and intensity. Their classic human sexual response cycle included four predictable phases: excitement, plateau, orgasm, and resolution. Figure 8.5 shows the female physiological changes that occur during the human sexual response cycle. Their key

FIGURE 8.5 Female sexual response cycle

Excitement Vaginal lubrication begins within 10–15 seconds of stimulation. Labia majora and minora darken. Clitoris engorges with blood and increases in size and length. Uterus and cervix pull away from the vagina. Breasts swell and nipples become erect. Sexual tension heightens. Sex flush (darkening of the skin) may occur.

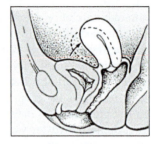

Plateau Vagina continues to expand and outer third fills with blood. Uterus elevates into abdomen. Tenting (distending of inner two-thirds of vagina) takes place. Cervix elevates. Clitoris retracts under clitoral hood. Secretion occurs from Bartholin's glands. Breasts continue to enlarge and areola engorges with blood. Sex flush may continue and spread.

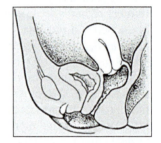

Orgasm Rhythmic contractions (3–15) of uterine walls, first 3–6 are most intense. Involuntary muscle spasms. Clitoris remains retracted under clitoral hood. Vasocongestion and myotonia (muscle tension) release. Respiration and heart rate increase frequency. Blood pressure increases.

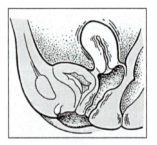

Resolution Vasocongestion and myotonia dissipate rapidly. Vaginal color returns shortly. Uterus returns to unaroused state. Labia major and minora return to normal size and shape. Swelling of breasts disappears.

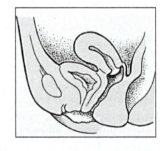

findings concluded that women differ from men in the experience of orgasm. Women experience a variety of different orgasmic responses and can experience multiple orgasms while men follow a consistent pattern through the four stages including a refractory period in the majority of males. The refractory period in males prevents them from experiencing multiple orgasms in a short period of time. They also found that for women, physiologically, orgasms are the same regardless of whether initiated by penile penetration or masturbation.[55] Their research has been used as the foundation for many studies of human sexual response.

More recently, researchers have suggested that sexual motivation comes from processing sexual stimuli, which leads to sexual arousal. These stimuli activate the humans sexual response cycle and sexual desire and sexual arousal are interrelated. A combination of events or circumstances must be present for excitement to lead to sexual functioning. Kaplan developed a triphasic model of sexual response consisting of (1) desire, (2) excitement, and (3) orgasm. She argued for the importance of sexual desire. Here, the brain plays the key role in determining whether the sexual response occurs and/or continues. The desire phase is triggered by some thought, emotion, fantasy, or sensation that activates the cerebral cortex.[56] Basson's model of female sexual response shows that biological and psychological factors determine how sexual stimuli are processed. When sexual stimuli are processed positively, sexual arousal and sexual desire lead to either non-sexual rewards or sexual satisfaction. The positive rewarding of the sexual experiences (context) leads to willingness to accept sexual stimuli. Sexual stimuli and a suitable context initiate the process again.[57] (See Figure 8.6.)

FIGURE 8.6 A sexual response to positive biological and psychological factors

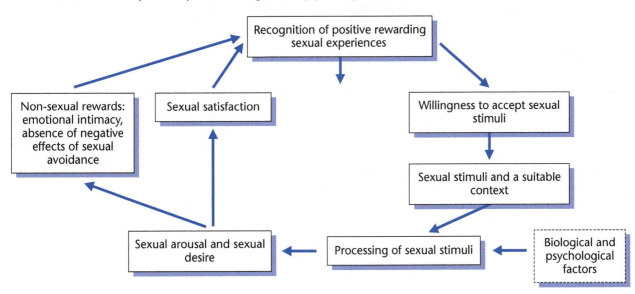

Basson, R. 2001. Using a different model for female sexual response to address women's problematic low sexual desire. *Journal of Sexual and Marital Therapy*, 27:395–403.

Meston and Buss found that while the top ten motives of men and women were closely matched, men were more inclined toward physical motives, such as seeing an attractive body, whereas women considered relational motives, such as showing love, to be more important.[58] Not surprisingly, intimacy was determined to be more significant than age and menopause in determining women's sexual desire and arousal.

Sexual Dysfunction   Sexual dysfunction is more common among women than men, with the most common female dysfunctions being low or no sexual desire. Twenty to 30 percent of all women express some concerns about sexual functioning. Sexual function is defined as "the ability to experience desire (positive anticipation and feelings deserving of sexual pleasure, arousal (receptivity and responsivity to erotic touch resulting in lubrication for women and erection for the man), orgasm (a voluntary response that is a natural culmination of high arousal), and satisfaction (feeling emotionally and sexually fulfilled and bonded)."[59]

Female sexual dysfunction is a classification included in the *DSM-IV-TR* and can include (1) inhibited sexual desire, (2) nonorgasmic response during partner sex, (3) painful intercourse (dyspareunia), (4) female arousal dysfunction, (5) primary nonorgasmic response, and (6) vaginismus (a painful spasmodic constriction of the vagina, rendering copulation impossible.[60] The *DSM-IV-TR* classification of sexual disorders and dysfunctions has been criticized for focusing on disturbances of the genital response (vascular engorgement and lubrication of the vagina) rather than the more common female complaints of pain during intercourse or the subjective component of reduced feelings of arousal.[61] The *DSM-IV* also has been criticized for being

based on a linear model of the sexual response, which is primarily determined by a physiological response. This model implies that sexual desire occurs spontaneously and is independent of the sexual arousal response. The separation of the sexual desire phase from the sexual arousal phase has been challenged by numerous researchers.

For women, the physical genital component is not necessarily connected to the subjective component. A triphasic model proposed by Kaplan (1974) is still used to class sexual dysfunctions as disorders of desire, arousal, and orgasm.[62] Baumeister and colleagues found that women exhibit lower and less frequent sexual motivation than men. They masturbate less, fantasize less about sex, have less frequent desire for sex, and report more complaints of a lack of sexual desire.[63]

Sexual dysfunctions can include orgasmic difficulties, vaginismus, and dyspareunia. Orgasmic disorders can be primary (never had an orgasm) and secondary (not currently experiencing orgasms). Orgasmic difficulties can result from physiological causes (primary) or psychological factors (secondary). Vaginismus is painful, involuntary contractions of the vaginal muscles. Vaginismus can be caused by past traumatic experiences, religious prohibitions, anxiety, or fear of penetration. It can make intercourse difficult and painful or impossible. Dyspareunia is pain that comes during or after intercourse. Physiological and psychological factors can cause dyspareunia. (See *FYI:* "Causes of Dyspareunia.")

Aging and Sexual Response

Researchers continue to study the hormonal, relationship, and life-event factors that contribute to sexual responsiveness in older women. The aging process brings physiological changes in the human sexual response cycle. Physiologically, the excitement phase takes longer because

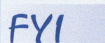 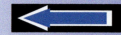

Causes of Dyspareunia[64]

- An improperly fitted diaphragm
- Hemorrhoids
- Herpes sores, genital warts, or other STIs
- Infections
- Inflammation due to irritants
- Intercourse too soon after surgery or childbirth
- Endometriosis
- Menopause
- Ovarian cysts
- Sexual abuse or rape
- UTIs
- Some medications
- Vaginismus
- Vaginal dryness or too little lubrication (for example, from not enough foreplay)

it takes more time to lubricate the vaginal area. The orgasmic phase is shorter in duration and contractions may be less intense. And the resolution phase has also been found to be longer.[65] The work of Masters and Johnson, as well as that of other sex researchers, has been criticized for focusing primarily on the biomedical changes that come with aging and menopause. A more woman-centered approach toward female sexuality focuses on the complex psychological and sociological factors that impact sexual functioning in later years. For instance, women tend to be more relationship and intimacy focused and less genitally and orgasm focused than men. While sexual desire continues in later years, a woman's perceptions of relationship qualities provide a strong indicator of the level of sexual desire she attains throughout the aging process. Nonhormonal factors that can have a negative impact on women's sexual responsiveness include career concerns, changing family relationships, a partner's incapacity to function sexually, not having a partner, and changing priorities. As women's health becomes a higher research priority, female sexual function and dysfunction receive more attention. As the baby boomer generation enters menopause, research can provide better information about the effects of aging and menopause on female sexual responsiveness.

Chapter Summary

- The vulva refers to the external genitalia, those parts that are outwardly visible.
- The hymen is a thin sheath that covers the vaginal opening.
- The perineum is the muscle tissue found between the vaginal opening and the anal canal.
- An episiotomy is a surgical incision that widens the vaginal opening during childbirth.
- The vaginal opening serves as the opening for menstrual flow and the birth canal during labor, and it receives the penis during intercourse.
- The endometrium is the inner lining of cells of the uterus that is sloughed off each month during the menstrual flow if fertilization does not occur.
- The ovaries produce and expel eggs each month and also the female sex hormones, progesterone and estrogen.
- Breasts can exhibit cyclic changes, including benign lumps or masses of overgrown breast tissue.
- The average age of menarche, the onset of the first menstrual cycle, is 12.8 years.
- The sex hormones involved in menstruation include follicle-stimulating hormone, luteinizing hormone, estrogen, and progesterone.

- A Pap test is the best method of detecting cervical cancer.
- Primary dysmenorrhea is painful menses without evidence of a physical abnormality.
- Secondary dysmenorrhea is usually due to anatomic abnormalities.
- Primary amenorrhea indicates a significant medical disorder.
- The causes of secondary amenorrhea remain unknown.
- The cause of endometriosis is unknown.
- Polycystic ovarian syndrome and ovarian failure are the most common causes of amenorrhea.
- PMS has physical and emotional symptoms that are associated with the luteal phase of menstruation.
- Uterine fibroids are common tumors of the uterus.
- Menopause is the time when ovulation and menstruation cease.
- The human sexual response cycle includes four phases: excitement, plateau, orgasm, and resolution.
- Sexual dysfunction is more common among women than men.

Review Questions

1. What are the anatomic parts of the vulva?
2. What are the anatomic parts of the internal genitalia?
3. How are the four sex hormones involved in the menstrual cycle?
4. What are the components of the female athlete triad?

5. Describe the differences between primary and secondary dysmenorrhea.
6. Describe the differences between primary and secondary amenorrhea.

7. What would you expect to occur during a pelvic examination?
8. What are some emotional and physical symptoms of PMS?
9. What are the changes that occur during the four phases of the human sexual response cycle?
10. Describe the most common female sexual dysfunctions.

Resources

Dr. Susan Love Research Foundation
866-569-0388
www.dslrf.org

Endometriosis Association
414-355-2200
www.endometriosisassn.org

Imaginis, The Women's Cancer Resource
864-209-1139
www.imaginis.com

National Women's Health Network
202-682-2640
www.nwhn.org

National Women's Health Resource Center
877-986-9472
www.healthywomen.org

North American Menopause Society
440-442-7550
www.menopause.org

Planned Parenthood Federation of America
800-230-PLAN
www.plannedparenthood.org

U.S. Department of Health and Human Services Office on Women's Health
800-994-9662
www.womenshealth.gov

References

1. Department of Health and Human Services, Office of Women's Health. 2008. *Urinary tract infections fact sheet.* http://www.womenshealth.gov/publications/our-publications/fact-sheet/urinary-tract-infection.cfm (retrieved November 16, 2011)
2. Department of Health and Human Services, Office of Women's Health. 2008. *Urinary incontinence fact sheet.* http://www.womenshealth.gov/publications/our-publications/fact-sheet/urinary-incontinence.cfm (retrieved November 16, 2011)
3. Ibid.
4. American Congress of Obstetricians and Gynecologists. *ACOG recommends restricted use of episiotomies.* http://www.acog.org/From_home/publications/press_releases/nr03-31-006-2.cfm (retrieved November 15, 2011)
5. Alperin,M, Keohn, MA Parvianinen, K. 2008. Episiotomy and increase in the risk of obstetric laceration in a subsequent vaginal delivery. *Obstetrics and Gynecology* 111: 1274–1278.
6. *New York Times.* November, 2011. *Evelyn H. Lauder, champion of breast cancer research, dies at 75.* http://www.nytimes.com/2011/11/13/nyregion/evelyn-h-lauder-champion-of-breast-cancer-research-dies-at-75.html (retrieved January 30, 2012)
7. American Cancer Society. 2011. *What are the key statistics about endometrial cancer?* http://www.cancer.org/Cancer/EndometrialCancer/DetailedGuide/endometrial-uterine-cancer-key-statistics (retrieved November 15, 2011)
8. Department of Health and Human Services, Office of Women's Health. 2010. *Uterine fibroids fact sheet.* http://www.womenshealth.gov/publications/our-publications/fact-sheet/urinary-incontinence.cfmhttp://www.womenshealth.gov/publications/our-publications/fact-sheet/urinary-incontinence.cfm (retrieved November 15, 2011)
9. Department of Health and Human Services, Office of Women's Health. 2010. *Polycystic ovarian syndrome fact sheet.* http://www.womenshealth.gov/publications/our-publications/fact-sheet/polycystic-ovary-syndrome.cfm (retrieved November 15, 2011)
10. National Institutes of Health. *Anatomy of the breast.* http://mammary.nih.gov/reviews/development/Human-breast001/ (retrieved November 15, 2011)
11. American Cancer Society. 2011. *Finding benign breast conditions.* http://www.cancer.org/Healthy/FindCancerEarly/WomensHealth/Non-CancerousBreastConditions/non-cancerous-breast-conditions-finding-benign-br-cond (retrieved November 15, 2011)
12. Imaginis. 2012. *Nipple discharge.* http://www.imaginis.com/breast-health/benign-breast-conditions-1 (retrieved November 15, 2011)
13. Ibid
14. Imaginis. 2009. *How are fibrocystic diseases treated?* http://www.imaginis.com/breast-health/fibrocystic-breasts-1#how-are-fibrocystic-breasts-treated (retrieved November 15, 2011)
15. American Cancer Society. 2011. *Screening mammography.* http://www.cancer.org/Healthy/FindCancerEarly/ExamandTestDescriptions/MammogramsandOtherBreastImagingProcedures/mammograms-and-other-breast-imaging-procedures-screening-mammogram (retrieved November 15, 2011)
16. American Cancer Society. 2011. *American Cancer Society recommendations for early breast cancer detection.* http://www.cancer.org/Healthy/FindCancerEarly/ExamandTestDescriptions/MammogramsandOtherBreastImagingProcedures/mammograms-and-other-breast-imaging-procedures-screening-mammogram (retrieved November 15, 2011)
17. Fingerson, L. 2005. *Adolescents' medicalization of menstruation.* Philadelphia, PA: American Sociological Association. http://research.allacademic.com/index.php?click_key=1&PHPSESSID=2bcd35ff3dbb43c24507b75d784f2148 (retrieved January 29, 2012)
18. Ibid.
19. National Women's Health Information Center. 2009. *Menstruation and the menstrual cycle fact sheet.* http://www.womenshealth.gov/publications/our-publications/fact-sheet/menstruation.cfm (retrieved October 4, 2006)
20. Chumlea, W. C., C. M. Schubert, A. F. Roche, H. E. Kulin, P. A. Lee, J. H. Himes, and S. S. Sun. 2003. Age at menarche and racial comparisons in U.S. girls. *Journal of Pediatrics* 111 (1): 110–13.
21. WebMD. 2011. *Normal menstrual cycle.* http://women.webmd.com/tc/normal-menstrual-cycle-normal-menstrual-cycle (retrieved November 17, 2011)

22. Ibid.

23. Merck Manual. 2007. *Female reproductive endocrinology.* http://www.merckmanuals.com/professional/gynecology_and_obstetrics/female_reproductive_endocrinology/female_reproductive_endocrinology.html#v1061583 (retrieved November 18, 2011)

24. Center for Young Women's Health. 2010. *Your first pelvic examination.* http://www.youngwomenshealth.org/pelvicinfo.html (retrieved November 18, 2011).

25. American Cancer Society. 2011. *Guidelines for cervical cancer screening.* http://www.cancer.org/Healthy/FindCancerEarly/CancerScreeningGuidelines/american-cancer-society-guidelines-for-the-early-detection-of-cancer (retrieved November 18, 2011)

26. Office of Women's Health, Department of Health and Human Services. 2009. *Pap test fact sheet.* http://www.womenshealth.gov/publications/our-publications/fact-sheet/pap-test.cfm#a (retrieved November 18, 2011)

27. Mayo Clinic. 2010. *Endometriosis – Definition.* http://www.mayoclinic.com/health/endometriosis/DS00289 (retrieved November 18, 2011)

28. A.D.A.M. 2011. *Endometriosis. Medical encyclopedia.* http://www.ncbi.nlm.nih.gov/pubmedhealth/PMH0001913/ (retrieved November 18, 2011)

29. WebMD. 2011. *Menstrual cramps.* http://www.medicinenet.com/menstrual_cramps/page4.htm (retrieved November 18, 2011)

30. National Institute of Child Health and Human Services, National Institutes of Health. 2011. *Amenorrhea.* http://www.nichd.nih.gov/health/topics/amenorrhea.cfm#causes (retrieved January 19, 2012)

31. Popat, V., et al. 2011. *Amenorrhea clinical presentation.* Medscape Reference. http://emedicine.medscape.com/article/252928-clinical (retrieved January 21, 2012)

32. Sports Tips and Advice for Female Athletes. *Female athlete triad statistics.* 2008. http://www.sportswomenfitness.com/female-athlete-triad/female-athlete-triad-statistics/ (retrieved January 21, 2012)

33. Scalise, D. 2010. *Types of PMS: An alphabet of choices.* http://www.netplaces.com/health-guide-to-pms/types-of-pmsan-alphabet-of-choices/ (retrieved January 21, 2012)

34. Lark, S. M. *Hormones.* http://www.drlark.com/MainSite/HealthCenter.aspx?Healthcenter=LARK_HC Hormones (retrieved January 21, 2012)

35. *Treating PMS.* 2006. www.pms.com/treating/Default.pmsx (Retrieved october 2, 2006)

36. Bhatia, S. C., and S. K. Bhatia. 2002. Diagnosis and treatment of premenstrual dysphoric disorder. *American Family Physician* 66(7): 1239–48.

37. Ibid.

38. National Uterine Fibroids Foundation. *Hysterectomy statistics.* http://www.nuff.org/health_hysterectomystatistics.htm (retrieved January 21, 2012)

39. Whiteman, M. K., Hillis, S. D., Jamieson, D. J., Morrow, B., Podgornik, M. N., Brett, K. M., and Marchbanks, P. A. Inpatient hysterectomy surveillance in the United States, 2000–2004. *American Journal of Obstetrics and Gynecology.* 198(1): 34.e1–7. http://www.cdc.gov/reproductivehealth/WomensRH/00-04-FS_Hysterectomy.htm (retrieved January 21, 2012)

40. WebMd. 2009. *Perimenopause.* http://www.webmd.com/menopause/guide/guide-perimenopause (retrieved January 21, 2012)

41. WebMd. 2010. *Understanding menopause: the basics.* http://www.webmd.com/menopause/guide/understanding-menopause-basics (retrieved January 21, 2012)

42. WebMd. 2009. *Your health in postmenopause.* http://www.webmd.com/menopause/guide/health-after-menopause (retrieved January 29, 2012)

43. WebMd. 2009. *Premature menopause.* http://www.webmd.com/menopause/guide/premature-menopause (retrieved January 29, 2012)

44. National Heart, Lung, and Blood Institute. 2008. *Why WHI?* http://www.nhlbi.nih.gov/whi/whywhi.htm (retrieved January 29, 2012)

45. National Heart, Blood, and Lung Institute. 2005. *Facts about menopause replacement therapy.* http://www.nhlbi.nih.gov/health/women/pht_facts.pdf (January 22, 2012)

46. Griffin, R. M. *Is hormone replacement therapy making a comeback?* WebMD. http://www.webmd.com/menopause/guide/hormone-replacement-therapy (January 22, 2012)

47. Heiss, G., R, Wallace, G. L. Anderson, et al. 2008. Health risks and benefits 3 years after stopping randomized treatment with estrogen and progestin. *JAMA* 299(9): 1036–1045.

48. Ibid.

49. Women's Health Initiative. 2008. *WHI follow-up study confirms health risks of long-term combination hormone therapy outweigh benefits for postmenopausal women* http://public.nhlbi.nih.gov/newsroom/home/GetPressRelease.aspx?id=2554 (retrieved January 29, 2012)

50. National Heart, Blood, and Lung Institute. 2005. *Facts about menopause replacement therapy.* http://www.nhlbi.nih.gov/health/women/pht_facts.pdf (January 22, 2012)

51. Thibodeau, G. A., and K. T. Patton. 2006. *Anatomy and physiology* (6th ed.) St. Louis, MO: Mosby.

52. Crooks, R., and K. Bauer. 2008. *Our sexuality* (10th ed.). Belmont, CA: Wadsworth.

53. Ibid.

54. Masters, W. H., and V. E. Johnson. 1970. *Human sexual response.* Boston: Little, Brown.

55. Ibid.

56. Kaplan, H. S. 1995. *Sexual desire disorders: dysfunctional regulation of sexual motivation.* New York: Brunner Routledge.

57. Basson, R. 2001. Using a different model for female sexual response to address women's problematic low sexual desire. *Journal of Sexual and Marital Therapy,* 27: 395–403.

58. Meston, C. M., and D. M. Buss. 2007. Why humans have sex. *Archives of Sexual Behavior,* 36: 477–507.

59. McCarthy, B. 2002. Sexuality, sexual dysfunction, and couple therapy. In A. S. Gurman and N. S. Jacobson (eds.), *Clinical handbook of couple therapy* (3rd ed., pp. 629–652). New York: Guilford Press.

60. Ibid.

61. Both, S., E. Laan, and W. W. Schultz. 2010. Disorders in sexual desire and sexual arousal in women, a 2010 state of the art. *Journal of Psychosomatic Obstetrics & Gynecology,* 31(4): 207–218.

62. Kaplan, H. S. 1995. *Sexual desire disorders: Dysfunctional regulation of sexual motivation.* New York: Brunner Routledge.

63. Baumeister, R. F., K. R. Cantenese, and K. D. Vohs. 2001. Is there a gender difference in strength of sex drive? Theoretical views, conceptual distinctions, and a review of relevant evidence. *Personal Sociology and Psychology Review,* 5: 242–273.

64. National Institutes of Health, U.S. National Library of Medicine. 2010. *Intercourse – Painful.* http://www.nlm.nih.gov/medlineplus/ency/article/003157.htm (retrieved January 29, 2012)

65. Masters, W. H., and V. E. Johnson. 1970. *Human sexual response.*

Designing Your Reproductive Life Plan

CHAPTER OBJECTIVES

When you complete this chapter, you will be able to do the following:

◇ Prepare your own reproductive life plan

◇ Describe the benefits and risks of the available contraceptive choices

◇ Describe how to plan for a pregnancy

◇ Describe the major fetal development stages during each trimester

◇ Describe the reasons for female and male infertility

◇ Differentiate between right to life and pro-choice positions

◇ Explain appropriate and inappropriate parenting styles

REPRODUCTIVE HEALTH

In an ideal world, all pregnancies would be planned and all children would be wanted. Yet annually in the United States, nearly half of all pregnancies are unplanned and nearly 1 million teenagers become pregnant. This rate is almost twice the rate of the United Kingdom which had the highest rate in Europe. The United States rate is nearly three times the rate of Canada, Spain and Greece, four times the rate of France, Germany and Norway, and ten times the rate of Japan and Switzerland.[1] The total number of pregnancies in the U.S. in 2001, the year for which statistics were available, was 6.4 million. Of the total pregnancies, 42 percent (2.7 million) of all planned pregnancies resulted in live births, while 21 percent (1.4 million) of all unplanned pregnancies resulted in live births. Ten percent (650,000) of all planned pregnancies ended in miscarriage while 20 percent (1.3 million) of unplanned pregnancies ended in abortion and seven percent (426,000) ended in miscarriage.[2] The landscape

for teen pregnancy in the United States changed between 1999 to 2009. Teens no longer had the highest rate of unplanned pregnancies. Teens constituted less than one-fourth of all unplanned pregnancies in the United States although eight in ten teens (82%) reported that their pregnancy was unplanned. Fifty percent of all unplanned pregnancies occurred to women with less than a high school diploma and one in six occurred to women who had graduated from college. The teen birth rate was at an all time low in 2009 having decreased 39 percent between 1991 and 2009 (61.8 per 1000 to 37.9 per 1000, respectively).[3] On the opposite end of the life spectrum, a growing number of women are postponing pregnancy until later in their life when risks for complications also increase and infertility is more common.

A woman's reproductive life begins during fetal development and ends with menopause, when ovarian follicular development ceases. A woman can control her own reproductive life only when she has access to, choice of, and affordability of contraceptive choices.

Viewpoint

The Benefits of Family Planning

The ability to plan the number, spacing, and timing of births is essential for the empowerment of women. Family planning has a number of benefits for women, including the following:

- Family planning contributes significantly to the decrease of women who live in poverty.
- Family planning provides women with more time to spend on education and employment opportunities.
- Family planning reduces the number of maternal and infant deaths.
- Family planning reduces the global population.
- Family planning reduces the number of teenagers who give birth, thus reducing overall premature and unintended pregnancies. Teenage childbirth is associated with greater risk of dying in pregnancy and complications during delivery.
- Family planning provides adolescents with more opportunities for a better education, jobs, and income and reduces the likelihood of divorce and separation.[5]

Given these benefits and more, what should the U.S. position be regarding family planning? What funding should the U.S. government provide to teenagers for contraceptives? How well does the United States support worldwide family planning efforts?

Governments throughout the world can reduce population overcrowding and improve the status of women by providing a wide variety of birth control methods, and by making birth control accessible and affordable. The ability to pay and a woman's status in society should not keep her from choosing the reproductive life plan that is right for her. This chapter addresses issues of reproductive health, including contraceptive choices, pregnancy, childbirth, birthing options, breast feeding, fetal health, infertility, abortion, and adoption.

BIRTH CONTROL METHODS

A landmark decision by the U.S. Supreme Court in 1967 created the present environment of contraceptive acceptance in the United States. *Griswold v. Connecticut* held that the state law prohibiting married couples from using birth control was unconstitutional. This decision afforded married couples the right of privacy in making choices regarding the use of birth control by placing the issue beyond state intervention.[6] Throughout this chapter, birth control and contraceptive choice are used interchangeably. While the courts have limited the definition, we define **birth control** methods as all the strategies used to keep from having a baby, including abstinence, contraceptive methods, IUDs, and emergency contraception (EC). Contraceptive choice includes those methods that prevent fertilization of the ovum such as hormonal methods, barrier methods, and sterilization.

Choosing an appropriate birth control method requires planning and informed decision making. The first consideration is whether to *involve a partner* in the decision. A partner can assist with the choice of the appropriate contraceptive, accompany the woman to scheduled physical examinations if a prescription is required, and share the cost for the contraceptive. (See Table 9.1.)

The second consideration is *acceptability*. The method a woman selects should be congruent with her personal values and beliefs (e.g., religious) about the likelihood of pregnancy or sexually transmitted infections (STIs). If she believes that premarital sex is not acceptable, her only choice is abstinence. If she is in a monogamous relationship and her partner is STI-free, she might choose hormonal methods. If she has had a previous ectopic (outside the uterus) pregnancy, she might want to consider a method other than an IUD. Another consideration is *availability* of the method she selects. If a prescription is required, she must have access to a health care provider who can prescribe the method. If she is a minor, she may need to secure parental consent. Fourth, she needs to consider the *cost* of the method. She must weigh the cost of the method against the cost of an unintended pregnancy or unwanted STI. Can she afford this method of protection (both monetarily and in terms of method and user effectiveness)? If she chooses to use the pill, she must remember to take it at the same time every day. If she forgets, she will need to use another method during the month. Is she knowledgeable about the method, and will she use it dependably? Can she afford (financially and emotionally) to become pregnant? Another factor to consider is *health risk*. A method may be contraindicated for medical reasons. For example, women smokers over age 35 or women who are breast feeding should choose a method other than the pill. If a woman has a family history of breast cancer, she may want to consider a nonhormonal method. If she had a previous pregnancy, the IUD may not be appropriate. If a partner has an STI, a woman may want to choose an appropriate method to reduce her risk of contracting it.

When making a decision about the choice of birth control, a couple must have adequate information about the available **contraceptive** methods, including the health benefits and drawbacks, the relative failure rates, and the cost estimate of each method. Birth control methods can be classified according to the method of protection, such as continuous abstinence, fertility awareness-based methods (periodic abstinence),

TABLE 9.1 Comparison of User Failure, Method Failure, and Cost

BIRTH CONTROL METHOD	USER FAILURE	METHOD FAILURE	COST
Fertility Awareness–Based Methods			
Cycle-based	20–25%	9%	Charts are free
Basal body temperature	20–25%	2–3%	Temperature kit $10–12
Cervical mucus	20–25%	2–3%	Free
Symptothermal	12–20%	2–3%	Temperature kit $10–12
No method	85%	85%	Free
Barrier			
Spermicides	29%	15%	$8–10 kit with 20–40 applications; refills $4–8
Male condom	15%	2%	Free at clinics to $6–12/dozen
Female condom	21%	5%	$4
Diaphragm	14–16%	6%	$15–75
		1–2%	
Cervical cap (FemCap)	14–29%	2–10%	$60–75
Lea's Shield	N/A	15%	
Sponge (Today Sponge)	16–32%	9–20%	$9–15 for 3 sponges
Hormonal Methods			
Oral contraceptives	6%	3%	$15–50, depending on site + visit
NuvaRing (ring)	8%	>1%	$15–80 a month + visit
OrthoEvra (patch)	8%	>1%	$15–80 a month + visit
Depo-Provera	3%	>1%	$35–75 every 3 months + visit
ECP (Plan B One Step and Next Choice)	10–25%	2–10% if within 3 days	$10–70 + visit for women under age 17 and no prescription for women age 17 and older
ECP (IUD)		1%	$175–500 + visit, lasts up to 12 years
Implanon		>1%	$400–800, lasts 3 years
Other Methods			
Intrauterine device	>1%	>1%	$500–1000 + visit, lasts up to 12 years
Tubal ligation		>1%	$1500–6000
Vasectomy		>1%	$350–1000
Lactational amenorrhea (LAM)	>1%	2%	Free, lasts up to 6 months

SOURCE: Planned Parenthood Federation of America, 2012.[7]

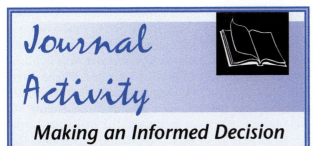

Journal Activity

Making an Informed Decision

The major factors to consider when choosing an appropriate contraceptive method (including abstinence) include whether or not to involve your partner, acceptability, accessibility, cost (money and effectiveness), and health risks. Choose a birth control method that is right for you at this time. Write about each major factor and how it affects your decision. Are there other factors you may need to consider?

barrier methods, hormonal methods, and other methods. Now complete *Journal Activity:* "Making an Informed Decision."

Continuous Abstinence

Continuous abstinence from sexual intercourse is the only sure way to prevent an unintended pregnancy and STIs. **Continuous abstinence,** as defined in abstinence-only programs and by those teenagers who sign virginity pledges, involves no sex play with a partner. Some teenagers describe themselves as abstinent but still engage in sex play without having sexual intercourse. This type of sex play might better be described as **outercourse.** Outercourse is effective in preventing unintended pregnancies if sperm is kept away from the vulva and vagina. It is also effective in preventing HIV and many other STIs if body fluid is not transmitted from one partner to another.

Viewpoint

Comprehensive or Abstinence-only Sexuality Education?

Statistics suggest that 13 percent of females have had sexual intercourse by age 15 and that 70 percent of all females have had sexual intercourse by age 19. Young men and women, particularly those at greatest risk for pregnancy and contracting HIV or other STIs, need to be well informed about the risks and strategies for preventing STIs and unwanted pregnancies. They need to hear messages regarding postponement of sexual behavior and proper protection when sexually active. Abstinence-only-until-marriage curricula are supported by parents and religious organizations who do not want teachers to address birth control, contraceptives, and sexual behaviors. For them, teaching sexuality education is a moral issue. During the Bush administration, Congress funneled $50 million per year for 5 years to states willing to match every $4 of federal monies with $3 of state monies. These programs have been supported by Focus on Family, Concerned Women for America, Moral Majority and the Eagle Forum. The curricula have never proven to be effective yet some in Congress want to continue funding only abstinence-only-until-marriage programs. Total federal taxpayer dollars spent on these programs has topped $1.1 billion.[8,9]

Comprehensive sexuality education is supported by parents, religious organizations and professionals who promote sexuality education for its medical/educational aspects. In 2012, the National Sexuality Education Standards for K-12 were released by Advocates for Youth and a number of national education organizations. The standards were developed to provide guidelines to schools for age appropriate instruction. The report stated there is "a pressing need to address harassment, bullying and relationship violence in our schools, which have a significant impact on a student's emotional and physical well-being as well as on academic success."[10] The debate regarding the moral versus medical/educational aspects of teaching sexuality education, particularly reproductive health, continues. What do you think about the moral and medical/educational arguments? Are schools, parents, churches, and communities doing everything they can to prevent unintended pregnancies in adolescents? How is sex defined by adolescents today (does it include oral sex)? What role should the federal government have in curricular decisions about sexuality education in the schools? What suggestions do you have for preventing or reducing STIs in adolescents? How will the current administration change the federal policy on sexuality education?

It may not be effective in preventing HPV or herpes if skin-to-skin contact occurs. Other teenagers describe themselves as abstinent when they refrain from sexual intercourse during the time of month during which a young woman might get pregnant. This type of restraint might better be called **periodic abstinence.** Periodic abstinence is sometimes referred to as fertility awareness.

Sexually transmitted diseases and teen pregnancy rates are at their lowest levels in decades for teenagers. Millions of federal and state dollars have been spent on abstinence-only-until-marriage with no federal dollars and limited state dollars spent on comprehensive sexuality education. Which policy will be most effective in the long term? (See *Viewpoint:* "Comprehensive or Abstinence-only Sexuality Education")

Fertility Awareness–Based Methods (Periodic Abstinence)

Fertility awareness–based methods (FAMs) of contraception are referred to as periodic abstinence and include the cycle-based method, the basal body temperature method, the cervical mucus method, and the symptothermal method, a combination of basal body temperature tracking, cycle monitoring, and mucosal sampling. Withdrawal, referred to as coitus interruptus, is common and is mentioned, but it is not a birth control method. Natural family planning methods or fertility awareness–based methods help women understand their menstrual cycle better but require high motivation and cooperation by both partners. These methods have high method and user failure rates, are not suggested for couples who cannot afford a pregnancy, and offer no protection against STIs. (See Figure 9.1.)

Cycle-Based Method   The **cycle-based method** (or calendar or rhythm) is a form of contraception that relies on abstinence during the period of time a woman is ovulating. It is the least user effective method of contraception and should be supplemented with another option if pregnancy cannot be tolerated. The average menstrual cycle is 21–35 days long, and **ovulation** can occur anytime between days 11 and 21 depending on cycle length. For some teenagers, the menstrual cycle can be as long as 45 days.[11] Ovulation occurs near the midpoint of a menstrual cycle or, put another way, approximately 14 days after ovulation, menses begins. The cycle-based method would be very effective if a woman knew the exact day of ovulation; however, pregnancy has occurred with isolated intercourse on virtually every day of the menstrual cycle. To use the cycle-based method, a woman determines the length of time between menstrual cycles, including the shortest and longest times between cycles. To be safe, a couple should

FIGURE 9.1 Fertility awareness, also known as natural family planning, can combine each method to identify when a woman is fertile. However, it must be remembered that the cycles for most women are not consistently 28-day cycles.

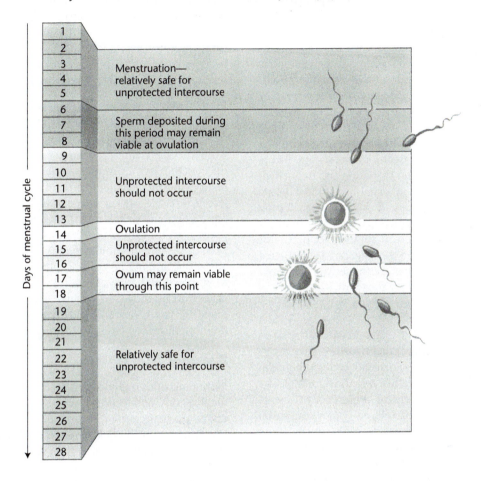

refrain from intercourse during the entire time that ovulation is possible, including 3–4 days prior to ovulation, the day of ovulation, and 2–3 days after ovulation. The egg can be fertilized anytime between its release by the ovary and its exit from the fallopian tube. Women with cycles shorter than 27 days should opt for another method.[12]

The cycle-based method has a 20–25 percent user failure rate, with higher rates for single women. With perfect use, 9 in 100 women will become pregnant within a year when using this method alone. The primary advantage of this method is its acceptance by most religious organizations. The primary disadvantage is the unpredictability of a woman's menstrual cycle, particularly during stress or illness. (See *FYI:* "Factors Known to Affect the Menstrual Cycle.") Most failures of the cycle-based method have more to do with the length of viability of sperm than the day of ovulation. Sperm can be found in the cervical mucus within 20 seconds and up to 7 days after ejaculation.[13]

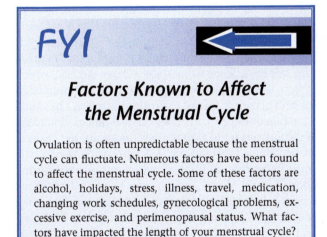

Factors Known to Affect the Menstrual Cycle

Ovulation is often unpredictable because the menstrual cycle can fluctuate. Numerous factors have been found to affect the menstrual cycle. Some of these factors are alcohol, holidays, stress, illness, travel, medication, changing work schedules, gynecological problems, excessive exercise, and perimenopausal status. What factors have impacted the length of your menstrual cycle?

Basal Body Temperature Method   The **basal body temperature (BBT) method** is designed to determine when a woman is ovulating. BBT is the temperature when the body is at complete rest. A woman's BBT is lower during the menstrual cycle prior to ovulation and may drop slightly 1 to 2 days before ovulation, typically 96–98° F. At ovulation, the BBT rises 1/10 to 1/2 a degree and remains elevated until menses begins. A woman who is using this method should take her BBT each morning before rising from bed. It is best to purchase a thermometer that only registers 96–100° F. Rectal thermometers are generally more reliable than those used by mouth. The thermometer should be read to within one-tenth of a degree. One problem with the BBT method, as with the calendar method, is that sexual activity should not occur 3–4 days before ovulation because the sperm can remain viable in the genital tract for several days. BBT is good at telling a couple when ovulation has happened, but not when it will happen. Sexual intercourse before ovulation carries a greater risk than intercourse during the post-ovulatory infertile phase, which is somewhat easier to determine. Intercourse should not occur for 2–3 days after ovulation, as the egg can be fertilized while it travels to the uterus. With perfect use, only 2–3 in 100 women will become pregnant within a year; however, perfect doesn't often happen.[14]

Cervical Mucus Method The **cervical mucus method** (or Billings method) distinguishes changes in cervical mucus during the menstrual cycle. When the egg begins to ripen, more cervical mucus is produced by the same hormones that control the menstrual cycle. This mucus is generally light colored (yellow or white) and cloudy. It feels sticky or tacky to the touch. These days are safe days in the cycle. The body produces the most mucus immediately before ovulation. This mucus is more clear, feels slippery to the touch, and can be stretched between two fingers. The period of time from increased mucus production through ovulation and until the mucus becomes light and cloudy again is not a safe time for intercourse. After menses, there may be several dry days when little or no mucus is produced. These are also safe days. Some women use a 2-day method, which is best used when a woman is certain that secretions haven't occurred. She asks two questions: Did I have cervical mucus today? Did I have cervical mucus yesterday? If she answers no to each of these questions, her chances of becoming pregnant are 3–4 percent. However, she must know that no cervical mucus was secreted during those 2 days! Mucus patterns can be altered by breast feeding, douches, recent use of hormonal contraceptives including EC, spermicides, STIs, and vaginitis. With perfect use of the cervical mucus method, only 2–3 in 100 women will become pregnant within a year.[15]

Symptothermal Method The **symptothermal method** is a combination of basal body temperature, cycle monitoring, and cervical mucus monitoring. In addition to monitoring basal body temperature, a woman can detect changes in consistency of the cervical mucus at ovulation. Monitoring basal body temperature, calendar, and mucus consistency is a better method than the cycle-based method for determining ovulation. This combination method still has a user failure rate of 12–20 percent but is preferred over any single fertility awareness method. Intercourse should be avoided or other methods considered until a woman becomes familiar with her menstrual cycle.[16]

Withdrawal Withdrawal, **coitus interruptus,** is not a contraceptive method; it is a method that leads to many unintended pregnancies. Some young teenage women believe that pregnancy cannot occur if the penis is withdrawn from the vagina before ejaculation. In reality, the pre-ejaculate carries sperm that may be released into the vagina before withdrawal. This method has an extremely high failure rate. If a woman wants to prevent an unwanted pregnancy or protect herself from STIs, this is one method to avoid! Women who are sexually active and use no contraceptive method have an 85 to 90 percent chance of becoming pregnant during the year. If unintended intercourse occurs, women can reduce the risk of an unwanted pregnancy by using EC (Plan B), discussed later in the chapter.

Barrier Methods

Barrier methods include spermicides, condoms, sponges, diaphragms, and cervical caps. Spermicides and condoms are inexpensive and available over-the-counter. Diaphragms and cervical caps require a prescription and are more difficult to use. Barrier methods have become increasingly popular because of the protection they provide against HIV and some STIs. However, their use as contraception for young women remains questionable because of high user failure rates. Many health care providers recommend using a combination of a barrier method and oral contraceptives to protect against unplanned pregnancy and some STIs.

Spermicides Vaginal **spermicides,** a chemical method of contraceptive use, come in a variety of forms: creams, gels, films, suppositories, and foams. (See Figure 9.2.) Spermicides provide a barrier over the cervix and prevent contraception by killing or immobilizing sperm before they reach the egg. They serve as a lubricant and can be used alone or with another barrier method, such as diaphragms or cervical caps. Spermicides are effective within 10 minutes of application and must be reapplied before each ejaculation to prevent loss of effectiveness. Douching should be avoided, or if practiced, should be delayed for 8–10 hours after intercourse because it could force sperm into the uterine cavity. (Contrary to the messages seen in advertisements, douching does not enhance feminine hygiene or provide health benefits.) Recommendations regarding the use of the spermicide nonoxynol-9

FIGURE 9.2 Vaginal spermicides are placed deep into the vagina no longer than 30 minutes before intercourse.

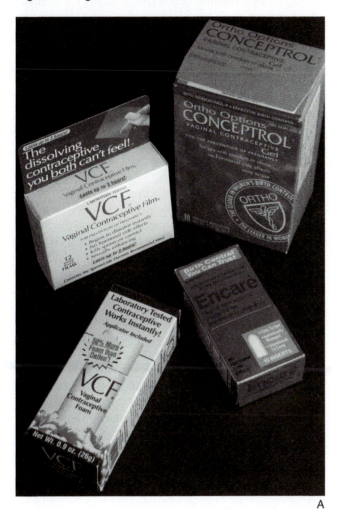

A

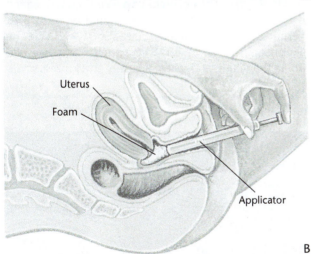

B

populations at high risk for HIV. In one study, women who used a condom and N-9 gel had a 50 percent higher HIV infection rate than women who used a condom and a placebo gel.[17] Method effectiveness is approximately 85 percent; user effectiveness is approximately 70 percent.

Condom, Male   The latex **condom** has increased in use, primarily because it helps to protect against HIV and other STIs such as herpes simplex 2 virus, chlamydia, and cytomegalovirus. Condoms also reduce transmission of gonorrhea, hepatitis B virus, and *Trichomonas vaginalis*.[18] The condom is a thin sheath (see Figure 9.3), and it is 85–90 percent effective when used alone.

Drawbacks to using a condom may include reduced spontaneity and possible allergic reactions. Using condoms as part of foreplay can help reduce a lack of spontaneity. The complaint of an allergic reaction can be addressed by a procedure called double bagging. If the male exhibits an allergy to latex condoms, he can roll a sheepskin condom onto the penis, followed by a latex condom to offer protection against HIV and other STIs. If the female exhibits an allergic reaction, the procedure can be reversed, with the latex condom applied first, followed by the sheepskin condom. Sheepskin condoms, made from lamb intestines, are not recommended for preventing HIV and other STIs because of their porousness. Polyurethane condoms could also be tried to avoid an allergic response. Regardless of the type of condom used—latex, sheepskins, or polyurethane, it must be applied before intercourse, and a new condom should be used before each act of intercourse. Condoms should be stored in a cool place to prevent deterioration, and Vaseline and other petroleum products that contribute to breakdown of the latex should be avoided. Proper application of the condom is essential for maximizing its effectiveness. The male condom should not be used concurrently with the female condom. If the condom breaks or semen spills into the vaginal area, a woman

FIGURE 9.3 Condoms.

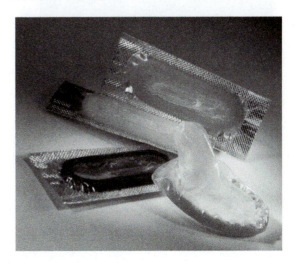

(N-9) have changed. The Centers for Disease Control and Prevention (CDC) recommends against the use of N-9 as an effective means for HIV or pregnancy prevention in

should consider EC as a safety measure. The sooner she starts, the better the outcome.[19]

Condom, Female

The **female condom** (Reality) is a one-size-fits-all barrier method. It is the first barrier contraceptive for women and offers protection against HIV and other STIs. Laboratory tests demonstrate that the HIV virus and other STI viruses cannot permeate the polyurethane material. The female condom consists of a prelubricated, soft, polyurethane pouch with two flexible rings, one inserted into the vagina to cover the cervix and the other ring partially covering the labia. It is approximately 6½ inches in length. (See Figure 9.4.) Polyurethane is strong, soft, and transfers heat, so it warms to body temperature soon after insertion. The advantage of the female condom is that it does not require fitting and its use is controlled by the woman. The major disadvantage seems to be its lack of aesthetic appeal. The female condom should be discarded in a wastebasket after one use, not flushed. The user failure rate is high, 12–22 percent, but approximately 5 percent when used correctly and consistently. The restrictive labeling suggests that this method is not as effective in protecting against HIV and other STIs as the male latex condom. If the partner ejaculates outside the condom, EC should be considered.[20]

Sponge

The sponge (Today) is made from polyurethane foam and contains spermicide. It is moistened with water and then inserted deep into the vagina, and has a nylon loop attached at the bottom for easy removal.

The sponge covers the cervix and blocks sperm from entering the uterus, and the spermicide immobilizes the sperm. Its user method effectiveness differs for women who have not given birth and for those who have given birth: 9 compared to 20 of 100 women will become pregnant during the first year of use. This method is easy to use once a woman learns, and the sponge can be worn for up to 30 hours without a need to be replaced and with repeated intercourse for up to 24 hours. It must be left in place for a minimum of 6 hours after last intercourse. The sponge cannot be used during any time of vaginal bleeding, including menstruation. It does not protect against STIs, so a condom should be considered.[21]

Diaphragm

The **diaphragm** is an oval, dome-shaped device with a flexible spring at the outer edge. (See Figure 9.5.) A spermicide is applied into the dome and a small amount is spread around the rim with the finger. Then the diaphragm is inserted with the back rim below and behind the cervix and held in place by the back of the pubic bone. (See Figure 9.6.) When the diaphragm is fitted properly, it is not felt by either partner. The diaphragm should be left in place for 6 hours after intercourse, and then removed. The diaphragm lowers the probability of contracting several STIs, including chlamydia and the human papilloma virus (HPV). It appears to lower the risk of cervical cancer, tubal infertility, and PID but increases the risk for urinary tract, bladder, and yeast infections.[22] The user failure rate ranges from 6 percent to 12 percent. The diaphragm must be initially fitted by a health care provider, and refitting may be necessary after weight change, childbirth, or pelvic surgery. The diaphragm comes in many sizes and designs.[23]

Cervical Cap

The **cervical cap** (FemCap) is designed to fit tightly over the cervix and should be filled with spermicide before intercourse. (See Figure 9.7.) Like the diaphragm, it must be fitted by a health care provider; unlike the diaphragm, there are only three sizes: small,

FIGURE 9.4 The female condom.

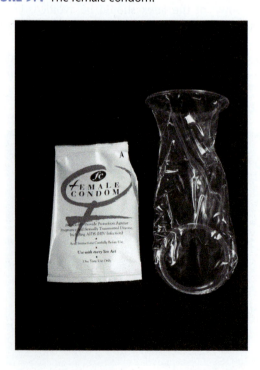

FIGURE 9.5 Diaphragm and contraceptive jelly.

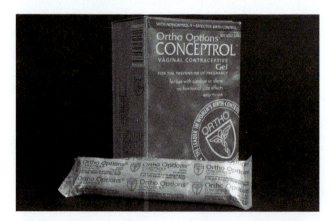

FIGURE 9.6 (*A*) Spermicidal cream or jelly is placed into the diaphragm. (*B*) The diaphragm is folded lengthwise and inserted into the vagina. (*C*) The diaphragm is then placed against the cervix so that the cup portion with the spermicide is facing the cervix. The outline of the cervix should be felt through the central part of the diaphragm.

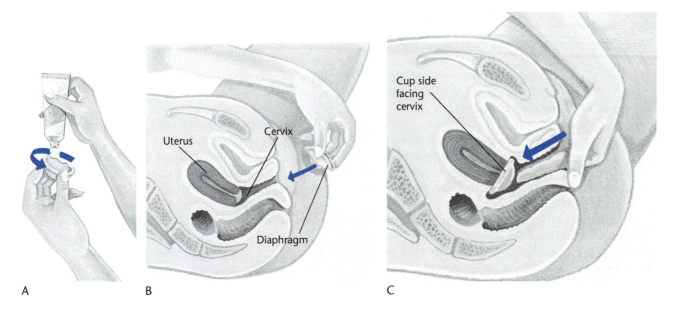

A   B   C

FIGURE 9.7 After the spermicidal cream or jelly is placed in the cervical cap, the cap is inserted into the vagina and placed against the cervix.

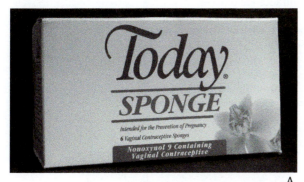

A

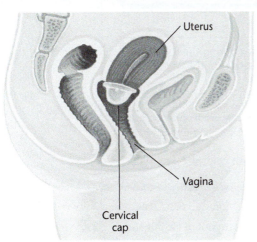

B

for nulliparous women; medium, for those who have not had an abortion or cesarean section; and large, for women who have given birth vaginally. The cervical cap can remain in place for 48 hours without spermicidal reapplication. User failure rates range from 14–29 percent, with higher rates in women who have given birth vaginally.[24] The advantages of the cervical cap include its smaller size and lower cost when compared to the diaphragm, and it can be left in place up to 48 hours with no need for additional spermicide. It also provides some protection against STIs. The disadvantage for many young women is that the smaller size makes it more difficult to ensure that the cervical cap is covering the cervix properly.

Hormonal Contraceptives

Every woman who chooses to use hormonal contraceptives should know the risks and benefits of use. Hormonal methods are convenient, effective, and reversible, but they provide *no* protection against HIV and other STIs and may cause health risks and side effects in some women. They are intended solely to prevent pregnancy. The primary methods available include oral contraceptives, transdermal patches, rings, injectables, hormonal intrauterine devices, emergency contraception, and implants. Hormonal methods act by preventing ovulation, thickening the cervical mucus making it difficult for sperm to reach an egg or thinning of the endometrium making it less likely for a fertilized egg to impact. A variety of hormonal methods are available to women.

The birth control products produce varying side effects in women including moodiness, weight gain, spotting, breast tenderness or swelling. Health care providers may prescribe a different hormonal product to alleviate potential side effects.

Oral Contraceptives **Oral contraceptives** (OCs) trail voluntary sterilization and IUDs in worldwide use among married women. OCs are the most popular form of birth control in the United States with more than 30 percent of all women choosing this method (see Figure 9.8). Nearly 100 million women worldwide use the pill. Among sexually active unmarried women and teens, OCs are the most widely used method of family planning because of their convenience, effectiveness, and reversibility. (See *Women Making a Difference:* "Margaret Sanger: Birth Control Activist.")

The idea of oral contraceptives dates back to the 1920s, but the pill was not approved by the U.S. Food and Drug Administration (FDA) until 1960. The first OC, Enovid-10, contained 150 micrograms of ethinyl estradiol and 10,000 micrograms progestin of noresthisterone (synthetic estrogen) compared to today's OCs of less than 50 micrograms of ethinyl estradiol and less than 150 micrograms of progestin.[26] Oral contraceptives act primarily by inhibiting ovulation through suppressing follicle stimulating harmone (FSH) and luteinizing harmone (LH). There are basically two types: the combination pills, which contain estrogen and progestin, and the progestin-only type (mini-pills). Most oral contraceptives come in 21- or 28-day packages

With the 21-day pack of combination pills, a woman takes one pill each day at the same time for 21 days. Withdrawal bleeding occurs during the 7 days that she is not taking the pill, and she begins taking the pills again after 7 days. Some women have a difficult time remembering to start taking the pills again after the seventh day, so a 28-day-cycle progestin-only pills are available where one pill is taken at the same time every day. The last seven pills do not contain hormones, and the woman will have withdrawal bleeding during that time. Some women prefer not to experience withdrawal

FIGURE 9.8 Chances of Pregnancy Based on Method of Birth Control

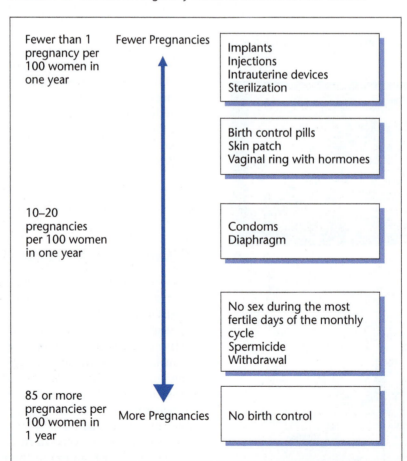

SOURCE: U.S. Food and Drug Administration, Department of Health and Human Services, 2008.

Women Making a Difference

Margaret Sanger: Birth Control Activist

Margaret Sanger (1879–1966) was acclaimed worldwide for her founding of the American birth control movement and the Planned Parenthood Federation of America, as well as for her international efforts to encourage family planning. She was responsible for opening the nation's first birth control clinic in the Brownsville section of Brooklyn, in 1916. Sanger established these important principles: that a woman's right to control her body is the foundation of her human rights, that every woman should be able to decide when and whether to have a child, and that volunteers could organize a network of family planning centers. Today, her grandson serves as the chair of the international Planned Parenthood council and carries on the cause of ensuring that all women have the right to decide whether, when, and how many children to have. For more information on Margaret Sanger, check out this Web site: www.nyu.edu/projects/sanger.

- What are some of the ways Sanger's detractors have attempted to discredit her?
- What obstacles did she face?
- How does Margaret Sanger's story parallel some stories of women today?

bleeding and use continuous hormonal contraception (or the NuvaRing) to control their menstrual cycles. This continuous birth control pill method has been used to relieve PMS, menstrual headaches, and anemia. Female athletes and those planning weddings or honeymoons have used monophasic pills for years. Some researchers believe that reduced ovulation and menstruation may reduce the likelihood of some cancers, particularly ovarian cancer. Women who use monophasic pills or continuous use of the Nuva Ring should continue to consult with their health care provider.[27] The pill is 94–97 percent effective in preventing pregnancy when used properly. However, a backup method should be used in the following circumstances:

- When a woman begins the first pill on any day other than the first day of her period (e.g. Sunday after the first day), she should use a backup method for the first 7 days that she takes the pill.
- When a woman is vomiting or has diarrhea, her body may not absorb the pill, and she should use a backup method for the rest of the cycle.
- When a woman forgets to take two or more pills during the cycle, she should contact her health care provider and ask for advice.
- When in doubt, use a backup.

When asked about the health benefits of OCs, most women cannot provide even one possible health benefit, yet research suggests that OCs provide several benefits. The health benefits of combination pills include protection against ovarian cysts, lowered risk for ectopic pregnancies and PID, lighter and less painful menstrual flow, decreased acne, premenstrual symptoms, and iron deficiency anemia.[28] Estrogen use has not been associated with increased breast cancer risk to date.

OCs may cause health risks and side effects for some women, however. Estrogen use is associated with a number of side effects including nausea, breast pain and soreness, and fluid retention. Progestin-only pills are associated with increased irregular menstrual cycles and vaginal bleeding, and must be taken exactly every 24 hours. If a woman becomes pregnant while on progestin-only pills, she has an increased risk of an ectopic pregnancy. Women should be advised against using hormonal methods if they are at risk for cardiovascular disease (particularly smokers over age 35) or if they have diabetes mellitus or hypertension. Rare, but serious, problems associated with the combination pill may include blood clots, strokes, changes in bone mineral density, and some reproductive cancers. Side effects from hormonal methods also may include headache, mood changes, dizziness, nervousness, depression, vaginal infections, and allergic skin reactions. Certain drugs may interact with hormonal methods to make them less effective. Some drugs used for epilepsy, herbal supplements such as St. John's wort, and certain antibiotics are a few examples of medications that may interfere with the effectiveness of hormonal contraceptives; however, progestin-only oral contraceptives may be used by women who smoke because they do not contain estrogen, and they may be better for women with diabetes or for those who are breast feeding.[29] The message is clear: Be aware and be informed! Make a wise consumer choice.

Transdermal (Skin) Patch The FDA approved Ortho Evra, the first **transdermal patch** for birth control, in 2001. Ortho Evra is a 1¾-inch square patch that releases norelgestromin (progestin) and ethinyl estradiol (estrogen) through the skin into the bloodstream.

The patch is applied to the lower abdomen, buttocks, upper outer arm, or upper body (not breasts) and is worn continuously for one week. The patch is worn a week at a time for 3 weeks and removed for the fourth week. A woman menstruates during the fourth week, as she would if she were using birth control pills. The patch prevents pregnancy by inhibiting ovulation and also causing the cervical mucus to thicken, making sperm less viable, and the endometrium to thin, reducing the changes of a fertilized egg attaching to it. If the patch becomes loose for more than 24 hours, an alternative, nonhormonal method should be used during the week. Clinical trials have demonstrated 99 percent effectiveness and risks similar to those of birth control pills. Women who use the patch need to know that there is an increased risk of blood clots, heart attack, high blood pressure, stroke, liver tumors, and gallbladder disease, and the label on the package includes a warning that cigarette smoking increases the risk of serious cardiovascular side effects. Five percent of the women in clinical trials had at least one patch that did not stay attached to the skin, and 2 percent withdrew from the trials due to skin irritations. The product was found to be less effective in women weighing more than 198 pounds. A higher risk of venous thromboembolisms (VTE) than with other combination birth control pills is associated with use of this product.[30]

The Vaginal Ring NuvaRing is a clear, flexible, thin polymer **ring** that provides a continuous low dose of etonogestrel (progestin) and ethinyl estradiol (estrogen) that inhibits ovulation and causes the cervical mucus to thicken, thus preventing pregnancy. The ring is inserted into the vagina, similarly to a diaphragm, and remains in place surrounding the cervix for 3 weeks. The ring is removed at the beginning of the fourth week, and a woman menstruates 2–3 days after its removal, similar to the cycle for birth control pills. The used ring should be wrapped and disposed of in the a wastebasket, not flushed. A new ring is inserted on the same day of the week as the previous one was removed. NuvaRing is available by prescription and is 98–99 percent effective when used correctly, but the user failure rate can be as high as 8 percent. Side effects and contraindications similar to those of birth control pills should be expected. If the ring slips (through improper placement or some exerting force), and it has been out of the vagina for less than 3 hours, the woman is still protected from pregnancy.[31, 32] However, using a condom as a backup for 7 days may be a wise decision.

Hormonal Injections **Depo-Provera** (DMPA) is the most widely used progestin injection. It is injected into the gluteal or deltoid muscle of a woman once every 3 months. Depo-Provera contains depot medroxyprogesterone acetate, which prevents the egg from ripening,

thus suppressing ovulation so that the egg cannot be fertilized by the sperm. It also thickens cervical mucus to keep sperm from fertilizing a viable egg. Depo-Provera lasts approximately 12 weeks and has high effectiveness (99.7 percent) and reversibility. Nearly 80 percent of women who stop using Depo-Provera because they want to get pregnant are expected to become pregnant within a year and 90 percent are expected to become pregnant within 2 years. The most common side effect is vaginal bleeding, and other side effects may include amenorrhea, weight gain, headache, nervousness, dizziness, stomach cramps, and decreased sex drive.[33] DMPA is not recommended for use of greater than 2 consecutive years, unless a woman cannot use another method, because of evidence of loss of bone mineral density. A new warning has been placed on this product that indicates that women who use Depo-Provera may lose significant bone mineral density. Bone loss is greater with longer use and may not be reversible.[34]

Emergency Contraception Postcoital contraception has been available since the early 1970s when a Canadian obstetrician/gynecologist, Dr. Albert Yuzpe, began prescribing an adaptation of the birth control pill for avoiding unintended pregnancies. Many physicians, particularly on college campuses, were prescribing the morning-after-pill (emergency contraception—EC) well before the 1998 FDA approval was given for use in the United States. Physicians used any number of different birth control pill combinations as EC. The number of pills in each dose depended on the brand of the pill. Today, Plan B One-Step, elle and Next Choice are the most common products for emergency contraception.

EC contains hormones that reduce the risk of pregnancy when taken within 72 hours of unprotected intercourse. EC can be taken in one or two doses, 12 hours apart, and is given to delay or inhibit ovulation, alter the tubal transport of sperm or ova to inhibit fertilization, and/or alter the endometrium to inhibit implantation.[35] The sooner the regimen is begun, the better the outcome. If taken within 72 hours of unprotected intercourse, birth control pills have been found to reduce the risk of pregnancy by 75 percent and Plan B One-Step and Next Choice by 89 percent. If taken within 24 hours of unprotected intercourse, Plan B One-Step and Next Choice have a 95 percent effectiveness rate. Emergency contraception is available without a prescription to women over age 17. Women younger than age 17 must have a prescription by a health care provider to purchase EC. This prescription requirement makes it difficult for some of the most vulnerable young women at risk of unwanted pregnancies to obtain EC.

Emergency IUD (intrauterine device) insertion is also a choice within 5 days of unprotected intercourse and reduces the risk of pregnancy by 99.9 percent. It must be inserted and removed by a health care provider. The

Copper T 380A IUD (ParaGard) can be left in place for up to 10 years or can be removed with the next menstrual cycle. The risks and benefits of IUDs are the same as when used for regular birth control. The cost of this method is greater than for other ECs, around $400 for the exam, IUD, and insertion, an average of about $40 a year over the 10-year period. EC does not induce a medical abortion or affect the developing pre-embryo or embryo. Rather, EC prevents pregnancy in cases of unanticipated sexual activity, contraceptive failure, or sexual assault. Side effects of the medication include nausea and vomiting and possible breast tenderness, irregular bleeding, abdominal pain, headaches, and dizziness. Progestin-only EC tends to have fewer side effects. The cost of the medication is minimal, and it has the potential to reduce the overall rate of abortion. EC is not intended to replace regular birth control, and does not prevent pregnancy during the remaining part of the cycle.

Unfortunately, distorted information provided by some religious groups has resulted in some health care providers' refusing to write prescriptions and some pharmacists refusing to fill prescriptions for women who request the pills. These health care providers and pharmacists believe the procedure is a form of medical abortion. However, the general medical definition of pregnancy endorsed by the American College of Obstetricians and Gynecologists in 1998 and by the U.S. Department of Health and Human Services in 1978 is that pregnancy begins when a pre-embryo completes implantation into the lining of the uterus. EC provides women with a viable alternative to unintended pregnancies. The best family planning methods involve pre-pregnancy planning and protected intercourse. When postcoital contraception is needed, it is now available. In the United States, a woman can call 1-800-230-PLAN to find a Planned Parenthood agency or 1-888-NOT-2-LATE for other sources of emergency contraception.

Implants In July 2006, the FDA approved another long-term birth control method, Implanon. Implanon is inserted subdermally on the inner side of the arm. Unlike an older implant called Norplant, which contained six matchstick-size rods, Implanon is a single-rod implantable contraceptive (etonogestrel, a progestin) that is 99 percent effective for up to 3 years. The risks associated with the implant are similar to those of other progestin-only contraceptives, including ectopic pregnancies, irregular bleeding, or ovarian cysts. It is not known if Implanon is as effective in overweight women since the number in the clinical trials were too low. Minimal local implant-site complications were noted in the clinical trials. As with all hormonal contraceptives, cigarette smoking increases the risk for serious cardiovascular and thromboembolic diseases. Implanon is currently available in 30 countries.[36]

Contraindications for Hormonal Methods A woman considering a hormonal method should be asked by her health care provider whether she is pregnant or if she has active liver disease, heart problems, breast cancer, diabetes, hypertension, migraine headaches, epilepsy, or a history of blood clotting. Research regarding the effect of hormonal methods on these conditions remains mixed, and a woman may choose another method if she has any of these conditions. A woman should be asked about her sexual history, including whether she or her partner has other sexual partners. Although hormonal methods are highly effective in preventing pregnancy, they provide no protection against HIV and other STIs.

Other Birth Control Methods

Other birth control methods include intrauterine devices and sterilization. Intrauterine devices have regained favor in the United States and remain one of the most common forms of birth control worldwide. Sterilization is the second leading form of birth control in the United States, with 27 percent of all women and 10 percent of all men choosing this method. Intrauterine devices are the fifth leading method of birth control with 6 percent of all women choosing this method.[37]

Intrauterine Devices (IUDs) and Contraception (IUCs) The World Health Organization (WHO) and the American Medical Association call **intrauterine devices** (IUDs) one of the safest, most effective, and least expensive reversible methods of birth control available to women.

The IUD works by preventing fertilization. The method works by reducing the number and viability of the sperm reaching the egg or impeding the number and movement of eggs in the uterus. Research does not support previous beliefs that IUDs work by preventing implantation of the fertilized egg into the uterus. This lack of evidence is important because it counters the pro-life view that IUD use is a form of abortion. Current IUDs such as Paragard and Mirena are more effective than oral contraceptives and similar in effectiveness to implants and injectables in preventing pregnancies.[38] (See Figure 9.9.)

Some women, particularly those exposed to STIs, may experience a higher incidence of pelvic inflammatory disease in the first month after IUD insertion. The risk of infection from IUD insertion depends more on the service provided than on the IUD itself. Health care providers should be trained to use sterile practices for inserting IUDs. Overall, IUDs are no longer associated with an increased risk of ectopic pregnancies or infertility resulting from PID. The T Cu-380A (ParaGard®) is FDA-approved for effective use for up to 12 years. ParaGard® was developed by the Population

FIGURE 9.9 Mirena IUD.

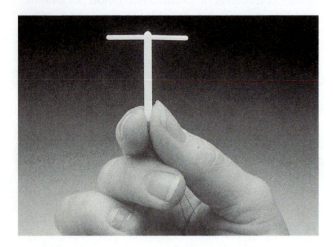

Council and introduced into the U.S. market in 1988. Method effectiveness is a 1 in 100 chance of pregnancy in the first year of use and 2.1 in 100 in 10 years of use. Mirena®, a hormonal IUC remains effective for 5 years and works by releasing small amounts of the hormone progestin into the uterus. Mirena® is made of a soft, flexible, ultralight plastic and results in a 90 percent reduction in menstrual bleeding. Nearly 20 percent of women using Mirena® experience no menstrual bleeding.[39]

If you should become pregnant, IUDs increase your risk of ectopic pregnancies, miscarriages, or premature births. Serious side effects are rare; however, contact your health care provider immediately if you

- find the length of the string tends to be shorter or longer than they were at first, or cannot feel the string ends when you reach for them with your fingers.
- feel the hard plastic bottom of the "T" part of the IUD against the cervix, when you check.
- think you might be pregnant.
- have periods that are much heavier than normal or last much longer than normal.
- have severe abdominal cramping, pain, or tenderness in the abdomen.
- have pain or bleeding during sex.
- have unexplained fever and/or chills.
- have flu-like symptoms, such as muscle aches or tiredness.
- have unusual vaginal discharge or unexplained vaginal bleeding.
- have a missed, late, or unusually light period.[40]

Sterilization Sterilization methods, *tubal ligation* and *vasectomy,* are the most common form of contraceptive method used by women over age 30 and by men. (See Figure 9.10.) In 2006–2008, 39.9 percent of African American, 33.5 percent of Hispanic, and 23.0 percent of white women chose sterilization for contraception. Tubal ligation remains more common than vasectomy (27 percent vs. 10 percent in 2006–2008).[41] These methods have low failure rates and low reversibility, so they should be considered only when voluntarily choosing to have no more children. Women with multiple partners or who have a partner with multiple partners still need to consider using a condom for protection against STIs and HIV/AIDS.

Tubal ligation can be performed on an outpatient basis or it can require hospitalization, depending on the type of procedure. It is the second most prevalent form of birth control used in the United States. The surgery involves closing the fallopian tubes—either by inserting microinserts or by cauterizing, tying, cutting, or clamping—thus preventing the egg from becoming

FIGURE 9.10 (*A*) Vasectomy. (*B*) Tubal ligation.

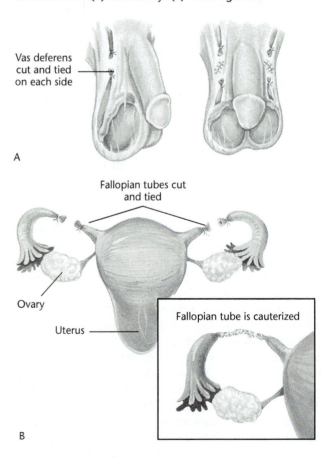

Vas deferens cut and tied on each side

A

Fallopian tubes cut and tied

Ovary

Uterus

Fallopian tube is cauterized

B

fertilized. A no-incision method (Essure) can be performed by a clinician who inserts two small, soft metallic coils into the fallopian tubes through the uterus. The coils cause scar tissue to grow, thus blocking the fallopian tubes. Three months after insertion, a test is performed to ensure the tubes are permanently blocked. Essure cannot be performed until 6 weeks after childbirth, miscarriage, or abortion. Advantages are numerous, but risks should be noted. Women should check with their health care provider about her or his expertise with this method. Laparoscopy, sometimes referred to as "Band-Aid" surgery, is completed through a small incision near the navel and is one of the most common methods of sterilization. Before the incision, the abdomen is inflated with a harmless gas to allow the organs to be seen more clearly.[42] A laparoscope is inserted into a small incision allowing the health care provider to locate the fallopian tube. Then, another incision is made through which the fallopian tubes are closed or an instrument is inserted through the laparoscope. This outpatient surgery takes 20–30 minutes to perform. Tubal ligation is most often performed immediately after childbirth. Mini-laparotomy does not require gas or a visualizing instrument. One incision is made into the abdomen through which both fallopian tubes are tied. Tubal ligation is a permanent procedure for a woman who is certain she does not want to have more children. Sterilization, as well as pregnancy or use of oral contraceptives, reduces the risk of ovarian cancer.[43] Women experiencing unusual symptoms (bleeding from the vagina, fever, or discharge, bleeding or redness at the surgical site) after tubal ligation should contact their health care provider immediately. The cost of sterilization ranges from $1,500 to $6,000.

Vasectomy is the fourth most popular form of contraception available. The traditional vasectomy is an office procedure, including one or two incisions by the surgeon to access each vas deferens. Each vas is then cauterized, tied, or sutured to prevent sperm from being ejaculated. An alternative is the no-scalpel, no-incision vasectomy (NSV) procedure in which the surgeon anesthetizes the vas deferens, makes a small puncture to access each vas, and then cauterizes, lasers, sutures, or hemoclips them. NSV, when compared to conventional vasectomy, reduces the psychological barrier for many men, the surgical time from 20 minutes to 10 minutes, and the risk for infection, bleeding, and pain.[44]

After vasectomy, couples should use another form of contraceptive control until all sperm have been cleared from the ampullar storage area, which can take several weeks. A semen sample should be examined by a health care provider to determine that the sperm count has reached zero. The advantages of vasectomy, whether conventional or NSV, include its greater safety and cost effectiveness compared to tubal ligation, its low failure rate, and better rates of reversibility than tubal ligation has. The cost of a vasectomy is nearly six times less than the cost of tubal ligation ($350–$1000). A common myth about vasectomy is that after the procedure males will lose their masculinity. Research shows no relationship between vasectomy and loss of masculinity or between vasectomy and prostate cancer, testicular cancer, or atherosclerosis, although studies are still being conducted.

Birth control and STI prevention are not just a woman's issue. Decisions regarding family planning and STI protection are a joint effort with both partners sharing responsibility. If a woman feels she is solely responsible for contraceptive choices, she may want to re-evaluate the relationship. We strongly encourage a woman to protect her body from unwanted diseases and unintended pregnancies. We encourage her to discuss birth control considerations with her partner. Her partner should be willing to take an active and supportive role in family planning. Remember, family planning is a joint venture.

Figure 9.11 shows that in 2006–2008, the most popular methods of contraception in the United States were the pill (28 percent), female sterilization (27 percent), the male condom (16 percent), and male sterilization (10 percent). Together, these four methods accounted for over 80 percent of contraceptive users.

- The condom is the leading method of contraception for first intercourse. Among women under 35 years of age, the pill is the leading method. After age 35, female sterilization is the leading method.
- Among college-educated contraceptive users, the pill is the leading method. Among those with a high school education or less, female sterilization is the leading method.[45]

MATERNAL AND INFANT MORTALITY

Family planning has health, social, and political implications for women and children. Women are impacted unfairly by governments that underfund birth control methods and family planning clinics; governments that determine and prescribe acceptable birth control methods; religious bodies that dictate reproductive choices; unavailable or limited health care options;

FIGURE 9.11 Percentage of current contraceptive users currently using each method: United States, 2006–2008

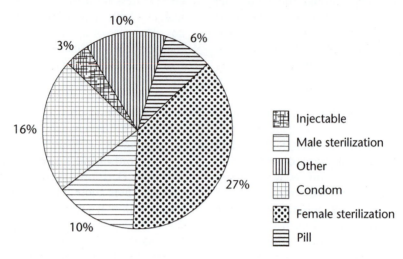

10%
6%
3%
16%
27%
10%

Injectable

Male sterilization

Other

Condom

Female sterilization

Pill

SOURCE: CDC/NCHS, *National Survey of Family Growth*, 2006–08.

and political agendas and laws that reduce women's options to choose.

In many developing countries, the leading causes of death for women are complications associated with pregnancy, childbirth, and abortion. Every minute of every day, somewhere in the world, a woman dies as a result of complications arising during pregnancy or childbirth. The majority of these deaths are avoidable. **Maternal mortality** is the best indicator of the status of women, particularly their health status. Maternal mortality is defined as the death of a woman while pregnant, regardless of the site or duration of the pregnancy, from any cause related to or aggravated by the pregnancy or its management and not from accidental or incidental causes. In 2005, the WHO estimated 358,000 maternal deaths worldwide, with 99 percent occurring in developing countries. Eleven countries account for 67 percent of these deaths including Afghanistan, Bangladesh, Democratic Republic of Congo, Ethiopia, India, Indonesia, Kenya, Nigeria, Pakistan, Sudan, and United Republic of Tanzania. While the statistics are staggering, they represent an estimated 34 percent decrease between 1990 and 2010. Estimates of maternal lifetime risk is 1 in 11 for Afghanistan, 1 in 31 in sub-Saharan countries, 1 in 2100 for the United States, 1 in 11,400 in Sweden and Switzerland, and 1 in 17,800 in Ireland. The U.S. maternal mortality ratio has double from 1990 to 2010, from 12 per 100,000 to 24 in 100,000. Potential reasons for declines in many countries included improvement in health systems and increased female education.[46]

The United Nations Declaration was signed in September 2000 by 189 heads of state. Two Millennium Development Goals were set as targets related to maternal health: (1) reduce the maternal mortality ratio by three quarters between 1990 and 2015 and (2) achieve universal access to reproductive health by 2015. If the 75 percent reduction target is to be met, developing countries will need to reduce their current maternal mortality ratio by 5.5 percent annually (current is 2.3 percent a year) until 2015.

Maternal deaths are classified as direct or indirect obstetric deaths. Direct obstetric deaths account for 80 percent of all maternal deaths and result from complications such as incorrect or inadequate treatment during pregnancy, labor, or postpartum. The most common complication is hemorrhage, usually during the postpartum phase. Infection, hypertensive disorders, prolonged or obstructive labor, and complications of unsafe abortions account for the remaining direct causes. Indirect obstetric deaths account for 20 percent of all maternal deaths and result from previous existing diseases (including HIV and AIDS) or diseases caused by the physiological complications of pregnancy.[47] Anemia is a significant indirect cause of death (and may be an underlying cause of hemorrhage and infection). Other causes include malaria, hepatitis, heart disease, and HIV/AIDS. In the United States, the maternal mortality rate is higher among African American women than among white women.

The WHO has determined that three interventions are essential to promote safe motherhood:

- Reducing the number of high-risk and unwanted pregnancies
- Reducing the number of obstetric complications
- Reducing deaths among women who develop complications[48]

The best mechanism for preventing maternal deaths is continuing to improve the status of women, including access to education, health care, and proper nutrition. The WHO acknowledges that maternal death is not only a health issue but also a matter of social justice. The long-term goal of bettering the status of women can be supplemented by the short-term goals of providing universal access to family planning and skilled health care.

Infant mortality, like maternal mortality, is an important indicator of a country's health status. Infant mortality is defined as the deaths of infants under 1 year old; neonatal mortality is deaths of infants under 28 days; and postneonatal mortality is deaths of infants aged 28 days to 11 months. Worldwide, nearly 8 million children under age 5 die annually with two-thirds of these deaths preventable. Three-fourths of the infant mortality rate is concentrated in two regions: 46 percent in the African region and 28 percent in Southeast Asia. The UN set a Millenium Development Goal to reduce childhood mortality by two-thirds by 2015. The goal is far from being reached by 2015 but the rate has dropped by one-third since 1990. In 2010, the infant mortality rate ranged from a high of 119 per 1000 infants in Africa to a low of 2 per 1000 in several developed countries. Worldwide, an infant's risk is highest in the neonatal period with birth asphyxias and infections accounting for 40 percent of mortalities. From the end of the neonatal period to age 5, the three leading causes of death are pneumonia, diarrhea, and malaria. The underlying contributing factor to over one-third of these deaths is malnutrition.[48] In the United States, the infant mortality rate remained 6.9 per 1000 infants, and, with the exception of 2002 and 2005, infant mortality has remained constant or decreased significantly. The health disparity among racial groups in 2008 remained significant with an infant mortality rate of 5.54 for white, 12.68 for black and 6.59 for all others.[49] Most infant deaths were concentrated primarily in the neonatal period and a key factor for the increase in neonatal deaths has been their increased low birth weight (LBW). This increase in LBW may be attributable to a number of factors, including an increase in multiple births, obstetric interventions, infertility therapies, and delayed childbearing. In addition, the percentage of black non-Hispanic infants born LBW (14 percent) was higher than for any other ethnic/race group. Congenital anomalies, LBW, and sudden infant death syndrome (SIDS) account for approximately 43 percent of all infant deaths in the United States.[50]

PROMOTING HEALTHY PREGNANCY OUTCOMES

Pre-Pregnancy Planning

When a woman decides to become pregnant, pre-pregnancy planning is the first step to promote the healthiest outcome. Pre-pregnancy planning encompasses not taking any drugs without the consent of a health care provider, nutritional planning, exercise, a time lapse of one menstrual cycle between contraceptive use and conception, immunizations, and folic acid supplements. These lifestyle changes should begin as soon as a childbearing woman is contemplating pregnancy—that is, before conception and before stopping birth control. If a woman smokes cigarettes, she should quit before getting pregnant because smoking during pregnancy increases the risks of LBW, a premature birth, or having a newborn with increased respiratory problems. If a woman drinks alcoholic beverages, she should stop drinking before getting pregnant because alcoholic beverages can cause infertility and birth defects, and no amount is safe for a pregnant woman and her baby. Any drugs, including over-the-counter drugs, should not be taken without the consent of a health care provider. Proper nutrition and exercise includes eating appropriately from MyPlate, avoiding megadoses of vitamins and minerals, and working out in moderation.[51] Folic acid is a nutritional supplement that provides protection against neural tube defects (defects of the brain and/or spinal cord) to the fetus. The U.S. Public Health Service recommends 4 milligrams (or 400 micrograms) of folic acid (the amount found in vitamin supplements) beginning 1 month before conception and through the first trimester. If a childbearing woman and her partner are contemplating pregnancy, it is important to discuss pre-pregnancy planning with a health care provider.[52]

Conception

Pregnancy begins with the union of the female egg, or ovum, and the male spermatozoan. These two gametes become fused into one cell, or **zygote,** that contains the characteristics of both the female and the male. The female ovum contains 23 chromosomes, and the sex chromosome of the mature ovum is always of the X type. The mature spermatozoan contains 23 chromosomes and may have an X type or Y type, thus determining the sex of the baby. The fertilized ovum again contains 46 chromosomes, 23 from the ovum and 23 from the spermatozoan. The fallopian tubes provide the environment in which fertilization occurs and cell division begins. After 3 days, the fertilized ovum is transported into the uterus. Premature expulsion from the fallopian tube could result in failure to implant, and prolonged retention in the tube could result in an ectopic pregnancy. The fertilized ovum spends another 4 days before implanting; thus, the process from fertilization to implantation is approximately 7 days. Once the chorionic villi cover the ovum, the villi begin producing hCG (the hormone tested for pregnancy). This hormone maintains the progesterone production by the corpus luteum, which supports endometrial growth. The villi decrease over time. Without hCG, the corpus

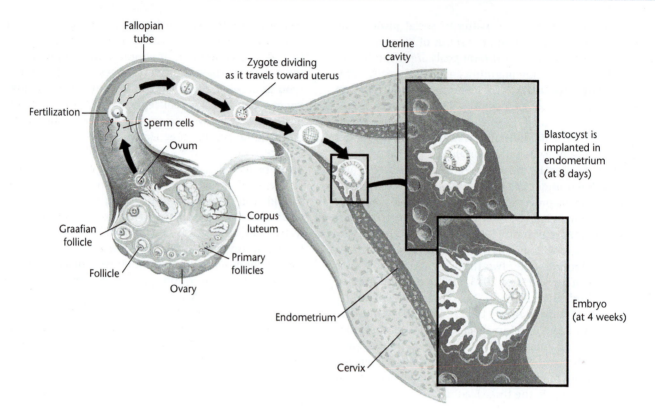

luteum would degenerate, as it does in menstruation, and the **embryo** would be aborted and the woman might not even know she had been pregnant.

Twins and Multiple Births   The inner cell mass, a small cluster of cells that projects into the cavity of a **blastocyst** (early embryonic cells before a cell layer has formed), may occasionally subdivide to form two separate groups of cells. Because the groups of cells have identical genes, they develop into identical twins. Fraternal twins develop when a woman ovulates two ova that are then fertilized by separate sperm. Because the sperm and ova have separate genetic codes, the fraternal twins are not identical and may be of the opposite sex. Fraternal twins are no more genetically similar than siblings from different births. Triplets and other multiple-birth babies may be either identical or fraternal, depending on whether they develop from a single ovum and sperm or multiple ova and sperm.

Amnion   The **amnion** (membranous sac) begins to develop even before the embryo evolves and eventually surrounds it. The amnion cavity, a fluid-filled space between the amnion and the embryo, then develops and provides the space in which the fetus moves. It keeps the fetus at an even temperature, cushions the fetus, and provides nourishment. By the end of the 4th month it can be sampled (amniocentesis) for prenatal diagnosis of genetic abnormalities.

Placenta   The **placenta** forms by the third month. It supplies food to the fetus and connects to the fetus through the umbilical cord. The placenta transfers gases and nutrients, excretes wastes, transports heat, and produces various proteins and hormones (including progesterone and estrogen). The placenta brings maternal and fetal blood close together, but the two circulatory systems are completely separate. The maternal blood provides nutrients and oxygen that the fetal blood transports throughout the body. The fetal blood passes the wastes to the maternal blood, and this waste is processed through the kidneys for disposal.

Early Signs of Pregnancy

A woman usually does not know she is pregnant until she misses a period because fertilization occurs approximately 2 weeks before menstruation. The major organs of the fetus develop before the eighth week of pregnancy. The importance of practicing positive health behaviors before conception and during the early pregnancy to prevent birth defects and LBW cannot be emphasized strongly enough. The early signs of pregnancy are one or more of the following: a missed period; a light period or spotting; tender, swollen breasts; fatigue; upset stomach or vomiting; feeling bloated; or frequent urination.[53]

Home Pregnancy Tests

A missed period is usually the first sign of pregnancy. When this happens, you may decide to buy a home pregnancy test to determine whether you are truly pregnant.

Most home pregnancy tests (HPTs) are urine tests that measure human chorionic gonadotropin (hCG). hCG is produced by the placenta when the embryo implants in the uterus. Some tests require urine to be combined with chemicals; others require placement of urine on a treated surface. Small traces of hCG can be detected as quickly as 6 days to as many as 15 days after conception. False negatives are much more common than false positives. False negatives often occur when the test is taken too early in the pregnancy, when hCG levels are undetectable. A positive test is usually accurate; however, some contaminants can create false positives.

A variety of HPTs such as e.p.t., First Response, Clearblue Easy, One Step Be Sure Pregnancy Test, and Fact Plus Pregnancy can be purchased without a prescription. Some home tests (First Response and e.p.t.) contain monoclonal antibodies that bond to hCG. Others (Clearblue Easy) give quick results by a testing method called rapid assay delivery system. These tests claim 99 percent accuracy in laboratory tests of the efficacy of the products. The cost for a HPT varies from $8 to $20 for a one-test kit. It is recommended that a woman re-test

the results so she will need at least two kits and must remember to check the expiration date. Test results can be obtained within several minutes depending on the product.

The following guidelines are suggested for proper use of a pregnancy test. First, the test kit instructions should be read thoroughly and the directions should be followed precisely. Second, the urine (preferably the first urine in the morning) sample should be collected in a clean, dry container. The test should be conducted in a well-lighted area with a cold water faucet and a watch or timer that measures time in seconds nearby. Last, the color of the test should be compared with the color chart on the package when the timing period has ended. These results should be recorded (time and date) so that you can discuss them with your health care provider.[53,54]

Fetal Development

The development of the fetus begins at conception. During the next 9 months, a sequence of changes occurs in the fetus and the mother. Table 9.2 shows the stages of

---

TABLE 9.2 Growth and Changes During Pregnancy

WOMAN	FETUS
0–14 Weeks (First Trimester)	**0–14 Weeks (First Trimester)**
• Your period stops or is light. • You may have nausea and vomiting. This usually goes away by the end of this time. • Your breasts become larger. They may be tender. • Your nipples may stick out more. • You may have to urinate more often.	• The heart begins to beat. • Bones have appeared—the head, arms, fingers, legs, and toes are formed. • The major organ and nervous systems are formed. • The placenta forms. • Hair is starting to grow. • 20 buds for future teeth have appeared. • By the end of this time, the fetus is 4 inches long and weighs just over 1 ounce.
14–28 Weeks (Second Trimester)	**14–28 Weeks (Second Trimester)**
• Your abdomen begins to swell—your uterus will be near your ribs by the end of this time. • The skin on your abdomen and breasts stretches. You may see stretch marks. • At about 16–20 weeks, you may start to feel the fetus move. • You may get a dark line from the navel down the middle of the abdomen or brown, uneven marks on the face. You may get a brown ring around your areolas.	• The fetus grows quickly from now until birth. • The organs are developing further. • Eyebrows and fingernails form. • The skin is wrinkled and covered with fine hair. • The fetus moves, kicks, sleeps and wakes, swallows, can hear, and can pass urine. • By the end of this time, the fetus is 11–14 inches long and weighs about 2–2½ pounds.
28–40 Weeks (Third Trimester)	**28–40 Weeks (Third Trimester)**
• The movements of the fetus are stronger. • You may have abdominal pains. These may be false or true labor pains. • You may feel short of breath as the uterus pushes against the diaphragm (a flat, strong muscle that aids in breathing). You will be able to breathe better when the baby drops. • When the baby drops, you may need to urinate more often. • Yellow, watery fluid (colostrum) may leak from the nipples. • Your navel may stick out. • Your cervix may begin to thin out and open slightly.	• The fetus kicks and stretches, but as it gets bigger it has less room to move. • Fine body hair disappears. • Bones harden, but bones of the head are soft and flexible for delivery. • The fetus usually settles into a good position for birth. • At 40 weeks, the fetus will be full term. It is about 20 inches long and weighs 6–9 pounds.

development during each trimester with descriptions of the changes for both.

Most health care providers say fetal development occurs after the 5th week of gestation, the time when human form begins. The sex can be distinguished by the 3rd month because external genitalia show signs of sex. At this time, movement begins but can't be felt. Hair (lanugo) appears by the end of the 5th month and **quickening,** or the perception of life, can be felt by the mother. The health care provider may also be able to hear the fetal heart beat for the first time. By the end of the 7th month, a premature infant may survive, but this is more likely after 8 months. The length of a normal pregnancy can vary from 240 to 300 days. Very few women actually give birth on their due date, but most give birth within 2 weeks of the due date. The American College of Obstetricians and Gynecologists recommends that scheduled births not be conducted before 39 weeks, unless medically necessary. Eighty percent of all births are full term. The March of Dimes has partnered with over 750 hospitals to further reduce medically unnecessary cesarean sections and inductions. Thirty-nine percent of these hospitals report an elective delivery rate of five percent or less.[55]

PRENATAL CARE AND DELIVERY

Prenatal care is extremely important to the health and well-being of mother and child. Young teenage women who unexpectedly get pregnant are at greatest risk for complications, especially if they lack prenatal care. They can usually receive services through local health department clinics or community health centers. These clinics offer low-prices or free services, depending on income. Pregnant women over age 35 were once labeled "high risk." Now 1 in 5 women has her first child after age 35. A review of several studies of pregnant women over age 35 found that most have healthy deliveries, however, their risks for complications such as gestational diabetes, high blood pressure, placental problems, premature birth, and stillbirth are greater than those under age 35.[56]

Primary Care Services

A primary care team may include an obstetrician/gynecologist, a certified nurse-midwife, and a childbirth educator. The initial visit may occur before conception and entails a discussion of maternal nutritional needs; exercise and weight management; current drug use including tobacco, alcohol, over-the-counter drugs, prescription drugs such as those for diabetes or hypertension control,

illegal drugs such as marijuana or crack cocaine, and other drugs; immunizations; and genetic counseling. The first prenatal visit includes a history of maternal, paternal, and family diseases and disorders; a physical examination to determine height, weight, and blood pressure; an examination of the reproductive organs including changes to the cervix and the size of the uterus; an estimation of the due date; blood, urine, and Pap tests; and a plan for future visits and tests. Routine tests during the first prenatal visit include screening for STIs and HIV, antibodies for immunity to rubella and chickenpox, blood type and Rh factor, and a urine test for presence of bacteria, glucose, or protein. A test for cystic fibrosis may be offered if both partners had not been prescreened prior to pregnancy.[57] Check Health Tip: Using Accurate and Reliable Information as one source for videos and podcasts related to pregnancy. Typically, visits occur monthly during the first 28 weeks, every 2 weeks during weeks 28–36, and weekly thereafter.

Each subsequent visit consists of a check of weight and blood pressure; fetal heartbeat, growth, and position; and a urine test for protein and sugar. In addition to routine tests, a health care provider may suggest special tests for birth defects or stress to the fetus. These tests include ultrasound, chorionic villus sampling (CVS), maternal serum screening, amniocentesis, a non-stress test, a contraction stress test, and a biophysical profile. Table 9.3 describes these tests, what they check for, who should have them, and when they should be given.

Weekly prenatal checkups are recommended after week 36. A woman will know that labor has begun when contractions

- are frequent, regular and evenly spaced apart (e.g., every 5–10 minutes),
- happen more than five times an hour,
- last for 30–70 seconds, and
- get worse as you move around.[58]

Health Tips

Using Accurate and Reliable Information

Check the Health Education Center at the March of Dimes for videos and podcasts on pre-pregnancy planning, pregnancy, newborn care, and postpartum changes. The Web site is www.marchofdimes.com/pnhec/39679 .asp. What other Web sites provide accurate and reliable information about childbirth and childcare?

TABLE 9.3 Special Pregnancy Tests

TEST	WHAT IT IS	WHAT IT LOOKS FOR	WHO SHOULD HAVE IT	WHEN
Ultrasound	Test that creates an image of the fetus from sound waves by either moving an instrument across the abdomen or placing a small device in the vagina.	Information about the fetus such as age; rate of growth; placement of the placenta; fetal position, movement, and heart rate; number of fetuses; some, but not all, fetal problems.	Women whose doctors want to tell how old the fetus is, confirm a condition, or check a suspected problem.	Depends on the reason for performing ultrasound.
Maternal serum screening	A blood test that tests for substances from the pregnancy that are also in the woman's blood.	Signs of birth defects such as open neural tube defects (NTDs) or Down syndrome.	Every woman should be offered maternal serum screening.	15–18 weeks
Chorionic villus sampling (CVS)	A sample of the chorionic villi is taken from the placenta, either through a needle passed through the abdomen and uterus or through a thin tube passed through the vagina and cervix.	Certain conditions, such as Down syndrome; other tests may be run depending on a woman's risk factors.	If available, test will be offered to women who already have a child with certain birth defects, who have a family history of birth defects, who will be 35 or older on their due date, or if they and their partner are at risk for certain genetic diseases.	10–12 weeks
Amniocentesis	A sample of amniotic fluid (the liquid around the fetus inside the uterus) is drawn through a thin needle that is inserted through the abdomen into the uterus. Ultrasound is used to guide the needle.	Certain conditions, such as Down syndrome and NTDs; other tests may be run on amniotic fluid depending on a woman's risk factors. May be used late in pregnancy to see if baby's lungs are likely to work if birth occurs soon.	Test may be offered to women who already have a child with certain birth defects, who have a family history of birth defects, who will be 35 or older on their due date, or if they and their partner are at risk for certain genetic diseases.	14–18 weeks
Nonstress test	Test that measures the fetal heart rate as the fetus moves. An instrument is attached to the woman's abdomen (an electronic fetal monitor). Fetal movements are felt by the woman or noted by the doctor or nurse.	Whether enough oxygen is getting to the fetus.	Women with diabetes or high blood pressure; who smoke or use drugs; who are carrying multiple fetures; or who have decreased fetal movements. Sometimes recommended in other circumstances.	As doctor recommends, usually in the last 10 weeks of pregnancy.
Contraction stress test	Test that measures how the fetal heart rate reacts to a uterine contraction. An electronic fetal monitor is used.	Whether the fetus is under stress.	Women with diabetes or high blood pressure; who smoke or use drugs; who are carrying multiple fetuses; or who have decreased fetal movements. Sometimes recommended in other circumstances.	As doctor recommends, usually in the last 10 weeks of pregnancy.
Biophysical profile	Combination of the nonstress test and ultrasound.	Checks the fetus's "breathing" movements, muscle action, movement, amount of amniotic fluid, and the result of the nonstress test.	Women with diabetes or high blood pressure; who smoke or use drugs; who are carrying multiple fetuses; or who have decreased fetal movements. Sometimes recommended in other circumstances.	Nonstress test results are not normal. Some doctors use this test instead of the nonstress test.

Labor and Delivery

Throughout the pregnancy, a woman will experience irregular contractions that increase in frequency and intensity as the pregnancy progresses. In the last trimester, contractions, known as **Braxton Hicks** (false labor), prepare the uterus for childbirth. Near the end of pregnancy, these contractions are difficult to distinguish from true labor. (See Table 9.4.) **Lightening** may occur 10–14 days before delivery, particularly in a woman's first delivery. Lightening, the descent of the head, relieves the upward pressure on the diaphragm and makes it easier to breathe. In subsequent pregnancies, it occurs at the onset of labor. A woman will know that it is time to go to the hospital, call the nurse-midwife, or prepare for home birth when contractions are 5 minutes or less apart, her "water breaks" (the amniotic sac ruptures), and the pain remains constant and more intense.[59]

True labor occurs in three stages. (See Figure 9.12.) Although the length and experience may vary among women, it also varies for a woman from the birth of her first child to ensuing births. The average length of time in labor for a first birth is approximately 12–14 hours and subsequent births average around 8 hours. *Stage 1* begins with regular, uterine contractions at 15- to 20-minute intervals, and throughout the first stage the contractions become longer and stronger. The signs of stage 1 include "show," a slight flow of bloody mucus; effacement (cervix flattens out and gets longer); and complete dilation (opening) of the cervix. *Stage 2* signs include a fully dilated cervix of approximately 10 centimeters and strong contractions (50–70 seconds) that facilitate the movement of the baby through the birth canal. This stage can last several hours. After dilation of the cervix, the presenting part of the baby and the exact position of the presenting part in relation to the pelvis can be determined by a health care provider. The position is described as the relationship of some arbitrary point to the right or left side of the mother's pelvis. Most often (97 percent), the presenting part of the baby is the head (cephalic presentation). In the cephalic position, the head becomes more visible and the vulva encircles the baby's head. This encirclement is known as "crowning." The next most common is breech presentation, which can be frank breech (thighs flexed and legs extended) or full breech (thighs and legs flexed) or foot breech (one or both feet at the lowest point). Shoulder presentation (transverse lie) is far less common. At this point in the delivery, the health care provider may perform an episiotomy, although this has become more controversial and less routine. Uterine contractions and intra-abdominal pressure (bearing-down efforts) are essential for the expulsion of the baby, which brings stage 2 to an end. Any mucus is cleared from the mouth and nose of the baby, and the umbilical cord is clamped. *Stage 3* occurs after the baby is born. It consists of two phases: placental separation and placental expulsion. Uterine contractions continue until the placenta is delivered. This stage usually lasts from 3 to 20 minutes. If an episiotomy was performed, the health care provider will suture the incision after the placenta has been delivered.[60]

Birthing Options

A wide variety of birthing options is available to women in the United States. Although the vast majority of births are still attended by a physician and delivered in a hospital, the number of births attended by certified nurse-midwives has been increasing in progressive locales and MDs have been replaced by DOs (doctors of osteopathy). More women are choosing natural birth options, and childbirth classes provide education on ways to become more actively involved in the decisions related to the childbirth process. These classes provide suggestions on available birthing options, breathing techniques, relaxation strategies, exercise, and methods to transition through labor. A misunderstanding of natural birth options is that medication and assistance by medical personnel are avoided, regardless of circumstances. Indeed, when labor is difficult or complications arise, additional support may be necessary. If a normal labor becomes high risk, the woman should remain flexible and may need to amend her choices.

Continuous Support Assistants The number of deliveries in hospitals has remained relatively constant over the past several decades, nearly 99 percent of all births. During this time, the number of birth or labor assistants has also remained relatively constant at about 8 percent of all births despite research to show the benefits to expectant mothers. Birth or labor assistants offer a wide variety of different supports for pregnancy, labor, and childcare to low-risk pregnant women. **Labor assistants** may be certified nurse *midwives*, certified midwives, lay midwives, *doulas,* or childbirth educators who assist the low-risk pregnant mother with prenatal care, childbirth and/or infant care. Mary Breckinridge

---

TABLE 9.4 True and False Labor Contractions: How Do You Know?

TRUE LABOR	FALSE LABOR
Regular intervals	Irregular intervals
Dilation of cervix	No dilation of cervix
Shortened intervals	Intervals remain longer
Increase in intensity	No increase in intensity
Back and abdominal discomfort	Minimal abdominal discomfort

FIGURE 9.12 The three stages of childbirth.

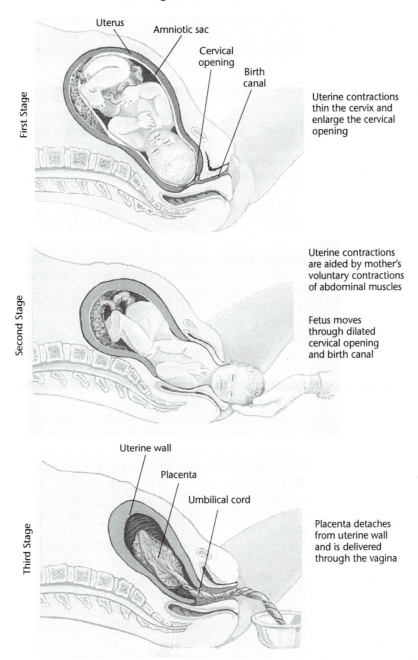

First Stage

Uterus   Amniotic sac
Cervical opening
Birth canal

Uterine contractions thin the cervix and enlarge the cervical opening

Second Stage

Uterine contractions are aided by mother's voluntary contractions of abdominal muscles

Fetus moves through dilated cervical opening and birth canal

Third Stage

Uterine wall
Placenta
Umbilical cord

Placenta detaches from uterine wall and is delivered through the vagina

established the first U.S. nurse-midwifery practice in 1925 in Hyden, Kentucky. Today, nurse midwifery practice is legal in all fifty states. A certified nurse-midwife (CNM) is a registered nurse with two additional years of training from a midwifery accredited program, such as the American College of Nurse-Midwives. Most CNMs list a hospital or physician practice as their place of employment and delivery occurs in the hospital. Most midwife-assisted births are conducted by CNMs (nearly 94 percent) and most midwife-assisted births occur in hospitals (nearly 96 percent).[61] Labor assistants offer special guidance and comfort during labor and childbirth. Doulas are certified by the Doulas of North America (DONA), Association of Labor Assistants and Childbirth Educators (ALACE), the International Childbirth Education Association (ICEA), or Birth Works.

The American College of Obstetricians, in an opinion on planned home births, stated that "although the absolute risk of planned home births is law, published medical evidence shows it does carry a two- to three-fold increase in the risk of newborn death compared with low risk births." ACOG does not support planned home births but does recommend that women who choose home births should be offered standard screenings and choose a certified birthing care provider who has access to consultation and emergency support.[61, 62]

Births to unmarried women

The number of babies born to unmarried women in 2007 was higher than ever before reported in the United States. The 2007 total (1.7 million) was 4 percent greater than in 2006 and 26 percent greater than 2002. The percentages were lowest for young teens and women 35–39 and highest for women in their 20s.[63] Since 1970, 50 percent of nonmarital births were to teenagers aged 19 and younger compared to 23 percent in 2007.

Unplanned Pregnancies

Unplanned pregnancies (3 million annually) are not just a teenage issue. The highest percentage of unmarried women ever reporting unplanned pregnancies in 2001, the year for most recent and reliable statistics, was in the age group 20–24 years (36 percent) followed by the under-20 age group (31 percent). Nearly 2 million of the unplanned pregnancies were unwanted. Over three-quarters occurred in teenaged women and those in their 20s; 69 percent of the unplanned pregnancies occurred in unmarried women compared to 31 percent in married women. Nearly 50 percent of single, non-cohabiting women and 44 percent of cohabiting women had abortions compared to 19 percent of married women. Unplanned pregnancies are particularly important to unmarried women who choose to have a baby because of their increased likelihood of poverty, father absence, school and health problems, and child neglect. The National Campaign has a goal of reducing all unplanned pregnancies.[64]

Cesarean Deliveries

The cesarean section delivery rate reached a record high of 32.9 percent in 2009 before stabilizing at 32.8 percent in 2010. The cesarean section rate had been increasing annually since the low of 21 percent in 1996. The rate has increased to 49.5 percent for women age 40 and older compared to about 25 percent in women age 20 and younger. Black women (35.4 percent) are 8 percent more likely than whites (32.8 percent) and 11 percent more likely than Hispanics (31.6 percent) to have a cesarean section delivery.

The continuing increase in the rate of cesarean deliveries prompted the National Institutes of Health to recommend that non–medically indicated cesareans should not be performed for pregnancies of less than 39 weeks of gestation and for women desiring several children. The rate of primary (first birth) cesarean deliveries rose sharply, as did the likelihood of the next birth being by cesarean (92 percent). The cesarean rates

ranged from under 23 percent for New Mexico and Utah to over 36 percent for Louisiana and New Jersey. While the rate of cesarean deliveries has increased, the percentage of infants delivered by forceps (less than 1 percent) or vacuum extraction (around 3.2 percent) remains relatively low.[65]

Multiple Births

In 2008, the unprecedented rise in multiple birth rates of the past decade seemed to stabilize. The twin birth rate was 32.6 per 1000 births, a 70 percent rise from 1980 to 2004 but stable from 2004 to 2008. The rate of triplet and higher multiple births reached an all-time high of 193.4 per 100,000 births in 1998 and then declined to 147.6 per 100,000 births in 2008. The increase in multiple births over the past decade has been attributed to the older age of women giving birth (women in their 30s are more likely to give birth to multiples) and the increase in fertility-enhanced therapies such as in vitro fertilization and ovulation-inducing drugs. Multiples do not compare favorably with singletons in preterm deliveries or LBWs. In singletons, 11 percent were preterm and 7 percent were LBW in 2008. In twins, nearly 60 percent were preterm and 57 percent were LBW. In triplets, nearly 93 percent were preterm and 95 percent were LBW. In quintuplets or higher, 90 percent were preterm and 96 percent were LBW. In 2008, the highest twin and triplet or higher birth rates occurred in New Jersey.[66] In January, 2009, a young, unmarried woman in California made history and the news when she gave birth to octuplets. (See *Viewpoint:* "Mother Gives Birth to Octuplets.")

BREAST FEEDING

Breast feeding and complementary feeding practices can save the lives of 1.5 million children under age 5 annually. The WHO recommends early initiation of breast feeding within 1 hour of birth, exclusive breast feeding for 6 months, and continued breast feeding with complementary foods at 6 months up for to 2 years. In 2010, WHO revised its recommendations for HIV-infected mothers. WHO supports HIV-positive women breast feeding their child for the first 6 months. If given antiretroviral medication, the risk of transmitting HIV to the infant is significantly reduced.[67]

The percentage of women in the United States who are breast feeding has been increasing, particularly among racial and ethnic minorities. Yet, while 75 percent of mothers start breast feeding, only 13 percent exclusively breast fed their infant for 6 months. And, the percentage is even lower for black mothers.[68] The advantages of breast milk over formula are well known and include its inexpensiveness, its better nutritional quality, its ability to act as a birth control measure to

Viewpoint

Mother Gives Birth to Octuplets

On January 27, 2009, 33-year-old Nadya Suleman, a young, unmarried woman gave birth to eight babies ranging in weight from 1 pound 8 ounces to 3 pounds 4 ounces. As the media began their investigative reporting, a number of controversies arose. The young mother already had six children between ages 2 and 7, three of whom had disabilities. She was unemployed and drawing disability insurance, although she indicated a desire to return to college. She was receiving food stamps and had filed for bankruptcy. Her mother was providing the home in which she and her children were living. The medical assistants apparently had not followed assistive reproductive therapy protocols. Estimates of the cost of delivery and keeping the neonates in intensive care range from $1 to $3 million. What's happening today in the lives of this young mother and her children? What emotional toll will raising fourteen children have on the children, on Nadya, and on her mother and relatives? How much intervention by governmental agencies do we want to see in reproductive technologies? What screening protocols should we expect fertility clinics to have in place? Should we focus on the extreme cases, or should we focus on all the positive outcomes? What are your thoughts regarding this scenario?

limit fertility, and its role in reducing ovarian and pre-menopausal breast cancer.[69]

Breast milk is unique and, because of its qualities, more women should be encouraged to breast feed their infants. Breast milk has been described as "dynamic," ever changing in content to meet the needs of a growing infant. It provides the perfect mix of nutrients, hormones, and proteins and cannot be duplicated. Lactose, the predominant sugar in milk, cannot be found in any other natural state. **Colostrum,** the initial milk produced by the mother, has numerous infection-fighting agents and is tailored to the needs of the infant. Colostrum is followed by transitional milk within a few days, then by mature milk. WHO and UNICEF recommend that every infant be breast fed exclusively for the first 6 months of life and then breast fed up to 2 years or longer.[70] Breast feeding plays a role in reducing obesity, helps prevent insulin-dependent diabetes and high cholesterol, and significantly decreases the risk of several acute and chronic diseases. It has been associated with better psychomotor and mental development and reduced risk of celiac disease (a malabsorption syndrome of the gastrointestinal tract), some childhood cancers, Crohn's

disease (a chronic inflammatory bowel disease affecting the digestive tract), urinary tract infections, and atopic disease (a genetic disorder related to allergies and asthma).[71]

Breast feeding has beneficial health results for the mother as well as the infant. Maternal benefits when Breast feeding begins immediately include reducing the risk of hemorrhage by helping the uterus contract; reducing the risk of breast and ovarian cancer, osteoporosis, and endometriosis; and assisting in family planning. The longer a woman Breast feeds her children, the lower is her risk of breast cancer. The Lactational Amenorrhea Method (LAM), a family planning method, uses three measures to determine a woman's fertility: the return of a menstrual period, the pattern of breast feeding, and the length of time since birth. The chance of getting pregnant is less than 2 percent if menstruation has not resumed, breast feeding is regular and on demand, and the infant is less than 6 months old.[72]

Breast feeding is awkward for some mothers and babies to learn. It is a specific learned skill and, given adequate assistance, both mother and infant will be successful unless unusual circumstances exist. Almost every mother can breast feed. The Baby-Friendly Hospital Initiative is a joint project of the WHO and UNICEF. Nearly 152 countries with 20,000 designated facilities participate in the program. *FYI:* "Ten Steps to Successful Breast Feeding" presents the criteria for successful breast feeding, which a facility must satisfy to qualify as a baby-friendly hospital.[73] In 2011, the U.S. Surgeon General released Call to Action as an effort to increase the number of mothers who exclusively breast fed their infants for 6 months. The report cited a study in *Pediatrics* that estimated if 90 percent of U.S. families exclusively breast fed for 6 months, the savings would be $13 billion in reduced medical costs. The Healthy People 2020 objective for breast feeding set goals of: 82 percent ever breast fed, 61 percent at 6 months, and 34 percent at 1 year.[74]

POTENTIAL PROBLEMS WITH PREGNANCY

Ectopic Pregnancy

Nearly 100,000 ectopic pregnancies occur every year, and they account for 9 percent of all pregnancy-related deaths in the United States. One in sixty pregnancies results in implantation of the embryo in a fallopian tube or other extrauterine site such as an ovary, abdominal cavity, or cervix. Ninety to 95 percent of ectopic pregnancies are tubal pregnancies, primarily in the ampulla (dilated segment).[75] The women at greatest risk include those with a prior history of ectopic pregnancy, a previous pelvic infection or surgery to the fallopian tubes, endometriosis,

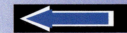

Ten Steps to Successful Breast Feeding

Every facility providing maternity services and care for newborn infants should

1. Have a written breast feeding policy that is routinely communicated to all health care staff.
2. Train all health care staff in skills necessary to implement this policy.
3. Inform all pregnant women about the benefits and management of breast feeding.
4. Help mothers initiate breast feeding within a half hour of birth.
5. Show mothers how to breast feed and how to maintain lactation even if they have to be separated from their infants, such as if they return to work.
6. Give newborn infants no food or drink other than breast milk, unless medically indicated.
7. Practice rooming-in: Allow mothers and infants to remain together 24 hours a day.
8. Encourage breast feeding on demand.
9. Give no artificial teats or pacifiers (also called dummies or soothers) to breast feeding infants.
10. Foster the establishment of breast feeding support groups and refer mothers to them on discharge from the hospital or clinic.

and uterine fibroids and those who used an intrauterine device before becoming pregnant. Some medical procedures, such as previous fallopian tube surgery for reversing sterilization or in vitro fertilization, tubal ligation failure, or infection (scarring) from surgery of the uterus or fallopian tubes may result in ectopic pregnancies.[76] Tubal pregnancies may be caused by any condition that narrows the fallopian tubes. An **ectopic pregnancy** presents a potential risk to a mother and can cause infertility and maternal mortality. The symptoms vary and may mimic those of various other pathologies such as appendicitis, salpingitis (inflammation of the fallopian tubes), or spontaneous abortion. The symptoms may include menstrual irregularities such as spotting or missed periods, pelvic pain on one side, elevated temperature, internal bleeding before tubal rupture, and external bleeding if rupture occurs. The degree of risk to a mother depends on the stage of diagnosis and the presenting symptoms. Health care providers who treat women of childbearing age should not assume that a history of tubal sterilization rules out the possibility of an ectopic pregnancy. Ectopic pregnancies can occur years later, particularly in women sterilized before age 30. Hospitalizations for ectopic pregnancies

have remained relatively stable over the past 10 years. Nearly one-half of all ectopic pregnancies are treated on an outpatient basis.[77]

Hypertensive Disorders

Preeclampsia and **eclampsia** describe pregnancy-induced or aggravated hypertension, usually associated with edema (swelling) and/or proteinuria (excess protein in the urine). They are the same processes, but eclampsia describes the condition when it has progressed to generalized convulsions and/or coma if preeclampsia is undiagnosed. Eclampsia is one of the top five causes of maternal and infant death. Hypertensive diseases are a common complication of pregnancy, seen in 5 to 8 percent of all pregnancies. This condition is a major complication of pregnancy (along with hemorrhage and uterine infection following delivery). Early detection of signs and symptoms can help in the prevention of negative outcomes, thus making ongoing prenatal care a necessity. The earliest warning signal is a sudden development of hypertension or sudden excessive weight gain.[78]

INFERTILITY

A growing number of couples are having difficulty conceiving. Some couples have delayed childbirth decisions until their late thirties to early forties, a time when women are less fertile. Others face the challenge of infertility at a younger age. Regardless of the age of the couple, advances in assisted reproductive technology have allowed couples who previously were childless to experience the joy of childbirth. The initial step for the health care provider is to determine the cause of the infertility. **Primary infertility** is the inability of a couple to conceive a pregnancy after at least 1 year of unprotected intercourse. **Secondary infertility** is difficulty conceiving after already having conceived and carried a normal pregnancy. In 10–15 percent of the cases, no cause for infertility can be established. Overall, women and men account equally for cases of primary infertility. The most common reasons for primary infertility in women are failure to ovulate or having a damaged uterus or fallopian tubes. In men, low sperm count or abnormal sperm development causes primary infertility. *FYI:* "Reasons for Infertility" presents some of the recognized reasons for infertility in women and men.[79] Also, see *Health Tips* for information on where to go for help.

Assisted Reproductive Technology

Louise Brown, the world's first "test tube" baby turned 34 in 2012. Since 1978, **in vitro fertilization (IVF)** has been practiced extensively. The number of cycles

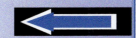

FYI

Reasons for Infertility

Failure to Ovulate

- Hormonal imbalance
- Obesity and/or weight gain
- Prolonged stress
- Ovarian tumor or cyst
- Abbreviated menstrual cycle
- Weight loss, including eating disorders
- Alcohol, tobacco, or other drug abuse, including caffeine

Damaged Fallopian Tubes or Uterus

- Pelvic inflammatory disease (PID) or other STI infection
- Birth defect
- Previous removal of ectopic pregnancy
- Endometriosis or uterine fibroids
- Irregularly shaped or tipped uterus

Low Sperm Count

- Alcohol, tobacco, or other drug abuse, including steroids and marijuana
- Prolonged stress
- Previous STI infection
- Exposure to toxic substances in the workplace

Health Tips

RESOLVE, Inc.

RESOLVE, Inc., is a national, nonprofit organization that provides resources for those facing infertility. It offers assistance, medical referral, emotional support, and education. RESOLVE provides immediate, compassionate, and informed help to people who are experiencing the infertility crisis and provides visibility of the issues through advocacy and public education. Contact RESOLVE, Inc., www.resolve.org.

performed and the number of live birth deliveries with some multiple births that are a result of **assisted reproductive technology (ART)** have increased steadily since that time. ART now accounts for slightly more than 1 percent of total U.S. births.

The CDC publishes the success rates of U.S. fertility clinics annually. The CDC report is a valuable resource for couples seeking infertility assistance by becoming better informed on the procedures, clinics, and factors contributing to success and failure. The most important factors affecting the chances of a live birth are the woman's age and the reason for infertility. The CDC reports are published with the cooperation of the Society for Assisted Reproductive Technology (SART) and the American Society for Reproductive Medicine (ASRM); 441 known U.S. fertility clinics provided data for the 2009 report. During 2009, 146,244 ART cycles were reported with 45,870 live birth deliveries and 60,190 live births.[80] Eighteen percent of ART pregnancies did not result in a live birth.

ART procedures include in vitro fertilization (IVF), GIFT (gamete intrafallopian transfer), and ZIFT (zygote intrafallopian transfer). The majority (72 percent) of these procedures are IVF with fresh, nondonor eggs or embryos. The remainder of the cycles are frozen-donor, frozen-nondonor, and combinations of GIFT, ZIFT, and IVF. These procedures are more common in women aged 40 and older. Figure 9.13 shows pregnancy and live birth rates for ART cycles.

An ART fresh, nondonor egg or embryo cycle begins when a woman takes medication or has her ovaries monitored (using ultrasound or blood tests) for egg production. Fertility drugs can be given to induce ovulation and function with the intent of stimulating a woman's ovaries to produce extra eggs. A woman may also receive a drug to suppress natural hormonal increases. When the eggs mature, an injection of human chorionic gonadotropin (hCG) is administered to facilitate the release of eggs. IVF involves the surgical retrieval of the eggs, fertilizing the egg with sperm in the laboratory, and then transferring the embryo(s) into the woman's uterus through the cervix. **Gamete intrafallopian transfer (GIFT)** involves the use of a laparoscope to guide the transfer of *unfertilized* eggs and sperm (gametes) into the woman's fallopian tubes through small incisions in her abdomen. **Zygote intrafallopian transfer (ZIFT)** involves fertilizing the eggs in the laboratory and using a laparoscope to guide the transfer of the *fertilized* eggs (zygotes) into the woman's fallopian tubes. If one or more of the embryos implant in the uterus, the cycle progresses to clinical pregnancy and then delivery of one or more liveborn infants.

An ART cycle may be discontinued for a variety of reasons, the primary reason being that no or inadequate egg production has occurred (84 percent of cases). In 2009, 11,296 of the total ART cycles using nondonor, fresh eggs performed in the United States (11 percent) were discontinued before egg retrieval. Most of the cycles (67 percent) did not produce a pregnancy, less than 1 percent resulted in an ectopic pregnancy, and 37 percent resulted in clinical pregnancy (23 percent in a single-fetus pregnancy and 12 percent

FIGURE 9.13 Fresh-nondonor cycles

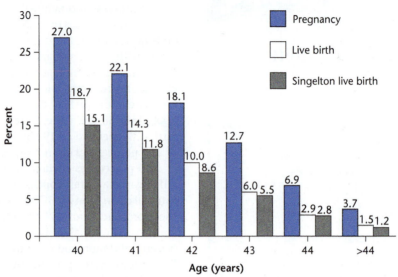

Centers for Disease Control and Prevention. 2011. *2009 Assisted reproductive technology success roles: National summary and fertility clinic reports.* www.cdc.gov/ART/ART2009/PDF/ART_2009_Full.pdf.

in a multiple-fetus pregnancy). Nearly 82 percent of the pregnancies resulted in a live birth (57 percent in a single birth and 25 percent in a multiple-infant birth). Approximately 18 percent resulted in miscarriage, induced abortion, or stillbirth.[81] Concerns have arisen regarding the use of fertility drugs. Do these hormones increase the woman's risk of ovarian cancer? What are the long-term risks from these procedures or drugs? What should be done with the frozen embryos that do not get used in ART cycles? How should the risks associated with multiple births be handled? The *Journal Activity:* "Medical and Ethical Issues" addresses another concern of ART.

Donor Eggs   The use of donor eggs provides a woman with the opportunity to experience pregnancy and childbirth. Egg donors are usually matched with the recipient regarding hair color and other physical features. Older recipients who no longer have viable, mature eggs may benefit from receiving a more viable, mature egg (often from a younger donor). Success rates for older recipients who use donor eggs are likely to be similar to success rates in younger women who use IVF and their own eggs.

Intracytoplasmic Sperm Injection (ICSI)   **ICSI** is a micromanipulation procedure that enables males with less viable sperm potentially to fertilize individual eggs. A single sperm is injected into an egg, and if the egg is fertilized, the embryo is inserted into the uterus. ICSI is often used for couples with a diagnosis of male factor infertility.

Journal Activity

Medical and Ethical Issues of Assisted Reproductive Technology

Multiple-infant births are associated with greater problems for both mothers and infants. It is not uncommon with ART to transfer multiple embryos (two to six) into the uterus of the woman. The 2009 rate of multiple-infant births was approximately 31 percent of all live births from fresh, nondonor embryos (29 percent twins and 2 percent triplets or more). This compares with a multiple-birth rate of less than 3 percent in the general U.S. population. However, there were more triplet (or more) pregnancies than triplet (or more) live births.[82] This can happen naturally (fetal death), or a woman and her doctor may choose to reduce the number of fetuses (multifetal pregnancy reduction). What are your feelings about the decisions to reduce the number of fetuses? How should the risks of multiple births be handled? What role do you think religion should play in these decisions? What role do you think the government should play in these decisions?

Vasovasostomy Microsurgical procedures have advanced the efforts to reverse what was once believed to be irreversible vasectomies. **Vasovasostomy** repairs a surgically removed section and other blockages of the vas deferens, thereby restoring fertility.

Epididymovasostomy This procedure is similar to vasovasostomy, but the technique creates a new connection between the epididymis and the end of the vas deferens. This technique is less successful than vasovasostomy, but pregnancy rates can still reach 30 percent.

Egg Retrieval Immature egg collection, a method similar to IVF, has received attention because it reduces or eliminates the need for fertility drugs. This method, first used in Australia, removes immature eggs from the follicles, matures the egg outside the ovary, fertilizes the egg with sperm, and places the fertilized egg in the uterus. The immature egg collection procedure raises issues such as whether retrieval and storage of eggs from aborted fetuses, accident victims, or women undergoing a hysterectomy should occur. Immature eggs, often four to seven viable eggs with each monthly cycle, can be removed from the follicle.[83]

Artificial Insemination

Artificial insemination (AI) involves the use of sperm from a donor or partner to fertilize an egg. AI is not considered an ART procedure because there is no manipulation of the egg. Couples with infertility due to male problems or female cervical mucus problems may fare well with this procedure. Sperm are collected and placed in the woman's vagina or uterus through a catheter. AI is the general term for several procedures named according to the location of sperm insemination: intracervical, intrauterine, or intrafollicular. The most common procedure is intrauterine insemination (IUI). IUI is a relatively simple procedure performed by passing a sterile catheter containing sperm through the cervix and directly into the uterine cavity. The major disadvantage of AI compared to IVF is that because fertilization occurs within the body, the health care provider cannot determine if other factors may be responsible for the infertility. The pregnancy rates for IUI are approximately 10–20 percent per cycle.[84]

Controversy still exists regarding whether single women should be permitted access to assisted conception. More and more lesbians and single women are deciding to have children. Some conservative groups would like to deny these women the opportunity to use donor sperm. Is it right to deny some women access to artificial insemination? If so, who should be denied access? (See *Her Story:* "Toni and Kelly: Lesbian Parents.")

Surrogacy

Surrogacy has been practiced throughout history and can be controversial and emotionally charged. How does this differ from selling babies? How will the non–egg donor woman feel about her partner providing sperm to impregnate another woman? In surrogacy, a woman, other than the partner, agrees to become pregnant and carry the fetus to full term. There are two types of surrogacy. Traditional surrogacy involves

Her Story

Toni and Kelly: Lesbian Parents

Toni and Kelly, a lesbian couple, chose artificial insemination as their route to having children. They have been together in a committed relationship for 8 years. When Toni decided she wanted to have a baby, she was 35 years old. Kelly thought it was a great idea and they immediately started asking friends about their options. Soon they found a health care provider who was willing to work with them and who informed them about a fertility clinic in California that would mail-order sperm to them. They contacted the clinic and received an information packet with the description and background information on a variety of sperm donors who were identified only by a code number. After careful consideration, they chose donor number 872. Toni got pregnant on the second try and gave birth to a beautiful girl, Jana.

The donor, 872, has provided a waiver to the clinic, giving permission to Jana to learn the identity of her father when she is 18 years old.

Although the birth of Jana occurred in a loving family, Toni and Kelly know that their child may face many challenges as she grows up. Not all people are going to share Toni and Kelly's joy and happiness. Not all people are going to understand their desire to be a family.

- What do you think about this couple's desire to create a family through artificial insemination?
- What are the difficulties that Jana may face as she grows up?
- What is the strength of this family unit?

the surrogate provides the egg and the intended father provides the sperm. In gestational surrogacy, the surrogate carries the pregnancy but genetic material (egg and sperm) are provided by donors, the intended parents or other donors.

Many states have banned or restricted the practice of commercial surrogacy. Others have restricted the amount of payment a surrogate mother can receive for medical expenses and have eliminated the expenses of a broker. If a couple is considering a surrogate, they should contact an attorney in their state to ensure that the protocol is legal and that their interests are covered. The cost of surrogacy can range from $40,000 to $65,000 for traditional surrogacy and $75,000 to $100,000 for the lawyer fees, medical costs, possible surrogate fee, and miscellaneous expenses. If a legal issue arises, the jurisdiction is in the state where the birth occurs. If a surrogate woman changes her mind and wants to keep the baby, do you think she should be allowed to do so? If the couple separates while the surrogate is carrying the fetus, who should have the right to the infant? (See *Viewpoint:* "Surrogate Grandmothers")

Stem Cell Issues

The use of human stem cells in medical therapy has unlimited and unknown possibilities. The research still creates controversy among medical scientists, bioethicists, clergy, and politicians. *Stem cells* are of three types: *adult* stem cells, *embryonic* stem cells, and induced pluripotent stem cells. Adult stem cells are undifferentiated cells found among human tissues and organs. These cells are renewable and can differentiate into the specialized cell types needed in a body's tissues and organs. A stem cell's primary role in a host organism is to repair and maintain the tissue in which they are found. Some scientists

prefer the use of the term *somatic stem cells* in describing these cells.

Somatic stem cells differ from embryonic stem cells as the term "embryonic" describes their origin. Embryonic stem cells are derived from embryos created through in vitro fertilization, which are then donated, with informed consent, for such research and are *not* drawn from an embryo already present in a woman's body. The embryos from which these cells derive are typically between 4 and 5 days old and are in the microscopic, hollow-ball stage called a *blastocyst*. The stem cells used in research are drawn from a blastocyst's inner cell mass.

The process for developing induced pluripotent stem cells (iPSCs) was discovered in 2006. Researchers created the conditions that allowed for some specialized cells to be "reprogrammed." These adult cells were genetically reprogrammed to an embryonic stem cell–like state. They are still trying to determine if iPSCs and embryonic stem cells differ in clinically significant ways. These adult cells are also capable of generating cell characteristics of all three germ layers. This discovery has provided a new technique to "de-differentiate" cells.[85]

Scientists and medical experts working in the field of stem cell therapy believe these discoveries have the potential to alleviate many kinds of human illness and debilitating conditions, including Alzheimer's disease, spinal cord injuries, blindness, deafness, birth defects, stroke, diabetes, arthritis, heart and cardiopulmonary diseases, and cancers. Stem cell therapy is used in replacing bone marrow stem cells into individuals undergoing chemotherapy for cancer. As chemotherapy often destroys bone marrow, these cells are harvested from the individual prior to treatment, then later re-injected where they are able to replenish and rebuild fresh bone marrow. Human stem cells are being used to test new drug therapies for cancer, to generate cells and tissues to replace destroyed or nonfunctional cells and tissue, such as cells destroyed by heart attacks. Stem cell research is still in its infancy. Technical and legal hurdles remain.[86]

For stem cells of any type to be used as medicinal therapy, they must be cultured, or grown, in a specific medium under highly controlled conditions. Large numbers of stem cells are needed for therapeutic use, and embryonic stem cells are more easily grown in laboratory culture than are mature, adult stem cells.

The international scientific, medical, and religious communities continue to debate stem cell use in medical therapy. Some persons see the destruction of human embryos as the destruction of potential human life, and argue no matter how noble the cause, embryonic stem cells should never be used for such purposes. Others argue that the rights and medical needs of human beings suffering from chronic or debilitating conditions must come before those of a microscopic cell colony. What

Viewpoint

Surrogate Grandmothers

A grandmother in England gave birth to her own grandchild. Her daughter was born without a uterus, and she wanted her daughter and son-in-law to have their own child. A grandmother in South Dakota gave birth to her own grandchild. Her daughter, a librarian, was unable to have children, so the grandmother carried the fertilized embryos for her daughter and gave birth to twins. Should surrogacy remain legal? When should the children be told about this event?

are your thoughts on the issues regarding stem cell research? Do you believe only adult stem cells should be used for research? Do you believe creating and using human embryos for medical research is never ethical or appropriate?

ABORTION

Not all pregnancies are planned and not all children are wanted. Worldwide, of the nearly 210 million women who become pregnant every year, not all will have live births. In fact, nearly 15 percent of pregnant women will spontaneously miscarry (usually in the second or third month) or experience a stillbirth. Another 22 percent will terminate the pregnancy by **abortion,** of which 20 million are obtained illegally. These illegal abortions place a woman's health in jeopardy. The vast majority of abortions are sought for personal, not medical, reasons and include social influences (value placed on premarital chastity or marital fidelity, disapproval of having children late in life, rape, genocide), financial concerns (insufficient funds to take care of existing children, career interruption, lack of educational opportunities), or religious beliefs (from tolerance to condemnation). Figure 9.14 reports the legal abortion rate for every 1000 women of childbearing age in the United States. Nearly 47,000 mothers worldwide lost their lives from abortion-related complications in 2008. The worldwide number of abortions decreased from 45.6 million in 1995 to 41.6 million in 2003. The number increased to 43.8 million in 2008, primarily because the United States decreased funding to U.N. agencies, making contraceptives and health care less available.[87] The WHO defines "unsafe abortion" as the termination of an unintended pregnancy by persons lacking the necessary skills or in an environment lacking the minimal medical standards, or both. While the likelihood of having an abortion to terminate an unintended pregnancy is about the same in developed and developing countries, the percentage of abortions performed in unsafe conditions is vastly different (8 percent in developed countries vs. 55 percent in developing countries). The good news is that the abortion rate worldwide dropped from 35 per 1000 women in 1995 to 29 per 1000 in 2003. The bad news is that the rate stalled between 2003 and 2008 with a rate of 28 per 1000 women. And, nearly 98 percent of the unsafe abortions still occur in developing countries. The lack of contraceptive availability and adequate health care prevent women from making safe choices.[88] Unsafe, illegal abortions remain a persistent public health problem. In 2009, President Obama rescinded the "global gag rule" and pledged U.S. support and funding to the United Nations Population Fund. His commitment to child and women's health was welcomed by the international and national human rights communities. The best strategy for reducing abortions is to decrease the number of unintended pregnancies. WHO remains committed to ending unsafe abortion practices and reducing the need for abortions by supporting increased contraceptive use in developing countries.

From 1996 to 2010, the teen pregnancy rate in the United States continued its decline, and with this came a concurrent decline in induced abortions. The major contributing factor for the decline in pregnancies was the increase in contraceptive use. Contributing factors to the decline in abortions included the steep decline in pregnancy rates, fewer teens choosing to have an abortion, and increased difficulty in finding clinics willing to perform abortions. The lack of access to abortion has been an increasing problem for teenagers and low-income women. Barriers include:

- a decline of abortion providers in the majority of all counties and states.
- a weakening of legal protections for women and physicians in many states
- increased restrictions including parental involvement requirements, mandatory counseling, and waiting periods

FIGURE 9.14 Facts on induced abortion in the United States.

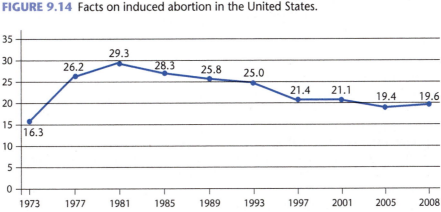

- limited public funding. Only seventeen states use their own funds to pay for abortions for poor women. Only about 3 percent of all abortions are paid with public funds. The federal government has banned the use of Medicaid dollars to pay for abortions, with the exception of a woman's life being in danger.[89]

Low-income women and teenagers often face fewer options for dealing with unwanted pregnancies than other women. Nearly 20 percent of the women who are denied public funded abortions go on to bear unwanted children at considerable emotional, physical, and financial hardship. In 2011, abortion rights was under attack. The number of bills submitted by states spiked to (See *FYI:* "The Status of Abortion in the United States")

Defining Abortion

"Abortion" is defined as the spontaneous or deliberate termination of a pregnancy. There are a number of different types of abortion including therapeutic, spontaneous, and voluntary. Spontaneous abortions (miscarriages) occur for a variety of reasons. These abortions can result from a chronic infection (i.e., PID or endometriosis), hormonal imbalances, fetal abnormalities, or problems with the uterus. Some women experience habitual abortions, which are defined as the abrupt end of three pregnancies in a row before the 20th week.

Therapeutic abortions are procedures conducted to terminate a pregnancy that threatens the life of the mother or fetus. An infected abortion is associated with an immature pregnancy that shows signs of infection of the genital tract. Fever is present and the uterus must be emptied. A septic abortion occurs when the womb is infected and the life of the mother is threatened. This abortion may be spontaneous or induced by the health care provider. A threatened abortion is a condition with symptoms of bleeding of the uterus and cramping before the 20th week. A woman with this condition requires rest and observation. Abortion may or may not occur, depending on the degree of vaginal bleeding and an undilated cervix. Figure 9.15 shows the percentages of pregnancies that end in miscarriages, stillbirths, induced abortions, and live births

A voluntary (elective) abortion is the ending of a pregnancy by choice. As of 2012, 37 states have adopted mandatory parental involvement laws for a minor seeking an abortion. Twenty-two states enforce parental consent, 11 states enforce parental notification, and four states require both parental consent and notification.[91] The procedures most often used in the United States for voluntary abortion include surgical techniques, vacuum aspiration or D&C, and more recently, a drug combination therapy. Forty-six states allow individual health

 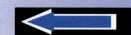

The Status of Abortion in the United States

Data from the Alan Guttmacher Institute[90] and the CDC provide information on the current status of abortion and abortion rights in the United States.

- Nearly 24 percent of all unintended pregnancies end in abortion.
- Nearly 2 percent of all women aged 15–44 have an abortion during their lifetime. Half have had a previous abortion.
- The majority of women having abortions are in their twenties, and nearly 93 percent of all abortions are conducted in clinics.
- Over half of women who have abortions consider themselves religious. Thirty-seven percent of women who have abortions identify as Protestant; 28 percent as Catholic.
- White women account for 36 percent of abortions, black women for 30 percent, and Hispanic women for 25 percent.
- There were 1819 abortion providers in 2000. The number remained stable between 2005 and 2008 at 1793 providers.
- Six in ten minors report that at least one parent knew about having the abortion.
- Eighty percent of large abortion provider services have experienced picketing as a form of harassment.
- More women are having abortions early in their pregnancy due to more sensitive technologies to detect pregnancy, the medical abortion option, and newer surgical techniques for early abortions.
- Nearly 60 percent of women who experienced a delay in getting an abortion cited making arrangments and raising money as primary reasons
- Abortion does not pose a risk to women's mental health
- There is no association between abortion and breast cancer or any other cancer
- Fewer than 0.3 percent of abortion patients experience a complication requiring hospitalization. Abortion is safe.
- The average cost for nonhospital abortion with local anesthesia at 10 weeks was $451.

care providers to refuse to participate in an abortion procedure.

Surgical Abortion **Vacuum aspiration,** also called suction aspiration, is the most common surgical method of first-trimester abortion. Early procedures—preemptive abortion and early uterine evacuation—can

FIGURE 9.15 Worldwide, more than a third of pregnancies do not end in the birth of a baby.

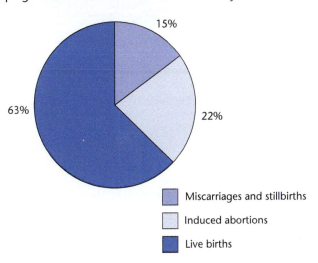

15%

63%

22%

- Miscarriages and stillbirths
- Induced abortions
- Live births

SOURCE: Alan Guttmacher Institute. 2012. Are You In the Know? www.guttmacher.org/in-the-know/abortion.html (retrieved February 21, 2012).

be performed in a clinic or a physician's office with a local anesthetic. These procedures are typically performed in the first 4–8 weeks, and the most common complications may be infection or heavy bleeding for a few days. Vacuum aspiration is the procedure used for abortions in the 6th–14th week. The cervix is dilated and a small plastic tube (or cannula) is inserted into the uterus. The cannula is attached to a pump that suctions the contents of the uterus. The procedure is completed within minutes; however, the clinical stay may be several hours to make sure there is no any unusual bleeding or any other complications. In some situations, the uterus may be scraped with a curette to loosen and remove tissue.[92] When a **dilation and curettage (D&C)** is performed, the cervix is dilated and the uterine lining is scraped with a curette to remove the contents. This procedure often requires general anesthesia and must be performed in a clinic or hospital. Possible complications include reaction to the anesthesia or cervical injuries. The use of D&C has declined sharply since the introduction of the vacuum aspiration procedure.[93]

After the 14th–15th week, abortion becomes more complicated because the fetus is larger and a greater blood supply goes to the uterus. Only 6 percent of abortions are performed between 13 and 15 weeks, and only 5 percent are performed at 16 weeks or later. A **dilation and evacuation (D&E)** procedure is an expansion of the vacuum aspiration, but a larger cervical opening is required. The method used by the health care provider determines the length of time required for dilation, from a few minutes to 2 days. The health care provider will use suction and forceps to remove the fetal parts. A curette is used to remove any

remaining tissue. The D&E is usually used in the first weeks of the second trimester but can be used through the 24th week of pregnancy. The procedure takes only 10–30 minutes, with either a local anesthetic or general anesthesia.[94]

Two late-term procedures, hysterotomy and intact dilation and extraction, can be performed during the end of the second trimester or during the third trimester. These procedures are major surgery and are reserved for life-threatening circumstances to the woman. All surgical abortions require an observation and recovery period. The length of time depends on the procedure and the time frame since the last menstrual period (LMP). The woman is given instructions for postoperative care, including a 24-hour number to call in case of an emergency, and an appointment for follow-up in 2 to 4 weeks.

Medical Abortion Mifepristone (trade name Mifeprex) was the first drug approved for the termination of an early pregnancy, defined as 49 days or less, counting from the beginning of the last menstrual period. Mifepristone, known to some as **RU-486,** was developed by a French pharmaceutical company and approved for use in France in 1988. A chronology of its development and introduction in the United States can be found at www.feminist.org/welcome/ru486two.html. Access to a medical abortion during the early stages of pregnancy has afforded women another option: the use of two medicines to end an early pregnancy. The regimen is effective in nearly 95 percent of women when used within 49 days from the beginning of their last menstrual period. In the United States several medicines are available. Misoprostol is a hormone that triggers uterine contractions. It is more effective when used with other drugs. Mifepristone blocks the effects of progesterone. Methotrexate interferes with the placenta's growth. It is usually used in combination with misoprostol, which starts the uterine contractions.

Medical abortion requires at least two visits to the health care provider over several week for the termination of a pregnancy over several weeks. The first visit includes thorough counseling, a physical examination, and determination of the length of the pregnancy. It is important that the health care provider be skilled in determining the length of pregnancy and ruling out an ectopic pregnancy. During the first visit, one medicine is given and a second one is taken at home. A second visit, 2–3 weeks later, is required as a follow-up examination to confirm that the abortion is complete. Nearly 75 percent of women abort within 24 hours after taking misoprostol. The side effects experienced by women are typically related to misoprostol and include headaches, nausea, diarrhea, vomiting, heavy bleeding, and cramping. The bleeding may include large blood clots, unrelated to the expulsion of the conception by-products.[95]

FYI

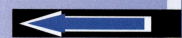

Comparison of Medical and Surgical Abortion

Medical Abortion

High success rate (about 95 percent)
Can be used in the earliest weeks following fertilization (up to 7 weeks LMP)
Requires no invasive procedure or surgery
Requires no anesthesia
Side effects other than bleeding tend to be short-lived
Does not carry risk of uterine perforation or injury to the cervix
Has the potential for greater privacy
Gives a woman greater control over her body

Surgical Abortion

High success rate (about 99 percent)
Requires only one office visit
Performed quickly (5–10 minutes)
Slightly more effective than medical abortion
Less blood loss
No awareness of the passing of the by-products of conception
Can be performed later than medical abortion (usually during the first trimester)

Postabortion Issues

Some groups would like to suggest that women who have abortions experience mental and emotional problems as a result of their decision. The most recent study, a 2011 population-based cohort study of Danish girls and women between 1995 and 2007 found no increased risk for any mental disorder within the 12 month postabortion period compared to the 9-month pre-abortion period.[96] Studies of women who choose abortion have found that the majority experience relief after the abortion, and the immediate feelings of guilt, loss, and/or depression usually pass quickly.[97] The circumstances leading to the decision to abort a pregnancy may include fear or threat of losing one's partner, financial hardship, missed educational opportunities or career advancement, loss of a job, detectable fetal defects, responsibility to other children, lack of social support, rape or incest, maternal age, and others.[98] A woman's feelings and emotions often are shaped by the political, religious, and social climate she experiences. Thus, support for the woman's right to choose can facilitate better recovery. (See *Her Story:* "Shelby: An Unintended Pregnancy and Choice.")

Like most major life events, a woman needs to handle her feelings after an abortion in her own way. She should reach a stage of accepting the loss (regardless of the reasons), rather than live in secrecy and guilt. If grief exists, the resolution of the process may be facilitated by sharing one's feelings with accepting friends and family members, health care providers, mental health professionals, or clergy. Guilt, depression, or other emotional trauma can linger if grief remains unresolved. Anti-abortion groups have attempted to document "postabortion syndrome" (PAS) with traits similar

Her Story

Shelby: An Unintended Pregnancy and Choice

Shelby had her first child at age 15. She stayed in school during the pregnancy, but once Jamie was born she needed a job and a place of her own. So she dropped out of high school and began working at the local restaurant. After 3 years of living paycheck to paycheck, she decided to finish her GED. She wanted to go to college and better her life. She met Justin in the class. He also wanted to go to college. They began dating, and 2 years later she completed her GED and was ready to apply for college—but she got pregnant. Neither Justin nor she was ready for a child.

- What should Shelby do?
- What options did she have?

Go to the Web site www.prochoice.org and read the self-assessment guide *What's Right for Me?*

to those for posttraumatic stress disorder (PTSD). However, mainstream medical positions have never supported this assertion. Research has found that the time of greatest distress is *before* the abortion. Also, the greatest predictor of emotional well-being after an abortion was the state of well-being before the abortion. For the vast majority of women who have had an abortion, a mixture of feelings occurs, with a predominance of positive feelings.[99]

Right to Life and Pro-Choice

Is it right to life, pro-life, or anti-choice? Is it pro-choice or pro-abortion? Even the terms we use to describe the stances toward abortion give some indication of a person's views. What do we know about the individuals who describe themselves as right to life or pro-choice advocates? Researchers have found that right to life advocates tend to have a more unified attitude structure than pro-choice advocates. Because attitude structures are more unified, right to life advocates tend to be more single-minded in their beliefs. This position can best be summarized as people advocating for the rights of the fetus and as people who believe that life begins at conception. Right to life advocates are more dogmatic than pro-choice advocates and conservative religiously, politically, and socially. They view abortion as a moral issue and often will vote for political candidates on the basis of this single issue.[100]

Pro-choice advocates tend to have less unified attitude structures, thus they are more open-minded to interpreting and organizing reality. The pro-choice position maintains that women should have control over their own bodies, including reproductive rights. The reasons pro-choice advocates give for choosing this stance are varied. They advocate for individual rights. Some may take a stance that the fetus is not a viable life, others may have strong feelings about a woman's right to choose, and still others may consider the circumstances of the pregnancy.[101] Right to life advocates sometimes appear to be more effective politically than pro-choice advocates, but this is due to their single-issue politics. This appearance should not suggest that pro-choice advocates are less committed to their values and beliefs. Rather, pro-choice advocates have a variety of issues on which to focus.

Another question we might ask is, How are children being influenced by a "moralistic" (right versus wrong) debate? Look at right to life and pro-choice rallies at which children often stand next to sign-carrying parents. At right to life rallies, young children carry signs with graphic pictures of aborted, discarded fetuses. These children are led to believe that the women who have abortions are murderers and baby killers. At pro-choice rallies, children tote signs saying KEEP CHOICE LEGAL. They are led to believe that individual rights and freedoms will be sacrificed if abortion isn't legal and that all right to life advocates are violent. At what age did you form your opinion about abortion? How did you reach this decision? Do you think it might change? Now complete *Assess Yourself:* "Attitudes toward Induced Abortion" to determine your attitudes toward abortion.

Assess Yourself

Attitudes toward Induced Abortion

For each statement about induced abortion, indicate your feelings based on the values in the following scale:

6—Strongly agree
5—Moderately agree
4—Slightly agree
3—Slightly disagree
2—Moderately disagree
1—Strongly disagree

_____ 1. Abortion is a moral issue.
_____ 2. The rights of a fetus should be protected because the unborn child can't protect herself.
_____ 3. A woman who has an abortion is selfish and self-centered.
_____ 4. Societies with high moral standards should prohibit abortions.
_____ 5. Life begins at conception.
_____ 6. If two people have unprotected sex, they should be willing to live with the consequences of their action.
_____ 7. Abortions are not an alternative when contraception has failed.
_____ 8. All abortions should be banned.
_____ 9. Parental consent should be required for all young girls under age 18 who seek an abortion.
_____10. Every young woman seeking an abortion should be required to watch a video about the procedure before making a final decision.

Total your score. Higher scores indicate a more right to life attitude and lower scores indicate a more pro-choice attitude.

ADOPTION

Adoption is an alternative to assisted reproduction or abortion. Adoption issues have changed because the rights of adoptees are now viewed as being equal to the rights of birth parents and adoptive parents. Couples who are making a decision on whether to adopt a child have a variety of issues to consider. First, they need to decide on the age, race, and health status of the child they want to adopt. Do they expect to raise a normal, healthy child from infancy? Does the child's background matter? Should they consider intercountry adoption or adopting a special needs child, a minority child, or an older child? Once they decide on the kind of child they desire, they need to find an appropriate agency to meet their needs. Agencies can vary from public agencies such as county social services to private adoption arranged a lawyer, physician, or church. Services can vary from matching children and adoptive parents to educational and support services throughout the parenting years. (See *FYI:* "Facts on Adoption.")

Adoptions can be closed or open. **Closed** (confidential) **adoption** means that there is no contact between birth parents and adoptive parents. **Open adoption** means that contact occurs between birth parents and adoptive parents. This contact can vary from occasional letters to regular contact with the child. Open adoption eliminates the need for children to fantasize about their birth parents; they get actual knowledge of their ancestry. However, open adoption also brings the inherent risk of birth parents' interfering or intruding on the life of the adoptive family. Bonding can become difficult if competition arises for the child's attention. Such attachment and identity issues in adopted children may not develop during the early years, especially if the child is adopted as an infant. Rather, these issues may develop during the adolescent years, when many young adults feel that they have a need to know their birth parents. This process can be difficult; the anticipation and expectation of being accepted by their birth parents are usually mixed with the fear of experiencing further rejection. The Internet has become a ready source for exchange of information between adopted children seeking birth parents and birth parents seeking information about the child they gave up for adoption years before. (See *FYI:* "National Adoption Registry, Inc.")

Foster Care

The U.S. foster care system had nearly 408,000 children, with more than 107,000 available for adoption in 2010. The courts terminated the parental rights for 64,000 children and during the year, only 55,000 were adopted.

With the passage of the Fostering Care Act of 2008, most states increased their focus on placing children with relatives. The number of children placed with relatives (24 percent of all placements) has continued to increase, as has the placements with non-relative foster families (48 percent). The placement of children in group homes and institutions remained around 16 percent overall, yet children age 16 and older disproportionately represented those placed in these settings (over 36 percent). The number of foster children aging out is also rising. In 2011, nearly 28,000 children aged out of foster care. These aged out foster children have high rates of incarceration, homelessness and unintended pregnancies. A number of myths exist regarding adoption.[102] Check FYI: Myths about Adoption to see several of the more common myths.

Costs of *adaption* vary depending upon the type of agency, state laws, whether travel is necessary, and attorney fees. Foster care can range from $0 to $2500; licensed private agencies and independent agencies can vary from $5000 to $40,000+; and intercountry agencies can range from $0 to $63,000. Adopt Us Kids, Adopt America Network, Children Awaiting Parents, and The Adoption Exchange are a few of the Web sites with photo listings of children waiting to be adopted. To evaluate your competence to be a parent, under any or most circumstances, check *Assess Yourself:* "How Do You Rate Your Competence to Be a Parent?"

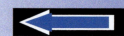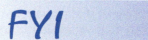

Myths about Adoption[103]

Myth: There are no orphans in the United States.
Fact: There are 107,000 children in foster care who are waiting for adoptive homes.
Myth: It's easier and faster to adopt internationally.
Fact: In 2010, 53,000 children were adopted in the U.S. while 11,058 were adopted from international sources.
Myth: You need lots of money to adopt a foster child.
Fact: You don't need a lot of money, your own home, other children, or to stay-at-home to adopt a child.
Myth: All children in foster care have special needs.
Fact: Many regular children are removed from their families due to abuse or neglect.
Myth: Only married couples with a stay-at-home parent can adopt a child from foster care.
Fact: In 2010, 33 percent of children were placed in single-parent households or with unmarried couples.

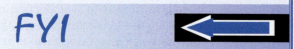

National Adoption Registry, Inc.

The National Adoption Registry is a private registry that accepts registrations from adoptees, birth parents, and other interested individuals. Vital statistics of the adoptee are entered in the database and matched with existing information in the file. A fee is assessed for registration.

Assess Yourself

How Do You Rate Your Competence to Be a Parent?

Rate each of the items below by indicating how competent you feel about your abilities according to the following scale:

a—Very competent
b—Fairly competent
c—Somewhat competent
d—Not very competent
e—Not at all competent

How do you feel about your competence and ability to

_____ 1. Care for a child when he or she is sick or upset?
_____ 2. Help a child solve problems?
_____ 3. Provide adequate time for a child?
_____ 4. Be a good parent?
_____ 5. Provide emotional support for a child?
_____ 6. Maintain a close relationship with a child?
_____ 7. Provide a good role model for a child?
_____ 8. Discipline a child?
_____ 9. Give advice to a child?
_____ 10. Meet the needs of a child (even special needs)?
_____ 11. Establish and enforce rules for a child's behavior?
_____ 12. Obtain needed resources for a child?

Using a rating of a = 5, b = 4, c = 3, d = 2, e = 1, total your score. Which competencies are you most comfortable doing? What skills would you need to improve some of the other competencies?

Chapter Summary

- Fertility awareness–based methods include the cycle-based method, basal body temperature method, cevical mucus method, and symptothermal method.
- Withdrawal, coitus interruptus, is not a birth control method.
- Barrier methods include spermicides, condoms, diaphragms and cervical caps.
- Hormonal methods include oral contraceptives, transdermal patches, injectables, Implanon, and NuvaRing.
- EC is most effective if given within 72 hours after unprotected intercourse or method failure.
- Intrauterine devices are the most popular worldwide forms of reversible birth control.
- Sterilization methods include tubal ligation and vasectomy and are the most common form of contraception used by women over age 30.
- Choosing a birth control method should be a joint decision between a woman and her partner, but women must take precautions to protect against unintended pregnancies and sexually transmitted infections.
- Nearly 45 percent of all pregnancies are unplanned.
- Lifestyle changes should begin before pregnancy. These changes include exercise, nutritional planning and necessary supplements, nondrug use without first consulting a health care provider, a time lapse if using oral contraceptives, and appropriate immunizations.
- Early signs of pregnancy include a missed period, a light period or spotting, tender or swollen breasts, fatigue, nausea and vomiting, and frequent urination.
- Home pregnancy tests are reliable when used properly. These tests are sensitive to the presence of hCG in the urine.

- A sequence of changes occurs to the fetus and the mother during the 40-week gestational period.
- The maternal mortality rate is higher among African American women than white women.
- Prenatal checkups are recommended monthly through the first 28 weeks, biweekly during weeks 28 to 36, and weekly thereafter.
- Certified nurse-midwives, lay midwives, and doulas provide primary care to women expecting low-risk pregnancies.
- Breast feeding is beneficial to both mother and infant.
- Primary infertility is recognized as the inability of a woman to conceive within 1 year of having unprotected sexual intercourse.
- Women and men account equally for cases of primary infertility.
- Artificial insemination involves the use of sperm from a donor or partner to fertilize an egg.
- In vitro fertilization involves the implantation of a fertilized egg into a woman's uterus.
- Multiple births are more likely to occur with assisted reproduction technology (ART).
- Categories of abortion include spontaneous, therapeutic, and voluntary.
- Closed adoption is confidential and eliminates contact between birth and adoptive parents.
- Open adoption means the possibility of contact between birth and adoptive parents.

Review Questions

1. Describe the techniques, benefits, and drawbacks for the fertility awareness–based methods.
2. What is the difference between method failure and user failure?
3. Discuss the procedures for applying a condom.
4. What is emergency contraception?
5. Discuss fetal development.
6. Discuss the stages of labor and delivery.
7. What are the advantages of Breast feeding?
8. What is the importance of maternal and infant mortality rates?
9. What are the arguments offered by pro-choice and right to life regarding abortion?
10. What components do couples need to consider with pre-pregnancy planning?
11. Discuss some advances in assisted reproductive technology.
12. Discuss the advantages and disadvantages of open and closed adoption.

Resources

Organizations, Hotlines, and Websites

Alan Guttmacher Institute
  800-355-0244
  www.guttmacher.org

American Association of Birth Centers (*to locate a birthing center*)
  866-54-BIRTH
  www.birthcenters.org

American College of Nurse-Midwives (directory of certified nurse-midwives)
  240-485-1800
  www.midwife.org

American Society for Reproductive Medicine (ASRM) (up-to-date report of fertility clinics in your region)
  www.asrm.com
  205-978-5000

Child Welfare Information Gateway (adoption resource)
  800-394-3366
  www.childwelfare.gov/

Childbirth.org

Dave Thomas Foundation for Adoption
  1-800-ASK-DTFA (1-800-275-3832)
  www.davethomasfoundation.org

Doulas of North America (DONA)
  888-788-DONA(3662)
  www.dona.org

Feminist Majority Foundation
  703-522-2214
  www.feminist.org

March of Dimes
  914-997-4488
  www.marchofdimes.org

NARAL Pro-Choice America
  202-973-3000
  www.naral.org

National Abortion Federation
  800-772-9100
  www.prochoice.org

National Adoption Registry, Inc.
  913-338-0800
  www.nationaladoptionregistry.com

National Right to Life Committee
  202-626-8800
  www.nrlc.org

Planned Parenthood Federation of America, Inc.
  800-230-PLAN (7526)
  www.plannedparenthood.org

Population Council
  212-339-0500
  www.popcouncil.org

RESOLVE: The National Infertility Association (services for fertility problems and adoption information)
  703-556-7172
  www.resolve.org

Resources for Adoptive Parents (a listing of agencies, facilitators, attorneys, and exchanges for adoption services and information)
  800-367-2367
  www.adoptionnetwork.com

Stars of David International, Inc. (services for Jewish and part-Jewish adoptive families)
  800-STAR-349 (800-782-7349)
  www.starsofdavid.org

UNICEF
  www.unicef.org
  212-686-5522

World Health Organization
  info@who.int (contact)
  www.who.int

References

1. National Campaign to Prevent Teen and Unplanned Pregnancy. *Teen birth rates: how does the United States compare?* http://www.thenationalcampaign.org/resources/pdf/TBR_InternationalComparison.pdf (retrieved January 23, 2012)

2. National Campaign to Prevent Teen Pregnancy. DCR report. http://www.thenationalcampaign.org/resources/dcr/SectionA/DCR_SectionA.pdf

3. National Campaign to Prevent Teen Pregnancy. *Counting it up: the public costs of teen childbearing: key data.* http://www.thenationalcampaign.org/costs/calculator.asp

4. Ibid.

5. World Health Organization. 2004. *Health benefits of family planning.* www.who.int/reproductive-health/publications/health_benefits_family_planning/health_benefits_fp.pdf (retrieved January 24, 2009).

6. Planned Parenthood. 2010. *The birth control pill: a history.* http://www.plannedparenthood.org/files/PPFA/pillhistory.pdf (retrieved January 27, 2012)

7. Planned Parenthood (comparison)

8. Guttmacher Institute. December 2011. *Facts on American teens' sexual and reproductive health.* http://www.guttmacher.org/pubs/FB-ATSRH.html

9. SIECUS. 2008. *Brief history of abstinence-only-until-marriage funding.* www.nomoremoney.org/index.cfm?pageid947 (retrieved January 26, 2009).

10. Advocates for Youth. 2012. *Future of sex education: national sexuality education standards.* http://www.advocatesforyouth.org/serced/951?task=view

11. WebMD. *Normal menstrual cycle.* http://women.webmd.com/tc/normal-menstrual-cycle-normal-menstrual-cycle (retrieved January 25, 2012)

12. Planned Parenthood Federation of America. (retrieved January 25, 2012)

13. Planned Parenthood. *What is the calendar method?* http://www.plannedparenthood.org/health-topics/birth-control/fertility-awareness-4217.htm (retrieved January 25, 2012)

14. Ibid.

15. Ibid.

16. Ibid.

17. Centers for Disease Control. December 17, 2010. Sexually transmitted diseases treatment guidelines, 2010. *MMRW* 59(RR12): 1–110.

18. Ibid.

19. Planned Parenthood. *What are condoms?* http://www.plannedparenthood.org/health-topics/birth-control/condom-10187.htm (retrieved January 25, 2012)

20. Planned Parenthood. *What are female condoms?* http://www.plannedparenthood.org/health-topics/birth-control/female-condom-4223.htm (retrieved January 25, 2012)

21. Planned Parenthood. *How effective is the sponge?* http://www.plannedparenthood.org/health-topics/birth-control/birth-control-sponge-today-sponge-4224.htm (retrieved January 25, 2012)

22. Centers for Disease Control and Prevention. 2010. *Sexually transmitted disease treatment guidelines.*

23. Planned Parenthood. *How effective is the diaphragm?* http://www.plannedparenthood.org/health-topics/birth-control/diaphragm-4244.htm (retrieved January 25, 2012)

24. Planned Parenthood. *How effective is the cervical cap?* http://www.plannedparenthood.org/health-topics/birth-control/cervical-cap-20487.htm (retrieved January 25, 2012)

25. *Drugs associated with birth control.* 2011. www.drugs.com/condition/contraception.html

26. Planned Parenthood. 2010. *The birth control pill: a history.* http://www.plannedparenthood.org/files/PPFA/pillhistory.pdf (retrieved January 27, 2012)

27. Feminist Women's Health Center. 2008. *Continuous hormonal birth control.* www.birth-control-comparison.info/continual-hormones.htm (retrieved January 27, 2009).

28. Planned Parenthood. 2010. *The birth control bill: a history.*

29. Ibid.

30. ORTHO Evra®. http://www.accessdata.fda.gov/drugsatfda_docs/label/2010/021180s035LBW.pdf

31. Organon. 2008. *NuvaRing®.* http://www.spfiles.com/pinuvaring.pdf

32. Merck. 2011. *NuvaRing®.* http://www.nuvaring.com/hcp/what-is-nuvaring/clinical-pharmacology/index.asp

33. Planned Parenthood. *Depo-Provera.*

34. FDA. 2010. *Highlights of prescribing information.* http://www.accessdata.fda.gov/drugsatfda_docs/label/2010/020246s036LBW.pdf

35. Planned Parenthood. 2011. *Morning after pill (emergency contraception).* http://www.plannedparenthood.org/health-topics/emergency-contraception-morning-after-pill-4363.asp?__utma=1.2032146722.1328378538.1328378538.13283 84837.2&__utmb=1.6.10.1328384837&__utmc=1&__utmx=-&__utmz=1.1328378538.1.1.utmcsr=(direct)|utmccn=(direct)|utmcmd=(none)&__utmv=-&__utmk=68634513

36. NV Organon (Merck & Co). 2011. *Implanon.* http://www.implanon-usa.com/en/consumer/about-it/compare-methods/index.asp

37. Mosher WD, Jones J. 2010. Use of contraceptives in the United States: 1982–2008. National Center for Health Statistics. *Vital and Health Statistics* 23 (29).

38. Planned Parenthood. 2012. *How effective is the IUD?* http://www.plannedparenthood.org/health-topics/birth-control/iud-4245.htm

39. Food and Drug Administration. 2008. *Mirena®.* http://www.accessdata.fda.gov/drugsatfda_docs/label/2008/021225s019LBW.pdf

40. Planned Parenthood. 2012. *The IUD at a glance.* http://www.plannedparenthood.org/health-topics/birth-control/iud-4245.htm

41. Mosher and Jones. 2010.

42. Planned Parenthood. What is sterilization? http://www.plannedparenthood.org/health-topics/birth-control/sterilization-women-4248.htm?__utma=1.2143074918.1328469625.1328469625.1328469625.1&__utmb=1.6.10.1328469625&__utmc=1&__utmx=-&__utmz=1.1328469625.1.1.utmcsr=(direct)|utmccn=(direct)|utmcmd=(none)&__utmv=-&__utmk=160697789

43. American Cancer Society. 2012. *Can ovarian cancer be prevented?* http://www.cancer.org/Cancer/OvarianCancer/DetailedGuide/ovarian-cancer-prevention

44. Planned Parenthood. What is *vasectomy?* http://www.plannedparenthood.org/health-topics/birth-control/vasectomy-4249.htm?__utma=1.2143074918.1328469625.13284

69625.1328469625.1&__utmb=1.14.9.1328469655568&__utmc=1&__utmx=-&__utmz=1.1328469625.1.1.utmcsr=(direct)|utmccn=(direct)|utmcmd=(none)&__utmv=-&__utmk=154856248

45. Mosher and Jones. 2010.

46. World Health Organization, UNICEF, UNFPA and World Bank. 2010. *Trends in maternal mortality: 1990 to 2008.* http://www.who.int/reproductivehealth/publications/monitoring/9789241500265/en/

47. Ibid.

48. World Health Organization. 2011. *Children: reducing mortality.* http://www.who.int/mediacentre/factsheets/fs178/en/

49. MacDorman MF, Mathews TJ. 2008. *Recent trends in infant mortality in the United States.* NCHS data brief (9). http://www.cdc.gov/nchs/data/databriefs/db09.pdf

50. Forum on child and Family Statistics. 2011. *America's children: key national indicators of well-being,* 2011. http://www.childstats.gov/americaschildren/health.asp

51. Planned Parenthood. 2011. *Pre-pregnancy planning.* http://www.plannedparenthood.org/health-topics/pregnancy/pre-pregnancy-planning-4254.htm

52. Centers for Disease Control and Prevention. 2011. *Facts about folic acid.* http://www.cdc.gov/ncbddd/folicacid/about.html

53. March of Dimes. 2007. *How will you know you are pregnant?* http://www.marchofdimes.com/pregnancy/trying_pregnant.html

54. Office of Women's Health. 2009. *Pregnancy tests.* http://womenshealth.gov/publications/our-publications/fact-sheet/pregnancy-tests.pdf

55. March of Dimes. 2012. *March of Dimes partnering with hospitals on quality improvement plans.* http://www.marchofdimes.com/news/10363.html

56. March of Dimes. 2009. *Pregnancy after 35.* http://www.marchofdimes.com/pregnancy/trying_after35.html

57. March of Dimes. 2011. *Prenatal care.* http://www.marchofdimes.com/pregnancy/prenatalcare_amniocentesis.html

58. March of Dimes. 2009. *Giving birth.* http://www.marchofdimes.com/pregnancy/labor_indepth.html

59. Ibid.

60. March of Dimes. 2009. *Stages of labor.* http://www.marchofdimes.com/pregnancy/vaginalbirth_indepth.html

61. American College of Nurse-Midwives. 2011. *Essential facts about midwives.* http://www.midwife.org/Essential-Facts-about-Midwives

62. American College of Obstetricians and Gynecologists. February 2011. *Committee Opinion #476: planned home births.* http://www.acog.org/About_ACOG/News_Room/News_Releases/2011/The_American_College_of_Obstetricians_and_Gynecologists_Issues_Opinion_on_Planned_Home_Births

63. Ventura SJ. 2009. *Changing patterns of nonmarital children in the United States.* NCHS data brief, no. 18. Hyattsville, MD: National Center for Health Statistics. http://www.cdc.gov/nchs/data/databriefs/db18.htm

64. National Campaign to Prevent Teen and Unplanned Pregnancies. May 2008. *Unplanned pregnancy in the United States.* http://www.thenationalcampaign.org/resources/pdf/briefly-unplanned-in-the-united-states.pdf

65. Hamilton BE, Martin JA, Ventura SJ. 2011. Births: *Preliminary data for 2010.* National Vital Statistics Report web release 60 (2), Hyattsville, MD: National Center for Health Statistics. http://www.cdc.gov/nchs/data/nvsr/nvsr60/nvsr60_02.pdf

66. Martin JA, Hamilton BE, Sutton PD, et al. 2010. *Births: Final data for 2008.* National vital statistics reports; vol 59 no 1. Hyattsville, MD: National Center for Health Statistics. http://www.cdc.gov/nchs/data/nvsr/nvsr59/nvsr59_01.pdf

67. World Health Organization. 2010. *Infant and young child feeding.* http://www.who.int/mediacentre/factsheets/fs342/en/

68. Health and Human Services, Office of the Surgeon General. 2011. *Breastfeeding: call to action.* http://www.cdc.gov/breastfeeding/promotion/calltoaction.htm

69. World Health Organization. 2009. *Baby friendly hospital initiative.* http://www.who.int/nutrition/publications/infantfeeding/9789241594950/en/index.html

70. Office of Women's Health. 2010. *Why breastfeeding is important.* http://www.womenshealth.gov/breastfeeding/why-breastfeeding-is-important/

71. Ibid.

72. Ibid.

73. World Health Organization. 2009. *Baby friendly hospital initiative.*

74. Health and Human Services, Office of the Surgeon General. 2011. *The Surgeon General's call to action to support breastfeeding.* http://www.surgeongeneral.gov/topics/breastfeeding/factsheet.html

75. Centers for Disease Control and Prevention. 2006. *Risk of ectopic pregnancy after tubal sterilization: women's reproductive health.* http://www.cdc.gov/reproductivehealth/Unintended Pregnancy/EctopicPreg_factsheet.htm

76. WebMD. 2011. *Ectopic pregnancy—what increases your risk?* http://www.webmd.com/baby/tc/ectopic-pregnancy-what-increases-your-risk

77. Ibid.

78. Preeclampsia Foundation. 2002. *Preeclampsia.* http://www.preeclampsia.org/pdf/Preeclampsia%20Fact%20sheet%20v2.pdf

79. National Institutes of Health. 2011. *Infertility.* http://www.nlm.nih.gov/medlineplus/ency/article/001191.htm

80. Centers for Disease Control and Prevention. 2011. *What is assisted reproductive technology?* http://www.cdc.gov/ART/

81. Centers for Disease Control and Prevention, American Society for Reproductive Medicine, Society for Assisted Reproductive Technology. 2009. *Assisted reproductive technology success rates: national summary and fertility clinic reports.* Atlanta: U.S. Department of Health and Human Services; 2011. http://www.cdc.gov/ART/ART2009/PDF/ART_2009_Full.pdf

82. Office of Women's Health. 2009. *Infertility fact sheet.* http://www.womenshealth.gov/publications/our-publications/fact-sheet/infertility.cfm

83. Ibid.

84. Adoption.com. 2010. *Surrogacy: how does it work?* http://adopting.adoption.com/child/surrogacy.html

85. National Institutes of Health. 2009. *Stem cell basics.* http://stemcells.nih.gov/staticresources/info/basics/SCprimer2009.pdf

86. Ibid.

87. Sedgh G, et al. 2012. *Induced abortion: incidence and trends worldwide from 1995 to 2008.* Lancet. http://www.guttmacher.org/pubs/fb_IAW.html

88. Guttmacher Institute. 2012. *Facts in induced abortion worldwide.* http://www.guttmacher.org/pubs/fb_IAW.html

89. Ibid.

90. Guttmacher Institute. 2011. *Facts on induced abortion in the United States.* http://www.guttmacher.org/pubs/fb_induced_abortion.html

91. Guttmacher Institute. 2012. *State polices in brief: an overview of abortion laws.* www.guttmacher.org/statecenter/spibs/spib_OAL.pdf

92. WebMd. *Manual and vacuum aspiration for abortion.* http://women.webmd.com/manual-and-vacuum-aspiration-for-abortion#tw1081

93. WebMd. *D&C (dilation and curettage).* http://women.webmd.com/guide/d-and-c-dilation-and-curettage

94. WebMd. *Dilation and evacuation for abortion.* http://women.webmd.com/dilation-and-evacuation-de-for-abortion

95. WebMd. *Abortion-choices: medical abortion.* http://women.webmd.com/tc/abortion-choices-medical-abortion

96. Munk-Olson T, et al. 2011. Induced first-trimester abortion and risk of mental disorder. *New England Journal of Medicine* 364:332–339.

97. Planned Parenthood. 2012. *The emotional effects of induced abortion.* http://www.plannedparenthood.org/files/PPFA/Emotional_Effects_of_Induced_Abortion.pdf

98. Henshaw SK, Kost K. 2008. *Trends in the characteristics of women obtaining abortions 1974–2004.* http://www.guttmacher.org/pubs/2008/09/18/Report_Trends_Women_Obtaining_Abortions.pdf

99. National Abortion Federation. 2003. Abortion myths: post abortion syndrome. http://www.prochoice.org/about_abortion/myths/post_abortion_syndrome.html

100. National Right to Life. 2012. *Defending the pro-life position & framing the issues by the language we use.* http://www.nrlc.org/abortion/facts/completeWhen%20They%20Say%20You%20Say%2012.11.09re.pdf

101. NARAL Pro-Choice America. 2012. *U.S. Supreme Court decisions concerning reproductive rights 1965–2007.* http://www.prochoiceamerica.org/media/fact-sheets/government-federal-courts-scotus-choice-cases.pdf

102. Health and Human Services. *Trends in foster care and adoption – FY 2002–FY2010.* http://www.acf.hhs.gov/programs/cb/stats_research/afcars/trends_june2011.pdf

103. AdoptUSKids. *Common myths about adoption.* http://www.adoptuskids.org/for-families/how-to-adopt/common-myths-about-adoption#special-needs

CONTEMPORARY LIFESTYLE AND SOCIAL ISSUES

Part Four

Chapter Ten

Eating Well

CHAPTER OBJECTIVES

When you complete this chapter, you will be able to do the following:

◇ Describe the factors to consider when making food choices

◇ Summarize the key concepts found in Dietary Guidelines for Americans 2010

◇ Explain the principles applied to eating patterns

◇ Summarize the nutritional requirements needed at different life stages: adolescence, pregnancy, the older years

◇ Discuss the Dietary Reference Intakes necessary for proper nutrition

EATING WELL AND EATING WISELY

In the United States today, nutrition generates more attention than all other health issues. There isn't a day that goes by that we don't hear about what we should or should not eat. We often hear the mantra "You are what you eat." We read the media messages about the "fattening of America." Indeed, researchers have found a strong relationship between the foods we eat and the quality of our lives. While many questions about food and nutrition are still being researched, scientists have determined that what we eat has a strong influence on our health status. Throughout this text, we will talk about how women can protect their health by what they *don't* do, such as not smoking cigarettes, avoiding excessive use of drugs and alcohol, and being physically inactive. We also want to strongly emphasize the positive behaviors women *can* do to protect their health.

Eating well is one of those positive behaviors we can do to protect our health. Perhaps no other health practice has a greater impact on our well-being than eating wisely. As an adult woman, you are faced with many nutritional choices every day. You either plan your meals or select from a menu of some sort every time you eat, day in and day out. In our culture, eating is often a ritual—something that brings us pleasure. Unlike so many women and children worldwide, we do not eat to prevent starvation or to ensure that we survive. Our choices are often not related to nutrition but, instead, related to the emotional pleasure and other factors associated with the meal. Do the *Assess Yourself:* "Determining Your Food Choices" exercise to decide the manner in which you make your food choices.

GUIDELINES TO GOOD EATING

What should an adult woman eat to stay healthy? Years of laboratory research and data collection from many segments of our population have revealed information that can help answer this question. Notably, research from organizations including The American Heart Association and the Nutrition Center at the Harvard School of Public Health indicate the healthiest diets are those which include the following:

1. Fruits and vegetables
2. Whole grains and high-fiber foods

Assess Yourself

Determining Your Food Choices[1]

Look at each of the associated factors below. Consider how much each one of them influences your food choices. As you consider each one, think of it in the role it plays *most* of the time. Circle the number that best reflects your perception of the factor.

Factor	Not significant			Very significant		
Family influences	0	1	2	3	4	5
Weight control	0	1	2	3	4	5
Health	0	1	2	3	4	5
Nutrition knowledge	0	1	2	3	4	5
Convenience/time	0	1	2	3	4	5
Advertisements	0	1	2	3	4	5
Emotions/stress	0	1	2	3	4	5
Peers (friends, coworkers)	0	1	2	3	4	5
Customs/ethnic background	0	1	2	3	4	5
Physical activity level	0	1	2	3	4	5
Food costs	0	1	2	3	4	5

Interpretation: The factors that you scored as 4 or 5 influence your food choices the most. Think about each one of those, and place a "+" or a "−" sign next to it, depending on whether you think the factor is a positive or negative influence on your eating habits and your health. The first step in a mature dietary program is to evaluate the things you eat and why you eat them. Is achieving good health a reason for your food choices? Should you make it a greater priority? Through thoughtful choices, your eating experiences can be rewarding for you.

3. Fish, especially seafood rich in omega-3 fatty acids, consumed twice weekly
4. Saturated fats limited to less than 7 percent and trans fats to less than 1 percent of daily energy needs; cholesterol limited to less than 300 mg per day
5. Fat-free (skim) or low-fat (1 percent) milk and dairy products
6. Small portions and lean meat and poultry
7. Minimal amounts of solid fats and foods with added sugar and salt
8. Alcoholic beverages consumed in moderation (not for everyone)[2]

It is no surprise that another key ingredient for healthy eating doesn't involve food at all. That key ingredient is exercise, and it's become an integral part of several dietary plans and recommendations. Physical activity will be discussed in detail in Chapter 11.

Dietary Guidelines for Americans 2010

With the 1977 release of *Dietary Guidelines for the United States,* the focus of federal guidelines for nutrition shifted from obtaining adequate nutrition to avoiding excessive intake of foods related to chronic diseases. Food industry producers and nutritionists voiced considerable disagreement with shifting the focus away from obtaining adequate nutrition, and eventually, the ensuing controversy led to the voluntary 1980, 1985, and 1990 joint publications of the Dietary Guidelines for Americans by the U.S. Department of Agriculture (USDA) and the U.S. Department of Health and Human Services (HSS). The published guidelines changed from voluntary to mandatory when the U.S. Congress passed the 1990 National Nutrition Monitoring and Related Research Act. This law mandated a review, update, and publication of the Guidelines every 5 years by the USDA and HSS. The most recent guidelines were published in 2010.

It is interesting to note that the 2010 Guidelines have recommendations that are quite similar to those published 40 years ago. The overarching concept in 1977 was to avoid overweight by having Americans consume only as much energy as they expended. The guidelines focused on increasing consumption of complex carbohydrates and "naturally occurring sugars" and reducing consumption of refined and processed sugars, total fat, saturated fat, cholesterol, and sodium. The recommendations advocated for an increased consumption of fruits, vegetables, and whole grains; decreased consumption of refined and processed sugars and foods high in such sugars, foods high in total fat and animal fat, and partially replace saturated fats with polyunsaturated fats, eggs, butterfat, and other high-cholesterol foods, salt and foods high in salt; and, choosing low-fat and non-fat dairy products instead of high-fat dairy products (except for young children).[3] Fast forward to the 2010 Dietary Guidelines and the two overarching concepts are "maintain calorie balance to achieve and sustain a healthy weight" and "focus on nutrient-dense foods and beverages."[4]

Unfortunately, as Americans, we've had a major disconnect between our knowledge and our actions. The prevalence of obesity and overweight are at epidemic levels. No community is immune. We have consumed too few fruits and vegetables, too few whole grains, too little low-fat milk and milk products, and too little fish and seafood. We have consumed too much sugar, solid fats, refined grains, and sodium. And, as a nation, we've been too sedentary.[5] Reversing this trend will take a concerted effort by our communities, our families, and us.

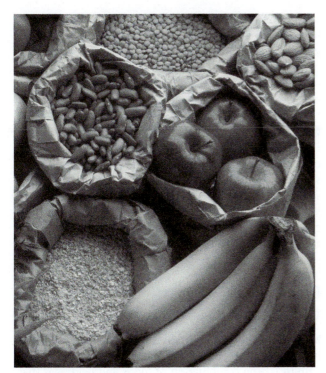

Eat a variety of foods.

Extensive nutrition research guides the recommended changes in the dietary guidelines and over several decades, the changes have been: a shift from the Basic 4 food group to the Food Guide Pyramid (1995) to the MyPyramid Food Guidance System (2005) to MyPlate (2010); new guidelines for safe food handling (2000); the preparation of a policy document (2005); numerical recommendations for intakes of dietary fat and saturated fat (1990); the issuance of separate guidelines for physical activity (2008); the establishment of the Nutrition Evidence Library (NEL) in 2009; and increased rigor and review of the science of nutrition across the forty-year period.[6] The 2010 federal call to action has four major foci:

- "Reduce the incidence and prevalence of overweight and obesity of the U.S. population by reducing overall calorie intake and increasing physical activity
- Shift food intake patterns to a more plant-based diet that emphasizes vegetables, cooked dry beans and peas, fruits, whole grains, nuts, and seeds. In addition, increase the intake of seafood and fat-free and low-fat milk and milk products and consume only moderate amounts of lean meat, poultry, and eggs.
- Significantly reduce intake of foods containing added sugars and solid fats because these dietary components contribute excess calories and few, if any, nutrients. In addition, reduce sodium intake and lower intake of refined grains, especially refined grains that are coupled with added sugar, solid fat, and sodium.
- Meet the 2008 Physical Activity Guidelines for American."[7]

Overweight and obesity are major contributors to morbidity and mortality in the United States and lifestyle factors, e.g. poor dietary behaviors and sedentary behavior, play a significant role. Specific diseases and conditions linked to poor diet include cardiovascular disease (CVD), hypertension, dyslipidemia (elevation of lipids, or fats, in the blood), overweight and obesity, osteoporosis, constipation, diverticular disease, iron deficiency anemia, oral disease, malnutrition, type 2 diabetes, and some cancers.[8] While our behavioral choices are important in reducing the risks of chronic disease, the current environment also plays a significant role by pushing overconsumption of calories and reduced physical activity. Schools, workplaces, foodservice, and food retail businesses impact individuals by the food policies and organizational environments they establish. Do children and adolescents have access to nutrient-dense foods in the school cafeteria? Are employees encouraged to choose water in vending machines? The health disparities among racial/ethnic groups and different socioeconomic groups can be greatly impacted by changes in diet and physical activity. African Americans have greater incidences of blood-pressure related diseases such as hypertension, stroke, and kidney failure. Mexican Americans, American Indians, and African Americans have higher prevalence of overweight and obesity. What role do social norms and values play within the community? Individuals with lower socioeconomic status consume fewer servings of vegetables and fruits. Is this related to cost and availability? Are community gardens and farmers' markets accessible? Are there "food deserts" in your community? What can be done to help reduce health disparities?[9]

These are some of the issues and questions we wrestle with when addressing obesity, overweight, and undernourishment. For the first time since Dietary Guideline reports have been issued, the majority of Americans are overweight or obese, yet undernourished in several key nutrients. Focusing on individual behavior change alone will not help Americans achieve healthy eating and physical activity guidelines. The Dietary Guidelines Advisory Committee (DGAC) recommended that a coordinated strategic plan be developed to find solutions. They highlighted the CDC's ecological (or systems-based) approach that emphasizes all sectors of society such as individuals, families, community groups, physicians, nurses, allied health professionals, public health and policy makers, scientists, business/industry, farmers, and all those impacted by policy and consumer decisions. This ecological approach pertains to all health-related behaviors, with a special focus on nutrition throughout this chapter. Your task is to be part of the solution: you can adopt the healthy eating and physical activity patterns that contribute to healthy living and reduced chronic diseases; you can avoid buying into advertising, social influences, and consumer products that lead to less productive choices; you can advocate for more accessible and less costly healthy food choices; and you can avoid being a statistic. Look for ways to help change the trend that Americans have been following for the past 40 years. This chapter focuses on the nutritional information you will need to be an informed consumer and a change agent for the next decade.

As you read the chapter, focus on a couple of key changes that we all need to consider. First, as you read the following sections, focus on issues related to energy balance and weight management. Nearly two-thirds of all Americans are overweight or obese. According to the DGAC, the average American gains about a pound a year between ages 20 and 60. Even more disturbing is the dramatic increase in overweight and obesity among children and adolescents. The prevalence of obesity and overweight has doubled in children ages 2–11 and tripled in adolescents ages 12–19. The DGAC considers obesity to be the single greatest threat to public health in this century, surpassing tobacco.[10] Second, focus on

why we overconsume calories and live a more sedentary lifestyle. What steps can you take to self-monitor your calorie intake and energy expenditure? What environmental changes can help you reduce consumption and increase physical activity? Third, focus on strategies to help you lower overall energy intake to match your energy needs. What energy-giving foods will you replace with nutrient-dense foods? Fourth, turn your focus to food safety (clean, separate, cook, and chill). What steps can you take to ensure that the foods you consume are safe from bacteria? And, last but not least, focus on the steps that need to occur to reverse the obesity epidemic. What can you, your family, and your community do to change the trend? (See *FYI:* "Reduce Overall Calorie Intake and Increase Physical Activity.")

Balancing Calories to Manage Weight

MyPlate. The Dietary Guidelines supports an "eating pattern" approach to achieving dietary goals. Eating pattern is "the combination of foods and beverages that provide energy and nutrients and constitute an individual's complete dietary intake, on average, over time."[12] The well-known MyPyramid Food Guidance System has been replaced by MyPlate to visually show the need for increases in fruits, vegetables, and whole grains, as well as other nutrient-dense foods. (See Figure 10.1.) Americans consume less than 20 percent of the recommended intake for whole grains, less than 60 percent for vegetables, less than 50 percent for fruits, and less than 60 percent for milk and milk products. These low intakes place Americans at risk for lower than recommended levels of some nutrients, such as vitamin D, calcium, potassium, and dietary fiber.[13]

Know your numbers. How many calories can you consume to achieve caloric intake and expenditure balance? Your age, gender, and physical activity level play a role in determining your caloric needs. For young women, ages 19–30, caloric intake between 1800–2400 calories is based on a sedentary, moderate or active level of physical activity. For women ages 31–50, caloric intake between 1800 and 2200 is based on your level of physical activity. Women who are pregnant and breastfeeding are not included in these numbers. Women who are pregnant need to eat foods high in heme-iron and/or consume iron-rich plant foods or iron-fortified foods with an enhancer of iron absorption, such as vitamin C–rich foods. They should also consume adequate folic acid daily.[14]

Consume smaller portions, especially of high-calorie foods. The top food sources may be energy-dense but not necessarily nutrient-dense. The National Health and Nutrition Examination Survey

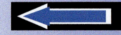

FYI

Reduce Overall Calorie Intake and Increase Physical Activity[11]

Our call to action is to:

- Know our calorie needs. In other words, we need to know how many calories we should consume each day based on our age, sex, and level of physical activity.
- Significantly lower excessive calorie intake from added sugars, solid fats, and some refined grain products.
- Increase our consumption of a variety of vegetables, fruits, and fiber-rich whole grains.
- Avoid sugar-sweetened beverages.
- Consume smaller portions, especially of high-calorie foods.
- Reduce your sodium intake.
- Choose lower-calorie options, especially when eating foods away from home.
- Increase our overall physical activity.
- Have access to improved, easy-to-understand labels listing calorie content and portion size on packaged foods and for restaurant meals (especially fast food restaurants, restaurant chains, and other places where standardized foods are served.

FIGURE 10.1 The USDA MyPlate

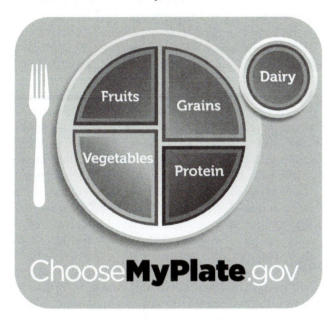

ChooseMyPlate.gov

Health Tips

Calculating Fat Intake

Adult women need an average of 2200 calories per day. This figure, of course, will vary depending on activity level. To find *your* total fat intake recommendation, multiply your daily calories by 0.30 (30 percent) and divide that figure by 9 (the number of calories in a gram of fat). For example:

2200 calories × 0.30 = 660 calories from fat
660 calories ÷ 9 = 73 grams of fat

(NHANES) reported the top five sources of energy consumed by Americans are grain-based desserts (cakes, cookies, doughnuts, granola bars, etc. (139 calories per day); yeast breads (129 calories per day); chicken and chicken mixed dishes (121 calories per day); soda/energy/sports drink (114 calories per day); and pizza (98 calories per day).[15] For children ages 2–3, whole milk (rather than low-fat milk) and, for adults, alcoholic beverages (106 calories per day) are other leading energy sources. These sources of energy have replaced nutrient-dense sources of energy. To reverse the trend in overweight and obesity, we need to move from energy-rich food sources to nutrient-dense food sources.

Significantly lower excessive calorie intake from added sugars. Excessive sugar consumption adds unnecessary calories and replaces nutrient-dense food choices. We should choose and prepare foods and beverages with little added sugar or caloric sweetener. We should avoid sugar-sweetened beverages and look for the different terms for sweeteners on food labels: sucrose (table sugar), fructose, honey, confectioners' sugar, corn syrup, maple syrup, dextrose, molasses, and glucose. The leading food sources of added sugars and percent of added sugars intake in American diets include soda (35.7 percent), grain-based desserts (12.9 percent), fruit drinks (10.5 percent), dairy-based desserts (6.5 percent), and candy (6.1 percent).[16]

Significantly lower excessive calorie intake from solid fats. Our fat consumption is lower than it was 20 years ago, but we are still consuming more solid fats than are needed for good health. Solid fat consumption should

be less than 10 percent of calories per day. Trans fatty acids should be kept as low as possible. We should concentrate on foods containing olive or plant oil and eat foods high in omega-3 fatty acids. Butter and cream should be replaced with margarine high in alpha-linolenic acid. Use the *Health Tips*: "Calculating Fat Intake" activity to determine your recommended fat intake. You can follow these tips for reducing fat in your diet:

- Use less salad dressing (one tablespoon may have 10–11 grams of fat).
- Use olive oil or plant oil when cooking.
- Check food labels for fat content.
- Trim fat from meat, and remove skin from poultry.
- Switch to a lower-fat milk (from whole milk or 2 percent milk)

If we are going to reverse the trend in overweight and obesity, we will need to reduce the consumption of solid fats. They should constitute a much smaller portion of our total caloric intake. Solid fats and added sugars (SoFAS) should constitute about 120 calories in a 1600-calorie pattern to 260 calories in a 2000-calorie pattern. Reducing SoFAS will allow for increases in nutrient dense foods without exceeding caloric intake.

Significantly lower excessive calorie intake from refined grain products. The typical American diet does not include a variety of whole grains, fruits, and vegetables. These products are usually lower in fats and richer in vitamins and minerals and contain dietary fiber. Starches added as filler to thicken foods tend to increase calories with limited/no nutritional value. These starches are particularly problematic when combined with solid fats, added sugars, and sodium. The five primary sources of refined grains in the diets of Americans are yeast breads (25.9 percent), pizza (11.4 percent), grain-based desserts (9.9 percent), tortillas, burritos, and tacos (8.0 percent), and pasta and pasta dishes (6.7 percent). These refined grains should be replaced with whole grains whenever possible. The recommended amount of refined grains is no more than 3 ounces daily.[17]

Choose lower calorie options, especially when eating out. The number of fast food restaurants has increased 147 percent since the late 1970s.[18] (See *FYI:* "What's Changed Since the 1970s?") The number of fast food choices has been paralleled by increased portion sizes in most restaurants. Portion size appears to reflect "value" to many Americans who have little regard for total calories consumed within one sitting. One can be more mindful of total calories by looking at labels listing calorie content and portion size for restaurant meals and beverages.

In addition to sources of energy, we must be mindful of portion control if we are to reverse the current over-consumption trend. And, we need to focus on reducing SoFAS, as they contribute approximately 35 percent of calories consumed by Americans. When saturated fats and cholesterol intakes are increased, intakes of dietary fiber and other nutrients are reduced.

Foods and Food Products to Reduce

Reduce sodium intake. Americans consume an average of 3400 mg of sodium each day, most of which is added to food during processing or food preparation. If only unprocessed foods were chosen and no table salt

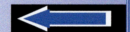

FYI

What's Changed since the 1970s?

Food supply and access have changed dramatically since the 1970s. Note the following:

- Number of fast food restaurants has increased 147 percent
- Portion sizes in restaurants and servings sizes on packaged food have increased
- Number of food items at the supermarket has increased from 10,500 to 47,000, with most contributing to SOFAS, refined grains, and sodium to the diet
- Average child now consumes 365 calories of added sugars and 433 calories of solid fats daily, more than one third of total caloric intake
- Average family spends 45 percent less time preparing food at home

Source: DGAC Report, 2010.

were added, a woman would consume about 500 mg of sodium naturally from the food—more than enough to prevent any dietary deficiency. Approximately 10–15 percent of adults with high blood pressure find their condition exacerbated by sodium sensitivity. The Institute of Medicine has not determined a recommended dietary allowance for sodium so they set Adequate Intake (AI) levels. The adequate intake level for individuals ages 9–50 is 1500 mg of sodium (approximately one teaspoon of edible salt) a day. The tolerable upper intake level is 2300 mg/day. Lower levels have been set for younger children and older adults because their caloric intake is less. In the Dietary Approaches to Stop Hypertension (DASH)—Sodium Trial, blood pressure was lowered as target sodium levels were reduced to 2300 mg/day and lowered further when sodium levels were reduced to 1200 mg/day.[19] Concurrently, potassium-rich foods, such as fruits and vegetables, should be consumed. Women with hypertension, African American women, and middle-aged and older adults should aim to consume no more than 1500 mg of sodium and at least 4700 mg of potassium a day. Fewer than 15 percent of Americans achieve these levels of sodium intake. The top six sources of sodium in the American diet include yeast breads (7.3 percent), chicken and chicken mixed dishes (6.8 percent), pizza (6.3 percent), pasta and pasta dishes (5.1 percent), cold cuts (4.5 percent), and condiments (4.4 percent).[20] Consider making a healthy adjustment to your eating habits by doing the following:

- Read labels of the foods you buy. Be sure to look for other sources of sodium, such as sodium citrate, monosodium glutamate, celery salt, and so forth.
- Experiment with herbs and spices to add flavor to food.
- Prepare your own salad dressings and sauces.
- Reduce the number of "shakes" you use to salt food.

Reduce solid fats. The body makes enough saturated fatty acids to meet the physiological and structural needs; therefore, we have no dietary need for saturated fatty acids. Limiting intake of fatty foods reduces the chance of being overweight or obese, developing heart disease, stroke, or diabetes, and suffering other health consequences of a high-fat diet. The 2010 DGAC states that solid fats need to be substantially reduced to reverse the current trend in overweight and obesity. The typical American total diet includes 35 percent of calories from SOFAS, and the recommendation is less than 10 percent of total caloric intake. Solid fats should be replaced with monounsaturated and/or polyunsaturated fatty acids that are associated with lower blood cholesterol. The leading solid fats and percent of solid fat intake of the American diet include grain-based desserts, including cakes, cookies, pies, doughnuts, and granola bars (10.8 percent), pizza (9.1 percent), regular cheese (7.6 percent), sausage, franks, bacon, and ribs (7.1 percent), and fried white potatoes, including French fries and hash browns (4.8 percent).[21] Concentrate on foods containing olive or plant oil, and eat foods high in omega-3 fatty acids. Focus on reducing solid fats by replacing butter with vegetable oils rich in monounsaturated fatty acids (canola, olive, safflower) and polyunsaturated fatty acids (soybean, corn, and cottonseed). Choose low-fat or fat-free milk and lean meats to reduce saturated fat intake.

Reduce dietary cholesterol. Individuals should consume less than 300 mg of cholesterol per day. Average cholesterol intake by women is 240 mg of cholesterol per day. The body produces sufficient cholesterol to meet physiological and structural functions, so we have no need to consume foods that contain cholesterol. Cholesterol is found only in animal products. The major sources of cholesterol in the American diet are eggs and egg dishes, chicken and chicken dishes, beef and beef dishes, and all types of burgers.[22] Women at high risk for CVD can benefit from consuming less than 200 mg of cholesterol per day, but the benefits of reducing saturated fat and trans fatty acids is greater.

Reduce calories from solid fats and added sugars (SOFAS). Solid fats and added sugars together contribute a significant portion of the calories consumed in the American diet. On average, 800 calories a day come from SoFAS. These calories are energy rich but not nutrient dense. As the amount of SoFAS increases in the diet, we tend to not meet the nutrient requirements of dietary fiber and essential vitamins and minerals and stay within the caloric limits per day. SoFAS should be reduced to no more than 5–15 percent of the total caloric intake per day. Focus on eating nutrient-dense foods, cooking with vegetable oils, and not adding sugar, and consume fewer and smaller portions of SoFAS.[23]

Reduce refined grains. The process of refining grains to give them a finer texture reduces vitamins, minerals, and dietary fiber. Products are then enriched to add back iron and B vitamins (thiamin, riboflavin, niacin, folic acid), but not all vitamins, minerals, and dietary fiber are recaptured. The average American consumes 6.3 ounces of refined grain daily, considerably more than the recommended amount of less than 3 ounces per day.[24] And, refined grain products are usually high in SoFAS (yeast breads, grain-based desserts and tortillas, burritos, and tacos), which adds unnecessary calories to the daily diet. We need to focus on replacing refined grains with whole grains so that half or more of our dietary fiber comes from whole grains.

Reduce alcohol consumption. For some, eating out or "chilling out" at home are also associated with having a few alcoholic drinks to relax. Alcohol (7 kcal/g) supplies "empty" calories that are devoid of nutrients, can be addicting, and contribute to annual violent crimes and serious automobile accidents. Alcohol contributes to five of the ten leading causes of death in the United States and to a variety of vitamin disorders because it interferes with vitamin absorption. For instance, alcohol may block the absorption of folate, an important nutrient necessary both for proper fetal development and the building of DNA.[25] One drink consists of 12 ounces of beer, 5 ounces of wine, or 1.5 ounces of 80-proof distilled spirits such as gin, vodka, whiskey, or other hard liquor. Moderate alcohol is defined as up to 1 drink per day for women. Heavy or high-risk drinking for women is the consumption of more than 3 drinks on one day or more than 7 drinks per week. Alcohol is not recommended for pregnant women or women who breastfeed. For women who are trying to manage weight, a reduction in alcohol consumption is very beneficial.

Foods and Nutrients to Increase

Increase vegetable and fruit intake. The typical American diet does not include a variety of grains, fruits, and vegetables. First, increasing the consumption of these foods can accomplish a number of objectives. Fruits, vegetables, and whole grains are generally low in fats, are rich in vitamins and minerals, and contain dietary fiber. To increase fiber intake, eat fewer processed foods, eat the skins on fruits and vegetables, and eat a variety of foods. Second, increased consumption of these foods is associated with reduced risk of some chronic diseases such as CVD and some types of cancer. Third, increased consumption of these foods can reduce caloric intake while satiating appetite. The majority of these calories should come from whole fruits and vegetables rather than juices.[26] You can select vegetables from all five subgroups (dark green, orange, legumes, starchy vegetables, and other vegetables) several times a week. Two cups of fruit and 2½ cups of vegetables per day are recommended for a 2000-calorie intake.

Increase whole grains. The entire seed, usually called the kernel, comprises a whole grain. If the seed is crushed or cracked, it must retain the proportions of the entire kernel to be considered whole grain. Whole grains can be a single food (popcorn, brown rice, flax seed) or an ingredient in foods (cereals, breads). The goal for healthy eating includes eating the equivalent of 3 ounces of whole grains, rather than the current less than 1 ounce per day. We need to increase our whole grain consumption to over half of all total grain consumption.[27]

Increase milk and milk product consumption. Milk and milk products are sources of calcium, potassium, and vitamin D. Milk and milk product consumption are associated with increased bone health in children and reduced CVD and type 2 diabetes and lower blood pressure in adults.[28] The recommended amount for adults is 3 cups per day of fat-free or low-fat milk and milk products. Cheese is a primary source of milk product consumption, and it would be beneficial to choose reduced fat or fat free cheese to reduce solid fat intake and calories. Replacing cheese with yogurt and milk improves intake of potassium, vitamin A, and vitamin D and reduces intake of sodium, cholesterol, and saturated fatty acids.[29]

Increase oils while reducing solid fats. Oils should replace solid fats whenever possible. Oils are concentrated calories and should be used in small amounts. Replacing saturated fats with unsaturated fats can have a positive impact on both total and DLD blood cholesterol. You can replace chicken and beef with seafood or unsalted nuts, butter with soft margarine, and butter in cooking with vegetable oils.

Positive effect of dietary change. Increasing the intake of fruits, vegetables, milk and milk products, and seafood can ensure that adults are meeting their needs for potassium, dietary fiber, calcium, and vitamin D. For some adults, it can also ensure adequate levels of iron, folate, and vitamin B12. Unless these changes are made within the diet, supplements may be needed to meet the recommended daily requirements. Potassium can lower blood pressure, reduce the risk of developing kidney stones, and decrease bone loss. Dietary fiber is important for increasing a sense of fullness and for promoting healthy laxation. Dietary fiber is associated with reduced risk of cardiovascular disease, obesity, and type 2 diabetes. Calcium and vitamin D are important for bone health and reducing the risk of osteoporosis. Sufficient iron and folate are important for women who may become or are pregnant, and foods fortified with vitamin B12 are important for adults aged 50 and older who have trouble absorbing the vitamin naturally.

Recommended Dietary Allowances

The Recommended Dietary Allowances (RDAs) are standards set by the Food and Nutrition Board of the National Academy of Sciences. The Dietary Reference Intakes (DRIs) further refine some of the RDA standards to improve clarity of dietary needs. Specific recommendations are incorporated in the following sections with reference to each nutrient.

NECESSARY NUTRIENTS

When we eat, we often give little thought to the real purpose of food in our bodies. Generally we know we are hungry or that we are full. We tend to make our food choices based on feelings of hunger and the availability of the foods we prefer to eat. Little thought is given to the role that food will play once it gets into our bodies. Once consumed, the food enters our digestive tract to be broken down into nutrients that are absorbed into the bloodstream so that they can be distributed to the body's cells. The nutrients come in many forms, each form serving specific roles in nourishing human beings by providing energy and materials for building body parts and regulating necessary chemical processes in the body.[30]

Carbohydrates

Carbohydrates are energy sources for the body. Each gram of carbohydrate yields about 4 calories. (See *FYI:* "Carbohydrates.") Both adults and children need to consume at least 130 grams of carbohydrates each day, the amount needed to provide enough glucose for the human brain to function. However, the majority of Americans consume much more.[31] Carbohydrates can be found in two forms: simple carbohydrates and complex carbohydrates. The simplest of the carbohydrates are the **monosaccharides**—the simple sugars. Glucose is a simple sugar and is the primary source of energy for body cells. The liver converts sugars from other foods to glucose, which provides immediate energy to the body. Fructose, a common sugar that comes mostly from fruit and honey, is sometimes added to certain soft drinks. Guidelines recommend that no more than 5–15 percent of total daily calories come from "added" sugars such as those found in candy, sodas, or pastries and solid fats. Fructose goes straight to the liver after it enters the small intestine and is quickly metabolized. Galactose is a monosaccharide that is similar to glucose. It is not found in the food we eat; rather, it occurs following digestion of lactose.

Disaccharides are also simple sugars, but they are formed by the combination of two monosaccharides. The most common disaccharides are sucrose, maltose, and lactose. Sucrose is ordinary table sugar made from sugarcane, sugar beets, maple sugar, or honey. Maltose is formed when grains are allowed to form malt. Lactose is a disaccharide found in milk products. As you may already have determined, disaccharides will take longer to be useful to the body than glucose because they must be broken down to glucose before they can be used by the cells. Therefore, a woman who is competing in athletics would find fruit to be a quicker form of energy than a candy bar.

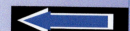

Dietary Guidelines for Americans 2010[32]

Key Recommendations of Foods and Food Components to Increase

- Increase vegetable and fruit intake.
- Eat a variety of vegetables, especially dark-green and red and orange vegetables and beans and peas.
- Consume at least half of all grains as whole grains. Increase whole-grain intake by replacing refined grains with whole grains.
- Increase intake of fat-free and low-fat milk and milk products, such as milk, yogurt, cheese, or soymilk.
- Choose a variety of protein foods, which include seafood, lean meat and poultry, eggs, beans and peas, soy products, and unsalted nuts and seeds.
- Increase the amount and variety of seafood consumed by choosing seafood in place of some meat and poultry.
- Replace protein foods that are higher in solid fats with choices that are lower in solid fats and calories and/or are sources of oils.
- Use oils to replace solid fats where possible.
- Choose foods that provide more potassium, dietary fiber, calcium, and vitamin D, which are nutrients of concern in American diets. These foods include vegetables, fruits, whole grains, and milk and milk products.

Complex carbohydrates are also known as starches. Whereas simple carbohydrates are known as monosaccharides and disaccharides, complex carbohydrates are **polysaccharides** because they are composed of numerous monosaccharide units. Some starches have as many as 3000 glucose units.[33] Complex carbohydrates are found in foods containing grains and in certain vegetables, including potatoes.

Recall that the current DRI recommends that children and adults consume at least 130 grams of carbohydrates each day. If a woman does not consume enough carbohydrates to meet the energy requirements of her body, for example, during long-term periods of starvation, her muscles, heart, liver, and other vital organs will begin to break down into amino acids, a metabolic process that is not healthy for a woman's body. Some of these amino acids will further convert to glucose to give energy to her body. Lack of carbohydrates will also interfere with fat metabolism resulting in the formation of **ketones.** Ketones may disrupt the acid–base balance of the body, a condition known as ketosis. It is, therefore, important that a woman consume sufficient amounts of carbohydrates to prevent energy supply problems in her body.[34]

Women also should be aware of **nutrient density** when making carbohydrate food choices. Foods that are high in energy value but contain few other nutrients lack nutrient density. These "empty calorie" foods do not contribute to a well-balanced diet. Soft drinks and sugary candies are examples of empty calorie foods. Alcohol is another substance that supplies the body with energy calories, 7 calories per gram of alcohol, but no nutritional value.

The **glycemic index (GI)** is an alternative system for classifying carbohydrate-containing foods, rather than as "simple" and "complex" carbohydrates. The GI is based on how foods affect the blood sugar level after a meal is consumed. The GI is calculated by comparing the blood glucose response to ingestion of 50 grams of available carbohydrate from a test food with that of a reference food (either glucose or white bread). Several studies have demonstrated efficacy of a low-GI diet in reducing obesity. Fruits, nuts, whole grains, and legumes tend to have low GI while refined grains, ready-to-eat cereals, and starchy vegetables tend to have high GI. Long-term benefits of a low-GI diet appear to be higher HDL (high-density lipoprotein, or "good") cholesterol, lower triglycerides (the chemical form of most fats in food and in the body), and less insulin demand.[35]

Protein

Proteins (4 kcal/g) serve very important functions in the body. Proteins build and repair body tissue including the blood, help regulate body processes, and provide some fuel for body cells.[36] Proteins are made from amino acids joined by chemical bonds. The proteins consumed from the food we eat are broken down into amino acids in the body and become the proteins needed to accomplish the tasks just listed. The human body uses twenty or so different amino acids. Nine of these amino acids are called *essential* amino acids because they must be consumed in the foods we eat. The remaining amino acids are referred to as *nonessential* because they can be manufactured by the other amino acids we consume.

Proteins in our diet come from two main categories. *Complete protein* comes from animal tissue. It is called complete because the food contains all the amino acids necessary to either make protein or make other necessary amino acids in our bodies. *Incomplete protein* is found in foods that come from plants. It is possible for a woman to gain the appropriate number of amino acids from combining one or more plant sources. For example, beans and rice each contain incomplete proteins, but when eaten together they complement each other by providing an amino acid from each that the other food lacks. Beans eaten with a flour tortilla would also provide all the essential amino acids.

How much protein does an individual need each day? Currently, dietary researchers disagree on the amount needed for optimal health, and answers to that question are still emerging. For most individuals, consuming 20–25 percent of daily calories in the form of protein may have health benefits, particularly if the protein comes from sources such as lean meat or fish or from those such as legumes.[37]

In recent years, much media attention has been focused on the theorized weight benefits from the consumption of high-protein diets. However, other attention has focused on whether or not high-protein diets may cause long-term harm to the heart and other organs. To receive the most benefit from the protein you eat while lowering your potential risk for illnesses such as colon cancer, it is best to limit your consumption of protein from sources such as red meats and processed meats while increasing your protein intake from lean meats, seafood (rich in omega-3 fatty acids as well as protein) and cooked dry beans and peas (rich in dietary fiber as well as vegetable protein).[38]

Fats

Fat is perhaps the most talked about but the least understood of all the nutrients. Fat is perceived as the villain among the food nutrients. It is linked with heart disease, cancer, and obesity. The concern may be somewhat valid because Americans have one of the fattiest diets in the world. In general, we consume more than 33 percent of our calories from fat. The recommended total fat intake is 20 to 30 percent of total calories, and it should be derived mostly from oils within a nutrient-rich diet. To achieve the recommended goal of less than 10 percent of calories from saturated fat, it is more likely to be achieved if total fat intake is less than 30 percent.[39] We are continually trying to assess the relative risks and benefits from fat consumption. Though their diets are high in fat, the people on the island of Crete have very low rates of heart disease. This is because most of their dietary fat comes from olive oil, a monounsaturated fat that tends to reduce levels of LDL (low-density lipoprotein) cholesterol and boost levels of HDL cholesterol. Eskimos also have high-fat diets, but their levels of heart disease are also low due to their intake of fish rich in omega-3 fatty acids. These fatty acids, found in salmon and mackerel (as well as canola and soybean oil), lower both LDL and triglyceride levels in the blood.[40]

Dietary fats come in many forms. Collectively they are referred to as *lipids*. Lipids contain carbon, hydrogen, and oxygen atoms. The simplest forms of lipids are the fatty acids. Fatty acids are joined together to form the fat molecule. Fats are a highly concentrated form of food energy, supplying 9–11 calories per gram (compared to the 4 calories in each gram of carbohydrate and 4 calories per gram of protein). Some lipids, such as butter and lard, are solid at room temperature. Other lipids, such as cooking oils, are liquid at room temperature. Whether or not a lipid is solid or liquid depends on how many hydrogen atoms there are on the molecule. A *saturated fat* is composed of fatty acid molecules that contain all the hydrogen atoms they can carry. All of the carbons are attached to each other with single bonds. Butter, milk fat, lard, and meat fat are examples of saturated fats. Palm oil and coconut oil are also saturated fats. Saturated fats and *trans*-fatty acid intake should be minimized.

Unsaturated fatty acids are classified according to the number of pairs of hydrogen atoms that are missing, leaving two carbon atoms attached by a double bond rather than a single bond. *Monounsaturated fats,* such as olive oil, peanut oil, and canola oil, lack only one pair of hydrogen atoms. Corn oil, safflower oil, and sesame oils lack two or more pairs of hydrogen atoms and are therefore said to be *polyunsaturated.* Unsaturated fats are generally liquid at room temperature. Both polyunsaturated and monounsaturated fats have been suggested as "healthy fats." Unsaturated fats, including omega-3 fatty acids from seafood sources, should constitute the majority of all fats consumed. However, limiting all fats contributes to healthier living. (See *Viewpoint:* "Where Is the Trans Fat?")

Not only are fats a source of energy in the body, they serve other purposes in our diet as well. Fats transport one of the essential fatty acids, linoleic acid, around the body. Fat-soluble vitamins A, D, E, and K are also carried by the fats in the bloodstream. To some degree, fats help contribute to our sense of fullness when we eat because fats take longer to leave the stomach than other nutrients. Fat is important for proper growth, development, and maintenance of good health. Fat also provides taste, consistency, and stability.

Vitamins

Until the beginning of the twentieth century, scientists believed the only things necessary for a good diet were proteins, carbohydrates, and fats, but studies in the late 1800s suggested that other elements in our foods were essential for health and preventing diseases thought to be infectious, such as beriberi and scurvy. The first of these elements to be identified was what we now know as vitamin B1, whose chemical composition included an "amine"; thus the word "vitamine" was created meaning "an amine needed for life."[41]

Vitamins are nutrients needed by the body to perform unique functions. These nutrients enable the body to use carbohydrates, proteins, and fats to build and maintain the tissues in the body. We generally need less than a gram of the various vitamins each day. Too

Viewpoint

Where Is the Trans Fat?

Because of all the concern about saturated fats, most fast-food chains and food manufacturers have switched from using beef fats and tropical oils to using vegetable oil. Vegetable oil is liquid. To give it a firmer consistency and reduce the likelihood of spoilage, food manufacturers pump hydrogen into the vegetable oil, producing a "hydrogenated oil." This oil is referred to as **trans fat** or *trans-fatty acid.* Trans fat has been associated with increasing the LDL (bad) cholesterol levels in the blood, just as saturated fats will. Trans fat has also been associated with *lowering* HDL (good) cholesterol. Trans-fatty acids have no known health benefits, and the safe level has not been established. You can get an idea of how much trans fat a food contains by reading the label. One clue is found in the list of ingredients. If you see something like "partially hydrogenated canola oil," you can count on that being a trans fat. If the label gives you the amount of other fats, such as saturated, polyunsaturated, and monounsaturated, add the figures for those fats and subtract them from the amount of total fat stated on the label.

Trans fats and saturated fats raise LDL cholesterol. Therefore, in an effort to provide better information to consumers, manufacturers are now required to list trans-fatty acids, or trans fat, on the Nutrition Facts panel of conventional foods and some dietary supplements. Trans fats are now listed on a separate line, immediately below saturated fats. Products high in trans fats include some margarines, shortenings, crackers, candies, baked goods, cookies, fried foods, salad dressings, and some energy bars. Trans fats **do not** need to be listed if the total fat in a food is less than 0.5 gram per serving. If trans fats are not listed, a footnote will state that the food is "not a significant source of trans fat." The Nutrition Facts panel does not have a percent Daily Value for trans fat because the FDA could not establish a Daily Value. Therefore, trans fat will be listed only as a gram amount.

Select two packaged foods from your food shelf or look at two items the next time you go shopping. What percentage of calories come from fat? from trans fat? Which of the two products contains the healthiest amount of fat? How might you reduce the trans fats and saturated fats in your diet?

---

often the term *trace nutrients* is misunderstood. Eating a variety of foods is important to ensuring that adequate vitamins are ingested. Thirteen vitamins are known to benefit human beings. Four of these vitamins (A, D, E, and K) are *fat-soluble;* that is, they are absorbed into and carried through the body along with dietary fat. The other nine vitamins are water-soluble. Because *water-soluble* vitamins dissolve in water, women should keep in mind that large amounts of these vitamins can be lost during food preparation. For example, steaming or boiling broccoli until it is light green and very soft will result in much of the vitamin C being left behind in the pan. For more information on vitamins, see Tables 10.1 and 10.2.

Antioxidants   Vitamin C, vitamin E, and beta-carotene are known as **antioxidants.** These compounds are believed to provide a defense against cancer and heart disease. We have known for some time now that our body cells use oxygen to "burn" the fuels inside them. As with any burning process, an "exhaust" will be given off as a by-product. This waste product comes in the form of oxidants, or *free radicals*. It is believed that these free radicals combine easily with cholesterol to damage the blood vessels, or with other chemicals to create the carcinogenic effects of cancer formation. The role of

antioxidants is a recent discovery, and the medical community has reported mixed reviews about the efficacy of antioxidants. Physicians suggest that women should consume fruits and vegetables rich in these antioxidants (e.g., beans, berries, apples) to reduce the likelihood of certain cancers and heart disease. So far we do not have any studies that conclusively demonstrate that taking these antioxidant vitamins in pill form will lead to a healthier life,[42] but it appears there is a protective effect if the antioxidants come from natural food sources. One research study, examining whether large doses of the antioxidants ascorbic acid (vitamin C), vitamin E, and beta-carotene lowered incidents of heart attacks, strokes, and related problems in women at high risk for cardiovascular disease, concluded that supplementation with these vitamins did not lower the women's risks for serious cardiovascular issues.[43] At this point it appears that consuming the appropriate foods and taking supplements are not harmful and are likely to be protective of our health.

Minerals

Like vitamins, minerals are needed in relatively small amounts. There are seven minerals included in the RDAs. Calcium, magnesium, and phosphorus are

TABLE 10.1 The Fat-Soluble Vitamins, Their Functions, Deficiency Conditions, Food Sources, and Dietary Reference Intakes (DRIs)

VITAMIN	MAJOR FUNCTIONS	DEFICIENCY SYMPTOMS	PEOPLE MOST AT RISK	DIETARY SOURCES	DRI	TOXICITY SYMPTOMS
Vitamin A (retinoids) and provitamin A (carotenoids)	Promote vision: light and color; Promote healthy skin, bone growth, and tooth development; Prevent drying of skin and eyes; Promote immune system health; Promote cell division	Night blindness; Xerophthalmia (dry eye); Poor growth; Diarrhea; Blindness in children; Dry skin (keratinization)	People in poverty, especially preschool children (still very rare in the United States)	Vitamin A: Liver, Fortified milk, Cheese, Cream, Butter, Eggs; Provitamin A: Sweet potatoes, Spinach greens, Carrots, Cantaloupe, Apricots, Broccoli, Winter squash, Pumpkin	Females 600–700 micrograms; Pregnant women 750–770 micrograms	Nausea, irritability, hair loss, skin changes, pain in bones, fetal malformations
D (chole- and ergocalciferol)	Facilitates absorption of calcium and phosphorus; Maintains optimal calcification of bone	Rickets in children; Osteomalacia in adults	Breast-fed infants, elderly shut-ins	Vitamin D–fortified milk; Fish oils; Sardines; Salmon; Egg yolks; Liver; Skin can make vitamin D when exposed to sunlight	Females 5–15 micrograms; Pregnant women 5 micrograms*	Growth and mental retardation, kidney damage, calcium deposits in soft tissue, weight loss
E (tocopherols, tocotrienols)	Acts as an antioxidant: prevents breakdown of vitamin A and unsaturated fatty acids; protects cell walls	Hemolysis of red blood cells; Nerve destruction	People with poor fat absorption (still very rare or impossible without starvation)	Vegetable oils; Some greens; Some fruits; Wheat germ; Nuts and seeds	Females 11–15 milligrams alpha-tocopherol equivalents; Pregnant women 15 milligrams alpha-tocopherol equivalents	Muscle weakness, headaches, fatigue, nausea, inhibition of vitamin K metabolism
K (phyllo- and menaquinone)	Helps form prothrombin and other factors for blood clotting	Hemorrhage, excessive bleeding	People taking antibiotics for months at a time (still quite rare)	Green, leafy vegetables; Liver; Milk	Females 60–90 micrograms; Pregnant women 15–90 micrograms	Anemia and jaundice

TABLE 10.2 The Water-Soluble Vitamins, Their Functions, Deficiency Conditions, and Food Sources Vitamin Toxicity

VITAMIN	MAJOR FUNCTIONS	DEFICIENCY SYMPTOMS	PEOPLE MOST AT RISK	DIETARY SOURCES	RDA OR ESADDI	TOXICITY
Thiamin (Vitamin B1)	Coenzyme involved with enzymes in carbohydrate metabolism nerve function	Beriberi, nervous tingling poor coordination, edema, heart changes, weakness	People with alcoholism, people in poverty,	Sunflower seed, pork, whole and enriched grains, dried beans, brewer's yeast	1.1–1.4 milligrams	None possible from food
Riboflavin (B2)	Coenzymes involved in energy metabolism; normal vision and skin health	Inflammation of mouth and tongue, cracks at corners of the mouth, eye disorders	Possibly people on certain medications if no dairy products consumed	Milk, mushrooms spinach, liver, enriched, grains and cereals	1.1–1.6 milligrams	None reported
Niacin (B3)	Coenzymes involved in energy metabolism, fat synthesis, fat breakdown, skin health	Pellagra, diarrhea, dermatitis, dementia	People in severe poverty for which corn is dominant food, people with alcoholism	Mushrooms, bran, tuna, salmon, chicken, meat, peanuts, enriched grains, peanut butter	14–17 milligrams	Flushing of skin at >100 milligrams
Pantothenic acid (B5)	Coenzyme involved in energy metabolism, fat synthesis, fat breakdown	Using an antagonist causes tingling in hands fatigue, headache, nausea	People with alcoholism	Mushrooms, liver, broccoli, eggs; most foods have some	5–7 milligrams	None
Biotin	Coenzyme involved in glucose production, fat synthesis	Dermatitis, sore tongue, anemia, depression	People with alcoholism	Cheese, egg yolks, cauliflower, peanut butter, liver; many foods have some	25–30 micrograms	Unknown
Vitamin B6, pyridoxine and other forms	Coenzyme involved in protein metabolism, neurotransmitter synthesis, hemoglobin synthesis, many other functions	Headache, anemia, convulsions, nausea, vomiting, flaky skin, sore tongue	Adolescent and adult women, people on certain medications, people with alcoholism	Animal protein foods, spinach, broccoli, bananas, salmon, sunflower seeds	1.3–2 milligrams	Nerve destruction at doses >100 milligrams
Folate	Coenzyme involved in DNA synthesis and making new cells	Megatoblastic anemia, inflammation of tongue, diarrhea, poor growth, mental disorders	People with alcoholism, pregnant women, people taking certain medications	Green leafy vegetables, orange juice, organ meats, sprouts, sunflower seeds; added to most refined grains	400–600 micrograms	None; nonprescription vitamin dosage is controlled by FDA
Vitamin B12 (cobalamins)	Coenzyme involved in folate metabolism, nerve function	Macrocytic anemia, poor nerve function	Elderly, because of poor absorption, vegans	Animal foods, especially organ meats, oysters, clams (B12 not naturally in plant foods)	2.4 micrograms	None
Vitamin C (ascorbic acid)	Immune system protection, iron absorption, protein metabolism	Scurvy: poor wound healing, pinpoint hemorrhages, bleeding gums, edema	People with alcoholism, elderly men living alone	Citrus fruits, strawberries, broccoli, greens, peppers, tomatoes	75 milligrams	Doses >1–2 grams cause diarrhea and can alter some diagnostic tests

macrominerals, or major minerals. Four other minerals, iron, zinc, iodine, and selenium, are trace minerals. We obtain minerals from both plant and animal sources. Minerals obtained from animal sources possess a greater level of *bioavailability;* that is, they become more readily available to a woman's body once they are consumed. Plant sources tend to have compounds that bind the minerals, thus reducing mineral bioavailability.

Minerals serve a variety of purposes within the body. No doubt you are familiar with the role of calcium in developing bone, and you know that iron helps to build good red blood cells. But other minerals serve many other very important functions. A healthy water balance requires appropriate levels of sodium, potassium, calcium, and phosphorus. Sodium, potassium, and calcium influence the movement of nerve impulses, and iodine is a key ingredient in the hormone thyroxin. Refer to Table 10.3 for more information about the major minerals. Two minerals of specific interest to women are calcium and iron, and these are discussed in the following sections.

Calcium   About 99 percent of the calcium in the body is found in bone and about 90 percent of adult bone mass is acquired by age 18 in girls. The remaining 1 percent is used to stimulate muscle contractions and nerve impulses, and to regulate blood clotting.[44] For the past decade, women have become increasingly more aware of their calcium needs. Yet, Americans still consume less than 60 percent of the recommended intake of milk and milk products. And, since nearly 90 percent of adult bone mass is acquired by age 18 in girls, adequate calcium intake at younger ages is essential. Medical research has uncovered a considerable amount of information about *osteoporosis,* an age-related condition characterized by demineralization of bone. In the United States, osteoporosis is a serious threat to the health of approximately 44 million Americans. Almost 34 million Americans are estimated to have low bone mass, and more than 10 million presently have osteoporosis. Of the 10 million who have the disease, 80 percent are women.[45] Menopause and aging increase the risk of developing osteoporosis, but it is not an inevitable disease of old age. In fact, it is now known that health behaviors can greatly reduce the risk of developing osteoporosis.

Osteoporosis is perceived as a disease that afflicts old people. Research indicates, however, that the quality of a woman's bones in old age, in the absence of risk factors, is related to what a woman is able to do for herself. The development of bone mineral density (BMD) is related to calcium intake over the woman's lifetime. Specifically, it appears that the greatest influence comes during childhood and the elderly years. The intake of calcium is very important in preventing osteoporosis, but other factors also affect the development of this disease.

A woman who has a family history of osteoporosis, drinks alcohol, smokes cigarettes, and/or has an eating disorder is at a greater risk for osteoporosis. If she has a diet that is low in calcium, she is at even greater risk. Although dairy products are good sources of calcium, there are other ways of getting calcium if the woman is lactose intolerant or if she does not like dairy products.[46] (See *FYI:* "Calcium Sources" for additional calcium sources.) Additional coverage of osteoporosis can be found in Chapter 15.

Iron   Humans need 10–12 mg of iron daily to manufacture **hemoglobin.** Hemoglobin is found in our red blood cells and is responsible for transporting oxygen to, and carbon dioxide away from, the body cells. Iron also helps build certain enzymes and proteins in the body. Because of the blood loss associated with menstruation, women have a greater need for iron during their reproductive years. A premenopausal woman may need as much as 18 mg/day, and even more if her menstrual flow is heavy while a postmenopausal woman needs only 8 mg daily. A typical adult diet contains 5–7 mg of iron per 1000 calories.[47] Women who consume fewer than 2000 calories per day may have trouble meeting RDA needs through their diet alone. Therefore, it is necessary for a woman to carefully evaluate the foods she eats to ensure sufficient iron consumption. There are two forms of iron found in our diet. **Heme iron** is found in animal tissue (e.g., in red meat) and is more rapidly absorbed than **nonheme iron,** which is found in plant sources such as spinach and grains. The amount of dietary iron will vary depending on the types and amounts of the various iron-containing foods. Not all of the dietary iron will be absorbed by the body, however. Many diet-related factors tend to interfere with absorption. Zinc competes with iron for absorption. Caffeine has a negative effect on iron

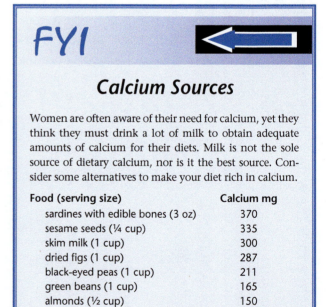

FYI

Calcium Sources

Women are often aware of their need for calcium, yet they think they must drink a lot of milk to obtain adequate amounts of calcium for their diets. Milk is not the sole source of dietary calcium, nor is it the best source. Consider some alternatives to make your diet rich in calcium.

Food (serving size)	Calcium mg
sardines with edible bones (3 oz)	370
sesame seeds (¼ cup)	335
skim milk (1 cup)	300
dried figs (1 cup)	287
black-eyed peas (1 cup)	211
green beans (1 cup)	165
almonds (½ cup)	150

TABLE 10.3 Water and Major Minerals

NAME	MAJOR FUNCTIONS	DEFICIENCY SYMPTOMS	PEOPLE MOST AT RISK	RDA OR MINIMUM REQUIREMENT	NUTRIENT-DENSE DIETARY SOURCES	RESULTS OF TOXICITY
Water	Medium for chemical reactions, removal of waste products, perspiration to cool the body	Thirst, muscle weakness, poor endurance, increased core temperature, decreased plasma volume	Infants with a fever, elderly persons in nursing homes	1.0–1.5 milliliter/kcal of energy expended*	As such and in foods	Seldom occurs and usually in those with mental disorders
Sodium	A major ion of the extracellular fluid; nerve impulse transmission	Muscle cramps	People who severely restrict sodium to lower blood pressure (250–500 mg/day)	500 mg/day	Table salt, processed foods	High blood pressure in susceptible individuals
Potassium	A major ion of intracellular fluid; nerve impulse transmission; fluid and electrolyte balance; muscle contraction	Unlikely to occur, irregular heartbeat, loss of appetite, muscle cramps	People who use potassium-wasting diuretics or have poor diets, as seen in poverty and alcoholism	750 mg/day	Spinach, squash, bananas, orange juice, other vegetables and fruits, milk and yogurt	Slowing of the heartbeat; raised blood pressure, paralysis
Calcium	Bone and tooth strength; blood clotting; nerve impulse transmission; muscle contractions; cell regulation	Poor intake increases the risk for osteoporosis	Women in general, especially those who constantly restrict their energy intake, consume few dairy products, or smoke	1000–1200 mg/day	Dairy products, canned fish, leafy vegetables, tofu, fortified orange juice	Very high intakes may cause kidney stones in susceptible people, poor mineral absorption in general, muscle rigor
Phosphorus	Bone and tooth strength; part of various metabolic compounds; major ion of intracellular fluid	Probably none; poor bone maintenance is a possibility	Elderly persons consuming very nutrient-poor diets; possibly total vegetarians and people with alcoholism	750–1200 mg/day	Dairy products, processed foods, fish, soft drinks	Hampers bone health in people with kidney failure; poor bone mineralization if calcium intakes are low
Magnesium	Bone strength; any enzyme function using ATP; nerve and heart function	Weakness, muscle pain, poor heart function	Women in general, people on thiazide diuretics	Women: 280–300 mg/day	Wheat bran, green vegetables, nuts, beans, milk	Causes weakness in people with kidney failure

*Dietary Reference Intakes (DRIs): Recommended Intakes for Individuals, Vitamins. Food and Nutrition Board, Institute of Medicine, National Academies, 2009.

absorption, whereas vitamin C has a positive effect on absorption. Substances called tannins found in tea interfere with iron absorption. If a woman wants to have good iron levels, red meat should *not* be completely avoided. Foods rich in vitamin C should be consumed to take advantage of nonheme iron sources. During pregnancy, iron supplements are a must because a woman will almost double her blood volume to accommodate the growing fetus.

Water Often overlooked as a nutrient, water is, without a doubt, our most important nutrient. Depending on our fat stores, we can live for extended periods of time without foods that supply vitamins, minerals, proteins, fats, and energy, but we can expect to live only a few days without water. Most of your body is composed of water—more than 60 percent of the body's weight. Water serves a number of very important functions in the body.

- Water helps to regulate the temperature of the body. Water in the blood collects heat generated by the body and transports it to the surface of the skin. Heat energy is taken from the body as perspiration evaporates.
- Water is necessary for many of the chemical reactions that take place in the body.
- Water serves as a vehicle for removing waste products from the body. Cellular by-products are picked up by the blood and transported to the kidneys for processing and excreting the by-products with the urine.

Thirst is regulated by the concentration of sodium in the blood. When water levels drop and the percent of sodium increases, the thirst sensation is triggered.[48] A woman needs to drink at least 6 cups of water each day. She will obtain an additional 4 cups from the foods she eats. It is advisable not to rely entirely on your thirst response, however. It is not unusual, especially in cool weather, to overlook the need for water. (See *FYI:* "Water: The Overpriced Nutrient.")

Phytochemicals **Phytochemicals** are substances in plant foods that act on the body's physiology in some positive way. More and more evidence is emerging that these components tend to have health-protective

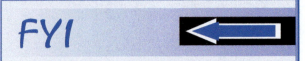

FYI

Water: The Overpriced Nutrient

Although the quality of our tap water is regulated by local law and the Environmental Protection Agency, many people are dissatisfied with water that comes from the faucet. In the quest to find drinking water that is believed to be safer, more palatable, and fresher, some consumers have turned to purchasing bottled water. Worldwide, individuals consumed more than 41 billion gallons of bottled water annually while spending over $100 billion on this important nutrient.[49] Compared to tap water, bottled water costs from 240 to 5000 times more per gallon to purchase, making it a very overpriced nutrient. If you're looking for transparency regarding the location of the source of the water, the treatment method, or the purity testing, very few companies share this information. A review of 173 bottled waters by the Environmental Working Group found that most companies will not share adequate information about their product. EWG contends that the majority of bottled water is municipal tap water and the plastic bottles are harmful because of leached chemical additives into the water itself and the pollution generated from all the plastic bottles. They recommend that we drink filtered tap water.[50]

qualities. Table 10.4 gives some of the phytochemicals and their functions. In the future, phytochemicals may become classified as essential nutrients.

PREGNANCY AND BREAST FEEDING

A woman's nutritional condition is always an important part of her life, but it takes on even greater importance when she becomes pregnant. The changes that occur within her reproductive system are profound. These changes require complex and challenging adaptations to the way she eats. In addition to her own well-being,

TABLE 10.4 Food Sources and Functions of Phytochemicals

PHYTOCHEMICAL	FOOD SOURCE	ACTION
Carotenoids	Yellow and orange fruits and vegetables, dark-green leafy vegetables	Provide protection against cancer and heart disease
Allylic sulfides	Garlic, onions, chives	Help reduce the production of some enzymes associated with cancer; cardiovascular protection
Phytosterols	Green and yellow vegetables	Block the uptake of cholesterol
Phytoestrogens	Cereals, grains	Prevent diseases and conditions related to aging and menopause

she is faced with the nutritional demands of the fetus. Many factors influence a successful pregnancy, but a healthy and balanced diet is a major factor that influences the health of the pregnant woman and the fetus.

Energy Needs during Pregnancy

The amount of weight that should be gained during pregnancy varies from woman to woman. No predetermined amount of weight gain is perfect for every pregnant woman. The average weight gain of a pregnant woman of normal weight is 25–35 pounds. Weight gain recommendations differ for underweight, overweight and obese women. Sixty percent of this weight pertains to the baby: approximately 6–8 pounds for the baby and 7.5 pounds for the placenta, amniotic fluid, breasts, and uterus. The remaining 40 percent relates to the mother's body fluids and accumulated fat.[51]

Nutrient Requirements during Pregnancy

Pregnant women need only 15 percent more calories, but up to 100 percent more nutrients, than women who are not pregnant. Ideally, a pregnant woman will make intelligent food choices that allow her to increase the intake of important nutrients without increasing her calorie intake to the point that she gains more weight than is necessary.

Protein A woman will produce about two additional pounds of protein during her pregnancy. About one-fourth of this increase will go to developing her blood supply, and one-half will be used to manufacture fetal tissue. The average woman, on a 2100 cal/day diet, normally needs about 46 grams of protein. During her pregnancy, she will need to increase daily protein consumption to 71 grams. The challenge will be in her ability to increase protein without increasing fat calories, typically found in many meat sources.

Iron The most common nutrient deficiency among pregnant women is iron. A woman in her childbearing years tends to have low iron stores to begin with, but during pregnancy her iron needs increase dramatically. In addition to the iron needed to build her increasing number of red blood cells, the fetus will demand iron as well. It is extremely unlikely that a woman will be able to consume enough iron in the foods she eats. It is therefore recommended that pregnant women take daily iron supplements. A pregnant woman needs 27 mg/day of iron.[52]

Folacin Folacin (also folate or folic acid) is very important during pregnancy and in women of child-bearing years who may become pregnant. Folacin is necessary for the formation of tissue. One can see how important this nutrient is, given the amount of tissue being

Assess Yourself

Foods for Folacin

Test your knowledge of the food choices. What are the best sources of folacin? Rank-order them with 1 being the highest source and 3 being the lowest source in the group. Answers appear below.

A. 10 Triscuit crackers _____
   Cap'n Crunch cereal, 1 cup _____
   oatmeal, 1 cup _____

B. 1 poached egg _____
   1 baked chicken breast _____
   chicken and rice soup, 1 cup _____

C. broccoli, 1 cup _____
   yellow beans, 1 cup _____
   asparagus, 1 cup _____

D. 1 hamburger _____
   1 steak _____
   ham, 1 cup _____

Answers: A. 3,1,2 B. 1,3,2 C. 3,1,2 D. All three low

generated by the mother and the fetus. Folate deficiency has been associated with neural tube birth defects, spina bifida, and anencephaly. Determine your knowledge of sources of folacin by completing *Assess Yourself:* "Foods for Folacin."

Calcium and Vitamin D Calcium is needed to support the mineralization of bone in the fetus. Much of the calcium required for this purpose is needed during the third trimester. It is important for a woman to increase the amount of calcium in her diet early in her pregnancy. A woman who doesn't like the foods found in the *FYI:* "Calcium Sources" is advised to take calcium supplements. Vitamin D is also important to the development of bone in the fetus. Vitamin D levels in the mother impact early bone strength and density in the newborn. The primary sources have typically been increased exposure to sunlight and use of supplements.

Vitamin and Mineral Supplements Many pregnant women, in an effort to help the growing fetus, will routinely take a complete vitamin/mineral supplement during pregnancy. The only nutrients that require supplementation are iron, folacin, vitamin D, and calcium (especially if the woman does not drink milk). All other nutrients can be obtained from the slight increase of 100–300 more calories in food consumption, if a woman eats a variety of foods.

Dietary Guideline Recommendations for Pregnancy

The dietary guidelines recommend that women who are capable of becoming pregnant should "choose foods that supply heme iron, which is more readily absorbed by the body, additional iron sources, and enhancers of iron absorption such as vitamin C-rich foods." She should also "consume 400 micrograms (mcg) per day of synthetic folic acid (from fortified foods and/or supplements) in addition to food forms of folate from a varied diet." Women who may be pregnant should refrain from drinking alcohol because no safe limit has been established and the consumption of alcohol may have detrimental behavioral and neurological consequences for her infant.

Women who are pregnant or breastfeeding should "consume 8–12 ounces of seafood per week from a variety of seafood types." Seafood types include fish such as salmon, trout, tuna and tilapia and shellfish such as shrimp, crab and oysters. She should limit white (albacore) tuna to 6 ounces per week and not eat tilefish, shark, swordfish, or king mackerel because of the methyl mercury content. She should take iron supplements as recommended by her health care provider. And, she should refrain from drinking alcohol throughout the pregnancy and may decide it is best to refrain from drinking alcohol during breastfeeding. If she chooses to drink a limited amount, she should wait 4 hours before breast feeding her infant.[53]

PHYSICAL ACTIVITY

Fitness activity levels will have an effect on a woman's nutritional needs. If a woman is a competitive athlete or happens to engage in vigorous activity for an hour or more at least 5 days per week, she could classify herself as *highly active*. As you might expect, high and low activity levels require differing food plans. The dietary guidelines call for Americans to maintain physical activity levels consistent with the *2008 Physical Activity Guidelines for Americans*. These guidelines recommend increasing physical activity and reducing time spent in sedentary behaviors. Chapter 11 provides specifics regarding a comprehensive physical activity program.

Caloric Intake

Energy requirements vary according to activity level. Energy consumption is a function of the intensity of the activity and the length of time you engage in that activity. Table 10.5 provides an estimate of calorie

---

TABLE 10.5 Estimated Calorie Requirements (in kilocalories) for Each Gender and Age Group at Three Levels of Physical Activity[a]

| | | ACTIVITY LEVEL[b,c,d] | | |
Gender	Age (years)	Sedentary[b]	Moderately Active[c]	Active[d]
Child	2–3	1000	1000–1400[e]	1000–1400[e]
Female	4–8	1200	1400–1600	1400–1800
	9–13	1600	1600–2000	1800–2200
	14–18	1800	2000	2400
	19–30	2000	2000–2200	2400
	31–50	1800	2000	2200
	51+	1600	1800	2000–2200
Male	4–8	1400	1400–1600	1600–2000
	9–13	1800	1800–2200	2000–2600
	14–18	2200	2400–2800	2800–3200
	19–30	2400	2600–2800	3000
	31–50	2200	2400–2600	2800–3000
	51+	2000	2200–2400	2400–2800

[a] These levels are based on Estimated Energy Requirements (EER) from the Institute of Medicine Dietary Reference Intakes macronutrients report, 2002, calculated by gender, age, and activity level for reference-sized individuals. "Reference size," as determined by IOM, is based on median height and weight for ages up to age 18 years of age and median height and weight for that height to give a BMI of 21.5 for adult females and 22.5 for adult males.
[b] Sedentary means a lifestyle that includes only the light physical activity associated with typical day-to-day life.
[c] Moderately active means a lifestyle that includes physical activity equivalent to walking about 1.5 to 3 miles per day at 3 to 4 miles per hour, in addition to the light physical activity associated with typical day-to-day life
[d] Active means a lifestyle that includes physical activity equivalent to walking more than 3 miles per day at 3 to 4 miles per hour, in addition to the light physical activity associated with typical day-to-day life.
[e] The calorie ranges shown are to accommodate needs of different ages within the group. For children and adolescents, more calories are needed at older ages. For adults, fewer calories are needed at older ages.

SOURCE: HHS/USDA *Dietary Guidelines for Americans 2010*.

requirements based on age group and levels of physical activity. These levels are based on estimated energy requirements for reference-sized individuals. "Reference size," as determined by the Institute of Medicine, is based on median height and weight for ages up to 18 years and median height and weight for the height to give a body mass index of 21.5 for adult females. *Sedentary* means a lifestyle that includes only the light physical activity associated with typical day-to-day life. *Moderately active* means a lifestyle that includes physical activity equivalent to walking about 1.5–3 miles per day at 3–4 miles per hour, in addition to the light physical activity associated with typical day-to-day life. *Active* means a lifestyle that includes physical activity equivalent to walking more than 3 miles per day at 3–4 miles per hour, in addition to the light physical activity associated with typical day-to-day life. If you are involved in some form of activity, your energy intake should match your energy expenditure unless you are attempting to lose weight.

Nutrients

It is generally believed that there is no need to increase the amount of nutrients beyond the DRIs as a person becomes physically active. Exercise increases the athlete's need for more energy and water, not for more protein, vitamins, or minerals. There are, however, some aspects of nutrition and athletic performance for women that deserve special mention.

Iron deficiency has been an area of interest for some time. Investigations have revealed that iron levels are not significantly different among female athletes versus non-athletes. Those studies that report differences attribute them to poor diet rather than to physical activity.[54] Also, one of the confounding factors in measuring iron levels is the menstrual cycle, which can influence the level of iron in the blood. Vegetarian athletes or those athletes who do not eat red meat are more vulnerable to low iron levels.[55] It is strongly recommended that women who are active or highly active get at least 18 mg of iron daily, either from their diet or through supplementation.

Calcium intake is another area that has been studied among female athletes. It appears that female athletes may not be getting all the calcium they need. Many female athletes, particularly those who are concerned with being thin, have been observed with calcium intake levels that are below DRI levels.[56] If calcium levels are low, and the woman develops amenorrhea, she is likely to experience demineralization of her bones, which in turn will increase her potential for leg injuries or stress fractures. If you are physically active and follow a vegetarian diet, you should be aware of potential problems. Because vitamin B-12 is found mainly in animal foods, vegetarians may become deficient in this vital nutrient, along with both iron and zinc. For those who choose to eschew meat, vitamin B-12 can be supplemented with the addition of dairy products including eggs and low-fat milk, yogurt and cheese; by consuming fortified cereals or soy products; or through vitamin supplements. If a woman is an athlete and chooses to become a vegetarian, she must pay particular attention to her diet to be sure it includes adequate amounts of these nutrients. Otherwise her performance, and her health, may suffer.[57,58] Vegetarians, because of high fiber intake, tend to lose estrogen. A vegetarian diet may also increase the likelihood of altering a woman's menstrual cycle, particularly if the diet is low in fat, low in protein, and high in fiber.

VEGETARIANISM

Women may choose to limit their diets to plant-based foods and eliminate or partially eliminate animal foods for a number of reasons: following religious beliefs, feeling that killing animals is unethical, using food resources that are low on the food chain, or eating less expensive foods. Vegetarian diet styles may vary. Vegetarians are grouped according to the animal-derived foods they eat. *Vegans* eat only plant foods; *lacto-vegetarians* eat plant foods and dairy products; *lacto-ovo-vegetarians* eat no meat, poultry, or fish, but do eat eggs and milk products; and *semivegetarians* include eggs, dairy products, and small amounts of poultry and seafood in the diet. First and foremost, nutritional health is dependent on balance, variety, and moderation in the diet. Whether the diet is **omnivorous** (consuming both plant and animal food sources) or vegetarian, attention must be paid to achieving the recommended DRIs. Women considering vegetarian diets should learn about the benefits and risks before starting a vegetarian diet. (See *Her Story:* "Deanne: Choosing Vegetarianism.")

Benefits of Vegetarianism

Numerous studies have been conducted on the benefits of a vegetarian meal plan. Most studies confirm that vegetarian eating patterns are lower in total fat, saturated fat, and cholesterol. Other beneficial outcomes of a vegetarian diet include:[59,60]

- *Leanness.* Vegetarians are more health conscious and more physically active. They typically have a lower body mass index.
- *Lower levels of serum cholesterol.* Vegans have lower levels than even lacto-vegetarians or nonvegetarians.
- *Reduced risk of cardiovascular disease.* Leaner body mass contributes to lower blood pressure. They

Her Story

Deanne: Choosing Vegetarianism

Deanne has always been interested in environmental responsibility, including compassion to animals. When she read about the animal suffering that happens with factory farming, like greater numbers of birds being put in smaller cages, reduced square feet for hog pens, fumes from manure causing eye and respiratory infections, and slaughtering of milk cows after 5–6 years of production, she decided to read about alternatives. She thought eating free–range meat might be okay, until she read that "free range" was a meaningless term. So, Deanne became a vegetarian. First, she made a list of all the meals she already ate that were meatless. Next, she made a list of the meals that could become meatless. She had a great start.

- What does Deanne need to know about eating healthy as a vegetarian?
- When Deanne takes meat out of her diet, what nutrients might she lose? What substitutes might she consider?
- What other reasons may people give for being vegetarian?

have a high unsaturated to saturated fatty acid ratio.
- Lower total mortality. They live longer. They consume fewer calories, more fiber, potassium and vitamin C.

Concerns of Vegetarianism

If a vegetarian encounters nutritional problems, it may be in the form of

- *Iron deficiency.* Iron levels are reportedly lower among lacto-ovo-vegetarians, and more so for women than men.
- *Insufficient levels of calcium.* Because dairy products are a good source of calcium, this nutrient can be erroneously omitted from the diet.
- *Vitamin D deficiency.* Vegans may have insufficient levels of this vitamin due to the absence of milk products and lack of sunlight. Vegans should try to get sunlight when possible and choose vitamin D–fortified products, such as orange juice and some cereals.
- *Vitamin B-12 deficiency.* Pernicious anemia develops in the absence of vitamin B-12. In fact, women can pass this deficiency on to their infants through

breast-feeding.[61] Cereals and breads fortified, not enriched, with B-12 should be considered, as well as fortified soy and rice drinks.

If you have an interest in following a vegetarian dietary regimen, there are certain principles you should follow for optimal health.

- No single plant food contains all essential amino acids, but combining a variety of grains and vegetables will help vegetarians get the essential amino acids. Vegans combine foods to form meals throughout the day that become complete with the essential amino acids. Suggested substitutes for dairy products and eggs include fortified soy milk, rice milk, and almond milk; using oils as substitutes for butter; and using egg substitutes.
- Plant proteins can provide all essential and nonessential amino acids, but varied sources and a high calorie intake are recommended for adequate energy needs.
- Animal foods contain zinc, calcium, and iron.[62] Attention should be paid to consuming plant foods that contain these nutrients. For example, whole grains, soy products, nuts, wheat germ, spinach, broccoli, dark-green vegetables, and dried fruit will serve as substitutes.
- Be aware that the iron in plant foods is not as well absorbed as the iron from meat sources. Be careful, too, about consuming too much grain, bran, and soy products. These foods contain phytates (a form of phosphorus that is not readily bioavailable), which inhibit the absorption of iron, calcium, and zinc.[63] The bottom line is that vegetarianism requires intelligent planning of meals, a working knowledge of how foods interact with one another, and knowledge of the factors that influence nutrient uptake.

NUTRITION AND THE CONSUMER

We are constantly confronted with food products that claim to do amazing things. There are claims that special foods can maintain our youth, cure or prevent cancer, and supply us with an endless amount of energy. Labels on special food products and dietary supplements are usually the means by which such products deliver their claims. Understanding terminology such as "health foods," "organic," and "natural," knowing which sources of information are reliable and trustworthy, interpreting food labels and practicing food safety can improve a woman's ability to become a healthier consumer.

Additives

Many women are concerned about the amount of additives found in their foods. We tend to think of food additives as chemicals that are unnatural and added to our foods unnecessarily. The truth is that food additives play very important roles in the food we consume. Food additives are used in foods for five principal reasons:

1. *To maintain product consistency.* Anti-caking agents help products like salt flow freely. Emulsifiers prevent products from separating.
2. *To improve or maintain nutritional value.* For instance, vitamin D is added to milk to help reduce the incidence of malnutrition. Vitamin D is necessary for the appropriate absorption of calcium in order to maintain bone density.
3. *To reduce spoilage.* Preservatives will prevent spoilage caused by mold, bacteria, and fungi.
4. *To provide leavening or control acidity/alkalinity.* Leavening agents are added to help baked goods rise during cooking. Some additives modify acidity and alkalinity to improve flavor, taste, and color.
5. *To enhance flavor or provide a desired color.*

Knowing that additives are placed in foods to maintain quality is one thing. However, concern that "unnatural chemicals" are added to our food is something else. The fear is that chemicals will harm us. Consider the ingredients in the following foods:

Product A: acetone, methyl acetate, furan, butanol, methyfuran, isoprene, methyl butanol, caffeine, essential oils, methanol, acetaldehyde, methyl formate, ethanol, dimethyl sulfide, and propionaldehyde.

Product B: actomycin, myogen, nucleoproteins, peptides, amino acids, myoglobin, lipids, linoleic acid, oleic acid, lecithin, cholesterol, sucrose, ATP, glucose, collagen, elastin, creatine, pytoligneous acid, sodium chloride, sodium nitrate, sodium nitrite, and sodium phosphate.

What do you think about these two products? Do you feel you could safely consume either of them over extended periods of time? Would you feel better knowing that product A is coffee and that product B is cured ham? The media and special interest groups have attempted to color our food supply as harmful, but the truth is that all foods we consume are made of chemicals. Calcium propionate is a common food additive. Although it may sound unnatural, it is actually a compound found naturally in Swiss cheese. It is added to food to prevent bacterial growth.

Food additives and food packaging are carefully regulated by the FDA and are permitted only after extensive testing. Additives can keep food wholesome and appealing, improve the nutritional value of some foods, and improve taste, color, and texture. Diets high in fat and alcohol actually pose greater risks to health than any of the additives found in our food supply.[64]

Organic Foods

Organic foods continue to be one of the fastest growing sectors of the U.S. food industry. Beginning in 2002, the USDA National Organic Standards required producers and food handlers to be certified by a USDA certifying agent to represent their products as 100 percent organic. Organic foods must be produced, grown, and processed without use of commercial chemicals such as fertilizers, pesticides, and synthetics such as color or flavor. Organic farming and production contribute to a more sustainable environment. Studies clearly shows that organic foods have less pesticide residual, but the levels of pesticide residual for all foods are heavily regulated by the EPA and USDA. Studies have not found any significant differences in flavor between organically grown and conventionally grown foods, and while vitamin C and some mineral content may be higher in organically grown foods, the level is insignificant to produce health effects.[65]

So why might a person consider purchasing organic foods? Are some organic products more beneficial than others? Meats, eggs, and dairy products labeled as organic come from animals that are given no growth

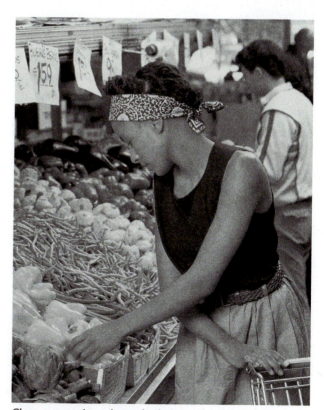

Choose organic and standard grown foods wisely.

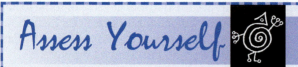

Assess Yourself

What Do You Know about the Foods You Eat?

Circle the answers that you think are correct, and then check your answers below.

1. The skins of fruits and vegetables are a significant source of nutrients and fiber, but pesticides may make them less healthy. From which of the following should you always trim the peel?
   a. carrots
   b. cucumbers
   c. pears
   d. apples

2. Which of the following foods should be avoided if mold appears?
   a. yogurt
   b. peanut butter
   c. individual cheese slices
   d. all of the above

3. How soon after a meal should leftovers be refrigerated?
   a. within 1/2 hour
   b. within 1 hour
   c. within 2 hours
   d. within 3 hours

Answers:
1. A—Peel apples and cucumbers only if they have been waxed.
2. D—If you can safely remove at least 1 inch of the food along with the mold, it may be safe to eat the food. It may not be possible to completely remove all mold from products like those above.
3. C—Prepared foods can safely sit at room temperature for up to 2 hours before needing refrigeration.

hormones or antibiotics. This difference between organically produced and conventionally produced may be important to you. If you must choose between organically grown and conventionally grown white potatoes, you may want to know that white potatoes grow beneath the surface in ground that may have considerable pesticides. On the other hand, sweet potatoes are grown with less pesticide application. Green leafy vegetables such as lettuce and spinach or more likely to absorb pesticides that cannot be washed off, so again, you may prefer to purchase organically grown green leafy vegetables. Products such as organic hair, cosmetic products and farm-raised fish or shellfish may have less beneficial outcomes. Your best bet is to read more about the differences between organically grown and conventionally grown foods to weigh the costs and benefits. Take

the short *Assess Yourself:* "What Do You Know about the Foods You Eat?" to determine your level of understanding about some of the foods you eat.

If you choose to purchase organically grown products, visit farmers' markets that sell organic foods and compare them to the supermarkets that advertise the same products. Buying locally can also help sustain the environment. Compare the claims, prices, and appearance of organically grown and conventionally grown foods. Does appearance matter to you? And, read *FYI:* "What Does a Food Label Mean?" to be sure you pay for products that deserve higher purchase prices and are a wise choice for you. The 2010 dietary guidelines call to action supports the development and expansion of "safe, effective, and sustainable agriculture and aquaculture practices to ensure availability of recommended amounts of healthy foods to all segments of the population."[66]

Food Labeling

When you purchase or use prepared foods, do you take the time to read the labels? If so, what do you look for? Brand names, ingredients, fat content, calories? Like all consumers, you are probably interested in specific things about the product. Reading food labels has become easier because there must now be consistency in information and terminology that describe the contents of food products. As a result of the 1990 Nutritional Labeling and Education Act and regulatory actions by the FDA and the U.S. Department of Agriculture, consumers can better determine the food products that meet their individual nutritional needs.

Food manufacturers are required to place labels on their products that offer complete, accurate, and useful nutritional information. Anyone who shops can make comparisons among all foods found in grocery stores everywhere.

Food labels provide information that help women make nutritious food choices to help meet recommended DRIs. The FDA mandates that the following must be included on food labels and packages: total calories, calories from fat, total fat, saturated fat, cholesterol, sodium, total carbohydrates, dietary fiber, sugars, vitamin A, protein, vitamin C, calcium, and iron.[67] Other dietary components can be voluntarily placed on the label. The daily value (DV), which is the daily nutrient intake level recommended by nutrition authorities, is stated in percentages and reveals how much of a day's ideal total of a particular nutrient a consumer is receiving based on a 2000-calorie-per-day diet. This reference quickly allows a woman to see how a packaged food product meets her nutritional needs.

Current food labels reveal a wealth of information by providing an easy-to-read format. The standardized

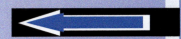

FYI

What Does a Food Label Mean?[68]

Food labels with so-called natural or organic names may not always be either "natural" or "organic." The following meaningful labels have U.S. government standards behind them while the meaningless labels do not.

Meaningful Labels
100% Organic. This designation means that, by law, no synthetic ingredients are allowed. Production processes must meet federal guidelines and have independent verification by accredited inspectors.

Organic. This means that at least 95 percent of the ingredients must meet federal standards for the term "organic." The remaining 5 percent may be inorganic or synthetic ingredients. The only exception is seafood, as no current government standards for "organic" exist when referring to seafood products.

Made with Organic Ingredients. At least 70 percent of the ingredients must meet the federal standards for the term "organic." The remaining 30 percent must be from the USDA's approved list of ingredients.

Meaningless Labels
"Free-range" or *"free-roaming."* Often stamped on eggs, chicken, and meat, these designations may mislead consumers into thinking a farm animal has spent much of its life outdoors. However, the U.S. government standards for these labels are weak. Such labeling may mean nothing more than that a farm animal had some limited access to the outdoors, not that it spent any significant time in a healthy, outdoor environment.

"Natural" or *"all natural."* These designations do not mean organic. Unless these terms are used on meat or poultry products, no standard definitions for either exist, and a food manufacturer or producer may use these terms at its own discretion. The exception is meat and poultry products, for which "natural" is defined by the USDA as containing no artificial coloring, flavoring, chemical preservatives, or other synthetic ingredients.

serving sizes allow comparison of nutrients on similar products. Labels provide uniform definitions for terms that describe a food's nutrient content ("low-fat" or "high-fiber"), and information about the relationship between a nutrient or a food and a health-related condition, such as low-saturated fat and heart disease. (See *FYI:* "What Does a Food Label Mean?")

Portion Distortion Portion size is extremely important to monitor when choosing any meal plan. Our society continues to place more value on receiving larger portions when dining out. The current trend in America is to "supersize it," "biggie size it," or "make it a grande." This, together with "all you can eat buffets" and "buy one, get one free" deals, encourages the food consumer to eat beyond meeting energy needs. Many food vendors, especially fast-food vendors, use larger portion sizes as a selling point by pricing the larger item at a better value. The perception of getting "more for less money" often keeps consumers eating or drinking more calories per meal than necessary. (See *Assess Yourself:* "What Do You Know about a Serving Size?")

Another way to test your knowledge about portion size is to try the interactive quiz prepared by the National Heart, Lung, and Blood Institute. Go to hp2010 .nhlbihin.net/portion to test your knowledge about portion distortion.

Assess Yourself

What Do You Know about a Serving Size?

One way to determine what constitutes an appropriate serving size per meal is to create a visual size comparison between a portion of food and an ordinary object. Some common comparisons are

1 ounce of cheese = size of four dice
3 ounces of meat = a deck of cards or a bar of soap
½ cup of mashed potatoes = the amount found in an ice cream scoop
1 medium potato = a computer mouse
1 fruit serving = a baseball

Fast-food restaurants, whether due to time, money or convenience, are often the restaurants of choice. A woman who wants to be healthy and keep her weight at a desired level can, however, still eat fast-food by making wiser choices from the offered menus for some healthier options at fast-food vendors. These choices may save money as well as calories.

Label Terminology Terms and their meanings are continually being revised. To better comprehend what you are buying, you must understand nutritional terms. Food label regulations require food manufacturers to use standardized terms when describing nutrient content of foods. Descriptors such as "less," "high-fiber," "low-fat," "free," "light," "lite," or "reduced calories" must meet FDA requirements. For meat, poultry, and fish, the terms "lean" and "extra lean" apply to the fat content of these products and must meet the established percentages for fat and lean content. Table 10.6 provides a review of the meanings for these terms that will increase your understanding of nutritional content of food products.[69]

Food labels have two distinct sections: a principal display panel (PDP) and an information panel. The PDP is usually on the front of the product and must contain the name of the product (not the name of the company), for example, "tuna packed in vegetable oil," and the net quantity of the product. The PDP may be where the manufacturer states certain claims, such as "low-fat," "fortified," and so forth. The information panel is the part of the label that is of greatest interest to consumers. Figure 10.2 is an example of a typical food label.

Labeling about Food Allergies Increasingly, the potential life-threatening outcomes from food allergies are being reported by the media. What exactly are they discussing, and why are food allergies more prevalent? Normally the body does not evoke an immune response. However, a food allergy is an abnormal response to a

---

TABLE 10.6 Common Food Label Terminology

The following are terms with brief explanations found on food product packaging.

Fat

- *Fat-free:* less than 0.5 gram (g)
- *Low-fat:* 3 g or less fat than found in the full-calorie product

Saturated Fat

- *Saturated fat–free:* less than 0.5 g and less than 0.5 g trans-fatty acid per serving. (Trans-fatty acid is found in solid vegetable fat products, like margarine. The FDA suggests that levels of trans-fatty acid be limited in products that claim to be "saturated fat–free.")
- *Low saturated fat:* 1 g or less per serving and not more than 15 percent of calories coming from saturated fatty acids
- *Reduced or less saturated fat:* at least 25 percent less each serving than the reference food (the same product that had the original level of fat)

Calories

- *Calorie-free:* fewer than 5 calories per serving
- *Low-calorie:* 40 or fewer calories per serving
- *Reduced or fewer calories:* at least 25 percent fewer calories per serving than the full-calorie food

Calories and Fat

Light (two meanings):

- One-third fewer calories or half the fat of the full-calorie food. (If food is composed of 59 percent or more of calories from fat, the reduction has to be 50 percent of fat.)
- A "low-calorie" or "low-fat" food, in which the fat amount has been reduced by 50 percent of the full-calorie food. "Light in sodium" means that the food product has 50 percent or less sodium than the full-sodium food.

Sugar

- *Sugar-free:* less than 0.5 g per serving
- *No added sugar, without added sugar, no sugar added:* Has no sugar or ingredients containing sugars, such as fruit or fruit juice added during processing or packing. Has no ingredients made with added sugars, such as jellies or fruit juice. (If a label states "sugar-free" or "no sugar added," this applies only to a reduction in calories related to sugar, not to calories from fat, protein, or other carbohydrates.)
- *Reduced sugar:* at least 25 percent less sugar than the full-calorie food

Fiber

Note: Any food claiming increased fiber content must also meet the definition for "low-fat," or the amount of total fat per serving must appear next to the claim.

- *High-fiber:* 5 g or more per serving
- *Good source of fiber:* 2.5 g–4.9 g per serving
- *More or added fiber:* at least 2.5 g more per serving than the full-calorie food

FIGURE 10.2 How to read the food label.

Serving size

Is your serving the same size as the one on the label? If you eat double the serving size listed, you need to double the nutrient and calorie values. If you eat one-half the serving size shown here, cut the nutrient and calorie in half. Pay attention to the serving size, including the number of servings in the food package.

Calories

Do you want to lose weight? Cut back a little on calories. Look here to see how one serving of the food adds to your daily total. The number of servings you consume determines the number of calories you have eaten.

Total carbohydrate

When you cut down on fat, you can eat more carbohydrates. Carbohydrates are in foods like whole-grain bread, fruits, and vegetables. Choose nutrient-dense carbs often. They give you nutrients and energy. Reduce sugars whenever possible.

Dietary fiber

Most Americans, including women, do not get enough fiber. That goes for both soluble and insoluble kinds of dietary fiber. Fruits, vegetables, whole-grain foods, beans, and peas are all good sources and can help reduce the risk of heart disease and cancer.

Protein

Most Americans get more protein than they need. Where there is animal protein there are also fat and cholesterol. Eat small servings of lean meat, fish, and poultry. Use skim or low-fat milk, yogurt, and cheese. Try vegetable proteins like beans, grains, and cereals.

Vitamins and minerals

Your goal here is 100 percent of each for the day. Don't count on one food to do it all. Most Americans don't get enough vitamin A, vitamin C, calcium, and iron in their diets.

Nutrition Facts

Serving Size 1 cup (228g)
Servings per Container 2

Amount per Serving

Calories 250 Calories from Fat 110

	% Daily Value*
Total Fat 12g	18%
Saturated Fat 3g	15%
Trans Fat 3g	
Cholesterol 30mg	10%
Sodium 470mg	20%
Total Carbohydrate 31g	10%
Dietary Fiber 0g	0%
Sugars 5g	
Protein 5g	
Vitamin A	4%
Vitamin C	2%
Calcium	20%
Iron	4%

*Percent Daily Values are based on a 2,000 calorie diet. Your Daily Values may be higher or lower depending on your calorie needs:

	Calories	2,000	2,500
Total Fat	Less than	65g	80
Sat Fat	Less than	20g	25g
Cholesterol	Less than	300mg	300mg
Sodium	Less than	2,400mg	2,400mg
Total Carbohydrate		300g	375g
Dietary Fiber		25g	30g

Total fat

Aim low: Most people need to cut back on fat. Too much fat may contribute to heart disease and cancer. Try to limit your calories from fat, particularly saturated and trans fat. For a healthy heart, choose foods with a big difference between the total number of calories and the number of calories from fat.

Saturated fat

Saturated fat is part of the total fat in food. It is listed separately because it's the key player in raising blood cholesterol and your risk of heart disease. Choose foods low in saturated fat to stay healthy.

Trans fat

Trans fat is formed when liquid oils are made into solid fats like shortening and hard margarine. Trans fat raises LDL cholesterol, which increases your risk of coronary heart disease. Choose foods low in trans fat to stay healthy.

Cholesterol

Too much cholesterol—a second cousin to fat—can lead to heart disease. Cholesterol occurs naturally in the tissues of the body, and there is no evidence that dietary cholesterol is needed. Challenge yourself to eat less than 300 mg each day.

Sodium

You call it "salt," the label calls it "sodium." Either way, it may add up to high blood pressure in some people. So, keep your sodium intake low—2,400 to 3,000 mg or less each day.

The DASH (Dietary Approaches to Stop Hypertension) recommends 1,500 mg per day.

Daily Values

Feel like you're drowning in numbers? Let the Daily Value (DV) be your guide. Daily Values are listed for people who eat 2,000 or 2,500 calories each day. DVs are recommended levels of intake. If you eat more, your personal daily value may be higher than what's listed on the label. If you eat less, your personal daily value may be lower.

For fat, saturated fat, cholesterol, and sodium, choose foods with a low % Daily Value. For total carbohydrate, dietary fiber, vitamins, and minerals, your daily value goal is to reach 100% of each.

g = grams (About 28 g = 1 ounce)
mg = milligrams (1,000 mg = 1 g)

---

perceived toxin that evokes an immune system response. If a food is perceived as harmful, an antibody called immunoglobulin E (IgE) is created and the next time it is eaten, high levels of histamine or other chemicals (called mediation) are released to protect the body. These symptoms can affect the respiratory system, gastrointestinal tract, skin, or cardiovascular system. Symptoms can range from tingling sensations to loss of consciousness, and death. The only way to avoid the reaction is to avoid the food. While some food allergies can be outgrown, foods like peanuts, nuts, fish, and shellfish are often lifelong allergies.

Some persons equate food allergies with food intolerance. Food intolerance is an adverse food-induced reaction that does not involve the immune system. Lactose intolerance is an example. Since January 1, 2006, the FDA has required food labels to state if food products contain ingredients derived from the eight major foods or food groups that account for 90 percent of all allergic reactions: milk, eggs, fish, crustacean shellfish, tree nuts (pecans, almonds, walnuts), peanuts, wheat, soybeans. The food label must list these ingredients or say "contains" followed by the name of the source of the food allergen.[70] Check the labels on some common food products that you eat to see if any of these ingredients are present.

A skin prick test or a blood test is commonly used to determine the presence of food allergies. The type of test used by the health care provider is determined by the patient's age or health symptoms. The test results along with a history of symptoms are used to determine whether a food allergy exists. Food allergies are skyrocketing, particularly in developed and developing countries. Nearly 2 percent of adults and 5 percent of infants and children in the United States have food allergies. Some studies suggest that growing up in large families or being exposed to others in daycare may actually *reduce* the potential for developing food allergies because increased exposure strengthens the immune system. An important consideration for persons with food allergies is the potential for cross contamination when eating at a restaurant or consuming a meal prepared by someone else.

Pathogens (bacteria, viruses), parasites, toxins, or chemical contaminants can cause foodborne illness. We are constantly at risk for serious illnesses from eating foods that have not been handled, cooked, or stored properly. (See *FYI:* "National Food Safety Warnings.") The contaminants that cause foodborne illness often cannot be seen, smelled, or tasted. Nearly 76 million individuals in the U.S. are impacted by foodborne illnesses with 325,000 hospitalizations and 5000 deaths annually.[71] Proper handling, cooking, and storage are essential for food safety. The USDA recommends the following "Fight BAC" guidelines: **Clean** hands, food surfaces, and utensils often. Meat and poultry should NOT be washed or rinsed prior to cooking. Fruits and vegetables should be thoroughly rinsed by running them under water before eating, cutting, or cooking. Precut, prepackaged foods will not need additional rinsing. **Separate** raw, cooked, and ready-to-eat food, even when shopping, preparing, or storing foods. Don't cross-contaminate foods such as raw meat, poultry, or eggs with other foods such as fruits and vegetables. Cutting boards, utensils, dishes, or preparation surfaces used for meat should be cleaned thoroughly with hot, soapy water before using with other kinds of foods. Reusable shopping bags should be cleaned regularly. **Cook** foods to proper temperatures to ensure that any illness-causing contaminants have been destroyed in the cooking process. Use of a meat thermometer helps ensure that meat reaches a safe internal temperature. Beef, veal, lamb, roasts or chops should be cooked to 140° F; pork (all cuts) to 160° F, ground beef, veal, or lamb to 160° F, all poultry to 165° F. **Chill** any unused food promptly at a temperature of 40° F or below. Frozen foods should be kept at a temperature of 0° F or below and should be thawed using appropriate methods. **Avoid** raw (unpasteurized) milk or any products made from unpasteurized milk, raw or partially cooked eggs or foods containing raw eggs, raw or undercooked meat and poultry, raw oysters, unpasteurized juices, and raw sprouts.[75]

Pregnant women, children, older adults and those with compromised immune systems are more susceptible to foodborne illnesses. Consult the U.S. food safety website for current information about food safety: www.foodsafety.gov.

MANAGING WEIGHT THROUGH NUTRITION

Few personal health topics have attracted the interests of the medical community as much as weight management. (See *FYI:* "Weight Management.") According to epidemiological data, women as a group are fatter now than they have ever been in our nation's history, and the percentage of overweight African American and Hispanic women is greater than that of white women.[76] At any given time, 50 percent of American women are spending billions of dollars to lose weight. Statistics like these are interesting, but what does all this mean to you? How much should you weigh? What is the best way to keep weight off?

Assessing one's risk involves using three key measures:

- Body mass index (BMI)
- Waist circumference
- Risk factors for diseases and conditions associated with obesity.[77]

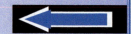

FYI

National Food Safety Warnings

No doubt you've heard about the nation's food supply problems in the past several years. Remember the 2008 food-borne outbreaks of a strain of *Salmonella typhimurium* traced to two peanut processing plants, one in Georgia and the other in Texas? These facilities processed peanuts into pastes and fillings used in cookies, cakes, snack bars, cereals, and other commercial foods sold to both institutions and individual consumers throughout the United States.[72] Remember the 2008 outbreak of *Escherichia coli* O157:H7 *(E coli)* that was traced to ground beef sold in grocery stores in seven states?[73] A 2006 outbreak of the same strain was traced to the consumption of fresh spinach packaged at a facility in California, in which it was believed sewage run-off from nearby animal farms had inadvertently contaminated a local growing field.[74] Each of these incidents led to large product recalls and serious outbreaks of both illnesses, with young children, the elderly, or those with compromised immune systems most at risk.

As consumers, we often do not find out about a hazardous situation until it is large enough to attract media attention. The Centers for Disease Control and Prevention and the Food and Drug Administration Web sites are frequently updated and provide accurate, timely information whenever problems occur with the nation's food supply. You can also peruse them if you simply have concerns or questions about the safety of food or other consumer products in your area.

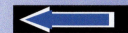

Weight Management

Key recommendations

- To maintain body weight in a healthy range, balance calories from foods and beverages with calories expended.
- To prevent gradual weight gain over time, make small decreases in food and beverage calories and increase physical activity.

Key recommendations for specific population groups

- *Those who need to lose weight.* Aim for a slow, steady weight loss by decreasing calorie intake while maintaining an adequate nutrient intake and increasing physical activity.
- *Overweight children.* Reduce the rate of body weight gain while allowing growth and development. Consult a health care provider before placing a child on a weight-reduction diet.
- *Pregnant women.* Ensure appropriate weight gain as specified by a health care provider.
- *Breast-feeding women.* Moderate weight reduction is safe and does not compromise weight gain of the nursing infant.
- *Overweight adults and overweight children with chronic diseases and/or on medication.* Consult a health care provider about weight-loss strategies prior to starting a weight-reduction program to ensure appropriate management of other health conditions.[78]

A combination of BMI and waist circumference is a better descriptor than a single measure of overweight, obesity, or extreme obesity. Other, related risk factors should also be considered when assessing risk for diabetes, cardiovascular disease, hypertension, stroke, and some cancers. These risk factors include high blood pressure, high LDL cholesterol, low HDL cholesterol, high triglycerides, high blood glucose, family history of premature heart disease, physical inactivity, and cigarette smoking. Weight loss is recommended for anyone with a BMI above 25.0, a waist measurement greater than 35 inches, and any two of the risk factors mentioned above. Even a small weight loss (merely 10 percent of a person's current weight) can provide significant benefits.

Underweight, Overweight, and Obesity

More than 64 percent of adult men and women in the United States are classified as overweight (BMI between 25.0 and 29.9) or obese (BMI > 30).[79] We know more about the consequences of obesity than we do about the causes. There seem to be conflicting explanations between nature (genetic and biological causes) and nurture (those factors in the environment) as the causes of obesity. The answer lies somewhere between the two theories. As with any other human condition, it is difficult to determine the exact and singular cause. Research has linked obesity to genetic, biochemical, metabolic, psychological, and physiological factors.

Weight Loss

The causes of obesity are many, and so are the ways of controlling it. millions of Americans are dieting at any given point in time and spending billions of dollars a year trying to lose weight. All of that money goes toward programs that are advertised as easy and successful, but the winners in the long run are the companies advertising their diet plans, not the women purchasing such plans. The Dietary Guidelines for Americans 2010 recommends balancing calories from foods and beverages with calories expended to maintain body weight and making small decreases in food and beverage calories and increasing physical activity to prevent gradual weight gain over time.

Popular Commercial Diets

High-carb, low-fat?

Low-carb, high-fat?

No fats?

All protein vs. low protein?

A stroll through the shelves of any bookstore chain reveals a slew of diet books bearing these and similar premises, with different titles or promoted by various "experts" in the fields of dietary health and nutrition. Often endorsed by celebrities or media hosts, these diets make claims based on dubious science, and once again, independent researchers are investigating how well they work or whether one commercial diet program holds an edge for greater weight loss.

A recent study compared four popular diets—the Zone, Atkins, Ornish, and Weight Watchers—for both weight and cardiovascular risk factor reduction. One hundred sixty participants, male and female, were randomized into each of the diet programs. Participants were measured at baseline for weight, blood pressure, and other metabolic factors and then examined again after 2 months and then, 1 year. Of the participants completing the full 12-month study, all lost a small but statistically significant amount of weight while lowering several cardiovascular risk factors. No diet was shown to be statistically better than another.[80]

Several studies to date have drawn similar conclusions. It appears that most commercial diet programs can produce clinically significant weight loss in *the short term*. Participants completing these studies lose nearly equal amounts of weight while lowering certain risk factors for cardiovascular disease, drawing dietary researchers to conclude it is the lower number of calories consumed, *not* the differences in the macronutrient content of a commercial diet or program that produces results.[81]

A major problem with many commercial diets is their extremity—it is often difficult and frequently expensive for people to follow such restricted ways of eating over long periods. Even within clinical studies, attrition rates are high. Participants frequently withdraw due to boredom with an eating plan or dissatisfaction with the diet to which they were assigned. Further, individuals participating in study follow-ups often report a regaining of some or even most of their initial weight loss, suggesting that both positive environmental factors and social support for health behavior change are needed for success.[82] Whether any commercial program results in long-term maintenance of weight loss has yet to be determined conclusively.[83]

While the causes of obesity are complex and may vary from individual to individual, current research indicates the best way to prevent extreme weight gain over time is to adopt an diet consisting mainly of fruits, vegetables, whole grains, low-fat dairy products, protein from lean meats or legumes; limiting intake of sugar, trans, and saturated fat, and, perhaps most important, to engage in sufficient amounts of daily physical activity.

The 2010 Dietary Guidelines suggests that healthy eating patterns can be found in the USDA Food Patterns with their lacto-ovo vegetarian or vegan adaptations or the DASH Eating Plan. The USDA Food Patterns plan was developed to give you a healthy eating plan that follows the Dietary Guidelines. The DASH Eating Plan was developed as a heart healthy eating plan to help individuals by preventing high blood pressure and other risks for cardiovascular disease. The USDA Food Patterns identify daily amounts of foods and beverages from the five major food groups: vegetables (dark-green, red and orange, beans and peas, starchy and other vegetables), fruits, grains (whole and enriched), dairy products and protein foods. The USDA Food Pattern provides weekly intake amounts for vegetables and recommends at least 8 ounces of seafood a week for adults, at least half of all grains as whole grains, fruits rather than fruit juices, and more low-fat or fat-free milk fortified with vitamin D. The Food Pattern also provided substitutions and changes for lacto-ovo and vegan patterns. The DASH Eating Plan limits saturated fatty acids and cholesterol and focuses food choices in increasing potassium, calcium, magnesium, protein and dietary fiber. Both plans recommend considerably less sodium, added sugars and

solid fats than the typical American diet and the substitution of water as a beverage for many of the current selections we made.[84]

Dieting versus Balanced Food Intake

The key to any "diet" is not to have to go on one to begin with. Regulating your weight must start when you are young. It involves a lifelong commitment to a lifestyle that balances the intake of calories with your calorie expenditure. Did you know that after your early twenties, you will require fewer calories as you age? Your **basal metabolic rate,** the amount of energy you need to maintain your body functions, will decline about 2 percent each decade after age 30.[85] If you consume a 2000-calorie diet now, and 10 years from now you are consuming the same number of calories, you can expect to gain weight. Expect that you will need about 40 fewer calories per day per decade as you age. This will be especially important if your activity level drops off. So you can also see the value of maintaining a physically active lifestyle in addition to monitoring your calorie intake.

The goal of any weight-loss program is to burn more calories than you consume. Once you reach a comfortable and healthy weight, the goal then becomes burning the calories you consume so that your weight is maintained. Keep the following points in mind to be successful with your weight management goals.

- *One pound of fat equals 3,500 calories.* To burn 1 pound of fat, a woman must either consume 3,500 fewer calories or perform some kind of physical activity that would use 3,500 calories more than she has consumed. Conversely, if a woman eats 3,500 calories more than she burns through activity, she will gain a pound of fat.
- *Exercise is crucial to a weight management program.* In fact, research has shown that, over the long term, exercise alone will contribute more to weight management than a regimen of calorie restriction and dieting.[86] This information is very important to women, because they are more likely than men to use food restriction to lose weight. Men are more likely to increase their exercise levels. Women say, "I need to quit eating so much." Men say, "I need to get to the gym."
- *Proper weight management is a lifetime lifestyle commitment.* It is not something undertaken because you want to fit into a particular bathing suit this summer or because you finally realize that you are 30 pounds over your ideal weight.
- *Weight management through medications does not work.* The medical community has attempted to use certain drug regimens to combat obesity. These regimens do not work for the long term.

In addition, a number of adverse side effects may come with drug therapy, ranging from depression to hypertension. Perhaps the most significant reason for avoiding drug therapy is that it results in the avoidance of responsibility. The dieter expects a "magic bullet" to take care of the "weakness" within the person who eats too much and exercises too little.

Nutrition and the Aging Population

Proper dietary intake is essential throughout the life span, and knowledge about nutritional needs after age 65 is the first step in healthy aging. Currently, people older than 65 account for 13 percent of the U.S. population, with life expectancy for men 74 years and 80 years for women. However, the over-65 age group accounts for 50 percent of the federal health budget; 85 percent of this group have nutrition-related problems such as hypertension, osteoporosis, heart disease, and type 2 diabetes.[87] Do dietary needs change for women as they age?

Older women usually have a diet containing about 1300 to 1600 calories per day. Most of the Dietary Reference Intakes (DRIs) can be met through this amount of calories, but women may need supplements to obtain additional amounts of essential nutrients including vitamin D, vitamin B-12, folate, and calcium.[88] There are differences in the DRIs for women over the age of 50. For example, women under the age of 50 need 1000 mg/day of calcium, but women over age 50 need 1200 mg/day; vitamin B-6 needs for women under the age of 50 are 1.3 mg/day, but 1.5 mg/day is required for women over 50; vitamin D is needed in the amount of 5 mg/dl (micrograms per deciliter) per day for women under the age of 50, but 10 mg/dl is needed between the ages of 50 and 70, with women over 70 needing 15 mg/dl.[89] Maintaining proper nutrition during a woman's later years can be achieved by adhering to the following suggestions.

- Use the USDA ChooseMyPlate to guide food and serving selections. Drink adequate, but not excessive, amounts of water to prevent constipation.
- Decrease fat consumption and increase consumption of nutrient-dense foods such as fruits and vegetables; use food intake to obtain the most nutrients possible (consume more bright-colored vegetables and deep-colored fruits).
- Take supplements to provide needed nutrients not consumed in food intake; reduced calorie intake can reduce the potential of obtaining critical nutrients.
- Obtain higher levels of specific nutrients such as vitamin D and calcium for stronger bones and folic acid to retain mental acuity and reduce potential of stroke and heart disease.
- Maintain a physician-approved exercise regimen to strengthen bones and muscles, promote sleep, and improve appetite.[90]

Chapter Summary

- A multitude of factors, such as family, knowledge, and emotions, influence the daily food choices we make.
- A typical American's energy values are derived from a number of sources.
- Dietary guidelines that assist American women in developing positive eating habits include the following: eat a variety of foods; balance food you consume with physical activity; select a diet with plenty of grain products, vegetables, and fruits; choose a diet low in fat, saturated fat, and cholesterol; select a diet that is lower in sugar, salt, and sodium; and if you drink, do so in moderation.
- The Web site choosemyplate.gov provides a visual account of the variety and amount of foods that should be consumed to ensure a balanced, healthy diet.
- The six major nutrients—carbohydrates, protein, fats, vitamins, minerals, and water—provide the chemicals our bodies need for energy, building and repairing tissue, and functioning effectively.
- Most food additives pose no threat to our well-being.
- Special conditions such as pregnancy, intense levels of exercise, or chronic disease often result in the need for special foods or increased amounts of certain nutrients.
- Being overweight may not mean that a woman is overfat; however, there are serious health consequences as a result of being overfat.
- The most effective way to lose weight is to monitor calorie consumption and maintain a physically active lifestyle.
- Good nutrition consumer skills can be an important asset when selecting food products that are both beneficial and assist with weight management.
- Nutritional needs in elderly women are more specific than in younger women.

Review Questions

1. Provide four key recommendations of the foods that Americans are encouraged to eat according to the Dietary Guidelines for Americans 2010.
2. What are the Dietary Reference Intakes and the current changes that are taking place with respect to their values?
3. What is the role of carbohydrates in the body, and what are the most healthful sources to choose from?
4. What is meant by the term *nutrient density?*
5. What are the sources of the water-soluble vitamins?
6. Other than milk, what are significant sources of calcium in the diet?

7. What are the specific nutritional needs that a woman has during pregnancy?
8. What are the specific cautions a woman must recognize if she chooses to follow a vegetarian diet?
9. What changes take place in a woman's nutrient needs during exercise?
10. What are the main components required by law to appear on the information panel of a food label?
11. List and explain the various ways of measuring the amount of fat a woman has in her body.

Resources

Academy of Nutrition and Dietetics
800-877-1600
www.eatright.org

American Society for Nutrition
301-634-7050
www.nutrition.org

Food and Nutrition Information Center
301-504-5414
fnic.nal.usda.gov

Jean Mayer USDA Human Nutrition Research Center on Aging (HNRCA) Tufts University
617-556-3000
www.hnrc.tufts.edu

Linus Pauling Institute
Corvallis, OR 97331-6512
541-737-5075
http://lpi.oregonstate.edu

National Dairy Council
312-240-2880
www.nationaldairycouncil.org/NationalDairyCouncil

Oldways Preservation Trust
617-421-5500
www.oldwayspt.org

Overeaters Anonymous
505-891-2664
www.oa.org/index.htm

Society for Nutrition Education and Behavior
317-328-4627 or 800-235-6690
www.sne.org

U.S. Food and Drug Administration (FDA)
888-INFO-FDA (1-888-463-6332)
www.fda.gov

The Vegetarian Resource Group (VRG)
410-366-VEGE (8343)
www.vrg.org/nutshell/about.htm

References

1. Wardlaw, G. .M, and A. M. Smith. 2008. *Contemporary nutrition.* 7th edition. New York: McGraw-Hill.
2. U.S. Department of Agriculture and U.S. Department of Health and Human Services. *Dietary guidelines for Americans, 2010.* 7th edition. Washington, DC: U.S. Government Printing Office, December, 2010.
3. Dietary Guidelines Advisory Committee. 2010. *Report of the Dietary Guidelines Advisory Committee on the Dietary Guidelines for Americans, 2010, to the Secretary of Agriculture and the Secretary of Health and Human Services.* Washington, DC: U.S. Department of Agriculture, Agricultural Research Service. p. 433.
4. Ibid., p. 62.
5. U.S. Department of Agriculture and U.S. Department of Health and Human Services. *Dietary guidelines for Americans, 2010.*
6. Ibid.

7. Ibid.
8. Ibid.
9. Dietary Guidelines Advisory Committee. 2010. *Report of the Dietary Guidelines Advisory Committee on the Dietary Guidelines for Americans, 2010, to the Secretary of Agriculture and the Secretary of Health and Human Services.*
10. Ibid.
11. U.S. Department of Agriculture and U.S. Department of Health and Human Services. *Dietary guidelines for Americans, 2010.*
12. Ibid.
13. Reedy, J., and S. M. Krebs-Smith. October 2010. Dietary sources of energy, solid fats and added sugar among children and adolescents in the United States. *Journal of American Dietetic Association* 110 (10), 1477–1484.

14. Dietary Guidelines Advisory Committee. 2010. *Report of the Dietary Guidelines Advisory Committee on the Dietary Guidelines for Americans, 2010, to the Secretary of Agriculture and the Secretary of Health and Human Services.*

15. Ibid.

16. National Cancer Institute. *Sources of added sugars in the diets of the U.S. population ages 2 years and older, NHANES 2005–06.* Risk Factor Monitoring and Methods. Cancer Control and Population Sciences, 2010.

17. National Cancer Institute. *Sources of refined grains in the diets of the U.S. population ages 2 years and older, NHANES 2005–06.*

18. U.S. Department of Agriculture and U.S. Department of Health and Human Services. *Dietary guidelines for Americans, 2010.*

19. Ibid.

20. National Cancer Institute. *Sources of sodium in the diets of the U.S. population ages 2 years and older, NHANES 2005–06.* Risk Factor Monitoring and Methods. Cancer Control and Population Sciences, 2010.

21. National Cancer Institute. *Sources of solid fats in the diets of the U.S. population ages 2 years and older, NHANES 2005–06.* Risk Factor Monitoring and Methods. Cancer Control and Population Sciences, 2010.

22. Dietary Guidelines Advisory Committee. 2010. *Report of the Dietary Guidelines Advisory Committee on the Dietary Guidelines for Americans, 2010, to the Secretary of Agriculture and the Secretary of Health and Human Services.* U.S. Department of Agriculture, Agricultural Research Service, Washington, DC.

23. Ibid.

24. Ibid.

25. Harvard School of Public Health. 2011. *The Nutrition Source. Alcohol: Balancing the risks and benefits.* http://www.hsph .harvard.edu/nutritionsource/what-should-you-eat/alcohol-full-story/index.html#Dark_side_alcohol

26. U.S. Department of Agriculture and U.S. Department of Health and Human Services. *Dietary guidelines for Americans, 2010.* 7th edition, Washington, DC: U.S. Government Printing Office, December, 2010.

27. Ibid.

28. Ibid.

29. Ibid.

30. Wardlaw and Smith. *Contemporary nutrition.*

31. Ibid.

32. U.S. Department of Agriculture and U.S. Department of Health and Human Services. *Dietary guidelines for Americans, 2010.*

33. Wardlaw and Smith. *Contemporary nutrition.*

34. Ibid.

35. Ebbling, C., M. Leidig, H. Feldman, M. Lovesky, and D. Ludwig. 2007. Effects of a low-glycemic load vs. low-fat diet in obese young adults. *Journal of the American Medical Association* 297 (19): 2092–2102.

36. Centers for Disease Control and Prevention. 2008. *Nutrition for everyone. Basics: Protein.* http://www.cdc.gov/nutrition/everyone/basics/protein.html

37. Harvard School of Public Health. 2011. *The Nutrition Source. Protein.* http://www.hsph.harvard.edu/nutritionsource/questions/protein-questions/index.html#howmuch

38. National Academies Press, Institute of Medicine. 2005. *Dietary references for energy, carbohydrate, fiber, fat, fatty acids, cholesterol, protein and amino acids (macronutrients) 2005.* http://www.nap.edu/openbook.php?record_id=10490&page=589

39. U.S. Department of Agriculture and U.S. Department of Health and Human Services. *Dietary guidelines for Americans, 2010.*

40. Harvard School of Public Health. 2011. *The Nutrition Source. Antioxidants: Beyond the hype.* http://www.hsph.harvard.edu/nutritionsource/what-should-you-eat/antioxidants

41. Gershoff S. 1996. *The Tufts University guide to total nutrition.* New York: HarperPerennial.

42. Harvard School of Public Health. 2011. *The Nutrition Source. Antioxidants.*

43. Cook, N., C. Albert, J. Gaziano, E. Zaharris, et al. 2007. A randomized factorial trail of vitamin C and E and beta carotene in the secondary prevention of cardiovascular events in women: Results from the Women's Antioxidant Cardiovascular Study. *Archives of Internal Medicine,* 167 (15): 1610.

44. Harvard School of Public Health. 2011. *The Nutrition Source. Calcium and milk: What's best for your bones and health?* http://www.hsph.harvard.edu/nutritionsource/what-should-you-eat/calcium-full-story/

45. National Osteoporosis Foundation. 2011. *Fast Facts.* http://www.nof.org/node/40

46. Ibid.

47. University of California-Davis. 2008. *Nutrition and health info sheet: Iron and iron deficiency anemia.* www.nutrition.ucdavid.edu/Infosheets/ANR/IronAndAnemiaFact.pdf

48. Blake J. 2008. *Nutrition and you.* San Francisco: Pearson Benjamin-Cummings.

49. Arnold, E., and J. Larson. 2006. *Bottled water: Pouring resources down the drain.* http://www.earth-policy.org/index.php?/plan_b_updates/2006/update51

50. Environmental Working Group (EWG). 2011. *What's in your bottled water—besides water?* http://www.ewg.org/bottled-water-2011-home

51. WebMD. 2011. *Pregnancy and weight gain.* http://www.webmd.com/baby/guide/healthy-weight-gain

52. Centers for Disease Control and Prevention. 2011. *Iron and iron deficiency.* http://www.cdc.gov/nutrition/everyone/basics/vitamins/iron.html

53. U.S. Department of Agriculture and U.S. Department of Health and Human Services. *Dietary guidelines for Americans, 2010.*

54. Blake, J. 2008. *Nutrition and you.*

55. Ibid.

56. Ibid.

57. Ibid.

58. Barr, S., and C. Rideout. 2004. Nutritional concerns for vegetarian athletes. *Nutrition* 20:696–703.

59. Dingott, S., and J. Dwyer. 2003. *Vegetarianism: Healthful but unnecessary.* http://www.quackwatch.org/03HealthPromotion/vegetarian.html

60. U.S. Department of Agriculture and U.S. Department of Health and Human Services. *Dietary guidelines for Americans, 2010.*

61. Dingott, S., and J. Dwyer. *Vegetarianism: Healthful but unnecessary.*

62. U.S. Department of Agriculture. 2011. *Tips for vegetarians.* http://www.choosemyplate.gov/healthy-eating-tips/tips-for-vegetarian.html

63. Ibid.

64. Food and Drug Administration. 2012. *Food additives.* http://www.fda.gov/Food/FoodIngredientsPackaging/ucm082463.htm

65. Curtis, C. S., and S. Misner. 2006. *Pesticides vs organically grown food.* University of Arizona Cooperative Extension. Department of Nutritional Sciences. http://ag.arizona.edu/pubs/health/foodsafety/az1079.html

66. U.S. Department of Agriculture and U.S. Department of Health and Human Services. *Dietary guidelines for Americans, 2010.*

67. Food and Drug Administration. 2011. *Guidance for Industry: A food labeling guide.* http://www.fda.gov/Food/Guidance ComplianceRegulatoryInformation/GuidanceDocuments/FoodLabelingNutrition/FoodLabelingGuide/ucm064872.htm

68. Curtis, C. S., and S. Misner. *Pesticides vs organically grown food.*

69. Food and Drug Administration. 2011. *Definitions of nutrient content claims.* http://www.fda.gov/Food/Guidance ComplianceRegulatoryInformation/GuidanceDocuments/FoodLabelingNutrition/FoodLabelingGuide/ucm064911.htm

70. Food and Drug Administration. 2012. *Have food allergies? Read the label.* http://www.fda.gov/ForConsumers/Consumer Updates/ucm254504.htm

71. Centers for Disease Control and Prevention. *Food safety.* http://www.cdc.gov/foodsafety/

72. Food and Drug Administration. 2009. *Peanut product recalls: Salmonella typhimurium.* http://www.fda.gov/Safety/Recalls/MajorProductRecalls/Peanut/default.htm

73. Centers for Disease Control and Prevention. 2009. *Investigation of multistate outbreak of E. coli.* http://www.cdc.gov/ecoli/2012/O26-02-12/

74. Food and Drug Administration. 2009. *FDA finalizes report on 2006 spinach outbreak.* http://www.fda.gov/NewsEvents/Newsroom/PressAnnouncements/2007/ucm108873.htm

75. U.S. Department of Agriculture. *Be food safe.* http://www.fsis.usda.gov/Be_FoodSafe/index.asp

76. Shields, M., M. D. Caroll, and C. L. Ogden. *Adult obesity prevalence in Canada and the United States,* No. 56. Hyattsville, MD: National Center for Health Statistics, 2011.

77. National Heart, Lung, and Blood Institute. 2011. *Assessing your weight and health risk.* http://www.nhlbi.nih.gov/health/public/heart/obesity/lose_wt/risk.htm

78. U.S. Department of Agriculture and U.S. Department of Health and Human Services. *Dietary guidelines for Americans, 2005.* 6th edition, Washington, DC: U.S. Government Printing Office, 2005.

79. Shields, M., M. D. Caroll, and C. L. Ogden. *Adult obesity prevalence in Canada and the United States.*

80. Danziger, M., J. Gleason, J. Griffith, H. Seckler, and E. Schaefer. 2005. Comparison of the Atkins, Ornish, Weight Watchers, and Zone diets for weight loss and heart disease risk reduction. *Journal of the American Medical Association* 298 (2), p. 173.

81. Sacks, F., G. Bray, V. Carey, S. Smith, D. Ryan, et al. 2009. Comparison of weight-loss diets with different compositions of fat, protein, and carbohydrates. *New England Journal of Medicine* 360 (9), 859–873.

82. Ibid.

83. Freedman, M., J. King, and E. Kennedy. Popular diets: A scientific review. *Obesity Research* 9(suppl 1), 1s–40s. 2001.

84. U.S. Department of Agriculture and U.S. Department of Health and Human Services. *Dietary guidelines for Americans, 2010.*

85. Wardlaw and Smith. *Contemporary nutrition.*

86. Harvard School of Public Health. 2009. *The Nutrition Source. The benefits of physical activity.* http://www.hsph.harvard.edu/nutritionsource/staying-active/staying-active-full-story/#exercise-for-weight-maintenance

87. Wardlaw and Smith. *Contemporary nutrition.*

88. Ibid.

89. Institute of Medicine, Food and Nutrition Board. 2001. *Dietary reference intakes for vitamin A, vitamin K, arsenic, baron, chromium, copper, iodine, iron, manganese, molybdenum, nickel, silicon, vanadium and zinc.* http://www.iom.edu/Reports/2001/Dietary-Reference-Intakes-for-Vitamin-A-Vitamin-K-Arsenic-Boron-Chromium-Copper-Iodine-Iron-Manganese-Molybdenum-Nickel-Silicon-Vanadium-and-Zinc.aspx

90. U.S. Department of Health and Human Services. 2008. *2008 Physical activity guidelines for Americans.* http://www.health.gov/paguidelines/pdf/paguide.pdf

Keeping Fit

CHAPTER OBJECTIVES

When you complete this chapter, you will be able to do the following:

◇ Describe the physical, psychological, and social benefits of fitness activities

◇ Distinguish between the four health-related components of fitness and explain the specifics of each component

◇ Analyze the relationships between chronic diseases and physical fitness programs

◇ Explain the importance of warm-up and cool-down activities

◇ Describe the methods to assess physical fitness levels

◇ Identify ways to create successful physical fitness programs

◇ Develop a comprehensive fitness program using the four health-related components of fitness

◇ Identify special considerations for exercise during pregnancy and menstruation

◇ Explain the issues which evolve from compulsive exercising

◇ Describe the advantages of weight maintenance through fitness workouts

◇ Summarize the advantages of fitness programs for women throughout the life span

BENEFITS OF FITNESS

One does not have to venture far to observe people of every age, size, and culture walking, biking, or swimming their way toward improved physical condition. Today we are more aware of the increased role that fitness plays in enhancing each dimension of our health than in past decades. It could be considered both a miracle drug and a fountain of youth that is *free* for the taking! Fitness not only plays a part in reducing the risks of developing heart disease and stroke, diabetes, osteoporosis, and obesity but also promotes the development of positive attitudes, increased energy, and general well-being.

Physiological benefits are well documented in hundreds of research studies conducted over many years. Often the physical benefits, such as weight loss or disease prevention, are the initial reason for engaging in fitness activities, but the multitude of additional benefits a woman gains is usually the reason for continuing the program. A fitness program can produce many positive outcomes including prevention of the diseases that cause illness and death in women. (See Table 11.1.)

Psychological benefits gained from participating in a regular fitness program can be somewhat subjective and may vary from research study to study. These benefits are not limited to any age or either sex, and may be achieved by all participants. Craft[1] suggests that

TABLE 11.1 Fitness and Disease

Cardiovascular diseases	Aerobic exercise (walking, jumping rope, cross-country/downhill skiing, swimming) strengthens and tones the heart muscle, improves blood circulation, helps control hypertension, lowers cholesterol, increases levels of high-density lipoproteins (HDLs), increases the number of red blood cells, and reduces weight, which lessens the risk of heart disease caused by obesity.
Stroke	Involvement in greater leisure-time activity is associated with reduced risk of stroke in women. Varying levels of physical activity provide varying levels of reduction in total and ischemic stroke. Walking has been shown to significantly reduce incidence of stroke.[2]
Osteoporosis	Aerobic as well as weight-bearing exercise helps to strengthen bones and prevents bone-density loss in women, helps to strengthen and tone muscle, increases muscle mass needed to support the skeletal system, and reduces risks of fracture. In older women, exercise improves strength, flexibility, and balance, which can reduce the chance of falls and fractures.
Arthritis	Exercises for range of motion (stretching), as well as water aerobics, walking, biking, and swimming, can help joints maintain strength and flexibility, and may relieve some pain.
Diabetes	Following physician approval to exercise, benefits include: lower blood glucose due to more sensitivity to insulin and increased use of glucose; take less insulin or other diabetic meds; increase caloric burn and help maintain or reduce body weight; improve sleep and increase energy levels.[3]
Breast cancer	Engaging in physical activity lowers the risk of developing breast cancer. Women who had been diagnosed with breast cancer and who engaged in the equivalent of walking 3–5 hours per week, at an average pace, appeared to have the greatest benefits.[4] Physically active women have up to an average of 25 percent reduced risk of developing breast cancer.[5]

women who are more active have lower levels of anxiety and depression. The Physical Activity Guidelines for Americans[6] states that a total of 150 minutes (2 hours 30 minutes) a week of moderate-intensity aerobic activity consistently reduces the risk of many chronic diseases and other adverse health outcomes. Reducing the risk of depression, lowering risk of cognitive decline, such as declines in thinking, learning, and judgment skills, as well as improving sleep are all outcomes of regular physical activity. The degree and extent to which these benefits are attained will vary depending on the participant and her dedication to a regular fitness activity.

Obesity has become a major and growing concern for women, men, and children in the United States, with more than one-third of adults (35.7 percent) classified as obese. Obesity-related conditions include stroke, heart disease, certain types of cancer, and type 2 diabetes, each a leading cause of death in the United States.[7] A consistent, well-planned exercise program is a critical factor in maintaining and regaining a health body weight for women. Fitting exercise into a lifestyle routine helps improve overall health and fitness and reduces the risks for developing many chronic diseases.

Social benefits are certainly a part of the attractive package a fitness program can provide. These offer an opportunity to be a part of groups and organizations in which women not only enjoy the company of others but also gain a multitude of health benefits in the process. Health clubs offer a choice of activities, and often new friends with similar interests can be found. Community recreational programs often develop activity-related

programs such as biking clubs, hiking, walking, or running groups; and tennis leagues in which one can find associates with mutual interests and lifestyles. Women can also associate with individuals having similar goals and interests by participating in special activities such as yoga, Tai chi, meditation, and self-defense. (See *FYI:* "Mind–Body Exercise: Yoga.") The social benefits abound when participating in fitness-related activities whether in small- or large-group settings.

Achieving any one of these fitness benefits is a positive addition to our lifestyle. However, the good news is that we usually achieve many of them. Regardless of "why" you decide to participate in a fitness regimen, whether it is to reduce weight, relieve stress, or prevent

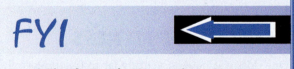

Mind–Body Exercise: Yoga

Yoga, either in mild and therapeutic form or in power form, can have multiple benefits for a woman's mind and body. This type of exercise has been practiced for centuries and supports a holistic approach to fitness, nutrition, and lifestyle. Yoga is a powerful method to reduce stress, improve concentration and balance, and increase muscular strength, endurance, and flexibility. A new study noted that participants reported a feeling of peace and calm, along with self-reported body weight improvement.[8]

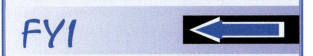

FYI

How Much Exercise Do Adults Need?

The *2008 Physical Activity Guidelines for Americans*[9] provides information regarding the amount and types of exercise needed by adult women and men. Two types of exercise are most important: health-aerobic exercise and muscle strengthening. To maximize health benefits:

- Adults need at least the following: 2 hours 30 minutes (150 minutes) of moderate-intensity aerobic activity (e.g., brisk walking) each week or 1 hour 15 minutes (75 minutes) of vigorous-intensity aerobic activity (e.g., jogging or running) every week.
- Aerobic activity can be broken up into smaller chunks of time; try a 10-minute brisk walk, three times a day, 5 days a week for a total of 150 minutes each week.
- For greater health benefits, try 5 hours per week (300 minutes) of moderate-intensity aerobic activity.
- Along with the aerobic level selected, add muscle-strengthening activities on 2 or more days each week that work all major muscle groups (legs, hips, back, abdomen, chest, shoulders, and arms).

For complete copy of the 2008 Physical Activity Guidelines, go to www.health.gov/PAGuidelines/guidelines/default.aspx

bone density loss, a woman still reaps a variety of the benefits. Fitness activities that improve your physical, psychological, and social well-being are worth your time, energy, and money (see *FYI: How Much Exercise Do Adults Need?*").

HEALTH-RELATED COMPONENTS OF FITNESS

Research firmly supports the concept of health promotion and disease prevention as a result of involvement in a regular fitness program. However, the fitness program must consist of several components. Do you have a friend who has no problem lifting, pushing, or carrying objects yet is out of breath after walking up two flights of stairs? Well, your friend has developed one component of fitness (strength) but is lacking in another (endurance). A well-designed and comprehensive physical fitness program consists of four **health-related components of fitness:** cardiorespiratory endurance, flexibility, muscular strength and endurance, and body composition. Other components of fitness can also be an important part of a fitness program. However, these components—agility, balance, power, and speed—are performance-related fitness components and are outside the scope of this book. In creating your own personal fitness program, the four health-related components of fitness need to be included. A brief explanation of each component follows.

Cardiorespiratory Endurance

Cardiorespiratory fitness is considered to be the most important component of a physical fitness program because it affects vital organs of the body—the heart and lungs—and the arterial system, which deliver life-giving oxygen to every cell in the body. Their health and fitness are essential to the basic life support of our bodies. **Cardiorespiratory endurance** is the ability to perform prolonged, large-muscle, dynamic exercise at moderate to high levels of intensity.[10]

Activities that produce this outcome, called **aerobic activities,** include cycling, swimming, jumping rope, cross-country skiing, walking, running, aerobic dancing, rollerblading, and jogging. Each of these calls for the use of large muscles and repetitive movements over a sustained period of time.

Principles of Condition
To benefit from participation in cardiorespiratory endurance activities, you need to include the principles of conditioning, which are represented by the acronym FITT: **F**requency, **I**ntensity, **T**ime, and **T**ype.[11]

Frequency relates to "how often" you engage in aerobic workouts, expressed in number of days. The minimum is three workout aerobic sessions per week up to a maximum of 6 days per week. Two to 3 days per week are prescribed for strength training, with stretching 2 to 7 days per week, or with each workout session. Workouts on a more frequent basis will result in greater and steadier improvement.

Intensity means "how hard" you should work out during the aerobic activity. Benefits of fitness activities take place when a person works out harder than her normal activity level. Intensity is determined by the number of times the heart beats in 1 minute during any given activity. To determine the level of intensity, you need to know how to calculate your target heart rate and then calculate it during the activity. (See *Access Yourself:* "Calculate Your Target Heart Rate.")

Time refers to duration or "how long" you spend in the aerobic phase of your fitness program. For minimal improvement, the workout should be continuous during the aerobic phase for at least 20 minutes at your target heart rate (THR). For great results and benefits, the aerobic phase should last 30–50 minutes. The American College of Sports Medicine (ACSM) recommends 150 minutes of aerobic workout per week.[12]

Type relates to the various types of aerobic activity from which you may choose. The activity must be continuous and involve large-muscle groups. Activities such as brisk walking, swimming, running, aerobic dancing, biking, jumping rope, and/or jogging performed in a continuous manner for the prescribed frequency, intensity and time, along with activities that increase muscle strength, endurance and flexibility should result in gaining all the benefits previously described in this chapter.

Flexibility

Flexibility allows an individual to use the full range of motion at a joint, which improves performance in fitness and recreational activities, and helps to reduce and prevent injuries and soreness. Flexibility has a genetic base; genetics determines how elastic the muscles and connective tissues will be and therefore makes individuals more or less flexible. This fitness component is joint specific and is affected by bulk and long arrangement of specific joints. Can you increase your flexibility? Absolutely! Stretching in one's exercise regimen helps reduce the rate that inflexibility occurs and reduces the shortening of muscles, tendons, and ligaments. At any age, flexibility can be greatly increased by using a variety of stretching exercises before and after fitness activities.

There are many stretching techniques that can improve one's flexibility. Following are three types of stretching techniques, with their specific benefits.[13]

- **Static stretching,** the safest way to stretch, involves stretching a specific muscle, usually for 10–30 seconds, until tension is felt. Remember, never "lock" a joint during stretching. (See Figure 11.1.)
- Active isolated stretching involves the same muscles as in the static stretch, but the position is held only for 1–2 seconds and repeated 8–10 times.
- The positive aspects of this type of stretch are that the individual does not force the muscle to stay contracted and the muscle is relaxed between each stretch. (See Figure 11.2.)
- Proprioceptive neuromuscular facilitation **(PNF)** is often done with the help of a partner who helps the exerciser to contract, release, and then stretch a particular muscle or muscle group. When a muscle is contracted and released, the resistance is less and you will be able to stretch the muscle farther. (See Figure 11.3.)
- **Dynamic stretching** incorporates movement with muscle tension and should be performed as active stretches. Dynamic stretches are similar to sport-or-function-specific warm-ups. TaeBo© or medicine ball exercises are examples of dynamic stretches.

Assess Yourself

Calculate Your Target Heart Rate

To determine intensity during the aerobic phase of the physical activity workout, follow these simple instructions:

1. Measure your pulse rate at either the radial artery (on the thumb side of the wrist) or the carotid artery (found in the neck groove by the "Eve's apple").
2. Count your pulse for 30 seconds and multiply this by 2 to find your 1-minute pulse rate. During the workout, count your pulse for 10 seconds and multiply this by 6, which also gives you the 1-minute pulse rate.
3. To determine your target heart beat (the intensity at which you want to exercise to attain benefits), complete the following calculation:

   a. Find your maximal heart rate (MHR) by subtracting your age from 220. (For example, 220 minus 20 equals 200.) You now have your personal MHR.
   b. Multiply MHR by 60, 70, and 80 percent to determine the target heart rate (THR) that is less intense, moderately intense, or highly intense for you. Select one of these percentages depending

on your initial physical condition, then increase the THR to 70 percent or 80 percent (or even 90 percent) as you become more fit.

Examples:

200	200	200
.60	.70	.80
120 beats/min	140 beats/min	160 beats/min

c. As you increase your fitness level, you may want to increase your THR to continue to improve your physical fitness.

Note: Women who have not engaged in fitness activities for a period of time should begin at 60 percent or less of their MHR. Women over the age of 50 should seek a physician's clearance prior to engaging in a **comprehensive fitness program,** a fitness program that includes all components essential to fitness: cardiorespiratory endurance, flexibility, muscular strength and endurance, and body composition.

Lack of flexibility reduces one's quality of life by limiting the enjoyable activities one can engage in as well as restricting the ability to carry out responsibilities. For example, Mary Jane, age 45, was restricted in her ability to play tennis with friends due to injuries to her skeletal system and subsequent weakening of the connective

FIGURE 11.1 Static stretch.

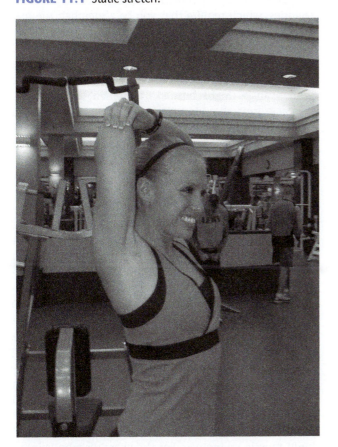

FIGURE 11.2 Isolated stretch.

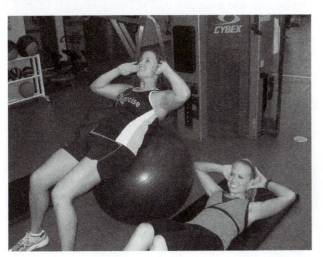

FIGURE 11.3 PNF stretch.

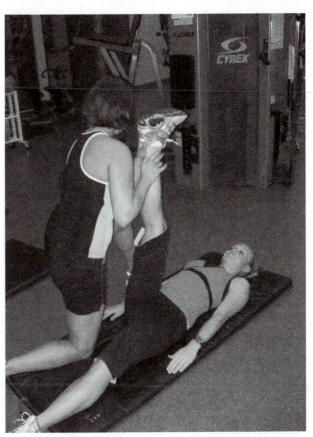

tissues. Additionally, not doing any flexibility exercises resulted in further weakening of connective tissues to her skeletal system. As a teacher, Mary Jane found that she had difficulty writing on the board and putting up classroom displays. Worse yet, she found it difficult to lift, carry, and play with her new grandchild. Upon consultation, Mary Jane's physician suggested a variety of stretching exercises to be done four or five times per week as well as simple muscle-strengthening activities. Mary Jane noticed an improvement after about 6 weeks and is determined to continue these activities to keep her connective tissue flexible and her muscles strengthened.

Flexibility training three to seven times per week improves physical performance; improves circulation as the temperature of the muscle tissue increases; improves posture through incorporating short, frequent stretch breaks throughout the day; and improves coordination and balance. Stretching has also been shown to provide relief from stress, improve mood, and increase alertness during the day.[14]

How many hours per day do you spend at a computer or sitting at a desk? Most of us spend several hours each day, which can lead to muscle tension and fatigue. By using a number of simple stretching exercises for

5–10 minutes, your entire body (and mind) can be revitalized and tension can be relieved.

Keep these suggestions in mind as you go through the stretches:

- Only stretch to the limit where you feel mild tension and then hold according to the number of seconds suggested.
- Do not stretch to the point of feeling pain.
- Do not bounce into or during the stretch.
- Breathe in a low and rhythmic manner.
- When you have finished stretching, close your eyes and breathe slowly for about 10 seconds.

Muscular Strength and Endurance

Muscular strength is the ability of a muscle to generate force against some type of resistance; **muscular endurance** is the ability to continue to generate a force over a period of time or for a number of repetitions. As a result of muscular strength and endurance, a woman can improve her performance in physical activities, reduce the possibility of injury, improve physical appearance, and improve the ratio of lean body mass to fatty tissue. This is an essential component of effective weight-loss programs due to the "burning" of calories during weight training.

Increasing muscle strength can be achieved by participating in weight-bearing exercise such as free weights (barbells) and weight machines (such as Nautilus), performing exercises such as push-ups or pull-ups, or using fitness aids such as Thera-Bands. Classification of weight-training exercises includes isometric exercise, isotonic exercise, and isokinetic exercise. **Isometric** weight training applies force without movement such as applying force in the muscle and holding the force (for example, tightening the buttocks while sitting at your desk). Hold the isometric contraction for a maximum of 6 seconds; do this for 5–10 repetitions for best results. A form of **isotonic** weight training uses force with movement, such as use of a barbell; both the muscle and the

weight move. Isotonic exercise is used more often than other forms of weight training because it better develops and utilizes strength in varied activities. Another type of weight training that can improve muscular strength is **isokinetic** weight training, an exertion of force (such as your leg) at a constant speed against an equal force exerted by a special strength-training machine. Although this type of exercise develops strength and endurance, strength-training machines are usually located in fitness facilities, which require that you be a member; the machinery is too expensive to purchase. (See Figure 11.4.)

You may need the help of an exercise professional in order to develop a strength- and endurance-training program that benefits all muscle groups. All areas of the body—calves, thighs, buttocks, abdomen, lower and upper back, arms, shoulders, and neck—should be included in a strength-enhancing workout. Determine your current level of fitness and the appropriate program needed to improve your strength and endurance. For example, lift approximately 80 percent of your maximum capacity to improve your strength. Choose less weight but increase repetitions to improve your endurance.[15]

Workouts to improve muscular strength and endurance should be done 2–4 days each week with rest between days to allow for recovery. However, you can train more than 4 days per week, if desired, by working out different muscle groups on different days. For example, work the lower-body muscles (legs, buttocks) one day, the upper-body muscles (upper back, arms, shoulders) on the next day, and then return to lower body on the third day. As you lift weights, select 8–10 exercises that focus on the muscle groups you want to develop. Using heavier weights, according to your strength level, and performing fewer repetitions (between 1 and 5) will build muscle strength; using lighter weights but performing a higher number of repetitions (15–20) will build muscle endurance. For the exerciser who is interested in building both strength and endurance, include eight to twelve repetitions for each strengthening exercise and use a weight that is heavy enough to create

FIGURE 11.4 (*A*) Isometric exercise. (*B*) Isotonic exercise. (*C*) Isokinetic exercise.

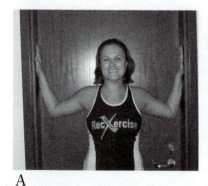
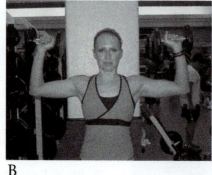
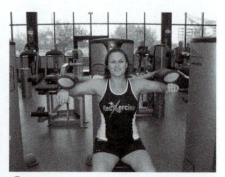

A   B   C

TABLE 11.2 Body Fat Standards for Women Recommended by Age Group[16]

CATEGORY	20–29	30–39	40–49	50–59	60+
Very low	<16%	<17%	<18%	<19%	<20%
Low	16–19%	17–20%	18–21%	19–22%	20–23%
Optimal	20–28%	21–29%	22–30%	23–31%	24–32%
Moderately high	29–31%	30–32%	31–33%	32–33%	33–35%
High	>31%	>32%	>33%	<34%	>35%

fatigue.[17] It is recommended that women over the age of 50 perform more repetitions (10–15 reps) but use lighter weights. This can reduce the chance of injury and rapid fatigue. Regardless of your age, be sure to include a warm-up stretch and a cool-down stretch routine with each weightlifting session.

Body Composition

Women with good to optimal body composition tend to be more active, healthier, and feel better about themselves. **Body composition** has two components: lean body mass that includes the muscles, bones, teeth, connective tissue, and organ tissue, and fat tissue that includes essential fat and nonessential fat. *Essential fat,* which makes up approximately 12 percent of total body fat in women, is just what the term implies—it is fatty tissue that is essential to normal, healthy functioning of the body. This particular type of fat is a component of our brain, nerves, mammary glands, and other important organs in the body and is necessary for proper body functioning. *Nonessential,* or storage, *fat* is located just below the skin within fat cells (adipose tissue) and around major organs. Although it offers cushioning for important body organs and stores energy for future needs, too much nonessential fat can be unhealthy and unsightly.

Measurement of body composition provides a better analysis of one's "body weight" than simply stepping on a scale and looking at the numbers. This measurement provides the weight for all the components of our body. The percentage of a woman's body weight that is fat, called percent body fat, is more important because too much fat is negatively associated with one's health status. Table 11.2 shows the range of percent body fat for women.

OTHER EXERCISE CONSIDERATIONS

A *warm-up* before engaging in the endurance component of a fitness program better prepares the body for a more effective workout and helps to reduce injury during the fitness activity.

As an individual begins the brief warm-up period (usually 5–10 minutes), the activity should be a slow general aerobic activity focusing on the muscles specific to the exercise plan. An increase in body temperature produces a number of beneficial outcomes, including the fact that warm muscles and tendons are less prone to injury and produce improved performance.[18] The warm-up period enables the person's body to receive sufficient blood and oxygen and prepares the muscle groups for more strenuous endurance activities.

The *cool-down* phase of the workout is similar to the warm-up period and is just as important. The major intent of the cool-down is to bring blood back to the heart for reoxygenation so that blood can supply essential oxygen to the brain, heart, and other major body organs, and not pool in major muscle groups. Additionally, during cool-down, the heart rate and breathing rate begin to return to normal and the body temperature begins to decrease. It aids the body in moving from an active state to a resting state. Engaging in a 5- to 10-minute cool-down stretching routine will reduce the probability of sore muscles and injury.

PERSONAL FITNESS PROGRAMMING

Having learned about the important components of a comprehensive fitness program, you can formulate a personal fitness program to meet your individual needs and interests. (See *Health Tips:* "Putting Together a Physical Activity Program.")

The Centers for Disease Control and Prevention (CDC) and other agencies recommend focusing on the frequency, rather than the intensity, of physical activity. According to the CDC, women should accumulate 30 minutes or more at least 5 days each week by engaging in physical activity that involves body movements and energy expenditure. A well-designed and regular fitness program is desirable and will yield positive results. However, some activity is better than no activity, and many women who do not participate in *exercise* programs can

Health Tips

Putting Together a Physical Activity Program

The major components of a physical fitness program are included in the following example. Additionally, suggestions are provided for making your workout work better for you.

Warm-Up Phase
- Spend 10–15 minutes in the warm-up phase.
- Move slowly into an activity that is similar to what your aerobic activity will be (for example, walk, do slow dance movements, etc.) for about 5 minutes. This will start to cause an increase in heart rate.
- Following this, use long stretching movements that stretch the muscles and take the joints through their full range of motion for 5–10 minutes. Stretch all areas and joints of the body: neck, shoulder, arms, trunk, hips, legs, thighs, calves, knees, and ankles.

Workout Phase
- Spend 20–60 minutes, depending on your fitness level. Women who are less physically fit should begin working out 20 minutes three times per week and increase the number of minutes as fitness level allows.

- Include flexibility movements, muscle-strengthening exercises, and endurance activities.
- Remember to watch for the intensity, duration, and frequency of the activities you do (a minimum of 60 percent of your target heart rate for 20 minutes at least three times per week).
- Check your target heart rate; decrease or increase the intensity accordingly.
- Slow down and/or rest as needed.
- Remember that "no pain, no gain" is *not* a true statement.

Cool-Down Phase
- Ease into a reduced-intensity level of activity. This is a very important component of a fitness program.
- Spend 5–10 minutes reducing the heart rate and "coming down" from your workout.
- Slow your movements, and stretch each area of the body as well as all your joints.
- Do relaxing forms of activity to slow down your heart and breathing rates.
- Check your heart rate. It should be reduced from the level it was during the workout phase.

---

still realize positive benefits by accumulating 30 minutes of physical activity (gardening, vacuuming, or walking) per day for 5 days each week.

Fitness Assessments

Deciding to participate in a fitness program is an important decision, but designing a personal fitness program is essential in order to derive the best results for your personal goals. It may require some professional assistance, especially in the area of assessments. Fitness assessments are designed to determine an individual's physical fitness condition as it relates to cardiorespiratory endurance, muscular strength and endurance, flexibility, and body composition. Assessments can be somewhat complicated, but the following information can assist you when deciding which assessments best fit the needs of your fitness goals.

1. *Cardiorespiratory endurance* measures the fitness level by engaging in an assessment test designed to calculating heartbeats per minute and comparing it established national norms developed by exercise physiologist. One easy and dependable method of determining your cardio endurance capacity is by using the 3-minute step test. Standing on the floor, use a bench that is 12 inches high; step up and down for 3 minutes. Upon completing the 3 minutes, sit

down and have your partner count your pulse for 1 minute. Compare the number of beats per minute to heart rates your age found on Table 11.3. Other methods of assess cardio fitness is the 1-mile walk test and the 1.5-mile run-walk test.

2. *Muscular strength and endurance*. To assess muscular strength and endurance, complete the following two activities:
   a. *Modified push-ups*. Lie face down on a mat and with your knees bent, raise your upper body, supported by your arms. Your back and arms need to be straight. Lower your upper body until your chest is about 3 inches off the floor. Then return to the starting position. Count the number of push-ups you can perform within 1 minute. Refer to Table 11.4 to determine your strength level.
   b. *Abdominal muscle strength (curl-ups)*. Lie flat on your back, cross your arms at the chest, and bend your knees at a 90-degree angle with your feet flat on the floor about 18 inches from the buttocks. If necessary, have someone hold your feet in place while you raise your head and chest off the floor or mat for 1 minute. Count the number of curl-ups you can do in 1 minute and compare this with Table 11.5. *Suggestion:* Keep your chin tucked in and sit up until your elbows touch your thighs.

3. *Flexibility*. Two ways to measure flexibility are
   a. *Shoulder flexibility*. Raise your left arm above your head and then bend it at the elbow and reach down your back as far as possible; at the same time, take your right arm and bend it behind your back and try to touch the fingers together from both arms. Finger overlap reflects fairly good flexibility; reverse the position and try to touch fingers again. You are usually more flexible on one side than the other.

   b. *Sit and reach*. Using a box that is 8–12 inches high with a ruler taped on top and extending 6 inches in front of it, sit on the floor with legs outstretched and feet flat against the box. Slowly stretch your fingers across the ruler to determine how far you can reach. Make three attempts to stretch across the ruler. Be sure you warm up first! Compare your results with those in Table 11.6.

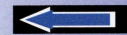

FYI

The Health Benefits of Physical Activity—Major Research Findings

The 2008 Physical Activity Guidelines provide a vast amount of information regarding multiple areas of physical education. A summary of physical activity research findings includes the following:[19]

- Regular physical activity reduces the risk of many adverse health outcomes.
- Some physical activity is better than none.
- For most health outcomes, additional benefits occur as the amount of physical activity increases through higher intensity, greater frequency, and/or longer duration.
- Most health benefits occur with at least 150 minutes a week of moderate-intensity physical activity, such as brisk walking. Additional benefits occur with more physical activity.
- Both aerobic (endurance) and muscle-strengthening (resistance) physical activities are beneficial.
- Health benefits occur for children and adolescents, young and middle-aged adults, older adults, and those in every studied racial and ethnic group.
- The health benefits of physical activity occur for people with disabilities.
- The benefits of physical activity far outweigh the possibility of adverse outcomes.

TABLE 11.4 Test Standards for Modified Push-Ups for Women[21]

Excellent	24 or more push-ups
Good	14–23 push-ups
Average	8–13 push-ups
Fair	2–7 push-ups
Poor	1 or 0

TABLE 11.5 Canadian Trunk Strength Test for Women: Number of Trunk Curl-Ups Completed[22]

STRENGTH CATEGORY	<35	35–44	>45
Excellent	50	40	30
Good	40	25	15
Marginal	25	15	10
Needs work	10	6	4

TABLE 11.6 Sit and Reach Scoring for Women[23]

Excellent	9.0–10.5 inches
Good	6.0–7.5 inches
Average	3.0–5.0 inches
Fair	0.5–2.0 inches
Poor	–2.5–0.0 inches

TABLE 11.3 Scoring Standards for 3-minute Step Test for Women (heart rate for 1 minute)[20]

AGE	18–25	26–35	36–45	46–55	56–65	65+
Category						
Excellent	<85	<88	<90	<94	<95	<90
Above Avg.	86–108	89–111	91–110	95–115	99–112	91–115
Average	109–117	112–119	111–118	116–120	113–118	116–122
Below Avg.	118–126	120–126	119–128	121–126	119–128	119–128
Poor	127–140	127–138	129–140	127–135	129–139	129–134
Very Poor	<141	>139	>141	>136	>140	>135

FIGURE 11.5 Body fat determination using skinfold calipers.

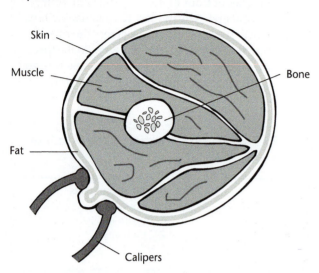

TABLE 11.7   Desirable Body Mass Index for Women

CATEGORY	BMI (kg/m²)
Underweight	<18.5
Normal	18.5–24.9
Overweight	25–29.9
Obese	30–34.9
Extreme obesity	35–39.9
Morbid obesity	>40

4. *Body composition.* Rather than "weighing in" each day to determine body weight, a much better measure is to determine healthy body weight by calculating body composition and comparing lean tissue to fat tissue. There are several methods of doing this, including skin-fold measurement and calculating body mass index (BMI).

a. *Skin-fold measurement.* Using **calipers,** we can measure the thickness of skin at certain sites on the body and apply this measurement to a formula which will give us the percentage of fat. (See Figure 11.5.) These skin-fold measurements have been compared to laboratory techniques that research studies have shown to be an accurate measure to determine body composition.

b. *Bioelectrical impedance analysis (BIA).* This measures the electrical resistance of small currents directed through the body. Electrical impulses pass more freely through tissues containing water, such as muscle tissue. Fatty tissue, containing less water, is not a good conductor of electricity; therefore, the more resistance measured during BIA, the larger the percentage of fat in the body. To measure bio-electrical impedance, electrodes are attached to the body and then to a computer that provides feedback. The electrical current is harmless and painless, and the feedback regarding body composition is rapid. The accuracy of BIA is about the same as for skin-fold measurement.

c. *Hydrostatic weighing.* Considered the "gold standard" of calculating body composition, this system measures the relative amount of fat and lean body mass while the person is submerged under water. Through the use of a special scale, a woman's underwater body weight is compared to her body weight out of the water, and then calculations are made to determine percentage of body fat. Some find this procedure uncomfortable because of the need to be submerged under water for a brief period of time.

d. *The body pod.* The body pod resembles a small chamber with computerized sensors. The procedure can be completed in 5 minutes. While the measurement principle is the same as for underwater weighing, this method uses air displacement rather than water displacement to determine the amount of air that is displaced by the person sitting in the chamber. The overall composition of the body can be measured by calculating the percentage of fat and lean tissue.

e. *Body mass index (BMI)* is a method of expressing the relationship of body weight (expressed in kilograms) to height (expressed in meters) for men and women. Although the BMI does not determine body composition, it is quite accurate in determining healthy body weight. To calculate your BMI, go to cdc.gov/healthyweight/assessing/bmi/adult_bmi/english_bmi_calculator/bmi_calculator.html. See Table 11.7 to determine your category for BMI.

DESIGN YOUR PERSONAL FITNESS PROGRAM

Knowing the benefits and "how-to" of fitness workouts is one thing. We usually have a motivating factor (such as a wedding, spring break, or more energy) for beginning the program. However, keeping the program successful enough to remain involved, called **exercise adherence,** creates a need for additional information and know-how.

Getting Started

How do you establish a fitness program that includes the necessary components, meets your needs, and safely helps you achieve the benefits you want to see? To answer this question, consider the following as an entry into a fitness program that can provide healthy and satisfactory rewards.

Should you get a physical checkup? Ask yourself the following questions to determine whether you should see a physician before embarking on your potential change of lifestyle program.

- Do I have any medical condition that might need special attention before starting a fitness program, such as heart problems, chest pains or pressure, dizziness or fainting spells, or high blood pressure?
- Have I experienced any shortness of breath after any type of exertion?
- Are my joints painful or my muscles overly sore following activity?
- Has my mother, father, brother, sister, or a grandparent had a heart attack before age 50?
- Have I had a physical exam within the past year, other than for an ailment (such as flu, cold, or other communicable disease)?
- Do I have any serious problems with my menstrual cycle?
- Am I bothered by breathing problems as a result of asthma or allergies?

If you answered "yes" to any of these questions, you should see your physician; if not, you are probably ready to engage in a sensible, fun, and comprehensive fitness program.

Another aspect of starting a fitness program is to assess your present physical condition to determine where you need to begin your program. The assessments found on pages 294–296 can assist you in this aspect of starting a fitness program.

The next step involves writing a personal contract about what you want to achieve as well as how and when you will carry out your plan. A contract not only will assist you in getting started but also will help you stay involved as well as achieve progress toward your objectives. *Journal Activity:* "My Personal Fitness Contract" provides an example of how to develop a fitness program contract.

Pacing yourself in the initial phase of your fitness program will allow you to build your fitness level gradually and avoid injury as well as burnout. Consider the information in the *Health Tips:* "Putting Together a Physical Activity Program" on page 308 and use this information to begin at the lower part of your target heart rate (around the 60 percent range). Over a period of several weeks, increase the intensity, duration, and perhaps frequency. After a month or so, you may want to change your routine as well as some of your goals. Consider a different environment, perhaps changing from an indoor facility like a health club to activities that take you outside and into a park or track facility, providing weather permits.

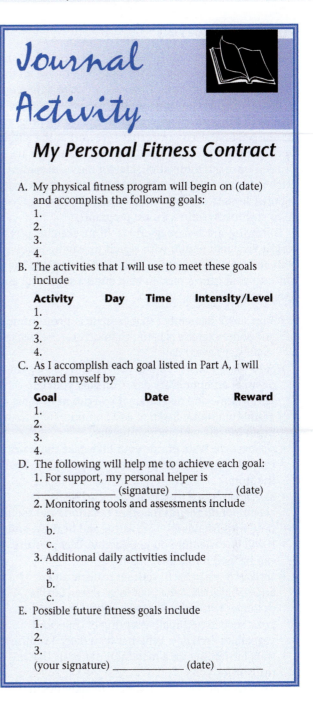

Journal Activity

My Personal Fitness Contract

A. My physical fitness program will begin on (date) and accomplish the following goals:
1.
2.
3.
4.

B. The activities that I will use to meet these goals include

Activity	Day	Time	Intensity/Level
1.			
2.			
3.			
4.			

C. As I accomplish each goal listed in Part A, I will reward myself by

Goal	Date	Reward
1.		
2.		
3.		
4.		

D. The following will help me to achieve each goal:
1. For support, my personal helper is
_____ (signature) _____ (date)
2. Monitoring tools and assessments include
  a.
  b.
  c.
3. Additional daily activities include
  a.
  b.
  c.

E. Possible future fitness goals include
1.
2.
3.

(your signature) _____ (date) _____

In summary, check with your physician, if necessary, then assess your current fitness level, develop a contract, and remember your personal goals of being involved in a fitness program (e.g., losing weight, looking better, having more energy, improving your mood, or preventing disease). Be sure to include the steps that assist you in staying with your program: making a commitment, finding a partner, setting a schedule, checking your progress, varying your routine, and rewarding yourself.

Staying Involved

Starting a fitness program is usually easy to do because we have some knowledge of the benefits or have an impetus to begin a program. However, exercise adherence is often more of a challenge. Sometimes we don't have a structured program, or we engage in the wrong program for our personal needs, or perhaps we start at the wrong level and then proceed at too fast or too slow a pace. Usually, once our motivational factor has been achieved (such as losing weight, toning muscles, etc.), our activity regimen lessens or may stop altogether. What can you do to stay involved in a fitness program?

Following are ten suggestions from exercise physiologist Elizabeth Quinn with regard to staying involved with an exercise program. Consider incorporating these tips into your fitness plan to help build a successful and long-lasting program.[24]

- *Start small:* Remember that exercise is a continuum and some exercise is better than no exercise. Make small steps every day.
- *Start where you are:* You do not have to join a gym or sweat an hour every day. Consider your current routine and determine if you can fit in short 15-minute walks; begin to add 5 minutes and then begin to walk with more intensity.
- *Go low tech:* Walk or ride your bike, take the stairs, mow the lawn with a push mower, park away from the store.
- *Surround yourself with good role models:* Save the couch potato friends for other occasions and spend time with friends who are active and healthy, and it will be easier for you to be active. Peer pressure can be used for positive habits.
- *Set weekly goals:* Each week set realistic and attainable goals. Set a plan to go faster, farther, or longer with your fitness routine. Set nutrition goals such as getting five serving of fruits and vegetables each day. Whether it's a daily 15-minute walk or training for a marathon, set goals that are realistic for you.
- *Try something new:* Try a variety of activities in order to find one you really like and want to do long-term. Suggestions include joining a yoga class, snowboarding lessons, going with others, exercising at different times of day, finding activities you enjoy.
- *Write it down:* Keep an exercise log book; write down what you did, for how long, and how you felt. You can view your progress, plan ahead, and make important decisions about where to go with your exercise program.
- *Make exercise part of your routine:* Aim to add exercise to what you already do. Walk the dog, the children, bike to the store or work, do crunches, push-ups, be active during TV commercials, meet friends for a walk. You may not need to change your routine so much in order to exercise.
- *Find a buddy:* Find someone to exercise with you and/or support your exercise efforts. Make yourself accountable to someone with regard to your fitness activities.
- *Make exercise a priority:* You never reach your exercise goals if they are at the bottom of your priority list. Talk about being active and work to include an active lifestyle in your routine. Put your energy into action, rather than making excuses.

Avoiding Injuries

Women who participate in sports and other fitness activities need to be aware of and take precautions to avoid injuries that hinder or suspend the continuation of their fitness program. Engaging in exercise too frequently or too intensely can result in a variety of injuries that are usually preventable. In general, most fitness-related injuries can be avoided simply by a warm-up and a cool-down stretching routine before and after every workout and by varying your fitness activities.

What are some of the more common injuries that women sustain during fitness activities, and what can be done about them? One of the more common and serious injuries is a tear of the **anterior cruciate ligament (ACL),** which is a major support structure of the knee. This injury occurs more often in active women than in active men and is usually an injury caused by contact of the knee with another object or when the leg is planted and then turned in another direction. If you experience swelling and pain of the knee, you should see a physician. This type of injury calls for rehabilitation exercises under the guidance of a physical therapist. Sometimes surgery is necessary. Another type of knee injury is called **patellofemoral knee pain,** which can result from, for example, repetitive jumping, improper stretching, or joint surface degeneration. Symptoms include inflammation with swelling, tenderness, and pain during movement.

Shin splints are recognized because of the pain that occurs in the shins and are usually caused by too much activity performed on hard surfaces such as gym floors or hard-surfaced roads. This may occur because of strains in the muscles that move the ankle and foot at the attachment points in the shin. Arch supports, either over-the-counter or, if needed, custom-made by a sports podiatrist, will usually cure the problem of shin splints. It may be necessary to reduce or temporarily discontinue your fitness activity until the injury is healed.

Low back pain can result from weak back or abdominal muscles, especially if you begin exercising with too much intensity or too frequently. Preventing low back pain can be accomplished in a number of ways: First, try reducing strenuous activity to a level that your body can safely accommodate. Second, improve your back muscles by carefully engaging in abdominal- and back-strengthening exercises. However, if back pain persists, see a physician for an evaluation of the problem.

Persistent inflammation and pain near the tip of the shoulder is called shoulder impingement and is caused by a continual forceful overhead motion of the shoulder.

Activities such as serving a tennis ball, swimming, weightlifting, or throwing can cause this injury. Strengthening the shoulder muscles with light weight-bearing exercises or eliminating activities that strain this area can help with this injury.

The simple **RICE** plan (rest, ice, compression, and elevation) can be most useful for temporary relief. *Rest* the injured area and apply an *ice* pack on the injury for 10–20 minutes three times a day for 72 hours after the injury. *Compress* the injured area with an elastic bandage and then *elevate* it several times a day. RICE should reduce pain and swelling of the injured area. If there is no improvement within a week, then it is time to see a physician.[25]

JOINING A FITNESS CLUB

There are more than 29,750 health and sports clubs in the United States, sustaining more than 45.3 million health club members.[26] Health clubs offer a number of advantages: an energetic environment with women who have some of the same goals; state-of-the-art equipment; trained and certified personnel to lead and assist exercisers; personal trainers for more one-on-one attention; an all-weather facility that often is open long hours; and opportunities to interact socially in a safe environment.

Selecting a health club that is appropriate for one's fitness needs and goals can take some important consumer skills. If you choose to join a health club, *FYI:* "Choosing a Fitness Club" can be used in determining if the club is right for you.

Female-only clubs have become popular because they often provide an environment of reduced anxiety and intimidation and offer special classes that appeal to women, such as classes for pregnant women. Strength machines and other equipment are often sized for women clients, and facility hours accommodate the needs of women, with child care available during these periods. If you are considering joining a health club, it may be wise to consider women-only clubs for the programs and conveniences provided to members.

SPECIAL CONSIDERATIONS
Exercise and the Menstrual Cycle

History tells us that women once went to bed during their menstrual period. In more recent years, menstruating women were told not to swim and not to participate in activity classes, and they were even excused from

---

FYI

Choosing a Fitness Club[27]

Having structure and guidance in a personal fitness program is beneficial to many women. Health clubs with properly trained fitness instructors can be the answer. How do you know which health club to join? Use the following checklist to help you make this important choice.

Consider whether the club provides:	Yes	No
An attractive, safe, effective environment or facility	_____	_____
A clean and convenient facility	_____	_____
Certified staff current with CPR training	_____	_____
State-of-the-art exercise equipment that meets your needs	_____	_____
Individualized fitness and health assessments	_____	_____
Cost of membership within your budget	_____	_____
Contracts that are understandable/staff who provide explanations	_____	_____
Membership fees and services that are equivalent	_____	_____
Class size that is small enough for individual attention	_____	_____
Child care on the premises, if needed	_____	_____
Staff that is friendly and helpful and open to questions	_____	_____
Adequate parking for all members	_____	_____

participation on sports teams. Today it is recognized that menstruation usually presents no problems to women who participate in active events.

However, a number of symptoms may interfere with a woman's participation in physical activities. Varying degrees of pain and cramping, which may be accompanied by pain in the lower back or legs, can curtail one's ability and desire to be physically active during the menstrual period. Painful menstrual periods, called dysmenorrhea, can be so severe that some women are incapacitated for several days. Certainly, women with this type of pain should seek and follow the advice of their physician.

Premenstrual syndrome (PMS) affects some women and is characterized by feelings of irritability, depression, bloating, headaches, tender breasts, and possible weight gain. Although most women who experience PMS can maintain normal functioning, some may need a variety of treatments and professional medical help. As a result of these monthly hormonal changes, a woman's motivation to continue her fitness activities may subside. Yet, engaging in a reduced-intensity level activity has been shown to reduce the symptoms of PMS and produce a feeling of well-being.

Amenorrhea, the cessation of the menstrual period, is related to overexercising, which can be the case with long-distance running, cycling, gymnastics, or swimming. When a woman's body fat drops below 12 percent, which often occurs in highly fit female athletes, irregular or absent menstrual periods often are the result.

If discomfort during the menstrual period is a problem for you, consider reducing the frequency, duration, and intensity of your fitness activity rather than eliminating it. Pamper yourself after a workout by enjoying a soothing, warm shower or time in a hot tub, or briefly relaxing to pleasant music. It is also beneficial during the menstrual period to incorporate relaxing activities that promote a good night's sleep.

Exercise and Pregnancy

Pregnancy may be compared to preparing for and running a marathon, as far as the physical stress it can have on a woman's body is concerned. Therefore, a woman needs to prepare her muscles, increase her stamina, and boost the immune system in case of infection as she moves toward the big finish line: the birthing process. If a woman is exercising prior to pregnancy, then it is usually healthy to continue exercising during pregnancy, with her physician's approval, though perhaps with some modifications.

What are the benefits of exercising during pregnancy? Through research studies, numerous benefits have been determined for women who exercise during pregnancy. Appropriate exercise can relieve back pain and help improve posture by strengthening and toning muscles prevent joint injury, help prevent gestational diabetes improve mood, and ease labor because of stronger muscles, a healthier heart, and increased endurance.[28] Pregnant women who exercise are also less likely to have hemorrhoids, low back pain, fatigue, or varicose veins than those who don't exercise.

The cardiovascular system must circulate about 30 percent more blood during the 267+ days of pregnancy. Exercise can aid in increased and more efficient circulation and can reduce the likelihood of swelling in the feet and legs. Controlling weight gain, avoiding low back pain, and improving the efficiency of the cardiorespiratory system can lead to an important psychological benefit during pregnancy. Exercise can give pregnant women a measure of control over their expanding bodies and enhance their chances to feel good, look good, and have a positive self-image.

The American College of Obstetricians and Gynecologists (ACOG)[29] offers exercise guidelines for pregnant women. This organization suggests that women not exercise if they are at risk for pregnancy-induced hypertension. Additionally, stop exercising if you feel faint, have chest pains, headaches, uterine contractions, decreased fetal movement, or have fluid leaking from the vagina.

However, women who have none of these risks are encouraged to exercise in moderation, with the supervision of their physician. ACOG offers the following suggestions to help pregnant women exercise safely: monitor your heart rate during exercise; a wear/bra that gives support; consume daily extra calories; drink plenty of liquids throughout the workout period; do not exercise during hot, humid weather to avoid overheating; and after the third month, avoid exercises that require lying on the back to perform. (See *Viewpoint:* "Should I Continue My Usual Exercise Level during Pregnancy?")

If you want to exercise during pregnancy, you may want to use less strenuous exercises, which can achieve positive results. Your fitness level before becoming pregnant will dictate to a major degree the intensity, frequency, and duration of your exercise program. (*Do not* exercise during pregnancy without the consent of your physician.) Here are two less strenuous exercises:

- Swimming, one of the best exercises for pregnant women because swimming in a prone position promotes optimum blood flow. The water acts as a support cushion for both mother and fetus. The pressure of the water also encourages water loss, which can prevent edema, and does not place extra strain on joints and ligaments for women in their third trimester.

Viewpoint

Should I Continue My Usual Exercise Level during Pregnancy?

Janene has been involved in an intense aerobic exercise routine throughout college. She married and became pregnant during her senior year. The energy, stress relief, and weight management that her aerobic running produced was something Janene wanted to continue to experience. She consulted her physician, who suggested reducing the frequency and intensity of her workout and changing the running to a walking program. Janene was not happy with that idea and discussed this suggestion with the members of her running club, many of whom were knowledgeable in the area of exercise physiology. Their opinion was that because Janene had been in excellent aerobic condition before the pregnancy, she would not have problems maintaining her previous fitness activities.

Consider the following:

- The fetus is in a "built-in" safe environment, surrounded by amniotic fluid that serves as a shock absorber.

- Exercise causes an increase in body temperature that results in an increase of temperature in the fetal environment that may not be safe for the fetus.
- A reduced sense of balance and coordination following the seventh month may increase the chances for accidents during activity.
- Aerobic activity such as bouncing, running, and step aerobics should not be undertaken during the third trimester.
- The heart rate should not exceed 140 beats per minute, depending on one's fitness level.
- After the third month of pregnancy, exercises that require lying flat on the back should be avoided.

What would you recommend that Janene do about her level of fitness and her fitness activities during her pregnancy? Who should she consult to make a decision about how much to exercise during pregnancy?

- Walking, maintaining a heart rate of under 140 beats per minute for approximately 15 minutes at least three times per week. If you exercised before pregnancy, you may increase the duration up to 30 minutes with physician approval. Supportive shoes and a pleasant and safe area in which to walk are additional benefits of this exercise.

Kegel exercises are movements that help strengthen the muscles of the pelvic floor, aiding in support of the extra weight of the baby. Conditioned muscles will make birth easier, and the perineum will more likely remain intact, with fewer tears and reduced need for an episiotomy, during childbirth. Kegels are performed by contracting and releasing muscles that are the same as the muscles that stop the flow of urine. Strengthening these muscles also helps stop urine leakage during a cough or sneeze and can also increase sexual pleasure during intercourse.

Here is how to perform Kegel exercises:[30]

- Empty your bladder.
- Relax muscles completely for ten counts.
- Suggestion: perform fifty contractions per day for 46 weeks.

COMPULSIVE EXERCISE

Too often, women incorporate health-diminishing behaviors into their lifestyles to attain an ideal image—an image that is usually dictated through external influences. Whereas too little exercise will not produce positive results, too much can be detrimental to your health. Ironically, exercise can be overused by women to reach an unnatural and unhealthy thin appearance. It is possible to exercise too much, too often. When we have a distorted view of ourselves (a perception of oneself that does not match society's or the media's portrayal of the desirable body), we tend to adopt measures, regardless of the health consequences, to achieve this ideal. As a result, we can become an appearance junkie and a fitness zealot. **Compulsive exercising** is the need to engage in fitness activities beyond the normal standards for good health and despite potentially negative consequences. Edward J. Cumella, an expert in eating disorders and compulsive behavior, equates compulsive exercising to *exercise addiction (EA)*, and states that EA can lead to medical complications such as stress fractures, osteoporosis, cessation of menstruation, heart arrhythmias, and disturbances in the electrical conduction of the heart that could lead to sudden death.[31]

Despite injury, neglect of other responsibilities, or inconvenience, a woman with an addiction to exercise will continue at an intensity that is considered excessive. Symptoms indicative of overtraining, as described by John Draeger, include chronic fatigue, decreased appetite, impaired concentration, apathy, and mood changes.[32] There is an apparent correlation between addictive behavior and poor self-concept, depression, stress, and eating disorders.

Researchers still do not understand all the factors that lead to addiction to exercise. What is the margin between gaining the benefits of a comprehensive fitness program and overdoing it? An exercise level equivalent to running 20 hours a week for 6 months appears to cause a stress response in our bodies. Feeling challenged, the body goes on the defensive and a number of negative physiological responses occur:

As a result of compulsive exercise, women may experience:

- Damaged tendons, ligaments, bone and joints
- If injuries are not allowed to heal due to continual exercise, short-term injuries may become long-term damage
- Imbalance of hormones resulting in change in the menstrual cycle and an increase in bone loss
- Too much stress on the heart, especially if food intake is restricted, such as anoxia or bulimia. In some cases, this combination can be fatal.
- Exercise addicts my experience depression and anxiety, leading to feelings of worthlessness and poor body image. As a result they may withdraw from family and friends and fixate on exercise.[33]

Ironically, many of the physical and psychological benefits that we gain from a well-designed and moderate fitness program are the ones we lose when we exercise to excess. Compulsive or addictive exercise patterns harm the health of a woman and eradicate any benefits that are intended to be gained through fitness activities. Professional medical help is usually needed to deal with compulsive behavior of any type. When it may be life-threatening, as excessive exercising can be, especially in combination with eating disorders, it is imperative that a woman seek professional help.

MANAGING WEIGHT THROUGH EXERCISE

Why do we all expect to look as if our bodies are ready for the fashion runway when, in reality, most of us can never achieve that physique? Nor is it necessarily healthy to achieve that look. Certainly, our concept of the ideal female body has changed over the decades.

For example, Marilyn Monroe, a sex symbol and actress born in 1926, was a curvy icon in the 1950s whose reported measurements were 37-23-36 with a 36D bra size; she was 5 feet 5 inches tall and weighed up to 140 pounds. She would almost be considered a plus-size model by today's "ideal" body image, wearing a size 10 to 12.[35] Today, models weigh 23 percent less than the average-sized women; only 20 years

---

Assess Yourself

Could You Be a Compulsive Exerciser?[34]

If you are concerned about your exercise habits, or one of your friend's, consider the following warning signs that could indicate that exercising is becoming a negative part of your lifestyle, rather than improving your well-being. After completing this assessment, consider if over exercising is or could become a problem for you.

Warning Signs	Yes	No
Become upset if you have to miss a workout		
How much you allow yourself to eat dictates how much you exercise		
You exercise even if you do not feel well		
Exercise takes preference over being with friends or family		
Have trouble being still because you feel you are not burning calories		
Concerned about weight gain if you're not exercising on a daily basis.		

ago, the models weighed 8 percent less. What is the average-size American woman today? According to the Centers for Disease Control and Prevention (CDC),[36] she is 5 feet 3 inches tall, weighs 165 pounds, and has a waist circumference of 37 inches. Compare these measurements to one of today's top models, Gisele Bundchen, who is 5 feet 7 inches tall, measures 35-23-35.5, and weighs 130 pounds.[37] With tall, thin, and attractive women serving as the perfect and desirable image of today's women, is it any wonder that women want to manage weight to achieve the ideal image? Weight management needs to be achieved through healthy behaviors, including eating a healthy diet and participating in a well-planned and ongoing exercise program.

Maintaining healthy weight for a woman's body type and activity level can be achieved by participating in a comprehensive exercise program, as well as a healthy diet. A woman needs to expend at least the number of calories she consumes in her diet. Donnelly and Smith[38] determined that increasing exercise without nutritional changes did not result in effective weight loss. After a 16-month study, women who increased their exercise but did not monitor dietary practices experienced no weight change. This study was compared to other similar studies, where women participants increased exercise and monitored dietary practices and lost an average of 13 pounds after 12 weeks.

More than half of all ingested calories are used to keep our bodies and minds functioning. As we engage in fitness activities, not only do we expend additional calories at the time of the activity, but exercise increases our basal metabolic rate (the amount of energy needed to maintain normal body functions while at rest) even after the activity is over. Usually exercise alone (without dieting) will produce a weight loss; but even if you don't lose weight, it often helps you become thinner. The reason? A pound of muscle tissue will take up less space in your body than a pound of fat tissue. Building muscle and losing fat can cause a loss of inches without even losing a pound. The result is looking better and feeling better.

Once a woman has achieved the weight loss she desires, maintaining the new and healthy body then becomes the challenge. Successful long-term weight loss, defined as losing 10 percent of initial body weight and maintaining the loss for at least 1 year, was researched by Wing and Hill.[39] Common behavioral strategies of persons who maintained their weight loss included eating a low-fat diet, monitoring their own body weight and food intake, and engaging in high levels of regular physical activity. As these behaviors were continued and weight loss was maintained for 2–5 years, the chances increased for continued maintenance.

EXERCISING DURING THE LATER YEARS

Successful aging, rather than being determined by genetic factors, is largely shaped by individual lifestyle choices. Certainly a leading factor in successful aging is engaging in a physically active lifestyle. Research supports the multiple benefits of older women who participate in regular physical activity:

- Inactive, nonsmoking women, at age 65 have 12.7 years of active life expectancy, compared to highly active, nonsmoking women, who have 18.4 years of active life expectancy.[40]
- Exercise helps lower pressure, improves balance and helps with walking.[41]
- Older adults have improved quality of sleep and reduced stress when participating in regular physical activity.[42]
- Seniors who are active are less likely to develop chronic diseases, have fewer doctor visits, and use less medication.[43]
- Midlife to elderly women who participate in moderate aerobic activities have significant improvements in stress-induced blood pressure levels and improved quality of sleep.[44]

Evidence continues to mount that women who engage in regular physical activity have an improved quality of life, have the energy and strength to meet the demands of busy lifestyles, and have reduced costs of medical care compared to inactive women.[45] As the number of older adults is projected to increase from 13 percent of the population in 2000 to 20 percent in 2030, promoting long-term health and well-being in older women is a national health priority. To assist with this priority, fifty organizations developed the *National Blueprint: Increasing Physical Activity among Adults Age 50 and Older,* which provides sixty specific recommendations to achieve a more physically active older population. This document can be accessed at the Robert Wood Johnson Foundation Web site at www.rwjf.org/pr/product .jsp?id=15729.

Midlife to older women engaging in regular physical activities should consider the following guidelines for safer and more effective outcomes.

1. Engage in endurance, resistance, and flexibility exercises for better overall fitness.

2. Avoid extremes in temperatures and drink plenty of water.
3. Wear appropriate clothing for the weather.
4. Gradually increase intensity and duration over time and as condition permits.
5. Cool down slowly, do static stretching, and reduce heart rate to below 100 before stopping the cool-down/stretching segment of the exercise.
6. Set weekly goals.

Of course, all exercise programs for older women should be started only after a physical exam and clearance from a physician. Plan to engage in lifelong physical activities; your quality and enjoyment of life will benefit from it as well as that of your family.

As with many other health-related behaviors, knowing is not the same as doing. We have presented information in this chapter that will help you develop a comprehensive and effective fitness program. That's the easy part. Engaging in the program and, more important, staying with it will be the challenge. Look at the suggestions for success with your fitness program in *Health Tips:* "Make Exercise Fun!" Establish your goals, make a commitment, find yourself a partner, and begin to realize all the positive results from this type of program. And good luck!

Health Tips

Make Exercise Fun!⁴⁶

Here are a few suggestions:

- Exercise with a friend, especially someone who is active and whose company you enjoy.
- Find a group class with a knowledgeable instructor. This helps create a support system and offers guidance from a qualified, expert.
- Find a "sport" activity you enjoy, such as tennis, swimming, soccer, or softball and join a team.
- Include such aids as music or books on your listening device as you go through your exercise program; also, try using exercise DVDs or television programs as a change of pace.
- Create a way to measure your progress and put the information in a place that you can view on a regular basis.
- Change your activities—mix it up. If you walk, run, swim on your own, try an exercise class with others. Vary your routine.
- After an exercise activity, give yourself a few minutes of relaxation. Sit or lie down, close your eyes, and breathe deeply. Look forward to the relaxation you experience following the exercise.

Chapter Summary

- Participating in a comprehensive fitness program provides a multitude of physiological, psychological, and social benefits.
- A comprehensive physical fitness program consists of four major components: cardiorespiratory fitness, flexibility, muscular strength and endurance, and body composition.
- When developing a fitness program, warming up and cooling down should be included as essential components.
- Developing an exercise program to meet your individual fitness needs includes assessments conducted to determine your cardiorespiratory endurance, flexibility, muscular strength and endurance, and body composition.
- Determining what you want to achieve from your fitness program, developing a personal contract with a built-in incentive, and taking measures to stay involved will help your program to be more successful.

- Injuries related to knees and joints, shin splints, back pain, and inflammation can often be prevented through use of proper equipment, effective stretching, and a commonsense approach to personal workouts. Treatment of these injuries can be helped by using the RICE method (rest, ice, compression, and elevation).
- Exercising during pregnancy can be beneficial for women, but only when done under the supervision of a physician.
- Weight management can be best achieved through having sensible eating habits and engaging in a comprehensive fitness program.
- Addiction to exercise can be detrimental to a woman's well-being. Professional counseling may be needed for recovery from this compulsion.
- Exercising throughout the life span produces multiple benefits for midlife and older women.
- One of the most effective weight-control methods is participation in a comprehensive fitness program.

Review Questions

1. In what ways does a physical fitness program benefit someone physically, psychologically, and socially?
2. What are the components of a comprehensive physical fitness program?
3. What are the differences among isometric, isotonic, and isokinetic weight training?
4. Why is it important to include the warm-up and cool-down phases of a workout session?

5. What methods can help to make your fitness program successful? What are some strategies for staying involved with your program?
6. What are four types of physical fitness injuries? What are the methods to avoid or reduce injuries?
7. What are the benefits and precautions a woman should consider if she chooses to exercise during pregnancy?

8. What are the potential negative consequences of compulsive exercise?
9. Why is exercise a positive and effective method of managing weight?
10. What precautions should older women take as they begin an exercise program?
11. What are methods that help make exercise more fun?

Resources

Organizations, Hotlines, and Web Sites

American Alliance for Health, Physical Education, Recreation and Dance
> 703-476-3400
> www.aahperd.org

American College of Sports Medicine
> 317-637-9200
> www.acsm.org

American Council on Exercise
> 800-825-3636
> www.acefitness.org

American Volkssport Association
> 800-830–WALK
> www.ava.org

Centers for Disease Control and Prevention
cdc.gov/physicalactivity/
> 800-232-4636

President's Challenge
> www.adultfitnesstest.org

President's Council on Physical Fitness and Sport
> 202-690-9000
> www.fitness.gov

Women's Sport Foundation
> 800-227–3988
> www.womenssportsfoundation.org

References

1. Craft, L. L., K. M. Freund, L. Culpepper, and F. M. Perna. 2007. Intervention study of exercise for depressive symptoms in women. *Journal of Women's Health* 16(10): 1499–509.
2. Sattelmair, J. R., T. Kurth, J. E. Buring, and I.-M. Lee. 2010. Physical activity and risk of stroke in women. *Stroke* 41: 1243–50.
3. American Diabetes Association. 2011. *Top 10 benefits of being active.* http://www.diabetes.org/food-and-fitness/fitness/fitness-management/top-10-benefits-of-being.html (retrieved May 22, 2012).
4. Holmes, M. D., W. Y. Chen, D. Feskanich, C. H. Kroenke, and G. A. Colditz. 2005. Physical Activity and survival after breast cancer diagnosis. *Journal of the American Medical Association* 293 (20): 2479–86.
5. Lynch, B. M., H. K. Neilson, and C. M. Friedenreich. 2011. Physical activity and breast cancer prevention. *Physical Activity and Cancer* 186 (1): 13–42.
6. U.S. Department of Health and Human Services. 2008. *Physical activity guidelines for Americans.* Chapter 2: Physical activity has many benefits. www.health.gov/paguidelines/guidelines/chapter2.aspx (retrieved May 22, 2012).
7. Centers for Disease Control and Prevention. 2010. *Overweight and obesity: Adult obesity facts.* http://www.cdc.gov/obesity/data/adult.html (retrieved May 22, 2012).
8. American College of Sports Medicine. 2012. *Pilates and yoga news from ACSM Annual Meeting.* http://www.acsm.org/about-acsm/media-room/acsm-in-the-news/2011/08/01/pilates-and-yoga-news-from-acsm-annual-meeting (retrieved May 22, 2012).
9. U.S. Department of Health and Human Services. 2008. *Physical activity guidelines for Americans.* Chapter 4: Active Adults. http://www.health.gov/paguidelines/guidelines/chapter4.aspx (retrieved May 22, 2012).
10. Insel, P., & W. T. Roth. 2012. *Connect core concepts in health,* 12th ed. New York: McGraw-Hill, p. 374.
11. Ibid., p. 386.
12. American College of Sports Medicine. 2012. *Quantity and quality of exercise for developing and maintaining cardiorespiratory, musculoskeletal, and neuromotor fitness in apparently healthy adults: guidance for prescribing exercise.* http://www.acsm.org/access-public-information/position-stands/ (retrieved May 22, 2012).
13. American College of Sports Medicine. 2009. *ACSM's resources for personal trainer, Chapter 16: Resistance training programs.* Philadelphia, PA: Lippincott Williams & Wilkins.
14. Luebbers, P. 2002. Enhancing your flexibility. *Fit society Page: Quarterly Report of the American College of Sports Medicine* Spring, 5.
15. Fahey T. D., P. M. Insel, and W. T. Roth. 2007. *Fit and well,* 7th ed. Brief ed., New York: McGraw-Hill, p. 86.
16. From *The Active Women's Health and Fitness Handbook* by Nadya Swedan, Copyright 2003 by Nadya Swedan. Used by permission of Perigree Books, an imprint of Penguin Group (USA) Inc.
17. Fahey et al., *Fit and well,* p. 86–7.
18. Nadelen, M. D. 2012. *Basic injury prevention concepts.* American College of Sports Medicine. http://www.acsm.org/access-public-information/articles/2012/01/10/basic-injury-prevention-concepts (retrieved May 22, 2012).

19. U.S. Department of Health and Human Services. 2008. *Physical activity guidelines for Americans,* Chapter 2: Physical activity has many benefits.

20. American College of Sports Management. 2010. *ACSM's health-related fitness assessment manual.* Philadelphia, PA: Lippincott Williams & Wilkins.

21. Anspaugh, E. J., M. H. Hamrick, and F. D. Rosato. 2006. *Wellness: Concepts and application.* 6th ed. New York: McGraw-Hill, p. 97.

22. Ibid., p. 133.

23. Assessment activities: Physical activity labs-sit-and-reach-test. 2003. *Health and human performance online assessments.* McGraw-Hill. http://www.mhhe.com/catalogs/sem/hhp/faculty/labs/index.mhtml?file=/catalogs/sem/hhp/labs/activity/15 (retrieved May 23, 2012).

24. Quinn, E. 2009. *Getting started and sticking with exercise.* http://sportsmedicine.about.com/od/tipsandtricks/a/getting started.htm (retrieved May 23, 2012).

25. American College of Sports Medicine. 2012. *Ankle sprains and the athletic.* http://www.acsm.org/docs/current-comments/anklesprainstemp.pdf (Retrieved May 23, 2012).

26. Statistic Brain. 2012. *Exercise statistics.* http://www.statistic brain.com/exercise-statistics/ (retrieved May 23, 2012).

27. American College of Sports Management. 2005. Selecting and effectively using a health/fitness facility. *Fit Society Page: Quarterly Report of the American College of Sports Medicine* Spring: 9.

28. The American College of Obstetricians and Gynecologists. 2011. *Exercise during pregnancy.* http://www.acog.org/~/media/For%20Patients/faq119.pdf?dmc=1&ts=20120523T15243632 40 (retrieved May 23, 2012).

29. Ibid.

30. The American College of Obstetricians and Gynecologists. 2011. *Pelvic support problems.* http://www.acog.org/~/media/For%20Patients/faq012.pdf?dmc=1&ts=20120523T1538235897 (retrieved May 23, 2012).

31. Cumella, E. J. 2005. The heavy weight of exercise addiction. *Behavioral Health Management* 25 (5): 26–31.

32. Draeger, J. 2005. The obligatory exerciser. *Physician and Sportsmedicine* 33 (6): 13–23.

33. Kidshealth. 2010. *Compulsive exercise.* http://kidshealth.org/teen/food_fitness/exercise/compulsive_exercise.html# (retrieved May 23, 2012).

34. The new American body. 1993. *University of California at Berkeley Wellness Letter* 10 (3): 1–2.

35. Tooley, H. 2011. *Marilyn Monroe Size: Revealed measurements of actress Marilyn Monroe, true measurements and size.* http://voices.yahoo.com/marilyn-monroe-size-revealed-measurements-8297959.html?cat=2 (received May 23, 2012).

36. Anthropometric Reference Data for Children and Adults: United States, 2003–2006. 2008. *National Health Statistics Reports* (10). http://www.cdc.gov/nchs/data/nhsr/nhsr010.pdf (retrieved May 23, 2012).

37. Wikipedia. 2012. *Gisele Bundchen.* http://en.wikipedia.org/wiki/Gisele_B%C3%BCndchen *(retrieved May 23, 2012).*

38. Connelly, J., and B. Smith. 2005. Energy balance, compensation, and gender differences. Is exercise for weight loss with ad libitum diet? *Exercise and Sport Science Reviews* 33 (4): 169–74.

39. Wing, R. R., and J. O. Hill. 2001. Successful weight loss management. *Annual Reviews Nutrition* 21: 232–41.

40. Ferucchi, L., B. W. Henninx, S. C. Leveille, M. C. Cirti, M. Pahor, R. Wallace, et al. 2000. Characteristics of nondisabled older persons who perform poorly in objective test of lower extremity function. *Journal of the American Geriatric Society* 48 (9): 1102–10.

41. National Institutes of Health. 2012. *NIH Senior Health.* http://nihseniorhealth.gov/exerciseforolderadults/healthbenefits/01.html (retrieved May 25, 2012).

42. Ibid.

43. Ibid.

44. Schmitz, K. H., et al 2003. Strength training for obesity prevention in midlife women. *International Journal of Obesity* 27: 326–33.

45. Garrett, N. A., M. Brasure, K. H. Schmitz, M. M. Schultz, and M. R. Huber. 2004. Physical Inactivity: Direct costs to a health plan. *American Journal of Preventive Medicine* 27 (4): 304–9.

46. Stibich, M. 2008. *Top ten ways to make exercise fun.* http://longevity.about.com/od/lifelongfitness/a/exercise_fun.htm (retrieved May 25, 2012).

Chapter Twelve

Using Alcohol Responsibly

CHAPTER OBJECTIVES

When you complete this chapter, you will be able to do the following:

◇ Explain the relationship between women, especially college women, and the use of alcohol

◇ Identify and describe the various types of alcohol

◇ Identify negative effects resulting from alcohol abuse related to the physical, behavioral, psychological, and societal aspects as well as upon relationships in the lives of women

◇ Describe the serious consequences that may result from the use of alcohol during pregnancy and the negative effects on the fetus and infant

◇ Explain the process of addiction and alcoholism in women

◇ Identify the appropriate resources to assist alcoholic women and their families

◇ Suggest guidelines that can be used by colleges and universities to reduce alcohol abuse among college women

WOMEN AND ALCOHOL

Humans have been consuming alcohol, an intoxicating and toxic chemical, for thousands of years. Early writings about alcohol use are found in Hebrew script, Egyptian tablets, and Chinese laws in which the use of wine was either allowed or disallowed between 1100 B.C. and A.D. 1400.[1] Used for many purposes and reasons, alcohol is a drug of choice for present-day Americans. In purely economic terms, alcohol-related problems cost society approximately $223 billion each year, but in human terms, the costs are incalculable.[2] Excessive drinking causes loss in workplace productivity, increased health care expenses, and criminal justice system overload.

Societal attitudes regarding women's use of alcohol have been inconsistent and ambivalent. Roman laws did not allow women to drink alcoholic beverages because it was thought to make women aggressive and

promiscuous; the Talmud denounced the overconsumption of alcohol by women, stating,

> One cup of wine is good for a woman;
> Two are degrading;
> Three induce her to act like an immoral woman;
> And four cause her to lose all self-respect and sense of shame.[3]

However, in ancient Babylon, women were temple priestesses who brewed beer. In Greco-Roman cults, women were a part of ceremonies in which alcohol was consumed. Through the centuries, alcoholic beverages were used medicinally and ceremoniously, but usually not in recreational circumstances, as they are presently used. In early America, women played a significant role in the control of alcohol use as participants of the temperance movement, which was an attempt to "temper" or curtail the use of hard liquor (distilled spirits).

The Women's Christian Temperance Union was formed in the late 1800s in Cleveland, Ohio, and Carrie Nation, Mary H. Hunt, and Frances Willard were actively involved with this movement. In fact, Carrie Nation, with fervent activities, was arrested more than thirty times. Rather than advocating temperance, these women promoted complete prohibition—no sale or consumption of alcohol. In 1920 prohibition became law with the ratification of the Eighteenth Amendment to the U.S. Constitution prohibiting the manufacture, sale, and transportation of "intoxicating liquors." However, this law was difficult to enforce as even former abstainers, in rebellion, began to drink; personal freedom was lost and alcohol use became a "smart thing" to do. Alcohol was manufactured and provided outside the law, and bootlegging became big business. By 1931 the Commission of Law Enforcement branded prohibition as a failure, and in 1933, after 13 years of attempting to enforce prohibition, the Twenty-First Amendment was passed, which repealed the Eighteenth Amendment. Today, alcohol is a legal substance with certain restrictions and is regulated by state governments.

ALCOHOL ABSORPTION

Absorption of alcohol takes place through the stomach, where about 20 percent is absorbed directly into the bloodstream, and from the small intestine where 80 percent is absorbed and moves into the bloodstream and to all parts of the body.[4] The absorption of alcohol in the body is determined by a number of factors. These include the following:

- *Number of drinks consumed.* The greater the number of alcoholic beverages consumed by a female, the faster the alcohol will be absorbed into the bloodstream.
- *Strength of alcoholic beverage.* Beverages with higher concentrations of alcohol will increase the blood alcohol concentration (BAC). (See Figure 12.1.)
- *Rate of drinking.* Faster consumption of drinks will usually result in a higher blood alcohol level because more alcohol is absorbed into the system.
- *Mixture with other beverages.* Alcohol mixed with fruit juices or plain water will be absorbed at a slower rate; "straight" alcohol or alcohol mixed with carbonated beverages will be absorbed at a faster rate.
- *Foods in the stomach.* Foods with higher fat content will slow absorption of alcohol because there is less stomach area exposed and protein in the food retains the alcohol.
- *Emotional factors.* Absorption of alcohol into the bloodstream can be affected by such factors as

emotions (jealousy, anger, fear), illness, stress, and expectations of how it will make you feel (e.g., relaxed, high, sociable).
- *Blood chemistry.* Each of us is a biochemical individual; absorption may be quickened or slowed due to an individual's blood chemistry.
- *Body weight.* The more body weight a woman has, the lower will be the blood alcohol concentration.

Three additional types of alcohol are *methanol, isopropyl,* and *butyl,* each of which is toxic to human beings. (See Table 12.1.) Methyl alcohol, also called "wood alcohol," is an ingredient in such products as glass cleaners, turpentine, solvents, and antifreeze.

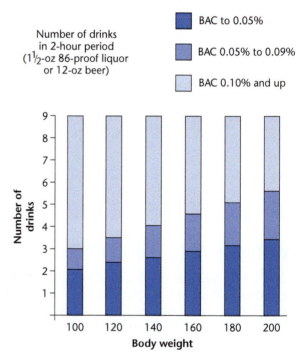

FIGURE 12.1 BAC is the level of alcohol contained in a person's blood volume. For example, a woman with a BAC of 0.10 percent has one part of alcohol for every 1000 parts of blood. A BAC of 0.08 and above is considered drunk in all states. However, a BAC as low as 0.05 percent can impair function enough to cause a serious accident.

TABLE 12.1	**Types of Alcohol**
Ethyl (Ethanol)	Alcohol beverages
	Over-the-counter drugs
Methyl (Methanol)	Antifreeze, solvents
Isopropyl	Disinfectant in rubbing alcohol
Butyl	Industrial and medical applications found in anesthesia

Isopropyl, a clear, colorless, bitter liquid, is a disinfectant used in rubbing alcohol. Butyl alcohol, obtained from petroleum, is used in industrial and medication applications and may be found in anesthesia. *None* of these should be ingested because doing so could cause serious illness or death.

Why Liquor Is Quicker for Women

The absorption of alcohol in the body influences to an extent the physical and behavioral effects experienced by the person ingesting it. An enzyme, **alcohol dehydrogenase (ADH),** in the liver and in the stomach (gastric) lining helps to break down the alcohol before it enters the bloodstream. The ADH activity in the stomach is lower in women than in men. As a result, about 30 percent more alcohol enters the female bloodstream, thus causing more alcohol to reach the female brain at a faster rate, creating an intoxicating effect; therefore, higher BAC is reached by women at a faster rate than for men. Over years of drinking, as frequency and consumption of alcohol increase the liver starts to fail, hence producing less ADH, causing the effectiveness of this enzyme to be impaired. Consequently, women who have been drinking heavily for many years will absorb almost all alcohol consumed without breaking it down, and the effect will be similar to alcohol being injected intravenously.

Drinking equivalent amounts of ethyl alcohol per pound of body weight will produce a higher peak of alcohol level for women than for men. This may be due to the higher percentage of body water in men (55–65 percent) than in women (45–55 percent), causing alcohol to be less diluted in women than in men. Ethyl alcohol is highly water- and fat-soluble. Because women have more body fat than men of the same weight and because alcohol is not diffused rapidly into body fat, females will have a higher amount of alcohol concentration in the blood than men. Considering each of these factors, a woman's ability to perform certain tasks (e.g., driving, speaking, decision making) will be impaired at a faster rate than a man's.

During the premenstrual stage of the menstrual cycle, alcohol is absorbed more quickly into the bloodstream. However, because of fluid retention during the premenstrual cycle, alcohol in the blood is more diluted and will have a reduced effect on the central nervous system, so a woman will not become intoxicated as quickly as at other stages of her cycle.

WOMEN AND ALCOHOL: A UNIQUE RELATIONSHIP

In the past, women have used alcohol medicinally to reduce menstrual cramps, to lessen pain associated with childbirth, and for fortification while breast feeding. It has been used in recreational settings to promote the "time away" environment and as a "social lubricant" to ease social interactions. Table 12.2 helps to explain the various classifications of alcohol consumers. This should provide you with what is meant by small, moderate, and heavy use of alcohol and foster a better perspective for alcohol use and its consequences.

Are there special concerns for use of this chemical by women? How much is too much? Alcohol, a depressant *psychoactive drug,* produces a number of unique qualities that are of special interest and concern for women. For example, a daily glass of wine with dinner can add as much as 10 pounds of body fat a year; it can increase the risk of developing breast cancer and osteoporosis. Women who drink large amounts of alcohol are more likely than men to develop cirrhosis of the liver and other alcohol-related diseases. The Centers for Disease Control and Prevention analyzed alcohol-related harmful effects of excessive alcohol use and estimated the number of alcohol-attributable deaths (AAD) and potential years of life lost (YPLL). Annually, 79,000 die from multiple causes (i.e., heart conditions, cancer, car crashes, homicide) related to alcohol abuse; the CDC calculated that all these equate to 23 million potential years of life lost.[5] Women who are heavy drinkers are more susceptible to depression and suicide attempts than women who do not drink or drink in moderation. Overconsumption of alcohol is less socially acceptable for women than for men. Society often considers women who drink too much more likely to engage in sexual activity.

Are women more vulnerable to alcohol's effects than men are? The physiological differences and effects from alcohol consumption discussed previously have some profound consequences for women. Consider the following:[6]

Medication interactions. Alcohol can cause a variety of consequences when consumed with both

TABLE 12.2 Drinking Classifications

CLASSIFICATION	ALCOHOL-RELATED BEHAVIORS
Abstainers	Do not drink; or may drink one time a year
Light drinkers	May drink one to two drinks once to two times per month
Moderate drinkers	Drink one to two drinks once a week
Heavy drinkers	Drink several drinks once a week
Binge drinkers	Drink five to six drinks or more per drinking occasion

prescription and over-the-counter medications. Alcohol is a depressant drug and may amplify the sedative effects of medicines that cause drowsiness, and treat anxiety and depression. It can reduce the effectiveness of some medications.

Breast cancer. As little as one drink per day can slightly raise the risk of breast cancer in some women, especially women who are menopausal or have a history of breast cancer in the family. Alcohol affecting breast cancer for all women cannot be predicted.

Fetal alcohol syndrome (FAS). Pregnant women who drink alcohol can harm the unborn baby and the results may result in FAS, which is a cluster of birth defects that affect the baby in various ways. A more extensive discussion of FAS is provided later in the chapter.

Drinking and driving. Ingestion of alcohol can impair a person's ability to drive and operate other types of machines. Obviously, as a woman drinks more alcohol, her blood alcohol level rises, and therefore increases her chances of having a car crash.

Heart disease. Heavy drinking on a long-term basis is a major risk factor in the development of cardiovascular diseases. Women who are heavy drinkers are more susceptible to alcohol-related heart disease than are men, even though women drink less alcohol than men over the lifespan.

Alcoholic liver disease. Women are more likely than men to develop alcoholic hepatitis and to die from cirrhosis of the liver.

Brain disease. Alcoholics have some loss of mental function, including reduced brain size, and modified function of brain cells. Women who abuse alcohol are more vulnerable to various types of brain disease than men.

Alcohol Consumption

According to the National Survey on Drug Use and Health (NSDUH),[7] over 50 percent of Americans over the age of 12, equating to about 131 million people, reported drinking alcohol prior to the survey, and more than 23 percent of persons over the age of 12 reported binge drinking in the 30 days prior to taking the NSDUH survey. Additionally, 7 percent over the age of 12 stated that they had engaged in heavy drinking. For females over the age of 12, 46 percent reported being current drinkers; of women between the ages of 18 and 25, 57 percent reported drinking within the last 30 days, compared to 65 percent of males who were current drinkers. Only 20 percent of all alcohol beverages are consumed by approximately 70 percent of the drinking public. The remaining 80 percent of alcohol beverages are consumed by 30 percent of people who drink and they can be categorized as heavy drinkers or even alcoholics. This information was explained in an interesting and understandable way by Kinney:

> Ten beers shared among ten individuals who follow adult drinking patterns would likely be divided in this way:
>
> Three persons abstain—representing the one-third who choose not to drink
>
> Five persons share two beers—70 percent of drinkers drink 20 percent of the alcohol
>
> Two persons share eight beers—30 percent of drinkers drink 80 percent of the alcohol. Of these two drinkers, one drinks two beers and the other drinks six beers.[8]

Drinkers may move from one type of drinking pattern to another during their lifetime. (To check your own drinking pattern, complete *Journal Activity:* "Alcohol Consumption Record.")

College-Age Women and Alcohol

The college years are a time of more freedom, independence, and important decision-making, with some decision resulting in life-long consequences and potential changes in long-term dreams and goals. Alcohol use in college-aged women is most prevalent; according to a research study conducted by the Harvard School of Public Health, 81 percent of college women reported drinking in the year previous to the survey with almost 19 percent reported abstaining from drinking alcohol.[9] Of concern is the increased practice of **binge drinking** among all college students, typically defined as consuming five or more drinks within 2–3 hours for men and four or more drinks within 2–3 hours for women. Binge drinking among college women students has risen dramatically in the past 25 years, and currently almost 40 percent of college-age females reported binge drinking on some occasions.[10] One recent study of 10,000 college-age women reported that more than 34 percent met or exceeded the binge drinking threshold at least once over a 2-week time period prior to the survey.[11] Consequences of binge drinking can be serious and undermine the opportunities that lie ahead for college women. Annually such tragic events as deaths due to drinking and driving, having unsafe sex, experiencing academic problems, being raped, encountering problems with law enforcement, and/or being injured occur and result in loss in life and quality of life.

Journal Activity

Alcohol Consumption Record

If you make the choice to drink, it is a wise idea to monitor your consumption. Below is a chart you can use to determine when, where, with whom, and how much you are drinking. If you find that you are experiencing problems as a result of alcohol consumption, it is important to seek professional help. The information recorded on this chart can help you determine if you do or do not have a drinking problem.

Date	Time	Where	With Whom	Number of Drinks

With the knowledge that abuse of alcohol can result in serious consequences, women still over consume a substance that can be a destructive force in their lives. (See *Her Story:* "Jessica: Driving Under the Influence." Then read *Women Making a Difference:* "Candace Lightner and Cindi Lamb: Founders of Mothers Against Drunk Driving – MADD.")

Why do college women drink? The following is a list provided by college women—if you drink, do these reasons compare to your reasons?

- To relieve stress and anxiety
- To feel more sociable
- To decrease inhibitions
- For the "high" that results
- To be part of the group
- To lessen sexual inhibitions
- To escape
- To relieve worrying
- To become less self-conscious
- To reduce depression

Colleges and universities are taking a closer look at the serious consequences that result from overconsumption of alcohol on campuses. *FYI:* "Reducing Alcohol Abuse on Campus" lists a number of measures that are being adopted on numerous campuses to curb the use of alcohol and the resulting consequences.

Health Tips: "Drinking Alcohol Responsibly" provides suggestions you can use as guidelines for drinking alcohol responsibly.

Her Story

Jessica: Driving Under the Influence

Jessica arrived for her freshman year in college and settled into her high-rise dorm room. She was invited by her roommates to go to the "Rooster House," a local bar frequented by college students. As a nondrinker, Jessica felt uneasy about this invitation, yet she also wanted to meet other students and become a part of the social scene. After deciding to join her new friends one evening, Jessica drove her own car to the bar so that she could leave when she chose. Having no former drinking experience, she began to feel the results of too many "drink specials" and decided it was time to go home. She drove back to the dorm under the influence and was stopped and given a Breathalyzer test. Having a BAC of 0.13, she was arrested and convicted of DUI. This became a part of her driving record for many years and resulted in an increase in her car insurance rates.

- How could Jessica have met people in her new college environment other than by going to a bar?
- Why did Jessica feel the effects of alcohol so quickly?
- What is the legal limit of alcohol consumption in your state?

Women Making a Difference

Candace Lightner and Cindi Lamb: Founders of Mothers Against Drunk Driving (MADD)

The death of Candy Lightner's 13-year-old daughter, Cari, in 1980, and the crippling of Cindi Lamb's 5½-month-old daughter, Laura, in 1979, both as a result of repeat drunk drivers, spurred these women to form the organization Mothers Against Drunk Drivers (MADD). This organization eventually was renamed Mothers Against Drunk Driving. From the time it was formed in 1981, MADD received donations from victims and concerned citizens, as well as grant funding, enabling it to expand to eleven chapters in four states. As a result of increased media attention, MADD began to develop in more states and to increase in the number of chapters across the United States. By its tenth anniversary in 1991, MADD had grown to 407 chapters, 53 community action teams, and 32 state offices with affiliates in Canada, England, New Zealand, and Australia. MADD's mission statement is "To stop drunk driving, support victims of this violent crime and prevent underage drinking."

Since MADD's inception, alcohol-related traffic fatalities have declined and thousands of people are safer today because of MADD. An untold number have received comfort, support, and assistance in dealing with the consequences of drunk driving. Candace Lightner and Cindi Lamb and other dedicated and action-oriented mothers across the United States are truly women who make a difference.

FYI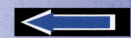

Reducing Alcohol Abuse on Campus

Colleges and universities across the nation are working to reduce alcohol abuse on campus. Here are some of the ways they are trying to achieve this:

- Banning alcohol from campus pubs
- Banning alcohol from college-sponsored activities (among sororities, in residence halls, and at sporting events)
- Avoiding social and commercial promotion of alcohol
- Consistently enforcing alcohol-related laws and policies
- Conducting student orientation about alcohol abuse
- Conducting seminars for women concerning alcohol and other drugs
- Training female resident hall advisors in alcohol abuse awareness
- Training university counselors about women who have alcohol-related problems

Associated Effects

Have you ever experienced negative consequences as the result of alcohol abuse? Overconsumption of alcohol can produce immediate and long-term negative physical, behavioral, psychological, social, and relational consequences. Although many of these negative outcomes are the result of chronic alcohol abuse, undesirable consequences can also result from occasional overconsumption of alcohol.

Hormonal Effects Physical effects resulting from alcohol consumption, especially long-term abuse of alcohol, can be serious and in some instances

life-threatening. Serious consequences, for example, include the impairment of proper functioning of essential hormones, briefly defined as chemical messengers that control and coordinate the operation of all tissues and organs. Hormone impairment results in a number of significant and severe medical consequences. One significant hormonal consequence of alcohol abuse causes low blood sugar levels, called hypoglycemia, and prevents an effective hormonal response to this condition. When blood sugar levels are too low to provide enough energy for the body's activities, symptoms such as hunger, shakiness, confusion, and/or weakness may occur.

Chronic heavy alcohol consumption can hamper a female's reproductive hormone functioning leading to a number of serious health issues. For example, breast development, distribution of body hair, regulation of the menstrual cycle, and disruption of a pregnancy can be the results of impaired hormone functioning caused by alcohol abuse. Long-term consequences include serious hormonal deficiencies, sexual dysfunction, and infertility. A study of healthy nonalcoholic women found that even in females who were just "social drinkers," small amounts of alcohol stopped normal menstrual cycling and they became temporarily infertile.[12]

College-age women can have menstruation cessation, menstrual cycle irregularities, failure to ovulate, and infertility. During pregnancy, alcohol use can increase

Health Tips

Drinking Alcohol Responsibly

- Drink no more than one drink per hour.
- Allow time to elapse between drinks.
- Intersperse alcoholic beverages with nonalcoholic drinks.
- Sip drinks; do not gulp them.
- Eat before drinking alcohol.
- Know your limits.
- Be comfortable choosing not to drink.
- Never encourage another woman to drink.
- Know when to say "no" when someone offers you a drink, and say it!

the likelihood of spontaneous abortion (miscarriage). Studies indicate a relationship between female alcoholism and sexual dysfunction, especially **anorgasmia.** The majority of female reproductive irregularities were found in studies of alcoholic women; however, a number of problems were also found in women who drank approximately three drinks per day.

Women, in general, are at increased risk for developing calcium-deficiency disorders, especially osteoporosis. However, alcohol consumption exacerbates this problem by causing hormone imbalances that reduce calcium absorption, excretion, and distribution. As a result, calcium metabolism is impaired and bone density is reduced. Additionally, an immediate effect of drinking alcohol is the prevention of proper utilization of calcium and a resultant increase in urinary calcium excretion. Because chronic drinking can disturb vitamin D metabolism, there is an increased risk of osteoporosis due to inadequate absorption of dietary calcium.

Studies have revealed a distinct link between alcohol intake and breast cancer. Increased production of estrogen has been linked to developing breast cancer. Dorgan[13] studied fifty-one postmenopausal women who were not taking hormone replacement therapy and followed them over three 8-week periods while they consumed 15 or 30 grams (½–1 ounce) of alcohol per day. The study found that even one drink per day increased the risk of developing breast cancer. Postmenopausal women with a history of alcohol use were found to be significantly more at risk for breast cancer when consuming the equivalent of two drinks each day.[14] To help explain this, if the risk for a female developing breast cancer is 1 in 10, the risk for a female drinker would be 1.5 in 10. In other words, 10 of 100 nondrinkers might get breast cancer, whereas 15 of 100 drinkers may develop breast cancer.

Medications containing estrogen, such as birth control pills and hormone replacement drugs, affect a woman's reaction to alcohol. Drinking alcohol in moderate amounts increases the estrogen levels in postmenopausal women. Light to moderate alcohol consumption may increase blood concentration of estrogen and the byproducts of estrogen metabolism, and the results can increase the risk of serious diseases for women.[15] (See *FYI:* "Are There Any Benefits to Drinking Alcohol?")

What should you do? Consultation with a physician should help you weigh the benefits versus the risks of taking medications with estrogen. Consider your family medical history related to cancer, heart disease, and osteoporosis, and your lifestyle as it relates to alcohol consumption, exercise, diet, and other health promotion or health risk behaviors. (See Table 12.3.)

Dieting Research studies have revealed the connection between use and abuse of alcohol, dieting, and disordered eating. A study by Cooley and Toray[16] found that freshmen women who used and/or abused alcohol tended to display signs of negative eating patterns. Peralta[17] discovered in his research related to alcohol use

FYI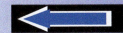

Are There Any Benefits to Drinking Alcohol?

Although the use and abuse of alcohol result in many negative consequences, studies have also determined that there are also a number of benefits from the *moderate* use of alcohol. Remember, moderate use of alcohol for women is one drink per day. (See Table 12.2.) These benefits include

- Decreased risk of heart attack
- Increases in high-density lipoprotein (HDL), the "good cholesterol"
- Decreased risk of coronary artery disease
- Decreased anxiety
- Relaxation
- Increased ease during social situations
- Increased life expectancy

Although these benefits have been reported in professional literature, it must also be noted that there are additional methods by which you can gain these benefits without using a potentially addicting and toxic drug. This is one of the many lifestyle decisions we must make by considering all potential alternatives and consequences.

TABLE 12.3 The Physical Consequences of Alcohol Abuse[18]

Reproductive system	Early menopause, amenorrhea, infertility, miscarriage, FAS
Sexuality	Reduced physiological arousal, decreased orgasmic intensity, sexual dysfunction.
Endocrine system	Increased possibility of osteoporosis, nutritional and metabolic disorders, poor absorption and utilization of essential nutrients.
Cardiovascular system	Hypertension, cardiomyopathy, dysrhythmias, coronary artery disease; slows manufacture of red blood cells; degenerates blood clotting ability.
Liver	Chemical imbalance: accumulation of fat in the liver, blood sugar imbalance, and altered protein production.
	Inflammation: impaired circulation, scar tissue formation, and alcohol-related hepatitis.
	Cirrhosis: poor circulation, kidney failure, and possibly death.
Digestive system	Oral: promotes possibility of cancer of the mouth, tongue, and throat.
	Esophagus: impaired swallowing.
	Stomach: irritation, gastritis, and ulceration.
	Pancreas: inflammation.
	Digestion: impaired absorption and possible malnutrition.
	Nausea: diarrhea and vomiting.

and the fear of weight gain that four specific categories of diet-related behaviors emerged. Students reported altering their eating patterns (limiting food consumption, thereby reducing calories from food in order to drink more), altering drinking patterns (drinking "lite" beer, shots, mixed drinks because of their perceived lower caloric content), engaging in self-induced purging (to rid body of excess calories from drinking and eating), or exercising to stave off unwanted weight gain believed to be caused by alcohol use. While exercising is a positive health-enhancing behavior, the other reported behaviors associated with alcohol use and abuse related to controlling weight are harmful and produce serious consequences for women who engage in these behaviors.

Disease When compared to men, women with alcohol-related problems are disabled more frequently and for longer periods of time. Alcohol-related liver damage in women develops after shorter periods of alcohol use and lower levels of consumption than it does in men. Studies have shown that alcohol-related diseases in women were comparable to those in men, even when the women had been drinking to excess for a significantly shorter period of time than had the men (14.2 years for women versus 20.2 years for men). Diseases and disorders such as pancreatitis, hepatitis, cardiomyopathy (degeneration of the heart muscle), and myopathy (a degenerative disease of the skeletal muscles) developed in a briefer period of time for alcohol-abusing women than alcohol-abusing men.[19]

Ethnicity The drinking pattern of women can be influences by cultural norms and practices of the ethnic

groups to which they belong. For both men and women, genetic heritage, occupational and social norms, and social class contribute to drinking patterns. However, women have greater propensity to have negative affective states, such as depression, and to experience negative life events, including childhood and adulthood victimization, increases women's risk for developing alcohol problems.

The National Institute on Alcohol Abuse and Alcoholism reported the differences of drinking status and heavy drinking for U.S. ethnic groups by gender.[20] Ethnic groups included in the study were *white, black, Native American, Asian,* and *Hispanic*. The findings revealed that white females (65 percent) were most likely to be current drinkers, while Asian females (36 percent) were least likely to drink. The findings related to heavy drinking, it was reported that white females (14 percent), black females (13 percent), Native American females (22 percent), Asian females (8 percent) and Hispanic females (9 percent) drank heavily on a weekly basis; for daily heavy drinking, Native American women (27 percent) were more likely to be heavy drinkers on a daily basis, while black women (19 percent) were least likely to drink heavily on a daily basis.

Collins and McNair examined influences that formed drinking behavior of women from four largest non-European ethnic groups in the United States: African Americans, Asian Americans, Latinas, and American Indians.[21] The study found that level of religious participation of African American women tended to serve a protective function and shielded them from higher rates of alcohol use. Drinking patterns among Asian

American women were influenced by their ethnic communities and by a biological factor: facial flushing. This affects their ability to metabolize alcohol, resulting in higher levels of alcohol in the blood, which tends to lower drinking behaviors in this ethnic group. Because Latino women who immigrated into the United States increased their level of drinking alcohol after three generations in this country, it is believed that acculturation caused this increase due to changes in income, education, and occupation. The drinking patterns of American Indian women seemed to reflect the norms of the tribal policies. These women tended to drink more alcohol if they lived on reservations where there were relatively high rates of drinking by American Indian men.[22]

It appears that drinking patterns of women among the four largest non-European ethnic groups in the United States display some similarity due to biological characteristics, social roles, and lower social status related to men. Drinking patterns, however, differ within and among the ethnic groups due to differences in ethnic norms.

Behavioral Effects Although long-term chronic alcohol abuse can cause a variety of negative physical consequences, a number of severe behavioral consequences can result from short-term or binge drinking. Alcohol-related behavior pertains not only to what women themselves do, but to what women may allow others to do to them. Because alcohol reduces a woman's inhibitions, or concerns about "what may happen if," she is more likely to act upon the immediate circumstances rather than considering the consequences of her actions. Examples include making a decision to leave a party or club or have sexual relations with some person she just met, driving after drinking, or being verbally abusive to friends or family. The more heavily a woman drinks, the greater the potential for problems at home, at work, with friends, and even with strangers.[23] Each of these situations can lead to negative societal and relationship-related consequences. In each instance, a woman would probably make a different decision if she were not disinhibited by alcohol consumption.

Additional indicators of behavioral effects of alcohol abuse include: impaired functioning in the social world such as financial irresponsibility, unusual accidents such as falling down stairs, impulsiveness, dysfunctional relationships, and poor parenting skills. Asocial behavior indicators include poor communication skills, irresponsibility regarding appointments or commitments, relinquishing former hobbies or activities, and even discarding friendships. Shoplifting and stealing from family or friends were cited as indicators of antisocial behavior of female alcohol abusers.

Psychological effects related to alcohol abuse can be serious. Women may experience anxiety, guilt, and stress; lose their inhibitions; display aggressiveness and other strong emotions; or have strong dependency needs. Women may become suspicious of others, grow defensive, or even demonstrate obsessive-compulsive behaviors such as being a "super student" or compulsively perfectionistic. Compared to male drinkers, female drinkers who chronically abuse alcohol are more likely to experience bouts of depression.

Social Effects Social consequences related to alcohol use and abuse are many. Alcohol often fosters relaxing effects that enable women to feel more confident, relaxed, and less inhibited in social situations. Although this may be perceived as a positive result of alcohol consumption, certainly being able to experience these qualities in social settings without the use of an intoxicating beverage would be an important skill to possess. In some instances, abuse of alcohol may become detrimental to our social well-being and to society at large. Negative situations can range from arguments to violent acts, from loss of a job to career destruction, from delinquent bills to financial ruin, from minor accidents in the home to deadly vehicular collisions, or from lousy dates to dysfunctional relationships. Alcohol abuse can be seriously detrimental to our personal, familial, and professional quality of life.

Economic Effects Economic issues related to alcohol consumption reveal the financial burden and costs to society Joseph Califano, former U.S. Secretary of Health, Education, and Welfare, states in his book, *High Society— How Substance Abuse Ravages America and What to Do About It,*[24] that overall drug abuse, including alcohol, costs approximately $1 trillion each year in America. Included in this cost is $1.9 billion yearly spent to care for infants born with FAS resulting from women who make the choice to drink during pregnancy. Over 1.7 million visits to emergency departments occur due to alcohol- or drug-related incidents add more than $4 billion to health care costs. Binge drinking on college campuses leads to 1700 alcohol- and drug-related deaths, 600,000 injuries, 700,000 assaults, and 400,000 college students engaging in unprotected sex, at an annual estimated cost per college of $80,000.[25]

Alcohol and crime seem to have a kinship because criminals often have problems with alcohol abuse. Studies have determined that in the majority of crimes, such as assault, robbery, homicide, or rape, alcohol is a factor. Prisoners frequently are alcoholics or have other drug problems. A large percentage of all crimes, both violent and non-violent, are committed under the influence of alcohol. The four leading causes of accidental death in this country are (1) transportation accidents, (2) falls, (3) drowning, and (4) fire and burns, and alcohol is known to be a contributing factor to each. (*FYI:* "Alcohol-Related Consequences" lists percentages of alcohol-related accidents.)

Women who commit suicide often have abused alcohol prior to the act. According to one study, alcoholic women are three times more likely to attempt suicide than alcoholic men.[26] Suicides tend to be more impulsive and more violent when alcohol is involved.

Effects on Relationships Relationship failure can be related to the abuse of alcohol in the partnership or family. Conflicts often arise from the consequences associated with the time, money, and energy spent on alcohol consumption. Because alcohol affects a person's ability to think rationally and respond appropriately, spouses, children, other family members, or friends can be neglected, abused, or abandoned. Nurturing, intimate relationships of all types often degenerate as a result of excessive alcohol consumption. Social occasions with friends, holidays or vacations with families, and special times such as birthdays or anniversaries can be sabotaged because of alcohol abuse.

Most people will admit that their thinking ability becomes distorted when they are drinking alcohol. Drinking by both men and women greatly increases the chance that sexual relations will occur. When this sexual encounter is forced on a woman by her date or an acquaintance while under the influence of alcohol,

it is called date or acquaintance rape. For a detailed discussion of alcohol and acquaintance rape, see Chapter 9.

Alcohol and Pregnancy

Would you, as a mother, get your baby drunk after she was born? Would you deliberately attempt to sabotage your baby's opportunity to have a healthy, productive life? Of course not! However, women who use alcohol, as well as other drugs, during pregnancy place their unborn child, and themselves, at risk for a reduced quality of life and reduced life expectancy. Pregnant women who consume alcohol are at greater risk for miscarriages. As a result of alcohol use during pregnancy, women may impair their personal health and increase the risk of the fetus developing serious and life-changing physical and mental health issues.

What does research reveal about the relationship between pregnancy and alcohol use? Alcohol crosses the placental barrier and decreases the amount of glucose and oxygen that is received by the fetal brain. The fetus may be more severely affected than the expectant mother because the fetus is unable to break down the alcohol as fast and efficiently as the mother. The fetus is most vulnerable during the first trimester of pregnancy. How much alcohol consumption do physicians and researchers recommend for pregnant females? *NONE!* Correct: not any! Research hasn't established a "safe" level of alcohol use during pregnancy; therefore, there is no way to know if the fetus will be affected by any alcohol consumption during pregnancy.

Scientist suspected a correlation between alcohol use and pregnancy complications as early as 1899, but it was not until 1973 that **FAS** was officially described in medical literature. Now referred to as **Fetal Alcohol Spectrum Disorders** (FASDs), it is a completely preventable cluster of birth defects including irreversible mental and physical disabilities that may develop as a result of expectant mothers consuming alcohol. Different terms are used to describe FASDs, depending on the type of symptoms:[30]

- **Fetal Alcohol Syndrome (FAS):** The severe end of the FASD spectrum with death being the most extreme outcome. Children with FAS may have abnormal facial features, growth issues, and central nervous system problems. They may also have problems with learning, memory, attention span, vision, and/or hearing, which can lead to difficulty in school and social interaction.
- **Alcohol-Related Neurodevelopmental Disorder (ARND):** Children with ARND might have intellectual disabilities and problems with behavior and learning. They often perform poorly in

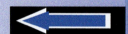

FYI

Annual Alcohol-Related Consequences for College Students[27]

- *Death:* 1825 college students between the ages of 18–24 die from alcohol-related unintentional injuries each year (i.e., motor vehicle crashes, drowning)
- *Injury:* 599,000 students between the ages of 18–24 are unintentionally injured while under the influence of alcohol
- *Assault:* 696,000 students between the ages of 18–24 are assaulted by another student who has been drinking
- *Sexual abuse:* 97,000 students between the ages of 18–24 are victims of alcohol-related sexual assault or date rape; of the 400,000 students who had unprotected sex, more than 100,000 stated they were too intoxicated to know if they gave consent.
- *Academic problems:* About 25 percent of college students report academic consequences due to drinking and missing class, falling behind, and doing poorly on exams and class work.
- *Drunk driving:* 3,360,000 students between the ages of 18 and 24 drive under the influence of alcohol.

FYI

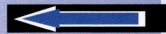

What's That in My Drink?[28]

The Drug Induced Rape Prevention and Punishment Act of 1996[29] states that it is a crime to give a controlled substance to anyone without his or her knowledge with the intent to commit a violent crime (such as rape). The punishment is severe, up to 20 years in prison and a large fine. Date rape drugs are sometimes used in sexual assault of women or in other types of sexual activity not agreed to by a woman. When ingested, these drugs produce helplessness, inability to refuse sex, and lack of memory of the event.

- *Rohypnol* (roofies) is NOT legal in the United States. It is legal in other countries and is even prescribed for sleep problems in Europe and Mexico. It is sold illegally in the United States. Initially, Rohypnol causes mild relaxation, slows psychomotor responses, and lowers inhibitions. Blackout periods may last from 8 to 12 hours, during which the victim may or may not appear "awake." Usually the potential rapist puts the small pill into the victim's drink. New Rohypnol pills turn blue when added to liquids; they are odorless and tasteless and easily dissolve in alcoholic or nonalcoholic beverages.
- *Gamma-hydroxybutyrate acid* (GHB) is a fast-acting central nervous system depressant, similar to Rohypnol. GHB is an odorless, colorless substance that is most often in liquid form, but it is also available in powder capsules. As with Rohypnol, the potential rapist puts the GHB into the victim's drink. Effects of GHB include an initial feeling of euphoria and calmness followed by drowsiness, respiratory distress, dizziness, seizures, and amnesia. It can also intensify the effects of alcohol and may increase sexual feelings. Unlike Rohypnol, GHB is legal in the United States.
- *Ketamine* (known as "Special K"), used as an anesthetic in veterinary practices, is a legal drug that blocks nerve paths and depresses the respiratory and circulatory functions. Ketamine is a popular substance in rave clubs and can create a hallucinogenic effect as well as increase sexual desires. Amnesic dreamlike memories make it difficult to remember if a sexual assault occurred. Ketamine is usually available in liquid form, easily slipped in someone's drink, and can cause the heart to stop.

To prevent becoming a victim of one of these drugs:

- Never leave a drink unattended or accept a drink from a stranger.
- Watch the behavior of your friends; anyone acting too drunk in relation to the amount of alcohol consumed may be in danger.

If you think you may have ingested any of these drugs, ask someone to take you to the emergency department or call 911. Try to keep a sample of the beverage for analysis.

---

school and have difficulties with memory, attention, judgment, math, and poor impulse control. This was formerly referred to as fetal alcohol effects (FAE).
- **Alcohol-Related Birth Defects (ARBD):** Children with ARBD may have problems with the heart, kidneys, bones, or hearing.

FASDs is considered the leading cause of developmental disabilities and birth defects in the United States, and each child with FASDs has one thing in common: a mother who consumed alcohol while pregnant. The 2007 *National Survey on Drug Use and Health*[31] revealed that 10.8 percent of pregnant women between the ages of 15–44 reported current alcohol use; 3.7 percent reported alcohol bingeing, and almost 1 percent reported heaving drinking. These rates are higher than in previous years, yet are significantly lower than the rates for nonpregnant women in the same age group.

Viewpoint

What Should Be Done About Pregnant Women Who Drink?

With all the information now available concerning FAS, what should be the legal consequences for women who consume alcohol during pregnancy and, as a result, have children with FAS? Does a woman have the right to choose unhealthy behaviors while pregnant with another human being? Should she be allowed to have more children and risk causing severe birth defects? Does the "right" to harm the fetus by drinking alcohol during pregnancy have any moral and legal ramifications?

Aren't you glad your mother took care of herself while she was pregnant with you? Do the same for your own children and return this morally and ethically correct courtesy should you ever become pregnant.

Research concerning paternal abuse of alcohol and resulting birth defects continues to be done. It is known that chronic alcohol abuse produces sexual dysfunction and impairs sperm production in both humans and animals. It appears that alcohol has a damaging effect on reproduction in males at all three levels of the male reproductive unit: the hypothalamus, pituitary, and testes.[32] Additionally, alcohol-related research using male rats indicates that paternal exposure to alcohol prior to mating has an adverse effect on normal development and behavior of their offspring. A possible explanation is that alcohol is toxic to the gonads and can have an adverse effect on synthesis and secretion of testosterone. One recent study in *Environmental Health Perspectives* reported that consumption of alcohol during pregnancy may increase the risk of cryptorchidism (undescended testicles) in sons.[33] Although research is inconclusive to some degree, it does indicate that paternal alcohol use must be researched to create a complete picture of alcohol abuse and fetal consequences.

ADDICTION AND DEPENDENCY

Addiction is a chronic relapsing condition characterized by compulsive drug-seeking and abuse and by long-lasting chemical changes in the brain. Addiction is the same whether the drug is alcohol, amphetamines, cocaine, heroin, marijuana, or nicotine.[34] Components of addiction include tolerance, physical dependence, and psychological dependence.

Dependency: What Is It?

Pharmacologically, alcohol is a depressant drug. With long-term continual use, it is capable of creating a physical and psychological dependence. **Physical dependency** means that body cells have come to depend on the presence of this depressant to maintain homeostasis (or balance). Once physically dependent, if the body is deprived of alcohol, an addict will experience **withdrawal symptoms.** Withdrawal symptoms can be extremely uncomfortable and even fatal. (See *FYI:* "Stages of Withdrawal from Alcohol.") Fatalities may be as high as one in seven. During the initial phase of withdrawal, called **detoxification,** or ridding the body of alcohol, women who have abused alcohol for a number of years may need to be hospitalized.

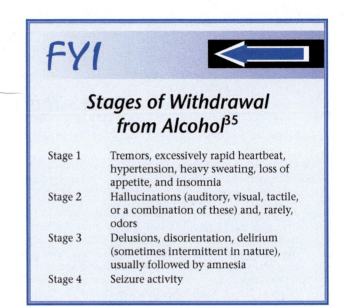

Stages of Withdrawal from Alcohol[35]

Stage 1	Tremors, excessively rapid heartbeat, hypertension, heavy sweating, loss of appetite, and insomnia
Stage 2	Hallucinations (auditory, visual, tactile, or a combination of these) and, rarely, odors
Stage 3	Delusions, disorientation, delirium (sometimes intermittent in nature), usually followed by amnesia
Stage 4	Seizure activity

Medically, withdrawal from alcohol is more severe and more likely to be fatal than is withdrawal from narcotic drugs.

Delirium tremens (DTs) are usually experienced in Stage 3 of alcohol withdrawal and are found mostly in serious cases of alcohol dependency. Although they often are manifested with shaking hands and jerky movements, DTs also produce vivid hallucinations and nausea. Withdrawal symptoms such as insomnia, panic attacks, irregular breathing, abnormal blood pressure, and/or anxiety may last for weeks, and the woman can feel an intense craving for alcohol. Aftercare programs, discussed later in this chapter, are important during this time to prevent the woman from returning to use of alcohol.

Psychological dependence, a learned process affecting the behavior of a long-term drinker, occurs when the drinker strongly desires, or craves, the feeling alcohol provides. Like the mother of a newborn infant who learns to function with less sleep, alcohol drinkers learn to function with the effects of alcohol. Learning what to expect from alcohol intake in varying circumstances, the woman learns to control her behavior and act accordingly. Psychological tolerance deceives a woman into believing she can perform certain tasks under the influence of alcohol. In reality, she will not be able to determine to what extent the alcohol affects her abilities. Even if she looks and acts sober, it does not mean that she is capable of skilled performance such as driving a car, using sharp instruments, or operating mechanical devices. Because of the psychological feelings (e.g., temporary escape, mood swings, relaxation, euphoria) sometimes resulting from the use of alcohol, the ability to recover from this type of dependency may be more difficult to achieve than recovery from physical dependency.

ALCOHOLISM

Quoting "Women Who Run with the Wolves":[36]

> When a woman is unconscious about her starvation, about the consequences of using death-dealing vehicles and substances, she is dancing, she is dancing. Whether these are such things as chronic negative thinking, poor relationships, abusive situations, drugs, or alcohol— they are like the red shoes: hard to pry a person away from once they've taken hold.

Demographics

Addiction to alcohol crosses all gender, economic, political, and social boundaries and generally is a well-established pattern of abuse by the time a male reaches his mid to late thirties or early forties, whereas women, if they develop alcoholism, generally do so at a later age and develop complications more easily and at a faster rate than males. **Alcoholism** is a chronic, progressive, and potentially fatal disease characterized by tolerance and by physical and psychological dependency; genetic, environmental, and psychosocial factors contribute to its development and progression. This disease is a direct or indirect result of ingesting alcohol and varies in the time it takes to develop. For some women the development can be somewhat rapid; for others, alcoholism may be years in the making. However long it takes to develop, this disease shortens life expectancy by an estimated 10–15 years. An estimated 5.3 million women in the United States drink in a way that threatens their health, safety, and general well-being.[37]

A myth about alcoholism is that a person has to be drinking or drunk all the time to be considered an alcoholic. The truth is that patterns of alcohol abuse vary. Regular daily intake of large amounts of alcohol, regular heavy drinking that is limited to weekends, or long periods of not drinking interspersed with binge drinking that can last from days to several weeks can each be typical of alcoholic drinking patterns. Another myth regarding alcoholism is that an alcoholic can resume drinking after remaining sober for a number of years without her drinking getting out of control. Although some researchers have tried to prove this is the case, no one in recovery from alcoholism would agree. Once a woman has developed the disease of alcoholism, she will always have the disease. She may not always be a drinking alcoholic, but she will be unable to ever control her drinking again; therefore, abstaining from any drinking is imperative. (Read *Her Story:* "Amanda: Portrait of an Alcoholic?" to see what you think.)

Her Story

Amanda: Portrait of an Alcoholic?

Amanda, a 22-year-old mother of one and a community college nursing major, maintains above-average grades. She rarely misses class and is a responsible parent Sunday through Thursday nights. However, after class is over each Friday, she takes Alissa, her 2-year-old daughter, to stay with her grandmother. Amanda spends the remainder of the weekend drinking with friends and out of control: partying, driving while drunk, engaging in sexual activity, and disregarding any responsibilities related to school or her daughter. Amanda refuses to stop spending her weekends in a drunken stupor and feels that as long as she is taking care of her responsibilities during the week, she can do as she pleases on the weekends.

- Does Amanda meet some of the criteria in the definition of alcoholism?
- Is she creating present or future problems as a result of continual overconsumption of alcohol?
- What consequences could result from her continual abuse of an addicting, toxic substance?

Is Alcoholism a Disease?

There is an ongoing controversy about whether alcoholism is truly a "disease" or if it is a willful abuse of a harmful and intoxicating substance. The American Medical Association classifies it as a disease, as does Alcoholics Anonymous, with millions of members whose "only requirement for membership is the desire to stop drinking." However, some professionals and researchers believe individuals should be responsible for their behavior under all circumstances and that it is wrong to "hide" behind the facade of disease to excuse any violent, antisocial, or illegal behavior because of alcohol abuse.

The cause of alcoholism is basically unknown, but studies have discovered that some of the following circumstances are revealed in the background of alcoholic women:

- Having an alcoholic parent or parents, which could mean that they have a genetic susceptibility or environmental influence to alcohol abuse; a large percentage of alcoholics have at least one alcoholic parent.
- Childhood abuse, of which almost half is the result of parental alcohol abuse. It may contribute to the abuse of a child and, as a result of this experience,

the abused child may become an alcoholic as well as a future child abuser.

- Excessive drinking as teens establishes the habit and social patterns, or even dependency.
- Social factors such as disappearance of the extended family, mobility of families, slackened family ties, and decline of religious affiliations.

Indicators of Alcoholism, and How to Help

If someone were to ask you about the signs that may indicate alcohol was becoming a problem or that signs of alcoholism were prevalent, would you know what they are? A progression of drinking alcohol more frequently and in larger amounts yielding ever-expanding negative consequences is indicative of alcoholism.

If someone you care about has a number of these indicators and continues to drink, what can you do? To better help the person(s) you care about and yourself through this serious situation, do the following:

- Learn the facts about alcohol and alcoholism, and find factual and unbiased resources.
- Develop a factual attitude rather than an emotional attitude toward the person and her drinking; avoid ridicule, criticism, and disgust.
- Do not use home remedies such as lecturing, hiding the liquor, soliciting promises the drinker won't or can't keep, saying, "If you loved me . . . ," or using a "holier than thou attitude."
- Find assistance for yourself and, if possible, the alcoholic such as your family doctor, minister, counselors, county agencies, and support groups (AA and Al-Anon).
- Talk with people who understand the illness, not just to friends and family.
- Allow the alcoholic to be responsible for her own behavior and the consequences of her drinking.
- Expect relapses and difficult days after recovery begins; immediate recovery will not happen.
- When protection from situations in which alcohol is present is not possible, the alcoholic has to learn to say "no, thanks" on her own.

Then complete *Assess Yourself:* "Do You Have a Drinking Problem?" to determine if you have a problem with alcohol.

A Family Disease

Growing up in a family in which alcohol was abused by one or both parents can produce lifelong negative consequences. Which would be a more difficult plight to endure: to be the daughter of alcoholic parents, to be the wife of an alcoholic, to be the mother of an alcoholic and having to see your child deal with alcoholism, or to be an alcoholic yourself? Each is hurtful, and many women experience all four circumstances.

Assess Yourself

Do You Have a Drinking Problem?

Use the following questions to determine if alcohol is a problem in your life. Check "yes" if the statement is true or "no" if the statement is not true about your drinking behaviors and patterns. Then consult the suggestions at the end of this survey.

Yes	No	Question
_____	_____	1. Do you drink more than three times a week?
_____	_____	2. Do you drink more than three drinks each time?
_____	_____	3. When everyone else is drinking, do you feel you should be drinking also?
_____	_____	4. Do you think it is acceptable for people to get drunk once in a while?
_____	_____	5. Do you find it difficult to say "no" when someone offers you an alcoholic drink even when you don't really want it?

Suggestions: If you answered "yes" more than "no" to these questions, it would be a good idea not only to reduce the amount and frequency of drinking, if you can, but also to talk with a counselor who specializes in alcohol treatment. If you suspect a friend or relative has a problem, encourage that person to take the assessment, too.

The physical and financial toll of alcoholism can to some degree be objectively calculated. However, the human loss to individuals, their families, communities, and society is incalculable. It is estimated that for every alcoholic, another four people are directly affected. The ripple effects from those four people then extend to numerous others.

Codependency Preoccupation with a particular individual and her or his problems to the point of self-neglect is an example of **codependency.** Eventually, the codependent's relationship with all others is affected. This results from prolonged association with the alcoholic and from the practice of oppressive "rules" that prevent the open expression of feelings, concerns, and problems. These rules, often developed subconsciously, include such things as it's not okay to talk about a problem; it's not okay to talk about feelings; do as I say, not as I do; don't rock the boat; it's not okay to play or be playful; be the best, but don't enjoy it! Codependent women often take care of their family's needs and wants. They tend to worry a lot; check on people; lose sleep over family problems; abandon their routine due to upset feelings about somebody or something; try to catch people in acts of misbehavior; control family members' behavior; think they know what is best for others; and try to control events and people through helplessness, guilt, coercion, threats, advice giving, manipulation, and/or domination. Codependency is unhealthy because the codependent woman tends to allow her physical, emotional, social, and mental quality of life to be dependent upon the quality of life of other people. Therefore, she feels as if she has little control over her own well-being. She is likely to develop stress-related disorders such as migraines, ulcers, arthritis, even heart disease and cancer. Women with codependent traits can obtain help through individual or family counseling with the alcoholic and other family members, involvement in twelve-step programs such as Al-Anon and Codependency Anonymous, and by reading the plethora of self-help material related to codependency and alcoholism.

Adult Children of Alcoholics *Adult children of alcoholics* (ACAs) grow up in a group of related people in which one or more members are alcoholic and cause stressful conditions, and continually create a dysfunctional environment. The family is the most significant social unit in our society and is responsible for the development of habits and beliefs that influence members' decisions throughout the life span. Yet children in the dysfunctional family often do not have role models who exhibit good habits or profess beliefs that help children develop important systems that can enhance

their life. The dysfunctional home environment places *children of alcoholics* (COAs) at risk for early alcohol and drug dependence, underachievement or unhealthy over-achievement, inappropriate classroom or social behaviors, lying, delinquency, unhealthy relationships with peers and adults, and emotional distress that can manifest itself in withdrawal, depression, or suicide attempts. As COAs become ACAs, unless they receive help, many continue to have these risk factors. Three rules, although not written, are learned by COAs: don't talk or tell (don't discuss the problem; pretend it doesn't exist); don't trust (nothing is consistent or predictable); and don't feel (numb out the anger and the pain; it hurts too much to feel). These rules lead to some serious consequences for ACAs. It sets the stage for shame and doubt, isolation, distrust of self and others, and uncertainty or numbing of feelings. Thus, there may be no pain but, also, there is no joy.

Strategies for overcoming the effects that are experienced by ACAs include

- going to ACA meetings,
- reading about the ACA experiences of others and writing about their own,
- using and incorporating information about methods and techniques of recovery,
- defining and enforcing boundaries, and
- building a personal support network.[38]

Effects of Growing Up in an Alcoholic Family
Surviving difficult family circumstances often means that family members develop coping mechanisms and roles that help them momentarily deal with the chaos of living in an alcoholic family. Four roles, identified by treatment providers, that COAs often develop to help them cope with problems related to parental alcoholism are the hero, the scapegoat, the lost child, and the mascot. The hero is the super-kid, caretaker, the "type E" female: everything to everybody; she is the cheerleader, honor student, and president of the class. Often irresponsible, disruptive, or antisocial, the scapegoat may become defiant and delinquent; she is vulnerable to unwholesome peer groups and drug abuse. The lost child (the loner) has her own private world of reading, television, computer, music, or any other refuge she can find that enables her to escape from the family chaos; she is at risk for poor health choices (e.g., smoking, drinking), early natural death, or suicide. Seemingly carefree, funny, the center of attention, the mascot (or clown) deals with the dysfunctional family by denying there is a problem. She diverts attention from the painful family situation by offering comic relief; she is at risk for physical and emotional problems and drug abuse.

Journal Activity

Who and What Does Alcohol Affect?

As you read the various events listed below, determine the area of greatest impact on one of the following: (a) the drinker (health effect), (b) the family (social effect), (c) or society (economic effect). For each event write the effect in the "Who or What?" column, and in the last column, explain why this effect has such a great impact. (*Hint:* It may affect more than one area!)

Event	Who or What?	Why?
1. Court system		
2. Auto death while DUI		
3. Increased welfare costs		
4. Injuring oneself in a fall		
5. Job loss		
6. Divorce		
7. Cirrhosis of the liver		
8. Neglect of one's children		
9. Heart disease		
10. Decreased work productivity		
11. Spousal abuse		
12. Passing out or vomiting at a party		
13. Increased medical costs		
14. Sexually transmitted diseases		
15. Abusing a child		
16. Depression		
17. Fighting at a sporting event		
18. Killing someone when driving drunk		

These roles help children (and often adults) survive the dysfunctional family situation. Their development may be thwarted without help, and these coping roles may prevent them from leading fulfilling lives outside the family system. Many of these behaviors do not serve them well as adults when they use the behaviors on the job or when interacting with family or friends. ACAs must be taught the four Cs of a dysfunctional family: You didn't *cause* it, you can't *control* it, you can't *cure* it, you *can help yourself.*

Fortunately, as alcoholics are being assisted in overcoming their disease and dysfunctions, the family members can also be assisted in overcoming risk factors generated by growing up in an alcoholic family. Twelve-step programs, such as Al-Anon, ACA meetings, Codependency Anonymous groups, as well as individual and group therapy have been successful in overcoming negative behaviors associated with alcoholic families, and moving ahead to productive and positive lives. Schools also have developed support programs for COAs that include such activities as building self-esteem, establishing consistency, providing a safe environment for expressing feelings openly, and learning to trust. This is an attempt to reduce risk factors that could lead to development of alcohol and drug abuse among children of alcoholics and to build protective factors that are traits or conditions intended to assist COAs in the development of healthy and productive lifestyles. (See *Journal Activity:* "Who and What Does Alcohol Affect?")

WHAT CAN BE DONE?

No one approach seems to be successful for recovery from alcoholism. Instead, greater success is found by utilizing a combination of treatment approaches. It is important to remember that the alcoholic will rarely move to "treat" herself and may need assistance in seeking help. However, no one can force another adult into treatment unless the legal system intercedes, and this happens only after some crime has been committed because of alcohol abuse.

Resources

Locating resources for the alcoholic and yourself is an important first step toward resolving this problem. Who, what, where, how, and how much are all questions that need to have answers prior to movement toward assisting the alcoholic.

Intervention

Intervention is a process by which the alcoholic is confronted by a person or persons each describing the "facts" associated with their concern for the alcoholic's drinking problem. Individuals close to the alcoholic (e.g., child, parent, sibling, spouse, friends, employer) can share in this calm, yet truthful process that is intended to assure the alcoholic of their concern for her, but also assertively express the situation as it is. If the intervention is successful, the alcoholic should be willing to move into inpatient or outpatient treatment. Betty Ford states that when her family intervened because of her abuse of prescription drugs and alcohol, she became angry and hurt. But, as she listened, she heard the love that came through their comments to her, and she realized they loved her too much to ignore the problem any longer. She decided to seek treatment and continues in recovery, which she says will be ongoing as long as she lives. The Betty Ford Center in Rancho Mirage, California, was created as a result of her efforts and continues to treat thousands of individuals in need of alcohol and other drug therapy.

Intervention actions include developing individual action plans, selecting treatment centers, facilitating an intervention meeting, and facilitating pre-interaction, family, and follow-up meetings.[39]

Types of Treatment

Various approaches are used in the treatment of alcoholism and include not only what precipitated the originating use but also the complex consequences of the disease. Women comprise about one-third of the population with alcohol problems and slightly less than half of those have problems with other drugs.[40] Lifestyle behavior change, stress management programs, individual counseling, spiritual renewal, hospitalization, drug therapy, support groups, and other therapies are often used in treatment for alcoholism.

Lifestyle Behavior Changes Lifestyle behavior changes include improved nutrition, engaging in exercise programs, developing stress management strategies, enhancement of self-worth, and recognizing a higher power. Treatment attempts to focus on making positive changes in one's life in addition to cessation of alcohol abuse.

Counseling Individual and/or group counseling assists the alcoholic in looking at issues related to the abusive behavior. It is important to determine whether alcohol abuse is the result of a variety of negative situations in one's life or the negative situations are the consequences of alcohol abuse. The counselor needs to be specifically trained in working with alcohol-dependent individuals as well as their families. Group therapy can provide an environment in which women feel safe discussing their alcohol-related problems and receive support from other women who understand and can relate to them. Realization that others have experienced the same pain, humiliation, or shame seems to bring relief because each woman no longer feels she is the only one.

Treatment Centers Use of hospitals or drug treatment centers has been beneficial for some women. In this environment women can go through detoxification under medical supervision, remove themselves from the surroundings in which they've had problems with alcohol, and begin to resolve the problems that caused this disease to develop. Treatment centers usually have a structured routine revolving around household duties, individual and group therapy, recreation, nutritious meals, and support group meetings, all of which help to reestablish routine, responsibility, and health. Many insurance companies provide for alcoholism treatment on both an inpatient and outpatient basis. Women in treatment often have different needs than men. Care of small children, finances, transportation, and even distrustfulness of male professionals hinder a woman's ability to engage in treatment programs. To promote recovery for women with these needs, treatment should include child care, female counselors, transportation, reduced fees, and women-only therapies.

Chemical Treatment Chemical treatment (drug therapy) occasionally becomes necessary if a woman cannot refrain from abusing alcohol through inpatient or outpatient treatment. Antabuse is a drug that inhibits an enzyme (acetaldehyde dehydrogenase) from breaking down acetaldehyde. As a result, a toxic effect to alcohol is created; therefore, if a woman who has taken Antabuse then drinks, extremely uncomfortable effects such as nausea, weakness, blurred vision, heart palpitations, and vomiting occur. These consequences are intended to impede the consumption of alcohol. Two drugs, nalmefene and naltrexone, both of which are opiate antagonists, block the brain's pleasurable response to drinking and help alcohol abusers to stop drinking compulsively. One research study discovered that only 15 percent of physicians, even among addiction specialists, prescribe naltrexone for alcohol abuse treatment.[41] Clinicians need to be better informed about drugs such as naltrexone so that patients can be prescribed the drugs and experience their positive effects. Drugs such as these can be beneficial in reducing a person's desire to drink and therefore decrease the high rates of alcoholics' relapse to heavy drinking, which occurs at a rate of about 80 percent.

Aftercare Aftercare, continuing care following treatment for alcohol or other drug abuse, needs to be comprehensive as well as attentive to individual needs. Provision of support groups and varied services can enable women to live drug-free lives and foster development of skills and abilities leading to self-confidence and independence. What services and support structures are most beneficial following treatment? Contact with other recovering women, recovery and personal growth literature, personal and family therapy sessions, life skills and job training, vocational training and job placement are all beneficial as women seek to move ahead to a healthy, productive lifestyle. Support and self-help groups such as twelve-step organizations, including *Alcoholics Anonymous (AA), Al-Anon (AA), Adult Children of Alcoholics (ACA), Codependency Anonymous (CODA),* and *Women for Sobriety,* offer emotional support and social interaction among women who can share experiences and solutions for a disease that is known best by individuals who have shared in its devastating effects. (See *FYI:* "Facts about Alcoholics Anonymous.")

Involving cultural and geographic community support, such as phone chains, hotlines, and recovery group gatherings, can keep recovering women in contact with one another so that the healing process will continue. Women who have just come out of treatment programs need to have follow-up contact for as long as the woman and her counselor and/or case manager deem it important and necessary. (See the resources and suggested readings at the end of the chapter.)

PREVENTION

Of course, the most effective way to prevent problems associated with alcohol abuse and the disease of alcoholism is to abstain from alcohol consumption. Because there are millions of women who drink, and many of them do develop alcohol dependency problems, it is important to look at how those problems can be avoided.

Primary prevention programs are aimed at women, especially young women, who have not begun to use

 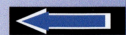

Facts about Alcoholics Anonymous[42]

- There are more than 114,000 AA groups worldwide in 170 countries.
- 35 percent of AA members are female.
- Approximately 36 percent of the members have been sober more thanr 10 years; 14 percent have been sober between 1 and 5 years.
- About 66 percent of AA members are between the ages of 21 and 50.
- Average member attends two meetings per week.
- Average age of members is 48 years.
- Other treatment programs follow the AA model (for example, Codependency Anonymous and Cocaine Anonymous).

alcohol, and they focus on reducing the rate of new alcohol users. This type of prevention program attempts to provide and promote activities that reduce the factors related to early use of alcohol. These factors include lack of awareness in school and community of alcohol-related problems, insufficient knowledge about alcohol and other drugs, lack of understanding about negative effects of alcohol abuse, students' need for life skills training, infrequent involvement of parents in their children's schools, lack of awareness of positive alternatives to using alcohol, and insufficient knowledge about regulations and laws pertaining to alcohol use/abuse.

Activities can be developed to combat each one of these factors and thus reduce the possibility that young women will begin to use alcohol. Suggested activities pertaining to these contributing factors include, but are not limited to, some of the following:

- Raising awareness through involvement of community organizations, church groups, or parent groups by developing a media campaign using local newspaper, television, and radio; promoting a community alcohol awareness day designated by wearing certain colors or driving with headlights on; or proclamations by community officials. The more segments of community involvement, the greater the opportunity to enhance awareness in school and community of alcohol-related problems.
- Accurate, current, and age-appropriate information can affect good communication between parents, teachers, and their children/

students. As part of a comprehensive approach to alcohol use prevention, purchasing materials and curricula and providing in-service programs for teachers, as well as providing opportunities for parents to become educated about alcohol use, can help to reduce the insufficient knowledge about alcohol and other drugs.

Young women often believe that alcohol use does not produce any negative consequences and therefore using this substance is okay. By developing strong anti-use policies in schools and communities and involving students in alcohol-free activities, young women are likely to behave accordingly and develop negative attitudes toward the use of alcohol.

Like all individuals, young women need life skills training. Activities and organizations that promote the resistance of peer influence enhance decision-making abilities, and aid young women in coping with personal and social issues, can provide a basis for choosing not to use alcohol. Developing leadership qualities and problem-solving skills can also reduce the likelihood of alcohol use by females.

Enhancing positive family influence and increasing involvement of parents and students in school can be accomplished by promoting parenting skills through parent-training programs in education systems or community organizations. More involvement in and allegiance to school means that students often adopt behaviors and values expounded by the school and have less time for alcohol-related activities or peers who may choose to drink. Club, sport, and other student–parent organizations not only involve the students but also provide reasons for parents to come to school events. Giving young women opportunities to engage in these activities can provide healthy alternatives to alcohol use. Youth centers, community and school recreation, and alcohol-free dances and parties can offer alternative activities to involvement with alcohol.

Regulations and laws can be useful in preventing abuse of alcohol and other drugs. Creating barriers to alcohol access and enforcing restrictions to curtail underage drinking and use of fake identification cards can be a deterrent to early use of alcohol. Increased supervision of youth and expanded security at places where young people congregate help prevent the influx of alcohol by underage consumers.

The majority of these suggestions are directed toward *young* women, because that is exactly when alcohol abuse prevention must begin. The younger the age at which females initially abuse alcohol, the greater the probability they will encounter negative consequences.

Prevention can yield the greatest benefit if initiated at an early age (e.g., preschool) and continued throughout the school years and into adulthood. During this process, many of the risk factors can be ameliorated and alcohol abuse prevented.

> Yes there is pain in being severed from the red shoes. But being cut away from the addiction all at once is our only hope. It is a severing that is filled with absolute blessing. The feet will grow back, we will find our way, we will recover, we will run and jump and skip again someday. By then our handmade life will be ready. We'll slip into it and marvel that we could be so lucky to have another chance.[43]

Chapter Summary

- Women and alcohol have a historical association that produced both positive and negative outcomes.
- Alcohol is the most commonly used psychoactive drug, and its use has a number of health benefits; the abuse of alcohol results in serious physical, psychological, social, and economic consequences.
- Women and men respond differently to alcohol, both physically and behaviorally.
- Alcohol and pregnancy do not mix; there is no safe level of alcohol ingestion for pregnant women; FAS can result from drinking alcohol during pregnancy.
- Alcohol is an addicting, depressant drug that can cause the disease of alcoholism and result in serious consequences for the addict, her family, and other important components of her life.

- There are indicators that can be utilized as a means of informal assessment to determine if someone is alcohol dependent.
- Children of alcoholics (COAs) develop family roles that enable them to attempt to cope with the chronic distress and chaos present in an alcoholic's family. Without assistance, COAs may take these roles into adulthood.
- Finding resources, intervention, seeking treatment, and changing lifestyle behaviors can all be beneficial when recovering from alcohol addiction.
- Prevention of alcohol abuse is important if women are to avoid the possible devastation that can occur from alcohol abuse and addiction.

Review Questions

1. What attitudes toward women and alcohol were held by society at different times in history?
2. What are the four different types of alcohol? What does the term *proof* mean?
3. What is the process of alcohol absorption in a woman's body?
4. Why does alcohol affect women differently than it affects men?
5. What are the criteria used to classify different levels of drinkers?
6. What are the possible consequences for the mother and her fetus and infant if she drinks alcohol during pregnancy?
7. How does the addiction process relate to alcohol dependency?
8. If alcohol is a disease, why don't we know exactly what causes it, how to successfully treat it, and how to prevent it?
9. What indications may be displayed by a woman who either is developing or has developed an addiction to alcohol?
10. What is codependency? How does it relate to alcohol abuse?
11. What characteristics may develop in children who grow up in homes where either one parent or both parents are alcoholic?
12. What are some approaches that can be taken to assist a woman in overcoming alcohol dependency?
13. What are some of the methods that can be used to prevent alcohol abuse in women?
14. What is the difference between fetal alcohol syndrome and fetal alcohol effects?

Resources

Web Sites for Alcohol-Related Organizations

Adult Children of Alcoholics (ACA)
    www.adultchildren.org
Al-Anon Family Group Headquarters
    www.al-anon.alateen.org
Alcoholics Anonymous (AA) World Services
    www.alcoholics-anonymous.org
Alcohol and Drug Information, U.S. Department of Health and Human Services
    http://ncadi.samhsa.gov/govpubs/rpo993
Centers for Disease Control and Prevention: Alcohol and Pregnancy
    www.cdc.gov/Features/AlcoholAndPregnancy

Higher Education Center for Alcohol and Other Drug Prevention
    www.higheredcenter.org
Mothers Against Drunk Driving (MADD)
    www.madd.org
National Council on Alcoholism and Drug Dependence (NCADD)
    www.ncadd.org
National Institute on Alcohol Abuse and Alcoholism
    www.niaaa.nih.gov
Substance Abuse and Mental Health Services
    http://www.samhsa.gov

References

1. Blume, S. 1990. Chemical dependency in women: Important issues. *American Journal of Drug and Alcohol Abuse* 16 (3&4): 297–307.
2. Centers for Disease Control and Prevention. 2011. *Excessive drinking costs U.S. $223.5 billion.* http://www.cdc.gov/Features/AlcoholConsumption/ (retrieved May 29, 2012).
3. Blume, Chemical dependency in women: Important issues.
4. Balentine, J. 2012. *Alcohol intoxication. E-medicine Health.* http://www.emedicinehealth.com/alcohol_intoxication/article_em.htm (retrieved May 30, 2012).
5. Centers for Disease Control and Prevention (CDC). 2008. *Alcohol-Related Disease Impact (ARDI).* Atlanta, GA: CDC. http://www.cdc.gov/alcohol/fact-sheets/alcohol-use.htm (retrieved May 30, 2012).
6. National Institute on Alcohol Abuse and Alcoholism. 2007. *Alcohol: A woman's health issue.* pubs.niaaa.nih.gov/publications/brochurewomen/women.htm (retrieved May 30, 2012).
7. Substance Abuse and Mental Health Services Administration. 2011. *Results from the 2010 National Survey on Drug Use and Health: Summary of National Findings*, NSDUH Series H-41, HHS Publication No. (SMA) 11-4658. Rockville, MD: Substance Abuse and Mental Health Services Administration.
8. Kinney, J. 2006. *Loosening the grip: A handbook of alcohol information.* 8th ed. New York: McGraw-Hill.
9. Wechsler, J., J. E. Lee, M. Kuo, M. Seibring, T. F. Nelson, and H. Lee. 2002. Trends in college binge drinking during a period of increased prevention efforts. *Journal of American College Health* 50 (5): 203–17.
10. News Editor, 2009. Dramatic increase in drinking among women college students. *Psych Central.* http://psychcentral.com/news/2009/06/23/dramatic-increase-in-drinking-among-women-college-students/6686.html (retrieved May 31, 2012).
11. Kelly-Wedder, S. and W. F. Connell. 2007. Binge drinking in college-aged women: Framing a gender-specific

prevention strategy. *Journal of the American Academy of Nurse Practitioners* 20 (12): 577–84.

12. Emanuele, M. A., F. Wezeman, and N. V. Emanuele. 2002. Alcohol's effects on female reproductive function. *Alcohol Research & Health* 26 (4): 274–81.

13. Dorgan, J., et al. 2001. Alcohol increases hormone levels, raising breast cancer risk. *Journal of the National Cancer Institute* 93 (9): 710–15.

14. Li, C. I., K. E. Malone, P. L. Porter, N. S. Weiss, M. C. Tang, and J. R. Darling. 2003. The relationship between alcohol use and risk of breast cancer by histology and hormone receptor status among women 65–79 years of age. *Cancer Epidemiology, Biomarkers and Prevention* 12: 1061–66.

15. Register, T. C., M. Cline, and C. A. Shively. 2002. Health issues in postmenopausal women who drink. *Alcohol Research & Health* 26 (4): 299–307.

16. Cooley, E. and T. Toray. 2001. Disordered eating in college freshman women: A prospective study. *Journal of American College Health* 49 (5): 229–35.

17. Peralta, R. I. 2005. Alcohol use and the fear of weight gain in college: Reconciling two social norms. *Gender Issues* 20 (4): 23–42.

18. Adapted from: Payne, W. A., D. B. Hahn, and E. Lucas. 2007. *Understanding Your Health.* 9th ed. New York: McGraw-Hill.

19. Center for Science in the Public Interest. 2000. *Alcohol policies project: Advocacy for the prevention of alcohol problems.* www.cspinet.org/booze/women.htm (retrieved May 31, 2012).

20. National Institute on Alcohol Abuse and Alcoholism. 2006. *Alcohol use and alcohol use disorders in the United States: Main findings from the 2001–2002 National Epidemiologic Survey on Alcohol and Related Conditions (NESARC).* Bethesda, MD: National Institutes of Health.

21. Collins, R. L., and L. D. McNair. 2003. *Minority women and alcohol use.* National Institute in Alcohol Abuse and Alcoholism. http://pubs.niaaa.nih.gov/publications/arh26-4/251-256.htm (retrieved May 31, 2012).

22. National Institutes of Health, National Institute on Alcohol Abuse and Alcoholism. *Percent distribution of the drinking levels of females 18 years of age and older according to selected characteristics: United States. NHIS, 1997–2004.*

23. National Institutes of Health, National Institute on Alcohol Abuse and Alcoholism. 2002. *Alcohol: What you don't know can harm you.* NIH Publication No. 99-4323.

24. Califano, J. 2007. *High society: How substance abuse ravages America and what to do about it.* New York: Public Affairs.

25. Ibid.

26. Preuss, U. W., et al. 2002. Comparison of 3,190 alcohol-dependent individuals with and without suicide attempts. *Alcoholism: Clinical and Experimental Research* 26 (4): 471–77.

27. National Institute on Alcoholism and Alcohol Abuse. 2010. *A snapshot of Annual High-risk College Drinking Consequences.* www.collegedrinkingprevention.gov/StatsSummaries/snapshot.aspx (retrieved May 31, 2012).

28. U.S. Department of Health and Human Services, Office on Women's Health. 2008. *Date rape drugs fact sheet.* http://www.womenshealth.gov/publications/our-publications/fact-sheet/date-rape-drugs.cfm#a (retrieved June 3, 2012).

29. Congressional Record: 104th Congress (1995–1996). 1996. *The Drug-Induced Rape Prevention and Punishment Act of 1996 (Senate – October 03, 1996).* http://thomas.loc.gov/cgi-bin/query/D?r104:4:./temp/&tidle;r104GsUqJX:: (retrieved June 3, 2012.

30. Centers for Disease Control and Prevention. 2010. *Facts about FASDs.* http://www.cdc.gov/ncbddd/fasd/facts.html (retrieved June 4, 2012).

31. Substance Abuse and Mental Health Administration, Office of Applied Studies. 2011. Results from the 2010 National Survey on Drug Use and Health: National findings. http://www.samhsa.gov/data/NSDUH/2k10NSDUH/2k10Results.htm#2.6 (retrieved June 4, 2012).

32. Emanuele, M. A. and N. Emanuele. 2001. Alcohol and the male reproductive system. *Alcohol Research and Health* 25 (4): 282–87.

33. Drinking during pregnancy may disrupt male reproductive development. 2007. In *Environment and Health Perspectives.* www.ehponline.org/press/20070201b.html (retrieved June 4, 2012).

34. National Institute of Drug Abuse. 2011. *The science of drug abuse and addiction.* http://www.drugabuse.gov/publications/media-guide/science-drug-abuse-addiction (retrieved on June 4, 2012).

35. Ksir, C., D. L. Hart and O. Ray. 2006. *Drugs, society and human behavior.* 11th ed. New York: McGraw-Hill, p. 227.

36. Estes, C. P. 1995. *Women who run with the wolves.* New York: Ballantine, p. 248.

37. National Institute on Alcohol Abuse and Alcoholism. 2007. *Alcohol: A woman's health issue.* http://pubs.niaaa.nih.gov/publications/brochurewomen/women.htm (retrieved June 4, 2012).

38. *Adult children of alcoholics.* 2003. www.adultchildren.org/lit/Handbook.s (retrieved June 4, 2012).

39. Assistance in Recovery. 2011. *Interventions.* http://a-i-r.com/ (retrieved June 4, 2012).

40. Greenfield, S. F., D. E. Sugarman, L. R. Muenz, et al. 2003. Epidemiology of substance use disorders in women. *Obstetrics & Gynecology Clinics in North America* 30: 413–46.

41. Thomas, C.P. et al. 2003. Research to practice: Adoption of naltrexone in alcoholism treatment. *Journal of Substance Abuse Treatment* 24: 1–11.

42. Alcoholics Anonymous Worldwide. 2012. http://www.aa.org/lang/en/en_pdfs/smf-53_en.pdf (retrieved June 4, 2012).

43. Estes, *Women who run with the wolves,* p. 251.

Chapter Thirteen

Making Wise Decisions about Tobacco, Caffeine, and Drugs

CHAPTER OBJECTIVES

When you complete this chapter, you will be able to do the following:

◇ Explain why smoking-related deaths are the most preventable causes of morbity in women in this country

◇ Identify the substances in tobacco and the role each plays in the development of smoking-related diseases

◇ Analyze available methods that can be used for smoking cessation

◇ Clarify the relationship between the use of tobacco and the effects on reproduction in women

◇ Explain the importance of a smoke-free environment in the home, the workplace, and recreational facilities

◇ Describe the physiological effects of caffeine on women's health

◇ Explain the interaction between caffeine and pregnancy

◇ Discuss illegal drugs and their characteristics

◇ Determine the consequences of illegal drug use and its impact on a woman's lifestyle, health, and pregnancy

◇ Describe the social problems that women encounter as a result of illegal drug use

The chains of habit are too weak to be felt until they are too strong to be broken.

SAMUEL JOHNSON

TOBACCO: LOOKING BACK

More deaths could be prevented if individuals stopped using tobacco than by changing any other lifestyle behavior. Despite the overwhelming amount of research linking tobacco use to *morbidity* (illness) and *mortality* (death), more than 4000 persons under the age of 18 begin smoking every day in the United States, which is almost 1.5 million each year.[1] The Food and Drug Administration (FDA) can restrict and regulate access to tobacco products and control the labeling on tobacco packaging. However, the advertising of various forms of tobacco cannot be regulated by the FDA. The federal government, to some degree, has been reluctant to place major constraints on tobacco products because of the possible economic impact on the production, manufacturing, and selling of this product. Yet, as you will read in this chapter, the substances found in tobacco cause serious health consequences, resulting in high costs in

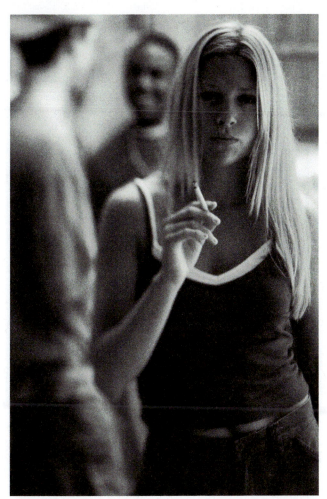

Unfortunately, the number of young female smokers is increasing.

WOMEN AND TOBACCO

Prevalence of Tobacco Use

The Centers for Disease Control and Prevention (CDC) states that one in six American women aged 18 or older (17 percent) smoke cigarettes. Women who smoke typically begin as teenagers. Among female high school students, approximately 17 percent reported smoking cigarettes and nearly 20% of women aged 25–44 smoke.[2] Presently, there are 46 million smokers in the United States, and approximately 21 million of them are female;[3] at least 1.5 million are adolescent girls. One-half of all long-term smokers will die because they choose to smoke tobacco. These are alarming statistics, as former surgeon general David Satcher points out:

> When calling attention to public health problems, we must not misuse the word "epidemic." But there is no better word to describe the 600-percent increase since 1950 in women's death rates for lung cancer, a disease primarily caused by cigarette smoking. Clearly, smoking-related disease among women is a full-blown epidemic.[4]

Increased risks of heart and lung diseases, cancers, and reproductive disorders are much more prevalent in women smokers than in men smokers accounting for 174,000 women who die each year from smoking-related illness.[5] Adult women who smoke lose almost 15 years of life; it is the most preventable cause of premature death in this country.[6] If women smoke, they usually initiate smoking as teenagers. Smoking rates for women who have less than a high school education are three times higher than for women who are college graduates.

Ethnicity is a factor in the prevalence of women who smoke. American Indian and Alaska Native women had the highest prevalence of smoking, followed by white and African American women; the lowest prevalence was found among Hispanic, Asian, and Pacific Islander women.[7]

Each of these factors plays a significant role in the probability that a woman will die prematurely from the use of tobacco: the earlier the age at which a woman starts to smoke, the longer she smokes, the more she inhales, and the higher the level of tar and nicotine in the tobacco product.

Why Women Smoke

Media influence is pervasive, compelling, and influential. There are thousands of television stations, radio stations, daily newspapers, and magazines and billboards, all of which reach millions of women on a daily, even hourly basis. Many thousands of these media avenues promote the concept that smoking relates to a desired image and lifestyle, fun times, attraction to others, athleticism, and quiet moments in beautiful surroundings. Mass media has certainly been used by the tobacco companies to zealously promote their product. In fact, cigarettes are one of the most widely advertised consumer products in this country even though this commodity has been banned from television and radio advertising since 1971. Emerson Foote, who was a well-known president of two large advertising agencies, states:

> The cigarette industry has been artfully maintaining that cigarette advertising has nothing to do with total sales. This is complete and utter nonsense. . . . I am

terms of poor health and an increased need for health care. Both the home and the workplace are negatively impacted.

always amused by the suggestion that advertising, a function that has been shown to increase consumption of virtually every other product, somehow miraculously fails to work for tobacco products.[8]

In 2008, the tobacco industry spent $9.94 billion on cigarette advertising and promotional expenses in the United States.[9] Including both cigarette and smokeless tobacco advertising, the tobacco companies spent $10.5 in 2008, or nearly $29 million each day.[10]

Through advertisements, the tobacco industry captured some of women's energy, perhaps unrest, and certainly their desire to make some of their own decisions. Using slogans, pictures, and scenarios, cigarette manufacturers promoted the idea of freedom, choice, and appeal. The billions of dollars the tobacco industry has spent in promoting its products through the years has influenced women to embrace tobacco use and, in the process, negatively affected their environment, their health, and even the well-being of their children.

Maintaining weight may be another reason that women choose to smoke. Have you heard the comment that women experience weight gain once they quit smoking? There is an explanation for this. Nicotine decreases the strength of hunger contractions in the stomach (e.g., inhaling the smoke of one cigarette can reduce "hunger pains" for almost an hour), increases blood sugar level, and deadens taste buds. As an oral habit, smokers associate hand-to-mouth activity with pleasure (or relief from anxiety); therefore, when smoking stops, hand-to-mouth objects (food) substitute for the former hand-to-mouth smoking behavior. With cessation of smoking, the senses of taste and smell increase; therefore, food becomes more appealing. It is important to remember that the average weight gain following smoking cessation is less than 10 pounds.[11] However, the amount of weight gain depends on the individual and her willingness to engage in behaviors that reduce the possibility of weight gain following the cessation of smoking. (See *Health Tips:* "Avoiding Weight Gain after Smoking Cessation" for suggestions to avoid weight gain.) Imagine this—a woman would need to gain between 50 and 100 pounds before she could come close to the equivalent health risks associated with tobacco smoking.

Parental smoking influences children to adopt this behavior; children whose parents smoke (especially if *both* parents smoke) are much more likely to become smokers themselves than are children whose parents do not smoke. We are certainly influenced by our peers; almost 90 percent of teens who smoke have friends who also smoke, and young women who smoke are more likely to have boyfriends who are also smokers. Additionally, if "your group" is composed of numerous smokers, there is a much greater chance that you will also become a smoker. For example, associating with coworkers who

Health Tips

Avoiding Weight Gain after Smoking Cessation

If you are a former smoker and want to control the possibility of weight gain, consider the following suggestions. You may even want to incorporate these suggestions into your lifestyle as a matter of improving your overall good health habits.

- Have low-fat, nutritious snacks easily accessible to help satisfy the hand-to-mouth habit.
- Keep a straw or other harmless object handy to chew on or use with your hands.
- Enlist the help of a significant other and try new activities together.
- Walk, jog, bike, or swim at least three times per week.
- Include in your diet your very favorite food (in moderation) at least once each week.
- Reward yourself at designated intervals for remaining smoke-free.

smoke and friends who smoke at clubs and parties, or engaging in an activity at which participants smoke, such as bowling, may increase your chances of smoking. The environment in which we work and recreate plays a part in the choice to use tobacco. Take *Assess Yourself:* "Could You Become a Smoker?" to determine which factors could influence you to become a smoker.

SUBSTANCES IN TOBACCO

With more than 4000 chemical components, at least 250 of which are harmful to human health, including 60 that are **carcinogenic,** adverse effects of tobacco use abound.[12] Compounds such as tar, carbon monoxide, hydrogen cyanide, ammonia, formaldehyde, benzene, and nicotine, among thousands of others, comprise the ingredients found in tobacco products.[13] **Nicotine,** which is physically and psychologically addicting, stimulates the central nervous system by the release of adrenalin, causing blood pressure and heart rate to increase. It also constricts the peripheral blood vessels and bronchial tubes. There is an increased need for oxygen *by* the heart, but not an increased oxygen supply *to* the heart. As you can imagine, the body's immediate response to nicotine can seriously affect the entire cardiovascular system.

Carbon monoxide, one of the 270 poisonous gases in tobacco smoke, increases the heart rate, elevates blood

Assess Yourself

Could You Become a Smoker?

Listed below are a number of factors you may have encountered that may influence you to become a smoker. Check those that apply to you. Obviously, the more checkmarks you have, the greater the likelihood that you could become a smoker.

Factors	Yes	No
1. Mother smokes(ed)	_____	_____
2. Father smokes(ed)	_____	_____
3. Siblings smoke(d)	_____	_____
4. Friends smoke(d)	_____	_____
5. Coworkers smoke	_____	_____
6. Boyfriend or husband smokes	_____	_____
7. Believe smoking is okay	_____	_____
8. Know the health consequences of smoking	_____	_____
9. Like the way someone looks when smoking	_____	_____
10. Believe that you can relax by smoking	_____	_____
Total points	_____	_____

The best advice is that if you don't smoke, *don't start!* If you do smoke, *quit!*

pressure, and impairs visual acuity. Carbon monoxide combines with oxygen to form *carboxyhemoglobin;* therefore, instead of oxygen being delivered to vital cells, tissues, and organs, a poisonous gas arrives and robs the body of life-giving healthy air.

Particulate matter, **tar**, is a mixture of ingredients that are inhaled into the lungs with use of cigarettes and it inhibits effective functioning of the respiratory system. More than 90 percent of particulate matter remains in a smoker's lungs. Imagine your lungs coated with a sticky, yellow-brown substance that contains cancer-causing chemicals such as pyrenes, benzo(a)pyrenes, and chyrsenes, which have been linked to lung cancer development.[14]

ADVERSE HEALTH EFFECTS

Smoking generates serious health problems for women just as it does for men, and long-term use of tobacco will cause various ill effects to become more discernible. Compared to nonsmokers, women who smoke more than double their annual risk of dying as a result of tobacco use.

Respiratory Concerns

Bronchiectasis is a condition that develops within the bronchial tree (the "branches" of the bronchi) and results in irreversible dilatation and destruction of the bronchial walls. Inflammation of airways and alveoli results in scarring and loss of elasticity in the airways of the lungs. Chronic bronchitis, characterized by long-term and persistent severe coughing, spitting, and excessive secretion of mucus, is a precursor to bronchiectasis. Smoking cigarettes causes the development of bronchitis or exacerbates the inflammation. This inflammation of the airways causes the passages to squeeze shut during exhalation, preventing the lungs from emptying completely.

Emphysema is a lung disease that occurs when tiny air sacs in the lungs are damaged, usually from long-term smoking. As airways lose their elasticity and trap unexpired air and toxins, the alveoli are destroyed and, thus, tear as a result of the pressure of inflation. Loss of alveoli will reduce the amount of surface area for gas exchange. This disease causes chronic shortness of breath due to the difficulty in exhaling and poor distribution of inhaled air in lungs. As a result, the heart must work harder to exchange and deliver oxygen-laden blood throughout the body.

Cardiovascular Diseases

Women who are smokers have a greater potential for developing heart disease and stroke than women who do not smoke. In fact, smoking is one major, if not *the* major, risk factor for the development of diseases of the cardiovascular system including hypertension, atherosclerosis, coronary heart disease, and aortic aneurysms. Smoking is linked to changes in blood chemistry. Cigarette smoking contributes to low levels of high-density lipoproteins (HDLs), which are considered to be beneficial components of the blood, and to an increase in low-density lipoproteins (LDLs). These two changes can lead to a buildup of plaque within the arterial system. The use of tobacco interferes with the production of red blood cells and reduces the blood's ability to clot, which can increase the possibility of hemorrhage during accidents or childbirth. Tobacco is a *vasoconstrictor,* and as such it can cause constriction of the coronary arteries. This condition is potentially dangerous because coronary arteries are the primary source of blood supply to the heart muscle; therefore, the reduction of blood supply to heart muscle tissue, even briefly, can at least damage the heart and at worst be fatal. Another detrimental effect of constricted blood vessels, combined with an increased heart rate, is the increase in blood pressure. The arterial system, therefore, endures more wear and tear as the heart works to force blood through smaller vessels, creating high blood pressure. Smokers are more susceptible to cerebral infarction, or "stroke," due to the above-mentioned factors.

Taking oral contraceptives *and* smoking cigarettes increases the risk of heart attack, stroke, and blood clots in women over age 25. In fact, a woman is more likely to have a *fatal* heart attack if she smokes and uses oral contraceptives than if she only smokes.[15] The very serious likelihood of having a heart attack or stroke if you smoke and take birth control pills prompted the FDA to mandate that all oral contraceptives must include labeling that reads, "Women who use oral contraceptives should not smoke."[16]

Smoking and Cancer

There is a strong relationship between cigarette smoking and the development of the vast majority of cancers at sites located throughout the body. Smoking is associated with cancers of the oral cavity, larynx, pharynx, esophagus, lungs, stomach, uterus, and kidney. Risk of developing smoking-attributable cancers increases with the number of cigarettes smoked and the number of years of smoking.[17]

Her Story

Sarah: Smoking and Lung Cancer

Sarah and her best friend, Betty, would sneak cigarettes from Sarah's mother's purse when they were very young. They pretended to smoke like her and the beautiful women they saw in their Saturday afternoon movie outings. In high school, Sarah smoked for real and developed an addiction to tobacco that she carried with her throughout college, marriage, and two pregnancies.

As Sarah "welcomed" her 40th year, she began to experience a persistent cough and one respiratory infection after another. Her lack of energy, which she attributed to possible early menopause, curtailed her activity with her tennis group. She became frightened when she saw blood in her sputum. After a number of visits to her physician, she was advised to see her gynecologist. Then she went to see one medical specialist after another: a cardiologist, a respiratory therapist, and finally a pulmonary specialist who put Sarah through a series of tests that revealed shadows on her lungs. She was sent to an oncologist's office where, after X rays and **computed tomography scans (CT scans)**, she was diagnosed with lung cancer.

Not believing this could happen to her, Sarah sought the medical opinions of two other oncologists who confirmed the diagnosis of lung cancer. Anger, then rage filled Sarah's hours and days. Not to her, not to Sarah with the supportive, loving husband and family, the intelligent and

well-liked children, the new house near friends and her tennis club! Yes, Sarah. Sarah of the 24-year smoking habit; the "I can quit when I want," Sarah.

Reality hit with the onset of her treatments: First, she received radiation to shrink the tumors, then surgery to remove all possible cancerous tissue, and then the series of chemotherapy treatments and the accompanying side effects. Amazingly, through all of this, Sarah still wanted a cigarette—she had a massive craving for nicotine and found the withdrawal from it one of the more difficult parts of the entire process.

Sarah's story does not end happily. She lost her battle against lung cancer 3 years after the original diagnosis. She lost the life she shared in her nice neighborhood with her loving husband and exceptional children. Sarah did quit smoking, but unfortunately she also quit everything else she loved and enjoyed.

- What symptoms did Sarah have that led her to the doctor?
- What suggestions do you have to prevent Sarah's tragedy from happening to other women?
- Have you ever thought that "this won't happen to me," and then lit up a cigarette and smoked anyway?
- What are your feelings about Sarah after reading her case study?

Smoking cigarettes accounts for 80 percent of the lung cancer deaths in women. The 72,590 annual lung cancer deaths have replaced the 39,510 annual breast cancer deaths as the leading cause of cancer death in women.[18] Due to the continual exposure of body cells and tissues to carcinogens in tobacco smoke, women greatly increase the probability of developing many types of cancers if they choose to smoke. (See *Her Story:* "Sarah: Smoking and Lung Cancer.")

Other Physical Consequences

In addition to the health conditions already described, there are other health effects related to tobacco smoking. Research in many of these problem areas is ongoing. Cataract formation in the eyes of women has been researched; although the exact relationship between smoking and cataract formation is not known, smokers are two to three times more likely to develop cataracts than are nonsmokers.[19] After surgery, smokers have more problems with wound healing and more respiratory complications.[20] Smoking causes peptic ulcers in smokers with *Helicobacter pylori* infections, and women smokers with ulcers usually develop complications of the ulcers.[21]

Conducting research on loss of bone density (e.g., osteoporosis) found that women who smoke have reduced bone density, which leads to an increased risk of hip fractures.[22] Female smokers often develop deeper facial wrinkles, sometimes called "smoker's face," at a faster rate than do females who do not smoke. A possible explanation of this phenomenon may be the reduced amount of blood flow to the skin because of constricted blood vessels. Research in a multitude of areas continues; however, it seems clearly evident that women who smoke tobacco harm their bodies in many ways and increase their likelihood of premature death.

ADDICTION

Tobacco users develop a strong physical and psychological dependence on the product. A woman who smokes 1½ packs of cigarettes a day will have about 110,000 "hits" of nicotine in 1 year.[23] Therefore, addiction and tolerance develop somewhat rapidly. Various studies have investigated the relationship between tobacco and addiction, and results indicate that between one-third and one-half of all individuals who experiment with smoking become addicted.

Over 90 percent of women who smoke develop a dependence on nicotine, the major addicting agent in tobacco. Most women experience withdrawal symptoms such as irritability, lack of concentration, sleep disorders, anxiety, hunger, headache, and craving for nicotine if

they stop smoking. A smoker's body cells adapt to a certain level of nicotine, and she is compelled to maintain that level. Nicotine levels peak within 10 seconds of inhalation. However, the acute effects of nicotine dissipate in a few minutes, which causes the smoker to continue dosing to keep the pleasurable effects and prevent withdrawal symptoms.[24]

Overcoming addiction is difficult, not only because of the physical and psychological dependency, but also because withdrawal symptoms are uncomfortable. Lifestyle rituals that accompany habitual smoking can also be difficult to change. Enjoying the morning cup of coffee, calling a friend, having a drink, riding in the car, or relaxing with a book may all be ritualistically tied to smoking a cigarette. Practices such as these bond the smoker to the substance and thus add to the difficulty of breaking the bonds between tobacco and user. (See *Viewpoint:* "What Rights Does the Smoker Have?")

Viewpoint

What Rights Does the Smoker Have?

As research continues to show that involuntary smoking is dangerous to women who breathe the chemical-laden smoke, more and more businesses, institutions, and schools are establishing a tobacco-free environment. Individuals spend the majority of their time indoors, which can lead to problems for smokers as well as nonsmokers. Designating smoking areas may not always protect the nonsmoker.

However, the individual who makes the choice to smoke does have a right to make that choice. Considering the rights of both smokers and nonsmokers creates a dilemma for businesses and institutions, as well as the personal environment of women in the home.

Consider the following questions and discuss the predicaments created by the situation:

- Does the person who smokes have a right to have a place to smoke?
- What can business and industry do to address the needs of both smokers and nonsmokers?
- If employers mandate a nonsmoking environment, should they pay for the assistance that the smoker may need to stop smoking?
- Where do individual rights and public rights begin and end in this situation?

ENVIRONMENTAL TOBACCO SMOKE

Environmental tobacco smoke (ETS), also referred to as *passive, involuntary,* or *secondhand* smoke, is inhaled from the surroundings in which we live and work. This smoke is discharged from the lighted end of the cigarette, called **side-stream smoke,** and accounts for about 85 percent of the smoke in a room where someone has a lighted cigarette. Side-stream smoke has two times as much tar and nicotine, three times as much carbon monoxide, and three times as much ammonia and benzopyrene as is found in **main-stream smoke,** which is the smoke drawn through the cigarette and inhaled and exhaled by the smoker.

The actual negative consequences from passive smoke are determined by the number of smokers in the room, as well as the number of cigarettes, ventilation, and amount of continual exposure.

Businesses, restaurants, schools and school events, airplanes, trains, and other entities have either banned smoking or segregated smokers into areas where nonsmokers will not be exposed to ETS. As tobacco smoke adds significantly to indoor pollution, women usually experience watery, itchy eyes, coughing, wheezing, increased levels of stress, and unpleasant odors that often stay in clothes, skin, and hair long after the nonsmoker has left the smoking environment.

Children and pets of smokers experience detrimental health effects from breathing air containing cigarette smoke. The more smoke to which a child is exposed, the greater will be the child's health problems. ETS increases the possibility of respiratory infections such as colds, bronchitis, and pneumonia, especially during the first 2 years of life. As children get older, if they continue to be exposed to passive smoke, they may develop a chronic cough and reduced lung function. Almost 60 percent of u.s. children, aged 3–11 years (22 million children), are exposed to ETS.[25] In addition to the physical consequences, the child of a smoker is more likely to become a smoker and to begin smoking at an early age.

ETS is not only harmful to women, children, and men but also has adverse effects on pets that live in the homes of smokers. ETS has been associated with oral cancer and lymphoma in cats, lung and nasal cancer in dogs, and lung cancer in birds, according to Dr. Carolynn MacAllister, Oklahoma State University Cooperative Extension Service veterinarian.[26] Additionally, curious pets may eat cigarettes and other tobacco products if cigarettes are not stored in a safe place. This, too, is dangerous to pets, as well as to children in the home or car.

Now that you have read about the effects of tobacco smoke, complete *Journal Activity:* "A Bill of Rights."

SMOKING AND PREGNANCY

Women who smoke while pregnant harm their babies in numerous ways, especially if they smoke throughout the gestation period. Despite knowledge that smoking during pregnancy has adverse health effects on the mother and the fetus, it is estimated that from 10 to 15 percent of pregnant women who smoke continue to do so *throughout* the pregnancy.[27] Negative consequences related to maternal smoking can be caused by nicotine's ability to constrict fetal blood vessels and breathing movements and by carbon monoxide reducing the oxygen supply to fetal blood. Nicotine easily crosses the placenta to the fetus, producing levels of nicotine as much as 15 percent higher than maternal levels. Nicotine concentrates in fetal blood, amniotic fluid, and breast milk.[28] A dose-related response has been found between smoking and infant birth weight: The more the mother smokes during pregnancy, the greater the infant weight reduction, and the possibility of infant illness and longer hospital stays. Children born to smoking mothers often will be shorter, have reduced reading and mathematical skills, exhibit hyperactivity, and have lessened social adjustment abilities than children born to nonsmoking mothers. Studies reveal that nicotine is found in breast milk; mothers who smoke while breast feeding will transfer this drug and its potential effects to the infant.[29] As a result, the health and well-being of the newborn are placed in jeopardy. Smoking-related low birth weight and the requisite consequences to the baby are 100 percent preventable—do

Journal Activity

A Bill of Rights

A "Bill of Rights" has been developed for nonsmokers. Briefly it includes guidelines related to the right to breathe clean air, to express one's discomfort around tobacco smoke, and to take legitimate action against tobacco pollution in one's personal environment. These are all fair and just ideas, as well as healthy suggestions. However, as discussed in the *Viewpoint:* "What Rights Does the Smoker Have?," there are also rights for people who choose to smoke. Even if you don't like the idea, write a "Bill of Rights for Smokers." Discuss these during a class period. Realistically, we must acknowledge that there are "rights" for both sides of this and many other issues.

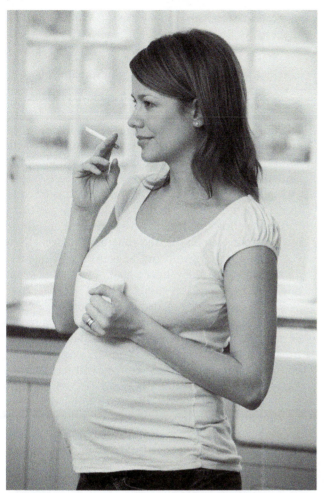

Pregnant women should avoid smoking as well as exposure to smoke to protect the health of the developing fetus.

not smoke during pregnancy and avoid exposure to secondhand smoke!

Babies born to women who smoke during pregnancy have an increased likelihood of dying of **sudden infant death syndrome (SIDS).** This devastating death of an infant is generally unexplainable because the cause of death usually cannot be determined in a postmortem examination. This finding may be related to an environment in which the pregnant woman is exposed too often to passive smoke or due to the infant's exposure to ETS. Studies have shown that two-thirds of women who quit smoking during pregnancy resume smoking once the baby is born.[30] Women who quit smoking during the first 3–4 months of pregnancy have healthier babies than those who keep smoking.[31]

During delivery, smoking mothers have an increased chance of hemorrhaging and an increased chance of delivering a stillborn infant or an infant who lives only for a brief time. Hospital stays are often longer for a smoking mother and her baby.

Following delivery, smoking mothers heal slower and often must spend more time caring for newborns who have more difficulties with feeding, digestion, sleeping, and restlessness than do newborns of nonsmoking mothers.

The bottom line is that there are serious health consequences for babies born to women who smoke during and after pregnancy. And there are also detrimental effects experienced by women who smoke during pregnancy. It is simple to avoid: do *not* smoke; if you smoke, it is time to quit.

SMOKING CESSATION

Why do women decide to quit smoking? According to one study, more than three-quarters of women who smoke want to quit, and almost one-half reported trying to quit.[32] Warnings of imminent health problems, becoming pregnant, having children, or working in a smoke-free environment can each provide the impetus to stop smoking. Smoking has become restricted in such areas as public buildings, domestic air flights, restaurants, and schools; the inconvenience of finding a place in which a person is allowed to smoke may lead to cessation of the habit. Most women quit several times before they are able to completely eliminate the habit. Each year, about 15 million smokers quit for at least one day, but fewer than 5 percent of them are able to stay tobacco-free for 3–12 months.[33] Therefore, smokers must be persistent in their attempts to stop. The benefits far outweigh the morbidity and mortality associated with smoking. Women may often need assistance in their attempts at smoking cessation, and a number of methods are available to assist women who want to quit.

Behavioral Changes

There appears to be no easy or right way to quit smoking, and those who have made the attempt, usually many times, will attest to that fact. Smoking cessation appears to be most successful for women who really want to quit and who consider all the beneficial reasons to quit and barriers that could make cessation unlikely.

Even though many women successfully quit on their own, **smoking cessation programs** that provide counseling and support groups may be more successful for women who smoke 25 or more cigarettes a day. Formal smoking cessation programs vary in their success rate, but about one-third of smokers who quit for a year often start again.[34] Research reveals that success in smoking cessation is more likely when a woman has a readiness to quit and believes that she will be successful.

Nicotine Replacement Products

In recent years, the FDA has approved products that assist in smoking cessation. The products usually deliver small, steady doses of nicotine and help relieve some of the withdrawal symptoms and avoid the "high" that keeps the smoker addicted. There are a number of nicotine replacement products available, either by prescription or as over-the-counter products, as well as non-nicotine medications. Consider the following information and determine the pros and cons of each product (Table 13.1).

Women must be aware of the serious consequences if they continue to smoke while using nicotine substitutes. Nicotine overdose symptoms include tremors, respiratory failure, low blood pressure, and fainting. Although these products provide a positive step toward smoking cessation, they are only one method. Drugs alone will not stop the smoker; a smoking cessation program needs to include support from family and friends and perhaps a formal stop-smoking program sponsored by the American Cancer Society (ACS) or the American Heart Association. (See *Health Tips:* "Choosing a Smoking Cessation Program.")

How to Stop Smoking!

The ACS has a variety of highly effective materials that individuals and groups can use to make the smart move and stop this life-destroying habit. The ACS suggests:[36]

- Make a decision to quit
- Set a quit date and choose a quit smoking plan
- Deal with withdrawal
- Stay tobacco-free

Looking at each of these suggestions in more detail and following the steps suggested increases the smoker's understanding and chances of stopping this addiction.

In developing a plan to quit smoking, it is essential to determine the triggers that result in the use of tobacco, meaning the links between an event and smoking a cigarette. When the trigger occurs, find something else to do instead of smoking. Suggestions include take a walk, chew on a straw, have a glass of water, call someone, and chew sugarless gum.

Plan a "stop day" and complete and sign a "Stop Smoking Contract." Ask a friend to sign it as a means of support. Throw all cigarettes and related items away from your home, your car, and any other place where you may be tempted to smoke. You will feel a strong desire to smoke, but use the "Four D" technique to quell this feeling: delay, deep breathing, drink water, and do something else. Other suggestions include keeping objects such as gum, straws, and low-calorie snacks near when you need/want something in your mouth; utilizing nicotine chewing gum or patches,

---

TABLE 13.1 Smoking Cessation Products[35]

OVER-THE-COUNTER NICOTINE REPLACEMENT PRODUCTS

Nicotine chewing gum *(Nicorette)*	Helps reduce the unpleasant effects of nicotine withdrawal; eliminates the harmful effects of other chemicals in tobacco; follow directions on package carefully.
Nicotine replacement patches *(Nicoderm, Habitrol, Nicotrol)*	Delivers a continuous flow of nicotine through the skin; replace daily on different part of skin; helps with withdrawal symptoms; follow package directions carefully.
Nicotine lozenge	Resembles small piece of hard candy; slowly releases nicotine as lozenge dissolves in the mouth; do not bite or chew as will cause heartburn and indigestion; follow package directions carefully.

Prescription Nicotine Replacement Products

Nicotine nasal spray	Inhalation through the nose to absorption through the blood stream; helps with withdrawal symptoms; nasal and sinus irritation are common side effects; follow package directions carefully.
Nicotine inhaler *(Nicotrol)*	Inhale into mouth where nicotine will be absorbed by the mucous membranes of the mouth to help relieve withdrawal symptoms; recommended only for 3 months' use; can cause cough and throat irritation and used cautiously by asthma patients.

Non-nicotine Medication (Prescription)

Bupropion *(Zyban)*	Helps abstain from smoking; helps nicotine withdrawal symptoms; not sure how product works and can be used in combination with nicotine replacement products; may experience some side affects.
Varenicline *(Chantix)*	Acts in the brain to provide some nicotine effects and reduce withdrawal symptoms; blocks the effects of nicotine from cigarettes if user resumes smoking; may experience numerous side effects.

Health Tips

Choosing a Smoking Cessation Program

Formal smoking cessation programs can provide structure, suggestions, and support for women who need a specialized "tool in their stop-smoking tool box." They are intended to help women who smoke recognize and cope with problems that arise during their attempt to stop. Here are some tips to finding a program that can lead to successful smoking cessation. Effective smoking cessation programs

- Offer group or individual counseling.
- Have intense program counseling and goals.
- Have a leader who is trained in smoking cessation.
- Have sessions that are at least 20–30 minutes in length.
- Have at least four to seven sessions.
- Last for at least 2 weeks.

Avoid smoking cessation programs that

- Use pills, injections, or "special" or "secret" cures.
- Promise easy success with little effort from the smoker.
- Require a lot of money to participate.
- Cannot or will not provide references from previous attendees.

SOURCE: Adapted from American Cancer Society. 2006. *Guide to quitting smoking.* www.cancer.org (retrieved April 18, 2007).

if needed; announcing that you are no longer going to smoke; placing "No Smoking" signs in important places; and treating yourself with something special when you stop.

Quitting smoking is one thing; remaining smoke-free may be more difficult. Some negative feelings may result within the first few days to weeks during withdrawal from nicotine. It is important to remember that these are normal and that they will go away. Find something else to do to cope with stressful situations other than falling back to a former bad habit—smoking! Include moderate exercise and nutritious, low-calorie food in your cessation program to avoid weight gain. Continue to remember all the very important reasons not to smoke. If you remain smoke-free for 3 months, you will probably be able to enjoy the rest of your life as a nonsmoker.

BENEFITS OF SMOKING CESSATION

Quitting smoking makes a big difference—and quickly. Food begins to smell and taste better, and the smoker also smells better. The cough disappears, and energy begins to return. Women who have stopped smoking are sick less often, miss fewer days at work and play, and have fewer complaints about their general health than women who continue to smoke. Women increase their chance of quitting smoking when they have a low level of stress, a supportive nonsmoking partner, a high education level, and a positive sense of well-being.[37]

Incentives for smoking cessation can be enhanced when women realize that within a few minutes of quitting, their health can be affected in many positive ways. Table 13.2 summarizes the short- and long-term benefits that can be gained when a woman quits smoking.

CAFFEINE

Due to the association of coffee and other caffeinated beverages with smoking, the coverage of caffeine is included in this chapter with smoking. A variety of beverages containing caffeine have become popular drinks in the United States and around the world. Teas of many types are served with meals or combined with a serene environment to provide a quiet, refreshing break from a stressful day. Cappuccino, latte, espresso, and café mocha are all flavorful specialty coffees that have gained widespread popularity. Nationwide, there are thousands of coffee houses brewing all varieties of coffee. Consider the current coffee drinking statistics:[38]

- 54 percent of Americans over the age of 18 drink coffee everyday
- 3.1 cups (9 oz each) is the average amount of coffee a coffee drinker consumes daily
- There are 100 million U.S. daily coffee drinkers
- There are 30 million U.S. daily coffee drinkers who drink specialty coffee
- $164.71 is the average amount of money spent on coffee each year by a coffee drinker
- 24 percent of coffee drinkers who drink 13 or more cups of coffee each week
- $18 million is spent yearly on specialty coffee in the United States

What Is Caffeine?

Caffeine is among a family of chemical compounds called **methylxanthines**, which stimulate particular neurotransmitters in the central nervous system (CNS).

TABLE 13.2   Short- and Long-Term Benefits of Smoking Cessation

As soon as 20 minutes after your last cigarette, your body will begin to benefit from not smoking. These benefits will continue as long as you do not smoke. However, you will lose each of these benefits even if you smoke only one cigarette a day.[39]

TIME SINCE SMOKING LAST CIGARETTE	BENEFIT
20 minutes	Reduced blood pressure and pulse rate; body temperature becomes normal
8 hours	Normal carbon monoxide levels in blood; blood oxygen level increases to normal
24 hours	Chance of heart attack decreases
48 hours	Senses of smell and taste improve; nerve endings start regrowing
2 weeks–3 months	Blood circulation improves; easier to engage in activities because lung function increases by 30 percent
1–9 months	Decrease in coughing, shortness of breath, fatigue; cilia regrow in lungs allowing cleansing dust and mucus from lungs; reduced chance of respiratory infection
1 year	Risk of coronary heart disease is half that of a smoker's
5 years	Lung cancer death rate for former one-pack-a-day smoker decreases by almost half; stroke risk is reduced to that of a nonsmoker 5–15 years after quitting; risk of cancer of throat, esophagus, and mouth is half that of a smoker
10 years	Death rate from lung cancer is half that of a continuing smoker; precancerous cells are replaced by healthy cells; decreased risk of developing cancer of the mouth, throat, esophagus, bladder, kidney, and pancreas
15 years	Risk of coronary heart disease is that of a nonsmoker

Found in more than sixty plants and trees, caffeine has a long history of use in many drinks such as colas, tea, coffee, and cocoa, as well as over-the-counter drugs.

Various types of coffee beans produce varying tastes and deliver different levels of caffeine. For example, high-quality arabica beans, which are often used in specialty coffees, have a stronger taste and less caffeine than robusta beans, which often are used in national name-brand coffees. The amount of caffeine in a drink is measured in milligrams, and the potency will vary according to the type of coffee bean used in the drink and the way the beverage is brewed.

Caffeine, taken into the body in a water-soluble form, is absorbed into the bloodstream principally through the small intestine. It takes about 30 minutes following ingestion for initial effects on the CNS to be felt. Along with all other organs of the body, caffeine is distributed to the brain. It may also be passed from the mother's blood through the placenta and to the fetus of any woman who is pregnant.

Effects of Caffeine

Why is the use of products containing caffeine so prevalent? Perhaps it is due to the wide variety of possible stimulating effects that caffeine produces. Among other reasons, millions of women use this drug to wake up and feel more energized each morning. It has been demonstrated to increase alertness, produce quicker reaction time, and reduce drowsiness. Coffee or colas are often the beverages that college women drink to help "pull an all-nighter." This is because studies have shown that caffeine can improve reading speed, produce better results on math and verbal tests, and increase the capacity for sustained intellectual activities. However, if one desires to sleep, caffeine, even in small amounts, can cause sleep disturbances and increase the amount of time it takes to go to sleep.

Some of the research on caffeine's effects is inconsistent. For example, some studies indicate that this drug may *not* improve verbal or math abilities or short-term memory. Caffeine purportedly enhances athletic performance by helping the body metabolize fats for use as energy, saving glycogen for long-term energy. Drinking caffeine also appears to delay the exhaustion that athletes feel following exertion. Yet other studies basically refute these findings because they found little or no link between caffeine consumption and enhanced performance.

Caffeine Products

Coffee was not always the popular beverage that it is in today's society. It has fallen in and out of favor with humans living throughout the world. English women, in 1674, published an anti-coffee pamphlet titled "The Women's Petition Against Coffee," because it was believed that men who drank too much coffee were "less lustful and more unfruitful."[40] Not true!

Coffee, in instant form, was introduced in the late 1800s and gained popularity during World War II. Instant coffee is less flavorful but more convenient in today's busy world. As women continue to take on more time-consuming responsibilities, a quicker avenue to an enjoyable product is most appealing. A healthier product appears to be appealing, as well, as evidenced by current widespread use of decaffeinated coffee. Americans today are consuming more decaffeinated coffee and less caffeinated coffee than ever before.

Tea in its early history was used medicinally but later came to be used more as a drink for social occasions. Pound for pound, tea has more caffeine than coffee, yet more cups of tea (about 200) are produced from a pound of dry tea leaves than cups of coffee (about 50–60) are made from a pound of coffee beans.[41] Therefore, less caffeine is found in an average cup of tea compared to an average cup of coffee. The caffeine content in a 5-oz cup of tea can range from 18 mg to 107 mg, depending on the brand and the type of brew. As with coffee, flavored teas, instant tea, and herbal teas (some with artificial sweeteners) have gained greater popularity at home and in restaurants in this country.

Colas today contain less than 6 mg of caffeine for each ounce of cola. These types of beverages, both caffeinated and decaffeinated, are consumed increasingly worldwide. The history of colas is basically the history of the Coca-Cola Company, and most cola products are a replication of this product. Colas are considered to be refreshing, stimulating, and in sync with today's active lifestyle. Caffeine is an added ingredient in colas, whereas it is found naturally in coffee, tea, and chocolate. Although sugar-free and caffeine-free cola products are available and widely consumed, the well-known classic cola with sugar and caffeine is still the most widely sold. In the United States, the consumption of all colas averages approximately 50 gallons per person per year.[42]

Chocolate was introduced in Europe before coffee or tea, but its use grew slowly because the method of preparing it was not widely known. One of the women of history, Maria Theresa of France, wife of Louis XIV, thoroughly enjoyed chocolate and was instrumental in the promotion of its consumption. From chocolate beans, ground chocolate kernels, chocolate liquor, or cocoa butter to the Nestlé milk chocolate of today, this substance has become one of the most widely consumed forms of caffeine. Caffeine in chocolate, though not as strong as caffeine in coffee, has similar physical effects. A cup of chocolate milk has about 4 mg of caffeine, whereas caffeine in denser baking chocolate ranges from 5 mg to 35 mg per ounce.

A number of over-the-counter (OTC) drugs containing caffeine produce a stimulating effect and suppress the appetite. They also may act as a stimulus for elimination of body fluids, called a diuretic. Products such as No Doz, Midol, Aqua-ban, and some cold remedies have from 30 to 200 mg of caffeine as an active ingredient. Although one product alone may not impact greatly on daily caffeine consumption, women often ingest beverages, food, and OTC drugs each containing varying amounts of caffeine, which, when added together, can cause a number of unwanted physiological effects. (See Table 13.3.)

Now complete *Journal Activity:* "Your Caffeine Consumption" to determine your daily caffeine intake.

Effects of Caffeine on Health

Consumption of this psychoactive drug is widespread and acceptable; therefore, research studies regarding caffeine use are numerous, varied, and to a large degree inconclusive. Data have been collected researching caffeine and its relationship to cancer, osteoporosis, pregnancy, benign breast disease, heart disease, nutrient absorption, cholesterol, gastrointestinal problems, and others. Let's consider the results of some of the studies as they pertain to women.

Osteoporosis and Caffeine   Osteoporosis is a loss of bone mass, especially in postmenopausal women, which can result in fractures and broken bones. Caffeine intake

TABLE 13.3 Comparison of Caffeine in Common Products

PRODUCT	CAFFEINE (MG)*
Coffee	
Starbucks coffee, grande (16 oz)	550
Starbucks, caffé latte (8 oz)	35
Starbucks coffee (8 oz)	250
Starbucks, caffé mocha (8 oz)	35
Maxwell House coffee (8 oz)	110
Decaf coffee (8 oz)	5
Energy drinks	
• Jolt shot (2 oz)	200
• 70-mg Energy drink (2 oz)	200
Medicine	
No Doz, max strength (1)	200
Excedrin (2)	130
Anacin (2)	65
Soft Drinks	
Cola (12 oz)	35
Mountain Dew (12 oz)	55
Cocoa or hot chocolate (8 oz)	5
Tea, leaf or bag (8 oz)	50

*The milligrams (mg) listed for these products are the average caffeine levels for drugs, foods, and beverages.

SOURCE: *The Caffeine Corner: Products ranked by amount. 1996. Nutrition Action Newsletter.* http://cspinet.org/nah/caffeine/caffeine_corner.htm (retrieved October 17, 2006).

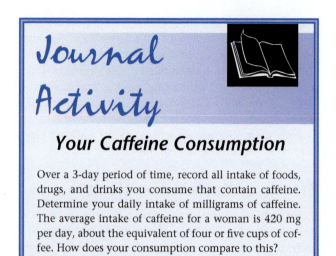

Journal Activity

Your Caffeine Consumption

Over a 3-day period of time, record all intake of foods, drugs, and drinks you consume that contain caffeine. Determine your daily intake of milligrams of caffeine. The average intake of caffeine for a woman is 420 mg per day, about the equivalent of four or five cups of coffee. How does your consumption compare to this?

does not appear to be a significant risk factor for osteoporosis, particularly in women who consume adequate calcium. Caffeine consumption causes a slight and temporary rise in the level of calcium excretion, leading to speculation that the use of caffeine could compromise bone health. Yet studies demonstrate that adequate calcium consumption offsets the potential negative effect of caffeine on bone health.[43] More than two servings of foods or drinks with caffeine appear to increase the risk of having osteoporosis.[44] In this same report, researchers found a negative correlation between caffeine intake and dairy product intake, which magnifies the possibility of bone loss if a woman consumes low-calcium beverages in place of high-calcium beverages. The problem with loss of bone mass in women may not be due to consumption of caffeine-containing beverages, but drinking caffeine products instead of calcium-containing beverages. Women who do not consume calcium-rich foods throughout their life will increase their risk of osteoporosis, whether they drink caffeine or not.

Absorption of nutrients may be inhibited not by caffeine but by other substances in coffee, such as polyphenols. Important minerals, particularly calcium and iron, may not be utilized properly by the body as a result of drinking too many cups of caffeinated drinks each day. Because women are prone to develop osteoporosis, this information should create an awareness to be moderate in the consumption of caffeine-containing products.

Pregnancy and Caffeine Pregnancy and caffeine intake has been the subject of numerous studies. The March of Dimes recommends that pregnant women limit consumption of caffeine to one to two cups per day.[45] The intake of caffeine during pregnancy may cause slower growth rate for the fetus and therefore result in reduced birth weight.[46] Additionally, studies

conclude that females who consume caffeine reduce their chance of conceiving and increase the risk of miscarriage. Nursing mothers who consume high levels of caffeine every day report irritable and restless babies. Research is inconclusive about the levels of caffeine consumption that are safe. Because of this inconclusiveness, women should reduce or eliminate caffeine consumption if they are pregnant or are considering becoming pregnant.

Breast Health and Caffeine Fibrocystic breast disease consists of benign lumps that form in a woman's breast. Although these lumps are sometimes tender and painful, they are not cancerous. A plethora of research studies have found no relationship between caffeine intake and fibrocystic breast disease. However, some physicians advise women with benign breast lumps to eliminate caffeine consumption or at least to consume it moderately. However, there is little scientific evidence to suggest that elimination of caffeine from the diet will improve conditions associated with fibrocystic breast disease.

Caffeinism

Caffeinism is the result of continual and excessive use of caffeine products and may lead to a number of uncomfortable consequences. Women can develop a dependency and a tolerance to caffeine and, upon cessation of use, may experience headaches, nausea, irritability, depression, heart palpitations, insomnia, and reduced attention span. Although these symptoms are uncomfortable, they are short-lived and can usually be avoided by reducing caffeine consumption gradually.

Caffeine Research

As we have seen, caffeine research is largely inconclusive. Why is this so? Consider these variables: Each woman is biochemically different and the response to caffeine varies with each person; tolerance to caffeine may not be taken into account because studies often fail to isolate caffeine consumers from noncaffeine consumers; and the lifestyle of the research population may not be taken into account. For example, individuals who drink excessive amounts of coffee are sometimes more likely to smoke, have a high-fat diet, and not engage in exercise; therefore, negative health problems may be due to other lifestyle habits, not to caffeine consumption.

It appears that moderate use of caffeine-containing products produces no major detrimental effect, except for pregnant women. However, as with many other issues, it is best to check with your physician if there is a concern.

ILLEGAL DRUGS

Although both women and men use and abuse illegal drugs, women's abuse of drugs can yield more health problems than men's and these problems may progress differently in women than in men. Reports from the National Survey on Drug Use and Health estimated that 12.5 million women used an illegal drug during the past year. Approximately 2 million women aged 18 or older met the criteria for abuse of or dependence on an illegal drug, including cocaine and marijuana.[47] In addition, hundreds of thousands of women have sniffed inhalants.

Many of today's illegal drugs were yesterday's legal drugs (such as cocaine and marijuana). Due to the potential for dependency and the devastating effects created by using these drugs, the federal government declared them illegal substances. They cannot legally be bought, sold, used, or possessed in any state in the United States.

Abuse of illicit drugs among women is of special concern. As women, we are responsible not only for our own personal health and well-being but also for the health and well-being of future generations. The discussion that follows explains how the abuse of drugs during pregnancy can produce devastating effects for both mother and fetus.

Drug Use and Pregnancy

According to National Survey on Drug Use and Health data, an estimated 4.4 percent of pregnant women aged 15–44 used illicit drugs in the month preceding the survey.[48]

Most drugs pass easily from the mother's blood through the placenta, the same route taken by oxygen and nutrients.[49] At least 90 percent of pregnant women take either prescription or nonprescription drugs, or use tobacco, alcohol, or illicit drugs sometime during their pregnancy. About 2–3 percent of all birth defects result from the use of drugs[50] (see Table 13.4). However, the time between drug intake and its transmission to the fetus varies with the type used. For example, marijuana can take hours to reach the fetal bloodstream, whereas opiates reach the fetus quickly. Data support the contention that alcohol causes fetal abnormalities, but research on the effects of various other illicit drugs on the fetus is inconclusive. Cocaine causes a decline in the delivery of oxygen and nutrients to the fetus because it is a *vasoconstrictor*. This results in an increase in blood pressure and heart rate. Marijuana increases the level of carbon monoxide in the blood, which decreases the amount of oxygen available to the fetus. Overall, drug use results in lower levels of oxygen and nutrients reaching the rapidly growing cells of the fetus.

TABLE 13.4 The Effects of Drug use on Mother and Baby[51]

ON MOTHER	ON BABY
Poor nutrition	Premature birth
High blood pressure	Low birth weight
Fast heart rate	Infections
Low weight gain	Small head size
Low self-esteem	Sudden infant death
Preterm labor	syndrome (SIDS)
Sexually transmitted diseases	Birth defects
Early delivery	Stunted growth
HIV/AIDS	Poor motor skills
Depression	HIV/AIDS
Physical abuse	Learning disabilities
	Neurological problems

Medical personnel should routinely ask pregnant women questions concerning their use of medications, alcohol, and other drugs. This information is important for administering proper medical care. Additional information regarding women and pregnancy can be found in Chapter 8.

If the outcome of the screening tests reveals that the woman is indeed using a particular drug, then immediate medical and antidrug treatment needs to be started. Additionally, drug therapy in the form of detoxification, support groups, and individual therapy should be sought. Upon delivery, the infant should be screened for drugs in the blood and, if the screening is positive, medical treatment as well as evaluation of the home environment is needed.

The following sections discuss the negative consequences of a woman's drug use on herself, her pregnancy, her fetus, and her newborn.

Cocaine and Crack

Cocaine is derived from a plant, *Erythroxylon coca*, which grows best in the mountains of South America. Substances in its leaves produce an exhilarating effect, providing quick energy, stimulation, and a sense of well-being. Early research in the 1800s led physicians to believe that cocaine was a new miracle drug. It appeared in patent medicines, tonics, and even leading soda drinks. Cocaine was found to be an effective topical anesthetic during surgery and beneficial for alleviating depression. As individuals became dependent on the products and medicines that contained this miracle drug, serious behavioral and health consequences resulted. Consequently, laws were enacted to put tight controls on the sale and use of cocaine. The Pure Food and Drugs Act in 1906 and the Harrison Act of 1914 reduced the legal availability of cocaine.

Crack is a rocklike substance that is the result of mixing cocaine with baking soda or ammonia. It is both easy to make and inexpensive to buy. Usually smoked in small pipes, it produces an almost immediate but brief high that is followed by depression and a strong longing for repeated use. The National Survey on Drug Use and Health (NSDUH) estimated that there were 1.9 million current cocaine users in 2008; of those, 359,000 were current crack users.[52] The 18–25 year old age group has the higher rate of current cocaine users.

Consequences of Use

The effects of cocaine on a woman's brain depend on the strength of the substance and the route of administration into the body. Cocaine can be inhaled by smoking, which requires only 8 seconds to reach the brain; absorbed by snorting, which requires 3 minutes to reach the brain; injected, which requires 14 seconds to reach the brain; or orally ingested, which requires 20 minutes to reach the brain.

Psychological and physical dependency develops with short- and long-term cocaine use. Research on both lab animals and humans reveals that the desire for cocaine effects is strong and that tolerance occurs with continual use. Tolerance is the capacity of the body to endure or become less responsive to a drug so that a larger amount is needed to obtain the same effect.

The short-term effects of cocaine use produce immediate bodily responses: increases in heart and respiratory rates and, coincidentally, an increase in blood pressure and elevated temperature. Appetite decreases, and the user feels more alert, excited, euphoric, and energized. The duration of cocaine's immediate effects depends on the manner in which it is taken. A faster route of administration, such as inhalation, will produce a more intense high and a shorter duration of action. However, due to lack of tolerance and experience and/or the high potency of cocaine, the user can also convulse, hemorrhage, or even experience heart failure.[53]

Long-time users of cocaine develop serious health consequences, including nasal inflammation, loss of appetite leading to malnourishment, a persistent cough, irregular heart rhythm, sleep disturbance, and even sexual dysfunction. Irritability, agitation, and paranoia can also result from continual use.[54] Psychological consequences can be as severe as paranoid psychosis. Fortunately, with the cessation of cocaine use, time seems to repair most of the physical and psychological damage.

Effects on Pregnancy

Among pregnant women 15–44 years of age, 4.4 percent reported using illicit drugs in the month prior to the survey. However, over 16.2 percent of pregnant girls who are 15–17 years of age reported using illicit drugs in the month prior to the survey.[55] As a result, the effects on women and the number of cocaine and crack-exposed infants have also increased. Research has found a variety of consequences that occur from cocaine and crack use during pregnancy:

- **Intrauterine growth retardation**, which is delay in the development and maturation of the fetus, appears to be an outcome of cocaine use during pregnancy.
- Sudden and severe pregnancy complications such as premature separation of the placenta from the uterus, and even fetal and maternal death, can result.
- Premature labor and spontaneous abortion can result.

Consequences to the Fetus and Newborn

The consequences of cocaine and crack use to the fetus and the newborn can be profound. While the full extent of the effects of pregnant women's cocaine use on their babies is not totally known, studies have determined that these babies are often born premature, have low birth weight, and have smaller head circumference. Fetal exposure to cocaine may lead to later deficits in cognitive performance and information processing and difficulty with attention to task, which reduces potential academic success.[56] Singer and Short studied the cognitive consequences of prenatal cocaine exposure to preschool children.[57] The research found that children scored significantly lower on some specific measures of intelligence; lower scores were especially significant in the areas of information, arithmetic, and reflecting visuospatial skills. However, in examining the home environment of these children, these researchers determined that effective child-rearing strategies may result in more positive outcomes for children affected by prenatal cocaine exposure.

Marijuana

Marijuana can produce sedating, hallucinating, intoxicating, and/or analgesic effects. The effects of smoked marijuana are felt immediately after the drug enters the brain within a matter of seconds and usually last from 1 to 3 hours. If marijuana is used with food or drink, the short-term effects begin more slowly, usually in ½ to 1 hour, and last for as long as 4 hours. Smoking marijuana yields several times more THC in the blood than does eating or drinking the substance.[58] Use of marijuana at moderate doses produces feelings of euphoria, relaxation, and peacefulness. Individuals may experience mood swings and an altered sense of time, space, and distance. There appear to be few immediate negative effects from short-term moderate marijuana use, but because of the altered sense of time, space, and distance, it is wise not to drive or use any type of power tools or devices.

Consequences of Use After decades of research, we know that a multitude of negative consequences can result from chronic, long-term use of marijuana. Consider the following effects that are concerns for the body systems:

- *Central nervous system.* Reduces short-term memory, alters judgment, increases chances of developing mental illness, reduces cognitive skills, blurs and impairs vision perception, produces personality change, and alters motor coordination.
- *Respiratory system.* Can cause lung cancer, lung damage, pulmonary diseases, chronic bronchitis, and may cause trachea damage due to inhalation.
- *Cardiovascular system.* Produces tachycardia (rapid heartbeat), increases blood pressure and concerns related to angina and diabetes, and aggravates high blood pressure in women who already have angina and diabetes.
- *Reproductive system.* Disrupts the menstrual cycle, impairs ovulation and fertility, increases levels of testosterone in females, and may cause irreversible damage to the female ova.

Effects on Pregnancy Research on the effects of marijuana use on pregnancy and the fetus is lacking. However, once inhaled, THC easily crosses the placenta of the mother to the fetus and causes similar levels of THC in both mother and fetus. Studies have shown that infants born to women who smoked marijuana during pregnancy are likely to weigh less and are shorter in length than infants born to nonsmoking women. Other studies revealed that babies who were chronically exposed to marijuana chemicals in their environment had poor nervous system responses and less response to visual stimulation. Additionally, THC is transported to nursing babies through breast milk.

Heroin and Methadone

Originally marketed as a cough suppressant, heroin is a very addictive, semisynthetic narcotic produced from chemically changed morphine, a naturally occurring opiate derived from the opium poppy plant. In its early history, heroin was thought to be safe and a substance that would aid in recovery from morphine addiction. Heroin was declared illegal in 1924 by the U.S. government when the addictive properties and negative consequences became clear, and it became unlawful to manufacture, import, or possess heroin.

Consequences of Use *Heroin* is a fast-acting narcotic that is injected directly into a vein or under the skin ("skin poppers") or snorted or smoked. It produces a dreamlike state and a feeling of euphoria in users, who often feel they have found the panacea for all their problems and a way to temporarily escape to paradise. Like most other narcotics, heroin creates a strong physical and psychological dependency. Addiction is fairly rapid; usually within just a few weeks the user feels the need to increase the amount used to achieve the "high" that she originally felt; thus tolerance is developed quickly. If the drug user stops taking heroin, she will experience unpleasant withdrawal symptoms—chills, nausea, tremors, diarrhea, and/or leg and abdominal pain—which can sometimes be severe and extremely uncomfortable though not life-threatening. Addiction to this chemical creates a situation in which women become so dependent on this drug that they may engage in life-threatening activities such as prostitution or stealing, in a never-ending pursuit to feed the addiction. As a result, their health and quality of life suffer as do those, especially children, who live with and around them.

Among the dangers associated with heroin use are factors related to the lifestyle of the user that result in accidents, injuries, diseases, infections, and sometimes death. The type of heroin, its potency, the contaminants in the heroin, the method of use (injection, smoking, snorting), and the risks of obtaining this illegal drug all contribute to its devastating effects. Adding to the concerns are the extended effects the use of this drug has on children, families, health care and judicial systems, the workforce, and the health of future generations.

Methadone is a synthetic narcotic that can be taken orally and provides a longer duration of its effects than heroin or morphine, usually lasting from 24 to 36 hours. It was developed during World War II as a substitute for morphine. Methadone can be used legally; with a doctor's prescription, to help avoid the negative effects of heroin and morphine withdrawal. It also produces physical and psychological dependency, as well as tolerance and withdrawal symptoms. Many of the same physical problems that result from the use of heroin and morphine can result from the use of methadone. However, because it is intended to be used as a legal, prescriptive replacement for heroin or morphine, the quality and dose of the drug are controlled.

Effects on Pregnancy A woman who uses heroin or methadone during pregnancy is putting herself and her fetus at risk for very serious consequences. **Toxemia**, also called blood poisoning, can occur in the blood of a pregnant woman, resulting in intrauterine growth retardation and even premature rupture of the amniotic membrane. Use of heroin or methadone can cause miscarriage and can also adversely affect delivery because these drugs may cause preterm labor or breech birth (delivery of the baby bottom-first). Of course, there also may be no effect from use of heroin or methadone during pregnancy. However, the risks are not worth the harmful effects the drugs *might* produce.

Newborns of heroin-addicted mothers tend to have low birth weight and smaller head circumference. These babies may be born either premature or stillborn and have a ten-fold increased risk of SIDS. Infants born to methadone-addicted women may have normal birth weight but soon may experience weight loss due to lack of sleep and hyperactivity and may have to go through withdrawal. Complications such as poor fetal growth, premature rupture of the membranes, and placental abruption can occur.[59] During the newborn period, serious prematurity-related health problems, such as breathing problems and brain bleeds, which may lead to lifelong disabilities, have been found among infants exposed to heroin in utero.[60] Lower levels of learning, difficult behavior, and poor adaptation abilities were found in preschool children who were born to women addicted to methadone and heroin.

The harmful effects of drug use notwithstanding, this lifestyle often creates negative outcomes during pregnancy for mother and child. Lack of prenatal care, poor nutrition, and vitamin and mineral deficiencies can occur due to the time, energy, and money the mother must spend engaged in finding, obtaining, and using heroin. Consequences of using dirty needles include bacterial infections, sores, and hepatitis, as well as the risk of contracting HIV infection. There is also a greater likelihood of contracting other sexually transmitted infections (STIs) such as chlamydia, herpes, and gonorrhea. Each of these, of course, can be passed on to the fetus in utero or during delivery.

Amphetamines and Methamphetamines

Stimulant drugs, which are completely synthetic, increase the activity of the central nervous system, resulting in increased alertness, euphoria, excitation, elevated blood pressure, insomnia, and loss of appetite. Amphetamines are used medically for weight reduction, narcolepsy, and attention-deficit/hyperactivity disorder (ADHD). Amphetamines used at low dosages produce increased energy, alertness, and elevated mood, but at higher dosages blood pressure and heart rate increase to near dangerous levels. Abuse of these drugs can yield strong psychological dependence, tolerance, and

possible psychosis, with periods of depression following discontinuation of use.

Methamphetamines—street names include *speed, crank, meth,* and *crystal meth*—are illegal and are often produced in home drug laboratories. The most dangerous form is crystal methamphetamine, or *ice;* when it is smoked, the effects can be felt within 7 seconds, producing powerful physical and psychological feelings of exhilaration. While there are immediate "good" feelings, long-term users often experience multiple consequences such as weight loss, malnutrition, immune system deficiencies, and damage to body systems. Women who abuse amphetamines or use methamphetamines reduce their quality of life and the lives of their children and family.

Effects on Pregnancy As with other drugs, amphetamines and methamphetamines can have profound effects if used during pregnancy. Potential effects include damage to the liver, heart, and brain of the fetus and abnormal bone and organ development. There is a greater risk of miscarriage, stillbirth, and premature birth. Use of all types of illegal drugs during pregnancy results in devastating effects for the fetus and usually long-term reduced quality of life.

ILLEGAL DRUGS AND SOCIETAL PROBLEMS FOR WOMEN

Women, Drugs, and HIV Infection

Although men still have the greatest number of AIDS cases, the number of women who contract HIV is increasing at a rate almost four times faster than that of men. Additionally, there is a chance that women will pass the virus to their unborn children, thereby doubling the tragic consequences. HIV is transmitted through direct exposure to body fluids (such as blood, semen, vaginal fluids, and mother's milk). Women can contract HIV as a result of vaginal or anal intercourse with an infected partner and by injecting an illegal drug with a needle that contains HIV-infected blood. Thirty percent of all new AIDS cases are women, many of whom contracted the virus via injection drug use.[61]

Researchers are looking at the use of psychoactive drugs that are not necessarily injected, such as alcohol, marijuana, and cocaine, but can cause activity that increases the risk of contracting HIV. Women are more likely to have unsafe sex while under the influence of alcohol and other drugs; therefore, women have an increased opportunity to contract or transmit HIV. Sexual activity increases the chances of contracting HIV and other pathogens that cause sexually transmitted diseases.

The association between contracting or transmitting HIV as well as other STIs while under the influence of drugs is a serious concern. Awareness, prevention, and support services are needed to help diminish the connection between and consequences of women, drugs and HIV. (See *FYI:* "What Are Designer Drugs?" to learn about other drugs that can cause problems for women.)

Women, Drugs, and Homelessness

Use of drugs, including alcohol, is a major risk for women and children as it relates to homelessness. Seeking, buying, and consuming illegal drugs can interfere with a woman's ability to locate employment and purchase essential resources such as housing, food, and medical services necessary for her and her children's well-being. Homeless women comprise a subpopulation at risk for substance abuse, and homeless substance-abusing women face severe barriers to drug abuse treatment.[62]

Even though homelessness is less prevalent among women than men, it is the woman who often has the responsibility for children. Therefore, if a mother is homeless, then her children are homeless as well. Although the effects of drugs themselves have serious consequences, abusing drugs has serious effects on the personal health of homeless women and children. In an attempt to "score" or purchase various drugs, women may engage in risky sexual activity that places them at risk for unintended pregnancy, STIs, including HIV, and street violence. Participating in criminal activities, such as prostitution, drug dealing, and theft, to buy drugs, or even basic necessities, increases the risk of jail, loss of work, and loss of her children.

Children of drug-abusing mothers also suffer greatly, sometimes even prior to birth due to the mother's drug abuse and illnesses. Substance-abusing women, especially homeless women, often have no prenatal care or postbirthing care and are prone to neglect, abuse, abandonment, and placing their children in dangerous circumstances and environments.

What barriers do these women face? Many! Too few substance-abuse treatment facilities to meet the special needs of addicted, homeless women is a serious problem, especially if they have children or are pregnant. Lack of money and insurance, often lack of family support, and inability to receive outpatient treatment because they do not have a place to live all present almost insurmountable barriers for homeless women and children.

Solving the complex issues related to drug abuse among homeless women with children is difficult. They need treatment programs that address a woman's drug addiction, her basic survival needs, health care, and care for her children.

The majority of drug-abusing women report histories of physical and sexual abuse, and they are more likely than men to report a parental history of alcohol and drug abuse. Many drug-abusing women refuse treatment because they are afraid of not being able to take care of or keep their children, fear reprisal from their partners, and fear punishment from authorities in the community. Usually the model for drug treatment programs has been directed toward recovery for the male addict. However, treatment specific to women who abuse substances is needed. Women receive the most benefit from drug treatment programs that provide comprehensive services for meeting their basic needs and programs that help them sustain their recovery and rejoin the community.

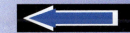

FYI

What Are Designer Drugs?

Designer drugs could be called *copycat drugs* because they are designed to mimic the effects of other illegal drugs but are different enough to avoid government control. You can imagine the risks involved in ingesting chemicals that are mixed and manufactured by persons using a clandestine drug lab such as a garage, a barn, or a basement where no regulations are required and ingredients are unknown and unclean. The potential for physical and psychological ill effects from using these designer drugs is enormous, creating the potential for injury and brain damage. Examples of designer drugs include

MDA (the "love drug"). This is a hallucinogenic amphetamine derivative that is slightly more potent than mescaline, a hallucinatory crystalline alkaloid that is the main active ingredient in peyote buttons.
DOM (STP). This is an amphetamine derivative with hallucinogenic effects that can sometimes be long-lasting.
MDMA ("ecstasy" or "XTC"). This drug produces hallucinogenic effects and strong psychological dependence; it can deplete serotonin levels, potentially leading to such concerns as depression, aggression, and anger.

Chapter Summary

- Use of highly addictive tobacco products is a very serious health behavior among American women, and deaths related to tobacco use continue to increase.
- A number of factors influence women to begin and continue smoking. These include media advertising, parental and peer smoking habits, and the work and recreation environments.
- A number of substances in tobacco are toxic in the human body and cause morbidity and mortality in women. Types of morbidity include heart disease, cancers, diseases of the respiratory system, osteoporosis, and aging skin.
- ETS produces an environment laden with toxic chemicals, and when breathed on a regular basis it can cause a number of very serious diseases in women and children.
- Pregnant women should not smoke because of the serious detrimental effects, not only to the woman but especially to the developing fetus. Young children exposed to ETS will suffer a number of negative consequences.
- Cessation of smoking is difficult because of the highly addictive nature of the substances in tobacco. However, there are a number of smoking cessation programs, prescriptive aids, and behavioral changes that can be beneficial in this endeavor.
- The benefits of smoking cessation are numerous, both for regaining one's physical health and for avoiding the high health care costs related to smoking.
- Caffeine is found in many popular and widely used products, and the health effects are still being researched.
- Caffeinated products such as colas, coffee, tea, and chocolate are sold all over the world and produce a number of concerns for the health of women.
- Women can develop a dependence on caffeine.
- Caffeine can produce negative health consequences for women and their children.
- Illegal drugs such as cocaine, marijuana, and heroin can produce devastating results for women and their unborn fetus or newborn infant.
- Designer drugs have effects similar to those of illegal drugs but are different enough to fall outside the purview of federal regulation.
- Social problems such as homelessness and sexually transmitted diseases often result for women who abuse drugs.

Review Questions

1. What are mortality and morbidity? How has the number of women who smoke affected mortality and morbidity rates in recent years?
2. How many women are current smokers? In the past few decades, has there been an increase or a decrease in the use of smoking tobacco among women? Why?
3. What are four factors that influence women to smoke?
4. What effects do nicotine, carbon monoxide, and tar have on the body?
5. What are three diseases that result from smoking tobacco? How has smoking contributed to the development of these diseases?
6. What component in tobacco causes addiction? What types of addiction patterns occur because of tobacco use?
7. What effects does environmental tobacco smoke have on the health of women and children who are exposed to it?
8. What are the risks for the fetus and for infants born to mothers who smoke during pregnancy?
9. What methods can be used to assist with smoking cessation?
10. In what ways can the Food and Drug Administration regulate tobacco use in the United States?
11. What are the benefits of quitting smoking? What is the length of time before a smoker can expect to experience these benefits?
12. In what ways can women's use of caffeine interfere with reproduction?
13. Does caffeine increase the risk of developing breast cancer? Why or why not?
14. What are the physiological and behavioral effects associated with the consumption of excessive caffeine?
15. What is the difference between the amount of caffeine found in a 12-oz can of Coca-Cola, one cup of brewed coffee, a bar of chocolate candy, and a cup of brewed tea?
16. What are the indications that a woman has developed a dependence upon caffeine, and what can she do to reverse the effects?

Resources

Web Sites

American Cancer Society
www.cancer.org

American Council for Drug Education
www.acde.org

American Lung Association
www.lungusa.org

ASH (Action on Smoking and Health)
www.ash.org/women.html

Caffeine Archives
www.caffeinearchive.com

Centers for Disease Control Office of Smoking and Health
www.cdc.gov/tobacco/quit_smoking/index.htm

Cocaine Anonymous
www.ca.org

Federal Trade Commission
www.ftc.gov/bcp/tobacco

Narcotics Anonymous (NA)
www.na.org

National Alliance for Hispanic Health
www.hispanichealth.org

National Coffee Association of the U.S.A., Inc.
www.ncausa.org

National Institute on Drug Abuse
www.drugabuse.gov

Smokefree.gov800-784-8669
www.smokefree.gov

Substance Abuse & Mental Health Services Administration
National Treatment Hotline: 800-662-HELP
www.samhsa.gov

U.S. Drug Enforcement Administration
www.usdoj.gov/dea/index.htm

U.S. Library of Medicine: Medline Plus
www.nlm.nih.gov/medlineplus/smokingcessation.html

Web of Addictions
www.well.com/user/woa

References

1. Centers for Disease Control and Prevention: Office of Smoking and Health. 2012. *Preventing tobacco use among youth and young adults.* http://www.cdc.gov/tobacco/data_statistics/sgr/2012/consumer_booklet/pdfs/consumer.pdf (retrieved June 5, 2012).

2. American Cancer Society. 2011. *Women and Smoking.* http://www.cancer.org/acs/groups/cid/documents/webcontent/002986-pdf.pdf (retrieved June 5, 2012).

3. American Cancer Society. 2011. *Cigarette Smoking.* http://www.cancer.org/Cancer/CancerCauses/TobaccoCancer/CigaretteSmoking/cigarette-smoking-who-and-how-affects-health (Retrieved on June 5, 2012.

4. Office on Smoking and Health, National Center for Chronic Disease Prevention and Health Promotion. 2001. *Smoking & Tobacco Use.* http://www.cdc.gov/tobacco/data_statistics/sgr/2001/highlights/ataglance/ (Retrieved June 5, 2012).

5. American Cancer Society. 2011. *Women and Smoking.*

6. American Cancer Society. 2011. *Cigarette Smoking.*

7. American Cancer Society. 2011. *Women and Smoking*

8. World Health Organization. 2000. *European Union directive banning tobacco advertising overturned: WHO urges concerted response.* Press release. www.who.int/inf-pr-2000/en/pr2000-64.htm (retrieved June 6, 2012).

9. Federal Trade Commission. 2011. *Cigarette report for 2007–2008.* http://www.ftc.gov/os/2011/07/110729cigarettereport.pdf (retrieved June 6, 2012).

10. Ibid.

11. National Institute of Diabetes, and Digestive and Kidney Diseases. 2010. *You can control your weight as you quit smoking.* http://win.niddk.nih.gov/publications/smoking.htm

12. Centers for Disease Control: National Center for Environmental Health. 2009. *CDC's Tobacco Laboratory.* http://www.cdc.gov/biomonitoring/pdf/tobacco_brochure.pdf (Retrieved June 6, 2012.

13. Centers for Disease Control and Prevention, Division of Laboratory Science. 2009. *Exposure to tobacco smoke and harmful substances in tobacco.* www.cdc.gov/nceh/dls/tobacco.htm (Retrieved June 6, 2012).

14. Carroll, C.R. 2001. *Drugs in modern society.* 5th ed. New York: McGraw-Hill.

15. American Heart Association. 2006. *Understanding your risk.* www.goredforwomen.org/understand_your_risks.aspx#smoking (Retrieved June 6, 2012).

16. Food and Drug Administration. 2003, April 1. *Title 21: Food and drugs—Patient inserts for oral contraceptives.* Code of Federal Regulations 21 (5): Sect.310-501.

17. Centers for Disease Control and Prevention. 2012. Smoking and Tobacco Use. http://www.cdc.gov/tobacco/basic_information/health_effects/cancer/index.htm (Retrieved June 6, 2012).

18. Ibid.

19. U.S Department of Health and Human Services. 2004. *The health consequences of smoking: A report of the surgeon general.* Washington, D.C.: U.S. Department of Health and Human Services, Centers for Disease Control and Prevention, National Center for Chronic Disease Prevention and Health Promotion, Office of Smoking and Health.

20. Ibid.

21. Ibid.

22. National Institute of Arthritis and Musculoskeletal and Skin Diseases. 2012. *Smoking and Bone Health.* http://www.niams.nih.gov/health_info/bone/Osteoporosis/Conditions_Behaviors/bone_smoking.asp (Retrieved June 6, 2012).

23. National Institute of Drug Abuse. 2009. *What is the extent and impact of tobacco use?* www.drugabuse.gov/researchreports/nicotine/nicotine2.html#impact (retrieved June 6, 2012).

24. Ibid.

25. U.S. Department of Health & Human Services: Surgeon General's Reports. 2006. *The health consequences of involuntary exposure to tobacco smoke: A report of the Surgeon General.* http://www.surgeongeneral.gov/library/reports/secondhandsmoke/ (retrieved June 6, 2012).

26. Science Daily. 2007. *Secondhand smoke is a health threat to pets.* http://www.sciencedaily.com/releases/2007/08/070831123420.htm (retrieved June 6, 2012).

27. American Cancer Society. 2011. *Smoking can affect your baby's health.* http://www.cancer.org/Cancer/CancerCauses/TobaccoCancer/WomenandSmoking/women-and-smoking-health-of-others (received June 6, 2012).

28. National Institute of Drug Abuse. 2009. *What is the extent and impact of tobacco use?*

29. U.S. Department of Health and Human Services. *The health consequences of smoking.*

30. American Cancer Society. 2011. *Smoking can affect your baby's health.*

31. Ibid.

32. American Cancer Society. 2011. Kicking the habit. http://www.cancer.org/Cancer/CancerCauses/TobaccoCancer/WomenandSmoking/women-and-smoking-quitting. (retrieved June 6, 2012).

33. U.S Department of Health and Human Services. 2004. *The health consequences of smoking: A report of the surgeon general.*

34. Ibid.

35. Food and Drug Administration. 2010. *FDA 101: Smoking Cessation Products.* http://www.fda.gov/ForConsumers/ConsumerUpdates/ucm198176.htm (retrieved June 7, 2012).

36. American Cancer Society. 2012. *Guide to quitting smoking: How to quit.* http://www.cancer.org/Healthy/StayAwayfromTobacco/GuidetoQuittingSmoking/guide-to-quitting-smoking-how-to-quit (retrieved June 7, 2012.

37. Klesges, L.M, K.C. Johnson, K.D. Ward, and M. Barnard. 2001. Smoking cessation in pregnant women. *Obstetrics and gynecology clinics of north America, 28:* 26982.

38. Statistic Brain. 2012. *Coffee Drinking Statistics.* http://www.statisticbrain.com/coffee-drinking-statistics/ (retrieved June 7, 2012).

39. American Cancer Society. 2012. *When smokers quit—What are the benefits over time?* http://www.cancer.org/Healthy/StayAwayfromTobacco/GuidetoQuittingSmoking/guide-to-quitting-smoking-benefits (retrieved June 7, 2012).

40. Ksir, C., C.L. Hart, and O. Ray. 2006. *Drugs, society, and human behavior.* 11th ed. New York: McGraw-Hill, p. 264.

41. Ibid., p. 270.

42. Ibid., p. 273.

43. International Food Information Council. 2006. *Setting the record straight on caffeine and health.* http://www.foodinsight.org/Portals/0/pdf/julaugfi406.pdf (retrieved June 7, 2012).

44. American College of Gastroenterology. 2006. *Osteoporosis: What you should know.* www.acg.gi.org/patients/women/osteo.asp (retrieved June 7, 2012).

45. March of Dimes. 2010. *Caffeine in pregnancy.* http://www.marchofdimes.com/pregnancy/nutrition_caffeine.html (retrieved June 9, 2010).

46. Ibid.

47. National Survey on Drug Use and Health. 2005. *Substance abuse and dependence among women.* http://store.samhsa.gov/product/Substance-Abuse-and-Dependence-among-Women/SR079 (retrieved June 7, 2012).

48. National Survey on Drug Use and Health. 2010. *National Survey on Drug Use and Health: National Findings.* http://www.samhsa.gov/data/NSDUH/2k10NSDUH/2k10Results.htm#3.1.3 (retrieved June 7, 2012).

49. Merck Manual Online Medical Library. 2007. *Drug use during pregnancy.* http://www.merckmanuals.com/home/womens_health_issues/drug_use_during_pregnancy/drug_use_during_pregnancy.html (retrieved June 7, 2007).

50. Ibid.

51. National Institute on Drug Abuse. 2009. *Medical consequences of drug abuse: Prenatal effects.* http://www.drugabuse.gov/related-topics/medical-consequences-drug-abuse/prenatal-effects (retrieved June 7, 2012).

52. National Institute of Drug Abuse. 2010. *What is the scope of cocaine use in the United States?* http://www.drugabuse.gov/publications/research-reports/cocaine-abuse-addiction/what-scope-cocaine-use-in-united-states (retrieved June 7, 2012)

53. National Institute of Drug Abuse. 2010. *What are the short-term effects of cocaine use?* http://www.drugabuse.gov/publications/research-reports/cocaine-abuse-addiction/what-are-short-term-effects-cocaine-use (retrieved June 7, 2012).

54. Ibid.

55. National Survey on Drug Use and Health. 2010. *National Survey on Drug Use and Health: National Findings.* http://www.samhsa.gov/data/NSDUH/2k10NSDUH/2k10Results.htm#2.6 (retrieved June 7, 2012).

56. National Institute on Drug Abuse. 2010. *What are the effects of maternal cocaine use?* http://www.drugabuse.gov/publications/research-reports/cocaine-abuse-addiction/what-are-effects-maternal-cocaine-use (retrieved on June 7, 2012).

57. Singer, L.T., S. Minnes, E. Short, et al. 2004. Cognitive outcomes of preschool children with prenatal cocaine exposure. *JAMA* 291(20): 2448–56.

58. NIDA Research Report Series. 2005. *Marijuana abuse.* NIH Publication No. 05-3859. Bethesda, MD: National Institutes of Health.

59. March of Dimes. 2007. *Drug use during pregnancy.* http://www.merckmanuals.com/home/womens_health_issues/drug_use_during_pregnancy/drug_use_during_pregnancy.html#v810428 (retrieved June 7, 2012).

60. Ibid.

61. U.S. Department of Health and Human Services, Health Resources and Services Administration. 2005. *Substance abuse and HIV/AIDS.* HIV/AIDS Bureau, Rockville, MD.

62. U.S. Department of Health and Human Services. 2000. *Health of Homeless Women.* http://www.jhsph.edu/wchpc/publications/homeless.PDF (retrieved June 7, 2012).

COMMUNICABLE AND CHRONIC CONDITIONS

Part Five

Chapter Fourteen

Preventing and Controlling Infectious Diseases

CHAPTER OBJECTIVES

When you complete this chapter, you will be able to do the following:

◇ Describe the consequences of untreated sexually transmitted infections (STIs) in women

◇ Compare and contrast the incidence and prevalence of various STIs

◇ Differentiate among the various forms of contraception that reduce the risk of transmitting STIs and HIV/AIDS

◇ Describe safer and riskier sexual behaviors

◇ Explain various ways to prevent the spread of STIs and HIV/AIDS among women and children

◇ Identify the highest risk groups for various STIs and HIV/AIDS

◇ Describe some strategies for preventing the spread of infectious diseases

◇ Identify signs and symptoms of some common infectious diseases

◇ Identify the trends in current infectious diseases

THE INCREASING THREAT POSED BY INFECTIOUS DISEASES

The significant advances in antibiotics and vaccines to fight infectious diseases during the twentieth century lulled many health officials and the public into thinking that the primary diseases of the twenty-first century would be chronic diseases caused primarily by lifestyle choices. The worldwide AIDS epidemic, the "bird flu," H1N1, drug-resistant strains of tuberculosis, and the reemergence of many infectious diseases believed to be close to eradication have sparked renewed focus by health care researchers and providers. The emergence and reemergence of many infectious disease agents have been fueled by unprecedented worldwide population growth, increased international travel, increased transport of animals and food products, changes in food processing and handling, human encroachment on wilderness habitats, and microbial evolution with resistance to antibiotics and other antimicrobial drugs.

Nearly fifty infectious diseases (including many sexually transmitted infections [STIs]) are notifiable at the national level. The current infectious diseases that state departments, physicians, and clinics are asked to report to the Centers for Disease Control and Prevention (CDC) are listed in Table 14.1. The CDC tracks the incidence and prevalence of these diseases and provides weekly and annual reports. Some of these diseases and a few other common infectious diseases affecting college students will be discussed in this chapter. We begin with STIs and later

TABLE 14.1 Infectious Diseases Designated as Notifiable at the National Level, 2009[1]

Anthrax	Malaria
Arboviral diseases,	Measles
neuroinvasive and non-neuroinvasive	Meningococcal disease, invasive
California serogroup	Mumps
Eastern equine	Novel influenza A virus infection
Powassan	Pertussis
St. Louis	Plague
Western equine	Poliomyelitis, paralytic
West Nile	Poliovirus infection, nonparalytic
Botulism	Psittacosis
Brucellosis	Q fever
Chancroid	Rabies, animal
Chlamydia trachomatis infections	Rabies, human
Cholera	Rocky Mountain spotted fever
Coccidioidomycosis	Rubella
Cryptosporidiosis	Rubella, congenital syndrome
Cyclosporiasis	Salmonellosis
Diphtheria	Severe acute respiratory syndrome–associated coronavirus
Ehrlichiosis/Anaplasmosis	(SARS-CoV) disease
Human granulocytic	Shiga toxin–producing *Escherichia coli* (STEC)
Human monocytic	Shigellosis
Human, other or unspecified agent	Smallpox
Giardiasis	Streptococcal disease, invasive, group A
Gonorrhea	Streptococcal toxic-shock syndrome
Haemophilus influenzae, invasive disease	*Streptococcus pneumoniae,* invasive disease
Hansen disease (leprosy)	drug resistant, all ages
Hantavirus pulmonary syndrome	non-drug resistant, children aged <5 years
Hemolytic uremic syndrome, postdiarrheal	Syphilis
Hepatitis, viral, acute	Syphilis, congenital
Hepatitis A, acute	Tetanus
Hepatitis B, acute	Toxic-shock syndrome (other than streptococcal)
Hepatitis B, perinatal infection	Trichinellosis
Hepatitis, viral, chronic	Tuberculosis
Chronic hepatitis B	Tularemia
Hepatitis C, infection (past or present)	Typhoid fever
Human immunodeficiency virus (HIV) diagnosis	Vancomycin-intermediate *Staphylococcus aureus* infection (VISA)
Influenza-associated pediatric mortality	Vancomycin-resistant *Staphylococcus aureus* infection (VRSA)
Legionellosis	Varicella (mobidity)
Listeriosis	Varicella (mortality)
Lyme disease	Vibriosis
	Yellow fever

address infectious diseases such as mononucleosis, influenza, hepatitis, tuberculosis, and streptococcal diseases.

THE PRIMARY BURDEN OF SEXUALLY TRANSMITTED INFECTIONS

STIs can be physically and emotionally devastating for women. The physical risks include potential serious and long-term complications such as pelvic inflammatory disease (PID), impaired fertility, ectopic pregnancies, chronic pain, cervical cancer, and chronic liver disease. The emotional impact may range from feelings of shame to fear of reprisal and feelings of isolation to disconnection from others. Ignorance is not bliss when it comes to STIs since the consequences may be permanent injury or death.

The stigma attached to many STIs can cause women to deny the possibility of having an STI and lead to a delay in testing and treatment. This stigma is perhaps more readily noticed in countries where women with STIs may be shunned, cast out, or physically harmed.

Discrimination can be found in the form of laws and regulations, such as those in developing countries that deny women the right to protect themselves from infected husbands or from gender-based violence, as well as more explicitly at community and individual levels. In addition, stigma associated with addiction and illicit drug use, persistent social and institutional racism, and gender and economic inequities prevent many women from seeking the treatment they need.[2]

Women need to become knowledgeable about the most common STIs and infectious diseases. Asking questions and seeking information are not equated with being sexually active. In fact, when given a choice, women who know the risks may choose less risky sexual behaviors. Abstinence is the first line of protection against future sterility, PID, and ectopic pregnancies, and it is the only way to absolutely prevent all unintended pregnancies and STIs. However, when a woman becomes sexually active, she should choose to act responsibly and protect her body as much as possible. (See *Assess Yourself:* "Assess Your STI Risk.") A woman should know the risks associated with STIs and practice assertiveness skills to prevent unprotected sex.

COMMON BACTERIAL SEXUALLY TRANSMITTED INFECTIONS

Chlamydia

Chlamydia infection is the most frequently reported infectious disease in the United States. The bacterium *Chlamydia trachomatis* causes chlamydial infection and can persist for long periods of time without causing symptoms. The exposure to chlamydia is usually sexual intercourse, and the site of infection is typically the cervix. Chlamydia infections range from lower genital tract infection and PID in women to conjunctivitis and pneumonitis syndromes in newborns. Approximately 75 percent of women with chlamydia are asymptomatic until they experience the fever and pain associated with pelvic inflammatory disease. Up to 40 percent of women infected with chlamydia develop PID if not adequately treated. Twenty percent of women with PID become infertile; 18 percent experience severe, chronic pelvic pain; and nearly 9 percent experience ectopic pregnancies. Recent studies have suggested that women infected with chlamydia and exposed to HIV have a three- to five-fold increased risk of acquiring the virus.[4]

Diagnosis Indicators such as PID and cervicitis are helpful in determining the incidence of chlamydia infections, but new diagnostic technology has allowed for more widespread screening. A variety of tests, including cell culture, antigen detection tests, and nucleic acid amplification tests (NAATs), are used to diagnose chlamydia infection. NAATs are the most sensitive tests for detecting chlamydia infections and are Food and Drug Administration (FDA)-cleared for use with urine testing. The CDC recommends annual screening of all sexually active women ages 25 or younger, and screening of older women with risk factors (e.g., a new sex partner or multiple sex partners). All pregnant women with **cervicitis** should be screened routinely because of the high rate of neonatal infection when chlamydia is left untreated. Symptomatic women may experience unexplained vaginal discharge, burning during urination, lower abdominal pain, bleeding between menstrual periods, fever, and nausea.[5]

Recurrence rates can be particularly disturbing because of increased risk of infertility due to scarring of the fallopian tubes. CDC recommends that women at risk for recurrence be retested for chlamydia at 3 months

Assess Yourself

Assess Your STI Risk

Answer the following questions by checking yes or no on the appropriate line.

Yes	No	
____	____	Do you have sex with men, women, or both?
____	____	Is it very important to you *not* to get pregnant in the near future?
____	____	Do you find it difficult to always use your current birth control method?
____	____	Has the recent change in a relationship caused a change in your method of birth control?
____	____	Do you wonder if your partner has ever had an STI?
____	____	Do you have difficulty discussing STIs with your partner?
____	____	Have you or your partner had sex with more than one person over the past several months?
____	____	Do you or your partner ever inject drugs?
____	____	Does it surprise you that some STIs have no symptoms?
____	____	Have you had a previous STI?

Having unprotected sex, even once, can put you at risk for STIs or unintended pregnancy. If you are sexually active and answered yes to any of the previous questions, you may want to discuss prevention and protection with your health care provider.[3]

and that antibiotic treatment prescriptions be provided for their male partners, if other strategies for treating their partners will not work.[6]

If the partner's infection goes untreated, the risk of recurrence through a repeat transmission exists. If the woman's infection goes untreated, serious complications, including hospitalization for PID, may result. Complications associated with chlamydia infection include cervicitis, infertility, chronic pain, salpingitis (inflammation of the fallopian tubes), increased risk of ectopic pregnancy, stillbirth, reactive arthritis, and neonatal conjunctivitis and pneumonia.[7]

Treatment   The treatment of chlamydia is relatively simple. Antibiotics are given to treat chlamydia, either in a 7-day or single-dose regimen, depending on the woman's compliance history and ability to pay. The single dose of azithromycin is three to five times more expensive than a 7-day regimen but has the advantage of one application. Many women who test positive for chlamydia infection may not comply with the treatment protocol, so a single dose may be more cost effective. Both treatment protocols are efficacious, with cure rates of 97–98 percent. Sex partners should also be treated to prevent reinfection. Partners should abstain from sex for 7 days after the single dose therapy. Despite better screening procedures, treatment compliance is difficult to ensure.[8]

Pregnancy   The CDC recommends that all pregnant women be screened for chlamydia at the first prenatal visit and that women who test positive be treated with azithromycin (or amoxicillin for women with intolerance to azithromycin). Infants can be protected from contracting chlamyida if this treatment is completed before delivery. A woman who tests positive for chlamydia infection risks severe complications if treatment isn't administered promptly.[9]

Epidemiology   Chlamydia affected an estimated 1.3 million persons (nearly 610.6 per 100,000 women in the United States in 2010). Consistently, the reported rate of chlamydia for women substantially exceeds the rate for men, suggesting that many male partners are not screened or treated. Nearly one in ten adolescent girls tested for chlamydia is infected. In all age groups except women 65 and older, the chlamydia rate increased between 2006 and 2010. The overall rate increased from 517.0 per 100,000 women in 2006 to 610.6 per 100,000 in 2010. (See Figure 14.1.)

Adolescent girls aged 15–19 and women aged 20–24 have the highest chlamydia rates. In 2010, the rate among blacks was eight times higher than that for whites. Case rates were higher in all racial/ethnic groups, with the exception of Pacific Islanders. The CDC estimates that annual screening and treatment programs may cost $175 million, and suggests that $12–$15 spent on complications from untreated chlamydia could be saved for every dollar spent on screening and treatment.[10]

Gonorrhea

Gonorrhea is caused by the *Neisseria gonorrhoeae* bacterium. Gonorrhea can affect any of the mucous membranes, including the vagina, cervix, anus, throat, and eyes. Symptomatic women may experience a thick yellow or white vaginal discharge; burning during urination, intercourse, and bowel movements; and severe

FIGURE 14.1 Chlamydia: Age- and sex-specific rates, United States, 2010.

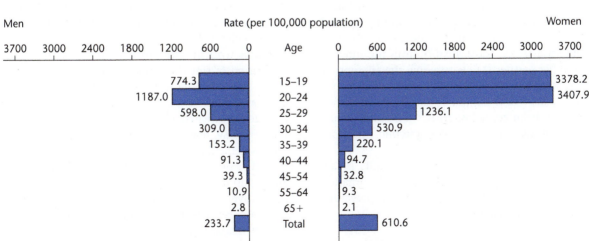

SOURCE: Centers for Disease Control and Prevention. 1. Sexually transmitted disease surveillance 2010. Atlanta: U.S. Department of Health and Human Services; 2011.

menstrual or abdominal cramps. The bacteria can move from the cervix, the site of first infection, into the uterus and fallopian tubes where they can remain indefinitely without causing symptoms and can begin to cause scarring and resultant chronic pain, ectopic pregnancy, or infertility. Nearly 50 percent of women who contract gonorrhea are initially asymptomatic. The first expressed symptoms may be those of PID rather than gonorrhea. Ten to 40 percent of women infected with gonorrhea develop PID if inadequately treated.[11] Among women, the infection often remains asymptomatic until complications such as PID occur. Because women are often asymptomatic, prevention efforts must include screening of women who are practicing high-risk behaviors. Many women who have gonorrhea are co-infected with chlamydia; thus routine dual therapy without testing for chlamydia infection is often conducted because the cost of therapy is less than the cost of testing.

Diagnosis A secretion is taken from the cervix, rectum, and throat for culturing or a urine specimen is used to determine whether a person has been infected. If a woman is infected, she and her partner must be treated concurrently to avoid reinfection, and they should abstain from intercourse during the treatment. Fortunately, most symptomatic men seek treatment quickly after gonococcal urethritis occurs because of pain with urination, and a man's partner(s) should be informed.

Treatment A large increase in resistant strains to first-line antibiotics such as ampicillin, penicillin, and tetracycline has caused a change in CDC treatment recommendations for gonorrhea. The most challenging aspect of controlling this disease may be the continuing spread of antimicrobial resistance in *N. gonorrhoeae*. The current U.S. protocol for dual therapy (gonorrhea and chlamydia) includes the administration of doxycycline, which may help prevent antimicrobial-resistant *N. gonorrhoeae*. Resistance of this bacterium is expected to continue to spread, necessitating that health care providers obtain a recent travel history from the infected person and her partner(s) to ensure that the appropriate therapy is administered. The only antimicrobial agents to which *N. gonorrhoeae* has not developed resistance are the broad-spectrum cephalosporins.[12] Untreated, acute gonorrhea can result in widespread, systemic, infection.

Pregnancy and Infancy Gonorrhea results in adverse outcomes of pregnancy, including inflammation of the newborn's eyes. This disease can be prevented with topical treatment at delivery.

Epidemiology Gonorrhea is the second most frequently reported infectious disease in the United States. The CDC reported rates of 106.5 cases per 100,000 in women in 2010. The south continued to have the highest gonorrhea rate (134.2 per 100,000 population). An estimated 700,000 new cases of gonococcal infections occur each year in the United States.[13] Risk factors for contracting gonorrhea include being a sexually active woman; being under age 25; having previous gonorrhea infections other STIs, or new or multiple sex partners; using condoms inconsistently or improperly; injecting drugs or being involved in commercial sex work. Pregnant women who have some of the risk factors should also be screened for gonococcal infection.[14]

Syphilis

Syphilis is caused by the spirochete *Treponema pallidum,* which spreads throughout the body within hours of infection. It is primarily transmitted through sexual contact, but it can also be passed from the infected mother to a fetus. Syphilis is characterized by active and latent phases, called primary, secondary, latent, and tertiary. The first symptom of primary syphilis, which occurs within 1–3 months (average 21 days) of contact with the infected partner, is a painless red or brown sore (chancre) or sores on the mouth, reproductive organs, or fingers. This chancre will last from 3 to 6 weeks and will heal on its own. In women, the chancre commonly appears on the labia but may develop on the cervix, making detection difficult or impossible. Even though the sore disappears, the person still has syphilis, with half of infected persons moving to the secondary phase and then the latent phase.[15]

Symptoms of the secondary phase appear within 1 week to 6 months after the sore has healed. The hallmark of this phase includes a rash that appears on the palms or soles and flu-like symptoms that disappear within 2–12 weeks. Some health care providers call secondary syphilis the "great imitator," because it may be mistaken for a rash from eczema, cutaneous drug reactions, psoriasis, measles, or even sunburn. The flu-like symptoms may be mistaken for influenza or infectious mononucleosis.[16]

Those who progress to the latent, hidden phases, the period of time between the secondary and tertiary phase, have no clinical signs or symptoms. They may remain asymptomatic, but they will still have syphilis unless they get treated. One-third will move to the tertiary phase. Today, few women progress to the tertiary phase due to penicillin therapy. The tertiary phase is characterized by destructive lesions, lymph node involvement, and organ destruction. The central nervous system may be involved, causing meningitis, spinal lesions, or cerebral vascular syphilis. Cardiac lesions may damage the cardiovascular system.

Syphilis has also been linked to increased susceptibility to HIV infection because the open sores remove the virus barrier and carry mononuclear cells that easily draw HIV. The symptoms of syphilis may manifest differently for HIV-infected persons, so experts suggest that women who test positive for syphilis also get tested for HIV. They should also be counseled about their increased risk for HIV infection and the importance of condom use.[17] All women who test positive for syphilis should be tested for HIV.

Diagnosis The gold standards for diagnosis of early syphilis are dark field microscopic examinations and direct fluorescent antibody tests of the lesion or tissue. Screening is also possible with serologic tests (nontreponemal and treponemal). Individuals who test positive with treponemal tests will often have positive tests for a lifetime, even when treatment has been effective. In many cases, nontreponemal tests will be conducted to follow the course of treatment.

Treatment Any woman with genital lesions should be tested for syphilis. Most primary, secondary, and early latent syphilis cases are treated with one injection of penicillin, which is the drug of choice. Women who are allergic to penicillin can be treated with alternative drugs. Those with tertiary syphilis will need a longer regimen of treatment. All persons must be monitored to determine the efficacy of the treatment.[18]

Infected persons receiving treatment must abstain from sexual contact until the syphilis sores are completely healed. Treated individuals may have a short period of protection from reinfection, but if they are exposed to syphilis sores, they may contract the disease again. Condoms are a good source of prevention; however, syphilis sores may occur outside the covered area, and a person may then become infected by coming in contact with the sores.[19] Treatment failure can occur as can reinfection. In all cases, follow-up is recommended.

Pregnancy Congenital syphilis is transmitted to the fetus during pregnancy and has a devastating impact on the newborn. It accounts for 40 percent of fetal and perinatal deaths in affected infants, and morbidity is even higher, with physical and mental developmental disabilities. Most cases of congenital syphilis are preventable if the pregnant woman is screened during the first prenatal visit and treated properly through early prenatal care. The CDC recommends expanded screening to all women of childbearing age during the early stages of pregnancy. Most states mandate screening. Pregnant women who are allergic to penicillin should be desensitized and treated with penicillin.[20]

If treated during the second half of pregnancy, the risk of premature labor or fetal distress may occur, so the health care provider should be involved in the treatment and follow-up protocol. Evaluation and treatment (if needed) of infants born to mothers who have reactive nontreponemal or treponemal test results are required until the infant tests negative. Children who have reactive serologic tests after the neonatal period (i.e., older than 1 month) should have the mother's records reviewed to determine whether syphilis was congenital or acquired. As with the mother, any child testing positive for syphilis should also be tested for HIV infection.

Epidemiology In 2000, the U.S. rate of primary and secondary syphilis was at its lowest since reporting began in 1941, 2.2 cases per 100,000. From 2001 to 2009, however, the rate of primary and secondary syphilis increased to 3.3 per 100,000, primarily resulting from an increase in cases among men who had sex with men (MSM). While syphilis continues to increase among this group, its rate among women also increased between 2000 and 2008. Primary and secondary syphilis increased from 0.8 women per 100,000 to 1.5 per 100,000 before declining again in 2010.

Serious racial and ethnic disparities persist in the number of reported cases of syphilis. Overall rates of primary and secondary syphilis for blacks was eight times higher than the rates for whites, 34.6 cases per 100,000 versus 4.3 cases per 100,000. In 2010, the rates of primary and secondary syphilis in black females was sixteen times higher than in white females.[21]

Chancroid

Chancroid is caused by the bacterium *H. ducreyi*. It is characterized by a painful genital ulceration. This STI is most prevalent in Africa and the Caribbean, although its prevalence has decreased steadily since 2001. There were only 24 reported cases of chancroid in the United States in 2010. It has been shown to be a risk factor for the transmission of HIV and is a difficult STI to culture or test, which can contribute to under reporting of the actual rate. Treatment for chancroid is a single dose or 7-day regimen of antibiotics. If successful, the genital ulcers begin improving within 3 days. The individual should be reexamined 3–7 days after the initiation of therapy. Sex partners should also be treated if they had sexual contact within 10 days of the onset of symptoms. Chancroid does not appear to have adverse effects on pregnancy.[22]

COMMON VIRAL SEXUALLY TRANSMITTED INFECTIONS

Herpes Simplex Virus (HSV)

Herpes simplex is one of a family of common viruses including varicella zoster virus (chickenpox and shingles) and Epstein-Barr virus (mononucleosis). Herpes simplex virus (HSV) is a contagious infection that spreads from direct skin-to-skin contact of an infected partner to the other partner, particularly in the oral and genital areas. The two primary types of herpes simplex viruses are HSV-1 and HSV-2. HSV-1 usually manifests as cold sores or fever blisters, primarily around the mouth. Once contracted, genital herpes is a life-long chronic infection.

The symptoms of genital herpes vary from one individual to another. Most infected women may not recognize the signs of genital herpes, and many who experience an initial outbreak will never have additional outbreaks. Symptomatic persons may experience the first episode within 2–30 days of contact with an infected partner. The first symptoms of the active phase may include itching, burning, and swelling at the site of infection. A woman can experience symptoms common to all viral infections: fever, headaches, muscle aches, and chills. Eventually, small painful blisters (lesions) appear on the genitalia (sometimes the mouth), then rupture, form a scab, and heal. The blisters disappear within 1–3 weeks, but some of the herpes simplex virus remains. The virus travels along a nerve to the ganglia (a cluster of nerve cells) near the spine and remains dormant until another outbreak occurs. Then the virus travels along the nerve to the surface of the skin.[23]

Diagnosis

Control efforts for HSV-2 are difficult because nearly 75 percent of individuals who transmit the virus are unaware of their infection. Often the infected person transmits the disease during periods of asymptomatic shedding of the virus. If a woman suspects that she has been exposed to HSV-2, she should consult a health care provider when she has lesions. The health care provider will take a sample from the lesions and request a culture to determine whether HSV-2 is present. However, the sensitivity of culture is low, unless lesions are detected early. Type-specific serologic tests are 80–98 percent accurate. Repeat tests may be necessary.

Treatment

There is no cure for herpes simplex, but the drug acyclovir (Zovirax) has effectively reduced the frequency and duration of recurrences in most people. Although acyclovir, an antiviral drug, prevents the herpes cells from replicating, it does not appear to reduce the transmission of the virus to one's partner. Acyclovir is available in pills, ointment, or injectable forms. The recommended regimen for the first episode of genital herpes is oral acyclovir taken three or five times a day for 7–10 days or until the active virus disappears. Valacyclovir (Valtrex) and famciclovir (Famvir) are two versions of acyclovir that absorb more readily and can also be prescribed.[24] Antiviral therapy can be administered when HSV recurs or daily as a suppressive therapy to reduce the frequency of outbreaks.

Prevention of Spread or Recurrence

Prevention depends on the management of outbreaks and preventing the spread of the virus to a partner. (See *Her Story:* "Kristin: Herpes and Sexual Activity.")

A young woman with herpes can prevent recurrences by maintaining a healthy diet, exercising regularly, getting plenty of rest, and managing her stress level. Intimate contact remains the primary mode of transmission, and there is no way to ensure that a partner will remain unaffected because the virus can be present on the skin without recognizable symptoms. Suppressive therapy, daily use of valacyclovir, decreases the risk of genital herpes transmission to an uninfected partner. The consistent and proper use of condoms are also recommended. If the infected partner notices itching or tingling at the primary site of the infection or has blisters, she should avoid sexual contact or use additional precautionary measures. Sexual contact should also be avoided when sores are active (infected), during the healing process, and for several days after the healing

Her Story

Kristin: Herpes and Sexual Activity

Kristin, a 19-year-old college sophomore, recently went to see Dr. Cox, a physician at the student health center. When Dr. Cox entered the room, she sat down and asked Kristin, "What brings you here today?" Kristin hesitated to answer, and Dr. Cox began to sense that something was bothering Kristin so she waited for her to speak. Finally, Kristin began, "Well, basically, I'm here to get some information from you. It is kind of hard to talk about it. I have been dating this really great guy for a long time now and, well, he is just so nice and considerate, and we really like each other. I have been thinking for a while that we might be ready to start getting sexually involved. I guessed he felt the same way so when we went out the other night I brought it up. Ben's reaction surprised me. He just looked down at the table and didn't say anything, and that is not like him, he usually is very willing to talk, even about hard things. I kept encouraging him to share his feelings. Finally, he did. And that is why I am here with you today. You see, Ben has herpes. I want to continue to be involved with Ben, but I am scared. Dr. Cox, I don't want to get herpes, and I don't want to overreact. So, what can I do?"

- Knowing the risks involved, is this a good time for Kristin to become sexually active?
- If Kristin chooses to become sexually active, what precautionary methods should she practice?

has occurred. A woman has about a 75 percent chance of becoming infected if her partner is actively shedding the virus.

A woman can spread herpes to other parts of her body. This transfer is referred to as **autoinoculation** and occurs by touching or scratching an area of shedding active cells and then touching another susceptible area. While the risk is low, to prevent autoinoculation, a woman should avoid touching active lesions or letting others touch the lesions. If her hands accidentally touch an active sore, she should wash them immediately to avoid spreading the virus to other susceptible parts.[25]

Pregnancy A pregnant woman who acquires genital herpes near delivery has a high risk of transmitting the virus to her infant (30–50 percent risk), whereas transmission is low (less than 1 percent) in a woman with recurrent herpes at term or when acquired in the first months of pregnancy. Preventing the transmission of herpes to the infant depends upon preventing, not acquiring, genital herpes during late pregnancy and ensuring the infant does not have contact with the lesions.

A pregnant woman should be asked about her history of genital herpes, during the first prenatal visit and prior to delivery. She should discuss prodromal symptoms and the risks to the neonate, and should be examined for lesions. If genital herpes was acquired late in the pregnancy, an infectious disease specialist should be consulted prior to delivery. Acyclovir and/or cesarean section may be recommended to reduce the risk for neonatal herpes.[26]

Epidemiology HSV-1 affects four in five adults, or approximately 80 percent of all adults. HSV-2, commonly referred to as genital herpes, infects one in six adults, or nearly 50 million American men and women.[27] Case reporting data of HSV-2 are not available so estimates are based on initial visits to physicians' offices. Evidence suggests that HSV-2 seroprevalence declined between 2000 and 2008. Although most persons with HSV-2 have not been diagnosed, about 19 percent of NHANES survey participants aged 20–49 years reported a diagnosis of genital herpes.[28] HSV-2 plays a major role in the transmission of heterosexual HIV, making the person infected with HSV-2 more susceptible and the HIV-infected person more infectious. HSV-1 and HSV-2 can manifest anywhere on the body, despite the common belief that HSV-1 is found only above the waist and that HSV-2 exists only below the waist.

Human Papilloma Virus

Human papilloma Virus (HPV) refers to a group of more than 100 viruses, one-third of which infect the genital mucosal sites. HPV is the most common STI and is nearly twice as high in women as in men. Genital warts, or condyloma, are usually spread by skin-to-skin contact with an infected person. The symptoms of genital warts include small, bumpy warts on the vaginal or anal area that vary from small to large, raised to flat, or single to clustered. Warts can appear several weeks to several months after contact with an infected person. They may remain undetected when located inside the vagina, on the cervix, or in the anus. Most warts are painless and flesh colored and will not disappear without medical attention. Some partners carry the virus without experiencing warts; others experience itching, pain, or bleeding.[29]

The relationship of genital HPV infection to cervical cancer is a significant concern for all women, particularly those infected with HPV and those who are sexually active and susceptible to HPV infection. In most cases, infected women do not know that they have HPV until an abnormal Pap smear is detected, and most of these women will not have experienced the external signs of genital warts. Genital HPV infections are generally characterized as either high-risk or low-risk types. High-risk types (e.g., HPV 16, 18, 31, 33, 35, 39, 45, 51, 52) are associated with low- and high-grade squamous intraepithelial lesions (LSIL and HSIL). Low-risk types (e.g., HPV 6, 11, 42, 43, 44) are associated with genital warts, LSIL, and recurrent respiratory papillomatosis.[30] (See *Viewpoint: "HPV Vaccine."*)

Viewpoint

HPV Vaccine

In 2006, all members of the FDA advisory committee recommended that Gardasil, an HPV vaccine, be approved for distribution in the United States. The vaccine, developed by Merck and Co., is effective in preventing two types of HPV known to cause about 70 percent of all cervical cancer cases worldwide. The vaccine is being recommended as most effective when given to young girls between the ages of 11 and 12 years, and as young as 9. The vaccine is also recommended for 13- to 26-year-old females who have not been vaccinated. It is ideally given before girls and young women become sexually active. The three-dose vaccine prevents four HPV types: HPV 16 and 18, which cause 70 percent of cervical cancers, and HPV 6 and 11, which cause 90 percent of genital warts. In 2009, Gardasil was recommended for boys between ages 9 to 26 and a second vaccine, Cevarix, was licensed for use by girls ages 9–25. These vaccines have been studied worldwide and have been found to be safe, with no serious side effects reported.

Diagnosis A woman should notify her health care provider if she detects any unusual growths, bumps, or skin changes in the vagina, mouth, or anus or if her partner has HPV. Visual inspection and confirmatory biopsy are used to diagnose HPV.

Treatment There is no cure for HPV, although lesions can be removed with proper treatment and follow-up. Usually, several treatments are needed to remove visible warts. The type of treatment prescribed by the health care provider depends on the location and size of the warts and the woman's preference of treatment. Current treatments of HPV include a conservative approach using cryotherapy with liquid nitrogen or a cryoprobe. Other treatments include chemicals such as podophyllin or trichloracetic acid and laser surgery. Podofilox, an FDA-approved prescription solution or gel, has the advantage of being a topical application that can be administered at home.

The decision to remove lesions located on the cervix depends on the severity and the risk of sexual transmission. They are usually removed by cryotherapy, laser, or excision. The goal of HPV treatment is the removal of external warts and the amelioration of signs and symptoms, not to cure the individual. Podophyllin, Imiquimod, and podofilox are not recommended treatment for pregnant women. Genital warts tend to proliferate during pregnancy, so experts recommend only the removal of visible warts.[31]

Prevention Most genital HPV infections are transmitted by sexual activity and are diagnosed on the basis of abnormal Pap smears. Studies have demonstrated that few (if any) cervical HPV infections have been found in females who have not yet been sexually active. The most commonly associated factors related to HPV infection are the number of sexual partners a woman has had and the number of sexual partners her partner has had. The most effective strategies to avoid HPV are abstinence or monogamy with a partner who is not infected. However, sexually active young women who do not have the HPV virus should consider the vaccination.

In 2006, the first vaccine for HPV, Gardasil, was approved for use in the United States in females aged 9–26. In 2009, the vaccine was licensed for use in males aged 9–26. Gardasil prevents HPV types 6, 11, 16, and 18. A second vaccine, Cervarix was approved later in 2009 for protection against types 16 and 18 in young women ages 9–26. Types 6 and 11 are associated with approximately 90 percent of anogenital warts, while types 16 and 18 are associated with anogenital cancers, including cervical cancers. Both vaccines protect against about 70 percent of the types that cause cancer and 90 percent against the types that cause genital warts. These vaccines are most effective when administered before any sexual activity and are given as a 3-dose series of intramuscular injections over a six month period. These vaccines have not been recommended for women over age 26.[32] (See Viewpoint: "HPV Vaccine")

Risk of Cancer Approximately one-third of the estimated 100 types of HPV are associated with infections of the genital area, and 13 are associated with cervical cancer. Some types of HPV, such as types 16, 18, 31, 33, and 35, cause cervical cancer or cervical dysplasia (precancerous changes in cell structure).[33] In fact, HPV types 11 and 16 account for nearly 90 percent of cervical cancer cases. The only effective treatment of cervical cancer is surgical removal of all or part of the cervix. In developing countries, cervical cancer surpasses breast cancer in mortality in women. The United States has reduced the mortality due to cervical cancer through early detection (Pap smear). It is recommended that women with HPV monitor their condition closely and have a Pap smear every 6 months. Other types of HPV have been linked to cancers of the oral cavity, larynx, pharynx, and lungs.[34]

Pregnancy HPV types 6 and 11 not only increase a woman's risk of cancer but are associated with potential disease in infants. An infant born to a woman with HPV type 6 or 11 can contract respiratory papillomatosis (small tumors that grow on the voice box, vocal cords, or air passages).

Epidemiology Some studies have suggested that the annual incidence of genital HPV infection is 5.5 million and that 20 million infected persons are currently living in the United States.

Worldwide, estimates of cervical cancer (the number-one cancer killer of women in many developing countries) may be 500,000 cases annually with nearly one-quarter dying each year. The prevalence of cervical cancer in the United States is approximately 12,000 cases with 4000 deaths annually. These morbidity and mortality occur despite nearly 50 million Pap smears a year. The annual Pap smear screenings detect an estimated 2.5 million low-grade abnormalities and 200,000–300,000 high-grade abnormalities. Most significantly, the annual estimated cost of treating HPV infection ranges from $1.6 billion to $6 billion a year, making genital HPV second only to HIV in total STI treatment costs.[35] With the introduction of Gardasil® and Cervirix® to prevent occurrence or protect against persistent infection, the prevalence of HPV infections and the need for treatment can decrease dramatically.

REPRODUCTIVE TRACT INFECTIONS

Vaginitis

Most women will have a vaginal infection during their lifetime and the majority will use OTC products before visiting a health care provider. Nearly 10 percent of health care visits by women involve complaints about vaginal discharge, a sign of **vaginitis,** or itching. Over 90 percent of vaginitis in women of reproductive age is classified as trichomoniasis, bacterial vaginosis (BV), or candidiasis. Nearly 45 percent have BV, 25 percent have trichomoniasis, and 25 percent have candidiasis. Cervicitis can also cause vaginal discharge. Your health care provider will ask a number of questions to determine whether you have vaginitis or some other infection. The information provided in *FYI:* "What to Tell Your Health Care Provider" will help you prepare for the visit to your health care provider. Diagnosis is determined by pH and microscopic examination of the discharge.

Bacterial Vaginosis (BV) formerly called nonspecific vaginitis, *Gardnerella*-associated vaginitis, or *Haemophilus*-associated vaginitis, is the most common cause of abnormal vaginal discharge or malodor. However, nearly 50 percent of women with BV are asymptomatic. BV occurs when bacteria usually found in the vagina multiply and replace the prevailing bacteria, changing the vaginal pH balance. It frequently affects women with multiple sexual partners and is sexually associated, but not sexually transmitted. BV can also be caused by a chemical imbalance in the vagina. It is recognized by a homogeneous, white, noninflammatory discharge with a fishy odor, either before or after a vaginal sample is examined with a drop of potassium hydroxide solution.

BV is associated with cervicitis, PID, and recurring urinary tract infections. In pregnant women, BV is associated with premature labor, lower birth weight, and postpartum endometritis. It can also increase the risk for HIV infections. Risk factors include having multiple sex partners, a new sex partner, douching, or lack of vaginal lactobacilli.

Treatment: Symptomatic women need treatment, but studies have not supported treating asymptomatic women. There is no recognized equivalent in male partners, and treatment appears contraindicated for preventing recurrences. The CDC recommends treating BV with a 2- to 7-day regimen of antibiotics. Some health care providers prefer antimicrobial creams over oral antibiotics because of fewer possible side effects. Pregnant women at high risk should be screened during the first prenatal visit. Pregnant women are treated with topical agents because some oral antibiotics are contraindicated.[36]

Trichomoniasis *Trichomonas vaginalis (T. vaginalis),* the protozoan that causes trichomoniasis, is found in both men and women. It remains dormant in many asymptomatic women and causes vaginal irritation, itching, and diffuse, malodorous discharge in symptomatic women. The discharge varies but typically is thin, frothy, homogeneous, and yellow-green or gray. Most infected women experience red spots on the vaginal walls or uterus; however, some have few or no symptoms.[37]

Treatment: Both partners need treatment for *T. vaginalis* to be effectively cured because *T. vaginalis* is sexually transmitted. **Trichomoniasis** is confirmed by the presence of trichomonads and a vaginal pH of 5 or higher. If confirmed, an oral antibiotic (metronidazole or tinidazote) is usually prescribed for the woman and her partner.[38] Clinical trials have resulted in cure rates of 90–95 percent. Follow-up is not necessary if symptoms disappear.

Candidiasis Vulvovaginal candidiasis (VVC), commonly known as yeast infection, is not a sexually transmitted infection but may coexist with STIs. *Candida* is the name of a single-celled fungus often present in the human body. When the balance of bacteria and yeast is altered, the yeast may overgrow. Symptomatic women will experience itching with vaginal discharge, burning, or irritation in the vulvovaginal area. Pregnant women and those who have significant changes in diet, have some type of immune suppression, and/or use broad-spectrum antibiotics commonly experience yeast infections. Nearly 75 percent of women will have one episode of VVC in their lifetime, and 40–45 percent have two or more episodes. Women with pelvic pain, a first-time yeast infection, multiple sexual partners, or unprotected sexual encounters and pregnant women should see a health care provider to get treatment.

Some women are more predisposed to recurrent yeast infections. The factors most often associated with repeat infections include diabetes, obesity, suppressed immunity, pregnancy, and using broad-spectrum antibiotics, corticosteroids, or birth control pills. Self-care

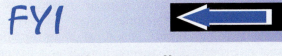

FYI

What to Tell Your Health Care Provider

- When the symptoms started
- Texture, color, and odor of discharge
- Burning, itching, pain, or redness
- Change in bowel movements, such as diarrhea
- Recent change in sexual partner or symptoms in current partner
- Problems in sexual intercourse such as pain with penetration during intercourse
- Anal intercourse
- Type of contraceptive used
- Use of home remedies or over-the-counter medications
- Number of pregnancies
- Previous pelvic infections, including during pregnancy

is appropriate for women who have recurrent yeast infections.

Treatment: Candida and other yeasts are found in the vagina of nearly 20 percent of all women, many of whom are asymptomatic and do not need treatment. Most symptomatic cases are uncomplicated and easy to treat. FDA-approved over-the-counter (OTC) medications that cure yeast infections include vaginal topical creams, tablets, suppositories, and combination packs. Familiar trade names include Monistat 7, Gyne-Lotrimin, Mycelex-7, and Fem Care. Prescription medications also come in topical creams, tablets, and suppositories. Another choice of treatment is a single-dose tablet of fluconazole. Treatment of partners does not appear to reduce the incidence of yeast infections.

Unfortunately, some women who self-diagnose a yeast infection may actually experience BV or another infection that cannot be cured by OTC medications. If a self-diagnosed infection does not appear to respond to treatment, a health care provider should be consulted.[39] When yeast infections recur without one of the causes mentioned earlier, the health care provider should suspect or rule out HIV. (See *Health Tips:* "Preventing Recurring Yeast Infections.")

Health Tips

Preventing Recurring Yeast Infections

- Use mild soaps and perfumes.
- Use unscented toilet paper and sanitary pads rather than tampons.
- Do not use feminine hygiene sprays.
- Double-rinse undergarments washed in harsh irritants.
- Use 100 percent cotton undergarments to keep the genital area dry.
- Wear loose rather than restrictive clothing.
- Limit hot-tub episodes.
- Change swimsuits immediately after a hot tub or swim to reduce exposure of the genital area to moisture.
- Wipe from front to back after a bowel movement to reduce possible infections.
- Male partners must wash their penis or change condoms when moving from anal to vaginal intercourse.
- Avoid sugar binges.
- Avoid drastic changes in dietary patterns.

Inflammatory Disorders

Pelvic inflammatory disease (PID) has one of the most severe outcomes of STIs. PID is a spectrum of inflammatory disorders of the upper portion of the female reproductive tract beyond the cervix. Common symptoms include severe pelvic pain, high fever, chills, nausea, and vomiting. Spotting or pelvic pain can occur between menstrual periods, and sometimes there is abnormal vaginal discharge.

Nearly one in eight sexually active adolescent girls will develop PID before the age of 20, with almost 1 million new cases of PID diagnosed annually.

Accurate estimates of PID rates are difficult to obtain because complex and invasive procedures are needed to diagnose this disease correctly. Interpretations of clinical findings are often used when reporting PID, and these interpretations vary depending on the health care provider. The rate of PID-related hospitalizations of women 15 to 44 years of age has continued to decline over the past 20 years; however, the declines may be misleading because they may point to a change in treatment protocol from inpatient to outpatient and better screening for chlamydia infections. Sexually active women can reduce the risk of PID by seeking annual STI screening exams.

PID is diagnosed by a health care provider through a pelvic examination or through analysis of cervical or vaginal secretions. If diagnosed, treatment includes antibiotics, rest, and sexual abstinence. The optimal treatment regimen for PID is unknown. Surgery may be required to remove any scars or abscesses or to repair injured reproductive organs. A single episode can damage the fallopian tubes. PID is the only cause of infertility that is preventable, accounting for as many as 30 percent of all infertility cases.[40]

Cervicitis is an inflammation of the cervix that is frequently asymptomatic. However, in some cases, women complain of abnormal vaginal discharge or vaginal bleeding between menstrual cycles or after sexual intercourse. The criterion for diagnosis has not been standardized, but leukorrhea (vaginal discharge) has been identified as an indicator of cervical inflammation. Cervicitis has been associated with chlamydial and gonoccocal infection. It can also accompany trichomoniasis, BV, or genital herpes. Many times there is no etiological organism. Cervicitis may be a sign of endometritis (upper-genital-tract infection) or PID. Women with persistent cervicitis should continue to be reevaluated for STIs and their sexual partner(s) should also be evaluated and treated for any identified STIs.[41]

HIV/AIDS

Human immunodeficiency virus (HIV) is a retrovirus that causes **acquired immune deficiency syndrome (AIDS),** a group of signs or symptoms that causes the immune system to function improperly. The virus is transmitted from person to person through blood, semen, or vaginal secretions. It can be transferred through sexual contact with an infected person, by sharing injecting drug needles, from mother to infant before or during childbirth, through breast feeding, and through receiving blood or blood products from someone infected with HIV. Persons receiving transfusions in the United States are virtually free from the possibility of blood or blood product transmission because all blood banks test for the virus.

Symptoms of AIDS may be similar to those of other diseases; however, they take longer to disappear and may recur. Some common early symptoms of AIDS are recurring fever including "night sweats"; rapid weight loss without diet or exercise; diarrhea lasting longer than several weeks; white, thick spots or coating in the mouth; a dry cough and shortness of breath; or purple bumps on the skin, inside the mouth, and in the rectum.

In the United States, women represent 24 percent of all HIV diagnoses. Women of color continue to be disproportionately represented. The rate of HIV infections in black women is over 15 times the rate for white women. The rate for Hispanic/Latina women is nearly four times that of white women. Lifetime diagnosis of HIV is 1 in 32 in black women, 1 in 106 in Hispanic/Latina women, and 1 in 526 for white and Asian women.[42] (See Figure 14.2). These increasing rates have placed an undue burden on an already impoverished group of women. These women are faced with an array of psychosocial, economic, cultural, and relational issues. HIV/AIDS is indeed a family issue because many of these women are the primary care providers for their children and themselves. African American and Hispanic women account for 83 percent of AIDS cases reported among women, yet constitute only one-fourth of all U.S. women. In 2008, HIV/AIDS was the third *leading cause of death* for African American women ages 35–44 years.

The most common methods for heterosexual women to contract HIV are through contact with bisexual or heterosexual men followed by injected drug use. (See Figure 14.3.) HIV is not transmitted through casual contact, tears, or saliva. HIV does not survive well in the environment. In laboratory settings, CDC studies have found that drying a high concentration of HIV reduces the infectious virus by 90–99 percent within several hours. In addition, HIV cannot reproduce outside the living host. In family households with an HIV-infected person, transmission to other family members is rare. Transmission usually occurs when skin or mucous membranes are exposed to infected blood.

Epidemiology

Nearly 95 percent of the global total of people with HIV live in developing countries. Women constitute nearly

FIGURE 14.2 Race/ethnicity of women with HIV/AIDS diagnosed during 2009.

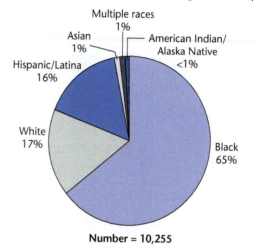

Race/ethnicity of women with HIV/AIDS diagnosed during 2009

Multiple races 1%
Asian 1%
American Indian/Alaska Native <1%
Hispanic/Latina 16%
White 17%
Black 65%

Number = 10,255

SOURCE: Centers for Disease Control and Prevention. 2011. HIV Surveillance—Epidemiology of HIV Infection (through 2009). http://www.cdc.gov/hiv/topics/surveillance/resources/slides/general/index.htm

46 percent of all people living with AIDS, further demonstrating that AIDS is not a disease for men only! The Joint United Nations Programme on HIV/AIDS (UNAIDS) and the World Health Organization (WHO) estimate that more than 34 million people were living with HIV at the end of 2010. HIV/AIDS accounted for 1.8 million deaths worldwide in 2010.

In 2009, of the 1.4 million pregnant women, more than 53 percent received antiretroviral treatment to prevent spread of the virus to the infant. The number of pregnant women who were tested for HIV rose from 8 percent in 2005 to 35 percent in 2010. The number of children who were newly infected with HIV dropped from 500,000 in 2001 to 370,000 in 2009; 456,000 children were receiving antiretroviral therapy in 2010, up from 71,500 in 2005. This increase represents only 25 percent of all children who need the therapy so efforts need to be enhanced. UNAID and UNICEF have called for the elimination of HIV infections in children by 2015. To reach this goal, funding efforts need to change. Funding decreased from $15.9 billion in 2009 to $15.0 billion in 2010. UNAID called for $24 billion by 2015 to reach the goal.[43]

More than 90 percent of the children (age 14 and younger) with HIV acquired the virus at birth, during pregnancy, or through their mother's breast milk. Poverty, limited access to adequate health care, and lack of prevention efforts remain the major factors in the continued spread of HIV/AIDS. (See *FYI:* "World AIDS Day National HIV Testing Day.")

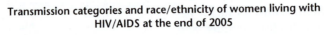

FIGURE 14.3 Transmission categories and race/ethnicity of women living with HIV/AIDS at the end of 2005.

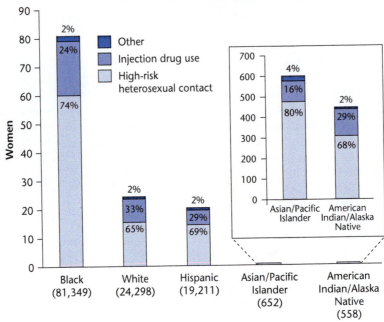

SOURCE: Centers for Disease Control and Prevention. 2008. *HIV/AIDS among women.* www.cdc.gov/hiv/topics/women/resources/factsheets/pdf/women.pdf.

FYI

World AIDS Day and National HIV Testing Day

The 2011 World AIDS Day theme was "Getting to Zero." The three primary aspects were: Zero new HIV infections, Zero discrimination, and Zero AIDS-related deaths. The goal is to eliminate new HIV infections by 2015. National HIV Testing Day is an annual campaign to encourage all at-risk individuals to get tested for HIV. The CDC estimates that 180,000–280,000 people nationwide are HIV-positive but do not know it. By going to www.hivtest.org a woman can find the nearest testing site by entering a zip code. Early detection is critical to decreasing the viral load of HIV, thus preventing or delaying AIDS. Are you at risk? Do you know your HIV status? The poster on page 370 challenges us to Take the Test: Take Control.

The World Health Organization suggests that biologic factors, epidemiologic factors, and social vulnerability cause women to be more susceptible to HIV than men. Women have increased biologic risk due to greater mucosal surface exposed during intercourse and high concentrations of HIV in seminal fluids. They have increased epidemiological risk because women date or marry older men who have often been with multiple partners. For instance, most teenage women date older males, many of whom have had several sexual partners. The more partners, the greater is the risk of contracting HIV or another STI. Social vulnerability is an issue when women are forced to be sexual with a partner who refuses to use a condom or when women must rely on a partner's saying he is monogamous when in fact he is not. This male behavior or "assumed right" increases a woman's risk of contracting HIV and other STIs.

Diagnosis of HIV

If a woman believes she has been infected with or exposed to HIV through sex, injected drug use, or other contact with contaminated blood, she should request an HIV antibody test. Because women can be infected more easily than men, they should request testing if they have the slightest suspicion of exposure. The testing center should offer pre- and post-test counseling, as well as confidentiality from employers and health insurance. Some centers offer anonymous testing. HIV infections are diagnosed through serologic tests and by virologic tests. Serologic tests are highly sensitive and can detect all known HIV-1 subtypes. The majority of HIV infections in the U.S. are HIV-1 subtypes. Rapid serologic testing allows clinicians to make an accurate first diagnosis within 20–30 minutes. Two tests have been used consistently for diagnosis: the **ELISA test** (enzyme-linked immunosorbent assay), a general screening test with high sensitivity, and the **Western blot test,** a less sensitive, more expensive but more specific test for the HIV antibody. If a person tests positive for the HIV antibody with the ELISA test, a second ELISA test is conducted on the same sample. If this test is positive, the Western blot test is conducted. Both tests must be positive to confirm a HIV infection. Nearly 90 percent of low-risk persons who test positive on the ELISA test will test negative on the Western blot test. Results for each test often take up to a week for reporting. If positive, other blood tests are conducted to determine the level of HIV in the bloodstream.[44]

A woman must wait nearly 6 weeks to 12 months from the time of the suspected exposure before getting tested because it takes time from the initial exposure until the body develops enough antibodies for detection. This period between infection and antibody development is called the window period. Experts recommend that two sets of antibody tests, approximately 6 months apart, be conducted for conclusive results. Repeat antibody testing may be necessary if antibodies have not developed. If a woman is unsure of where to go for HIV counseling and testing, she can contact the National AIDS Hotline (1-800-232-4636) or go to the CDC Web site for a listing of locations closest to her residence.

Home HIV Tests The FDA has approved only one home HIV test despite the numerous products advertised by companies on the Internet. Many people refuse to be tested at a health care facility because of concerns about breached confidentiality and potential loss of health insurance benefits. The home HIV test, Home Access HIV-1 Test, is marketed by the Illinois-based Home Access Health Corporation and has been clinically proved to be 99.9 percent accurate. It is available for purchase through a toll-free number (1-800-HIV-TEST) and the Internet (www.homeaccess.com) and at pharmacies nationwide. The test kit includes detailed instructions on how to collect a blood sample, ship the product, and call for results. The sample is screened at a lab using the ELISA test. If this screen is positive, a more specific confirmatory test (immunofluorescence assay [IFA]) is used. This test only gives results for HIV-1. An eleven-digit code (included in the kit) is all the individual needs to get the test results. The results are available within 1–7 days, and trained counselors at Home Access are available for confidential and anonymous support. If a woman does not have access to an anonymous testing site in her community, the FDA-approved home kit is beneficial. The earlier an HIV-positive woman knows her status, the earlier she can get treatment. Use of non-FDA-approved products is discouraged.[45]

Rapid Testing for HIV/AIDS The U.S. FDA has approved another HIV test, the OraQuick Rapid HIV-1 Antibody Test, manufactured by OraSure Technologies. When used correctly in an approved medical setting, OraQuick has a 99 percent accuracy rate. The advantage of rapid testing for HIV/AIDS is that the individual receives results in as little as 20 minutes. This is important because many persons who take HIV/AIDS tests through health departments and public clinics do not return to receive their results.

If a test result is positive, a second test using another method should be done to confirm the OraQuick results. Currently, OraQuick can be administered only by trained health care professionals and is not available for in-home use. Women should be aware of possible limitations: false negatives and delayed detection of exposure (the virus has not yet developed antibodies).[46]

No matter what type of test a woman chooses to confirm whether or not she is HIV-positive, it is important she receive test counseling throughout the procedure, as a positive diagnosis for HIV/AIDS can be both frightening and life-changing. The FDA provides an updated list of all approved screening assays for infectious agents and HIV diagnostic assays.

Treatment of HIV

Drug treatment typically focuses on reducing the viral load or reinforcing the immune system. The viral load can be lowered or kept low by blocking HIV attachment to the CDR cell, blocking antigens on the virus envelope, interfering with the uncoating of the virus as it enters the cell, disrupting the translation of virus RNA to cell DNA, and disrupting the assembly and maturation of virus particles in the CDR cell, and their release as a free-floating virus in the body. The four major classes of drugs include reverse transcriptase (RT) inhibitors, protease inhibitors, entry and fusion inhibitors, and integrase inhibitors. The FDA has approved nearly thirty antiretroviral drugs that often are combined into products from more than one class. These products suppress the virus, sometimes to undetectable levels, depending on when treatment began.[47] Now, complete *Journal Activity:* "Browsing the Internet for AIDS Research."

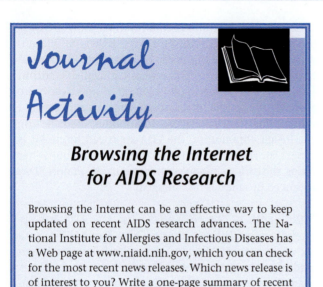

Journal Activity

Browsing the Internet for AIDS Research

Browsing the Internet can be an effective way to keep updated on recent AIDS research advances. The National Institute for Allergies and Infectious Diseases has a Web page at www.niaid.nih.gov, which you can check for the most recent news releases. Which news release is of interest to you? Write a one-page summary of recent events. Share your findings with classmates.

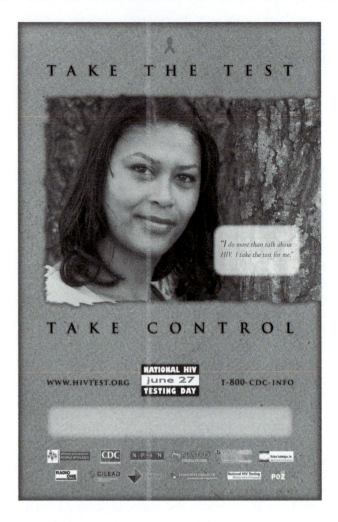

Pregnancy and HIV

All pregnant women should be tested for HIV infection as early in the pregnancy as possible. Testing is important for the health of the mother and for interventions to reduce perinatal transmission of HIV. In addition, all pregnant women should be tested for syphilis, hepatitis B surface antigen (HBsAg) and chlamydia at the first prenatal visit. Some states require further testing prior to delivery. All pregnant women at risk for gonorrhea or hepatitis C or living in a high-risk area for gonorrhea should also be screened for these STIs. Women who are HBsAg positive should be reported to the local and/or state department; partners and household residents should be tested and/or vaccinated, and notification should be sent to the health care providers at the hospital where delivery and care for the infant will occur.

Antiretroviral therapy or combination antiretroviral drug prophylaxis can substantially reduce the risk of infants contracting HIV during pregnancy and delivery. When combined with cesarean section and no breast feeding, the risk of HIV transmission to infants can be reduced to approximately 1–2 percent. The challenges in emerging countries are the low rate of testing of pregnant women, lack of resources for more effective drugs, and unwillingness to forego breastfeeding.[48]

SEXUAL ASSAULT AND STIs

Sexually assaulted children and women should be examined by an experienced clinician to reduce further trauma to the survivor. The STIs most frequently diagnosed include trichomoniasis, BV, gonorrhea, and chlamydia. Examination for STIs should be repeated 1–2 weeks after the assault, if possible. Postexposure HBV vaccine and emergency contraception (EC) may be recommended. The risk for HIV seroconversion is low, except in children who may be at higher risk if the abuser is HIV positive and exposes the child to repeated trauma.

STIs IN WOMEN WHO HAVE SEX WITH WOMEN (WSW)

Data are limited regarding the risk of STIs among lesbians, but if the infections are left untreated, the risks are similar to those for heterosexual women. Women who have sex with women (WSW) are a diverse group with differences in sexual identify, sexual orientation, sexual behaviors, and risk behaviors. Yeast infections and BV are the most common STIs in WSW and can be passed from partner to partner. WSW are also susceptible to HPV, HSV (often genital infection with HSV-1), and trichomoniasis. WSW who are not sexual with men are at low or no risk for gonorrhea, chlamydia, and PID. Female-to-female transmission of HIV is rare, with few cases reported. This transmission indicates that vaginal secretions and menstrual blood are potentially infectious, and mucous membrane (e.g., oral, vaginal) exposure to these secretions has the potential to lead to HIV infection. Since the beginning of reported AIDS cases in the 1980s, only a small percentage of HIV-infected women have reported having sex with women; however, the vast majority had other risks (injected drug use and sex with high-risk men). It is difficult to know the actual transmission rate for WSW because many health care providers fail to ask whether a woman had sex with women or the HIV-positive woman did not volunteer the information.[49,50] Reported same-sex behavior should not deter a health care provider from screening for STIs, including chlamydia and syphilis in women practicing risky behaviors.

Regarding female-to-female transmission, WSW need to know the following:

- Exposure of a mucous membrane to vaginal secretions and menstrual blood is potentially infectious.
- Condoms (cut-open), dental dams, or plastic wrap can help protect them from body fluids during oral sex.
- Condoms should be used consistently and correctly when having sex with men or using sex toys.
- Bacteria in the rectum can cause infections in the vagina and urethra.
- Self-contact after touching a partner's genitals can transmit some STIs.
- Some STIs can be transmitted from vulva-to-vulva contact.
- A woman's own and her partner's HIV status can increase the risk of HIV infection.

PREVENTION STRATEGIES

STIs have special implications for women because women are less symptomatic, more difficult to diagnose, less frequently tested, and suffer more severe consequences then men. Also, the transmission of STIs is easier from men to women. These factors make prevention efforts extremely important. What prevention strategies are available for women? What sexual behaviors are considered safer?

Preexposure Vaccination

Vaccines are available for several STIs, including hepatitis A virus (HAV), hepatitis B virus (HBV), and HPV. HAV vaccine is recommended for MSM and illicit drug users. HBV vaccine is recommended for all unvaccinated, uninfected persons being evaluated for STIs. HPV vaccines (HPV types 6, 11, 16, and 18) are recommended for females aged 9–26 years. Vaccine trials are currently under way for other STIs, including HSV and HIV. Every woman being treated for an STI should receive the HBV vaccine and, if practicing high-risk behavior (e.g., illegal drug use), the HAV vaccine as well.

Abstinence

Sexual abstinence (i.e., oral, vaginal, or anal) is the only 100 percent effective method to prevent STIs. Abstinence means no exchange of body fluids and no skin-to-skin exposure of the genital areas. Young people need to understand that being physically developed does not necessarily equate with psychological readiness for a sexual relationship.

When is abstinence appropriate? *Anytime you choose!* Abstinence is certainly an appropriate choice for women when they are not psychologically ready to be sexually active, when they have been drinking, if they have had unprotected sex with a different partner without subsequent testing, or if they do not have adequate protection (condoms). Can you think of other times when a woman might choose abstinence?

Monogamy

Many young women today are choosing to delay sexual intimacy until they have a committed relationship or until they are married. A committed relationship is not synonymous with "serial monogamy." Serial monogamy means having several relationships over time, with just one partner in each relationship. For teenagers, serial monogamy may mean having only one partner; however, the length of time for the relationship can vary from several days to several months. Reducing the number of sexual partners over one's lifetime and choosing a partner who has had fewer sexual partners translates into less exposure to the risk of contracting an STI.

Engaging in Less Risky Behaviors with Partners

STIs are not dependent on who the person is but rather on what the person does. Sexual behaviors can be considered safe (dry kissing) to dangerous (unprotected vaginal or anal sex). Review the list provided in *FYI:* "Playing It Safe with Sexual Behaviors."

Are there other behaviors you would add to the list? Where would you place these behaviors? Then complete *Journal Activity:* "Reasons for Unprotected Sex."

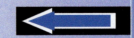

FYI

Playing It Safe with Sexual Behaviors[51]

Safe
Hugging
Dry kissing
Mutual masturbation on healthy skin
Oral sex with a latex barrier (condom, dams, gloves)
Touching, massage, fantasy

Less Safe
Vaginal intercourse or fingering with a latex condom or glove
Wet kissing
Anal intercourse or fingering with a latex condom or glove
Dildos with a condom

Risky
Oral sex without a latex barrier
Masturbation on skin that has cuts or abrasions
Exchanging sex toys without thorough cleaning
Anal-to-vaginal transmission

Dangerous
Vaginal intercourse without a condom
Anal intercourse without a condom
Sharing a needle or blood contact
Semen or urine in the mouth

Journal Activity

Reasons for Unprotected Sex

As a class assignment or an assignment with friends, brainstorm all the reasons that college women may give for putting themselves at risk for having unprotected sex with a partner. For each reason, write an alternative positive response in your journal.

Example
Reason: If I carry a condom with me, he could think that I'm planning to have sex.
Alternative response: I have a right to protect myself and the right to choose when and with whom I have sex.

Oral Contraceptives, Vaginal Spermicide, and Diaphragms

Oral contraceptives are *not* effective in preventing STIs but may reduce the risk of PID. Most health care providers recommend using oral contraceptives and condoms to reduce the risk of unwanted pregnancies *and* STIs. Studies have found that frequent use of **nonoxynol-9 (N-9)** can cause genital lesions in the vagina, which may increase the risk for HIV transmission. According to CDC guidelines, spermicides that contain N-9 should not be used for STI prevention and/or during anal intercourse. Spermicides are not effective in preventing gonorrhea, chlamydia or HIV infection. The diaphragm has been found to protect against gonorrhea, chlamydia, and trichomoniasis but not HIV infections. Vaginal spermicides and diaphragms have been associated with increased risk of urinary tract infections in women.[52]

Male Condoms

Male condoms are one of the most effective methods available for preventing STIs. Most viruses do not pass through the latex or polyurethane condom when properly and consistently used. A drawback of the polyurethane condom is higher breakage and slippage rates, and it is usually more costly. Natural membrane condoms (incorrectly called lambskin condoms) can allow passage of sperm and viral sexually transmitted diseases through the material. They are not recommended for prevention of sexually transmitted diseases or pregnancy. The problem for many young women is their difficulty in insisting that their partner use a condom. If the partner refuses to use a condom, the woman is faced with additional decisions. If her partner consents to using a condom, she cannot ensure that he will use the condom properly and consistently so she may want to consider not having sex with him.

In the past, STI prevention specialists recommended that condoms be latex with N-9. Those recommendations have changed. Condoms with N-9 have a shorter shelf life, cost more, and are associated with urinary tract infections in women. Males are still encouraged to use latex condoms consistently and correctly to significantly reduce the risk of HIV infection, chlamydia, gonorrhea, and trichomoniasis in women. They may also reduce the risk for HSV, PID, and HPV-associated diseases.[53]

Female Condoms

The female condom (Reality™) offers a woman another alternative contraceptive method and allows her to have more control over the sexual experience. She can insert it before intercourse, unlike the male condom, which requires an erect penis before it can be put on. Also, the female condom protects the outer labia, thus offering better protection against HPV or HSV. The female condom has been shown to be effective in providing protection against STIs, including HIV. It provides protection during receptive anal intercourse, but its efficacy is unknown.[54] Women have a variety of strategies available to prevent unwanted STIs and unintended pregnancies, from abstinence to proper protection. Keep informed! Stay assertive!

Promising Prevention Strategies

Antiretroviral (ARV) therapy is being explored as a potential method for reducing HIV transmission. ARVs suppress the viral load leading researchers to study whether ARVs can be sued as a prevention tool. Lower viral loads lead to reduced infectiousness of the HIV-infected person. **Pre-Exposure prophylaxis** (PrEP) could provide women with a method to protect themselves from contracting HIV from an HIV-infected partner.

Topical microbiocides (gels, creams, foams) could be applied vaginally and/or rectally to prevent HIV. They may kill or inactivate the virus, strengthen the body's immune system, block the virus from attaching to susceptible cells, or prevent viral spread to other cells.

Intervention strategies for injecting and noninjecting drug users could include providing sterile injecting equipment to intravenous drug abusers. Reducing other risks by using protection in situations when exchanging sex for drugs or money would also be a preventive strategy. Community and individual prevention strategies should continue to be researched.[55]

OTHER INFECTIOUS DISEASES

Epstein-Barr Virus (EBV)

EBV is a member of the herpes virus family and is a common human virus that infects nearly 95 percent of adults in the United States. When EBV occurs in teenagers or young adulthood, it causes infectious mononucleosis 35–50 percent of the time. Symptoms of mono include fever, sore throat, and swollen lymph glands. Although symptoms usually resolve in 1 or 2 months, the virus can reactivate (similar to other herpes viruses). Once a person has been infected with HBV, the virus remains in the body, usually dormant. Every once in a while, it may become active in the saliva. Usually, laboratory tests are used to confirm mono, including an elevated white blood cell count, an increased total number of lymphocytes, and a positive reaction to a "mono spot" test. Bed rest and reduced physical activity are recommended to overcome the fatigue, fever, and other symptoms of the disease. While unusual, spleen, liver, heart, or central nervous system involvement can occur, indicating the importance of self-care during the time one is symptomatic. Transmission of mononucleosis occurs through intimate contact with saliva (found in the mouth) of an infected person, hence its name "the kissing disease." Transmission of the virus is virtually impossible to prevent, because 95 percent of healthy people have the virus in their saliva. These individuals are the primary reservoir for person-to-person transmission. Researchers continue to explore a link between EBV and multiple sclerosis. Findings from a study of 7 million blood specimens found an association between the virus and MS. A combination of the virus and environmental factors may trigger MS in some susceptible individuals.[57]

Seasonal Influenza (Flu)

The flu virus infects the respiratory tract (nose, throat, and lungs) and can cause mild symptoms to severe illness and life-threatening complications (e.g. pneumonia). Typical symptoms of influenza include high fever, headache, extreme tiredness, dry cough, sore throat, runny or stuffy nose, and muscle aches; children may experience diarrhea or vomiting. The peak time for the "flu season" in the United States is late December through March, and the best way to prevent the illness is by getting a flu vaccination each fall. Transmission of the virus occurs person-to-person through respiratory droplets of coughs and sneezes. "Droplet spread" can be propelled up to 3 feet through the air and deposited in the nose or mouth of persons nearby. Hand washing is encouraged to prevent spread from respiratory droplets from one person to the nose or mouth of another person. An adult with the virus is usually contagious for 1 day prior to and up to 7 days after the first symptoms. Children may have longer periods of contagion. Once a person contracts the virus, she may develop some immunity to closely related viruses for one or more years. Persons with healthy immune systems have greater likelihood of immunity than persons with chronic diseases or weakened immune systems.[58] Therefore, children aged 6–23 months, pregnant women, persons over age 65, and persons with chronic medical conditions are at greatest risk for complications from the flu. A person can drastically reduce the risk of complications by receiving a flu shot, an inactive vaccine (containing killed virus). It is approved for use in children older than 6 months and in adults, including healthy people and those with chronic medical conditions. A nasal-spray flu vaccine contains live, weakened flu virus and is approved for healthy children 5 years and older and for adults up to age 49 who are not pregnant. Each year, nearly 36,000 Americans die and more than 100,000 are hospitalized from complications of the flu. The premature deaths and hospitalizations could be greatly reduced by annual vaccinations. Children and teenagers with flu symptoms need bed rest and should drink lots of fluids. They should not take OTC medications containing aspirin, especially if they have a fever. Taking aspirin may cause a rare, but serious illness called Reye's syndrome. Four antiviral drugs have been approved for treatment of the flu. Treatment of individuals at high risk for complications should begin within 2 days of initial symptoms and last for 5 days. Those individuals with mild symptoms can use OTC medications.[59] (Now take the *Health Tips:* "Adolescent and Adult Immunization Quiz: What Vaccines Do YOU Need?" to determine what vaccinations you should have. Then see *FYI:* "Telling the Difference between the Common Cold and the Flu.")

Hepatitis A

Hepatitis A virus (HAV) is a self-limited, nonchronic viral infection causing inflammation of the liver. Incubation is approximately 28 days. Peak infection occurs 2 weeks before jaundice sets in or liver enzymes increase. Signs and symptoms may include jaundice, fatigue, abdominal pain, loss of appetite, nausea, diarrhea, and fever. Once a person has had HAV, she cannot get it again, and there is no long-term chronic infection. Transmission of HAV is usually spread person-to-person by putting something in the mouth that has been contaminated by the stool (feces) of a person with hepatitis A. Persons who are at risk for contracting HAV include those who have household contact with an infected person or sexual contact with an infected person, those who live in or travel to areas with increased rates of HAV, MSM, and injecting and noninjecting drug users. The best protection against HAV is vaccination. Short-term protection can occur with immune globulin if given before and within 2 weeks of coming in contact with HAV. Hand washing with soap is also a preventive measure.[60]

Nearly one-third of Americans have evidence of past infection (immunity). The number of reported cases was 1987 in 2009, about 0.6 per 100,000 cases, the lowest ever reported.[61]

Health Tip

Adolescent and Adult Immunization Quiz: What Vaccines Do YOU Need?

The CDC provides an adult immunization quiz that allows you to determine the appropriate vaccinations for yourself. The quiz can be found at www2a.cdc.gov/nip/adultImmSched. Questions are related to gender, pregnancy, birth year, lifestyle and work, and health status. Based upon your input, the CDC will provide a list of suggested vaccinations. Print the page for your health records.

FYI

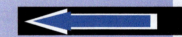

Telling the Difference between the Common Cold and the Flu

Symptoms	Common Cold	Influenza
Fever	Rare in adults and older children; may be as high as 102° F in infants and small children	Usually 102° F, but can be as high as 104° F, usually lasts for 3–4 days
Headache	Rare	Sudden onset and can be severe
Muscle aches	Mild	Usual, and often severe
Tiredness and weakness	Mild	Often extreme, and can last 2 or more weeks
Extreme exhaustion	Never	Sudden onset, and can be severe
Runny nose	Often	Sometimes
Sneezing	Often	Sometimes
Sore throat	Often	Sometimes
Cough	Mild hacking	Usual, and can be severe
Vaccination	Not at this time	Yes

SOURCE: National Institutes of Health. *Influenza.*
www.nlm.nih.gov/medlineplus/tutorials/influenza/htm/_no_50_no_0.htm

Hepatitis A Vaccination   Hepatitis A vaccine is prepared from inactivated cells and is available for children 12 months of age or older. A single dose is 94 to 100 percent effective. Immunoglobulin (Ig) is a sterile solution that induces protective antibodies in most all adults. A combined hepatitis A and hepatitis B vaccine can be administered as a three-dose series for adults 18 and older. Nearly one-third of U.S. adults have serologic evidence of previous hepatitis A infection, correlating positively with age.[60] The CDC updated the recommendations for vaccination to include all previously unvaccinated individuals who may come in close contact with international adoptees from a country with high endemic prevalence. The U.S. rate is usually 1.0 per 100,000 but can be as high as 106 per 100,000 in persons who come in contact with adoptees who are acutely infected with HAV (1–6 percent).[62] The first dose should be given 2 weeks prior to contact with an international adoptee.

Hepatitis B

Hepatitis B virus (HBV) is a viral infection causing inflammation of the liver. Transmission of HBV is similar to that of HIV, through exposure to infected blood and unprotected sexual intercourse, but HBV is more easily transmitted than HIV. In fact, HBV is a 100 times more contagious than HIV. The incubation period is 6 weeks to 6 months.[63] Persons at highest risk for contracting HBV include **hemodialysis** patients, injecting drug users, health care workers exposed to blood, infants born to HBV-positive women, gay men, and sexually active heterosexuals. Groups at highest risk for contracting HBV include Alaska Natives, Pacific Islanders, Asians, and others emigrating from high-incidence areas. International travelers to high-incidence areas may choose to receive the hepatitis B vaccine. In women, heterosexual activity is the most common risk factor, followed by injected drug use. The modes of transmission often overlooked by individuals include tattoos, ear piercing, non-medication injections of vitamins, minerals, or steroids, and acupuncture treatments.[64] HBV can be transmitted through menstrual blood or the sharing of razors, toothbrushes, or other items with blood on them. Sexually active women may reduce their risk of contracting HBV by using condoms and refraining from anal sex. The effectiveness of condoms in preventing the spread of HBV is unknown, but consistent and proper use is recommended.

Recognizing the risk factors for HBV is important; however, nearly one-half of adults with newly acquired hepatitis B have no identified risk factors. Symptoms of acute hepatitis B include **jaundice** and a tender liver upon palpation. Hepatitis B follows a predictable course through four phases: incubation, prodrome, icteric, and convalescence. The prodrome phase is characterized by generalized symptoms such as fever, fatigue, and discomfort. The icteric phase is recognized by jaundice and swelling of the liver, and the symptoms disappear during the convalescence phase.[65]

Nearly 95 percent of persons with hepatitis B recover, although a few persons develop fulminant hepatitis (acute liver failure) or experience persistent infections.

Diagnosis   The type of hepatitis can be determined only through serologic testing. Antibody and antigen presence are used to determine positive or negative results. HBsAg is evident in acute and chronic infection. Those with chronic hepatitis must have ongoing blood tests to monitor liver function and damage.[66]

Treatment   Persons with HBV should be evaluated for liver disease. Treatment is supportive for acute HBV, since no specific therapy is approved. All persons who test positive are reported to state and local health departments. Currently, five different drugs can be given to treat persons with chronic HBV. Drinking alcohol, because of its effect on the liver, can make the liver disease worse.

Hepatitis B Vaccination   The CDC recommends hepatitis B vaccine for infants, previously unvaccinated children and adolescents, and adults at increased risk for infection (including health care workers, dialysis patients, household contacts and sex partners of persons with chronic HBV infection, recipients of certain blood products, persons with a recent history of multiple sex partners or an STI, MSM, and injection-drug users). All pregnant women should be screened for HBV and immunoprophylaxis be given to infants born to infected women or to women of unknown infection status. After three intramuscular doses of hepatitis B vaccine, 90 percent of healthy adults and 95 percent of infants, children, and teenagers develop adequate antibody responses. The increased compliance with vaccination recommendations has greatly reduced the incidence of HBV, now at the lowest level of new cases since reporting to the CDC began.[67]

Epidemiology   An estimated 38,000 new cases of HBV occur each year in the United States, and about 2000–4000 infected persons will die of HBV-related complications such as fulminant hepatitis, cirrhosis, or liver cancer. The greatest decline in HBV has been among children and adolescents born since 1991 because of the vaccine. Nearly 1.4 million Americans are chronically infected with HBV, and about one-third acquired the infection during childhood. In 2009, the overall incidence of HBV reported was the lowest ever recorded, 1.5 per 100,000 population.[68]

Hepatitis C

Hepatitis C virus (HCV) is a viral infection affecting the liver. It is the most common chronic blood-borne infection in the United States. Signs and symptoms include jaundice, fatigue, dark urine, abdominal pain, loss of appetite, and nausea. The virus is transmitted through blood from an infected person. HCV is spread through sharing needles, through needle sticks or sharps exposures at work, and from an infected mother to the infant during childbirth. Persons using or injecting illegal drugs should be counseled to stop and enter an appropriate treatment program. If that does not occur, they can reduce risk by using only properly obtained needles; using new, sterile syringes; using sterile or clean water to prepare drugs; safely dispose of syringes; and properly clean the injection site before and after using a syringe.[69]

Persons at risk include injected drug users, hemodialysis patients, persons with undiagnosed liver problems, infants born to infected mothers, and health care/ public safety workers. There is no vaccine for HCV, but at-risk persons should be vaccinated for HAV and HBV. Prevention includes not using someone else's personal care items that might have blood on them (razors, toothbrushes), avoiding tattoos and body piercing or at least ensuring that all instruments have been sterilized, and following routine barrier precautions if you are a health care or public safety worker. Persons with HCV should not donate blood, organs, or tissue. High rates of coinfection with HIV are also prevalent so testing for HIV is important. Controversy persists regarding HCV transmission by sexual activity. It may be possible but is less likely than other risk behaviors.

The estimated number of HCV infections was approximately 16,000 in 2009, and most were due to the sharing of needles. Transfusion-associated cases and perinatal transfusions are relatively low. Of the estimated 3.2 million Americans who have been infected with HCV, about 2.7 million are chronically infected. Approximately 15 to 25 percent of persons who are infected will clear of the virus without treatment, although the reasons are not known. Diagnosis includes anti-HCV screening of asymptomatic persons based on risk factors. Anti-HCV positive persons should receive appropriate antiviral treatments.[70]

Tuberculosis (TB)

Tuberculosis is caused by the bacterium *Mycobacterium tuberculosis,* which usually attacks the lungs but can also attack other parts of the body such as the kidney, spine, and brain. TB, including resistant cases, is reported in every state in the United States. An estimated 10–15 million Americans are infected with *M. tuberculosis,* and about 10 percent will develop TB if intervention does not occur. Approximately 11,200 cases were reported in 2010, the lowest number recorded since reporting began in 1953. The TB bacterium is airborne, transmitted person-to-person by sneezing or coughing. It settles in the lungs, and when found in the lungs or throat, can be contagious. TB found in the kidneys, brain, or other parts of the body is usually not contagious. Latent TB infection occurs when a person has been infected, but the immune system is able to fight off the infection. The bacterium remains alive and can become active at a later time. A person with latent TB has no symptoms, is not infectious, and will usually have a positive skin test or serological test. This person will have a normal chest radiograph and sputum test. A person with latent TB may need to take medication to prevent getting TB later. If a person gets TB, it takes six months to a year of medication to kill all the TB germs.[71]

Active TB disease occurs when the immune system is unable to prevent the bacteria from multiplying. The bacteria attack and destroy tissue, and symptoms depend on where the bacteria are found. Symptoms of TB in the lungs may manifest as a bad cough that lasts 3 weeks or longer, pain in the chest, or coughing up blood or sputum. Other symptoms may include weakness and fatigue, weight loss, loss of appetite, fever, and night sweats. This person may spread TB to others, and can be diagnosed by a skin test or blood test.

Tuberculosis is a major global public health problem, particularly in low-income countries. Multidrug-resistant TB and HIV-associated TB pose challenges globally. The United States is affected by the worldwide TB epidemic as evidenced in 2010, when 60 percent of new U.S. cases occurred in persons born in other countries. The top five countries were Mexico, Philippines, Vietnam, India, and China. BCG vaccine is a widely administered vaccine in many high-incidence countries, but wide variation in vaccine efficacy, ranging from 80 percent to zero, has been found. Because of questions about efficacy and skin hypersensitivity, BCG is not routinely recommended for use in the United States.[72]

Methicillin-Resistant Staphylococcus Aureus (MRSA)

MRSA is a potentially dangerous type of staphylococcal bacterium that is resistant to certain antibiotics and may cause skin and other infections. MRSA is contracted through direct contact with an infected person or by sharing items, such as towels or razors, that have touched infected skin. Most staphylococcal skin infections, including MRSA, appear as a bump or infected area on the skin that may be red, swollen, painful, warm to the touch, full of pus or drainage, and fever.

Health Tip

Vaccine-Preventable Diseases

New vaccines are becoming available every year. The following diseases are now preventable, if persons would seek health care advice on the appropriateness of the vaccine for them.

Anthrax
Cervical cancer
Diphtheria
Hepatitis A
Hepatitis B
Haemophilus influenza type b (Hib)
Human papillomavirus (HPV)
Influenza (flu)
Japanese encephalitis (JE)
Measles
Meningococcal
Monkeypox
Mumps
Pertussis (whooping cough)
Pneumococcal
Poliomyelitis (polio)
Rabies
Rotavirus
Rubella (German measles)
Shingles (herpes zoster)
Smallpox
Tetanus (lockjaw)
Tuberculosis
Typhoid fever
Varicella (chickenpox)
Yellow fever

Check with your health care provider if you are planning to travel internationally, are planning to become pregnant, practice high-risk behaviors, live in a high-risk environment, are elderly, or are at risk for some other reason. See www.cdc.gov/vaccines/vpd-vac/default.htm for more information.

These skin infections commonly occur at sites of visible skin trauma, such as cuts and abrasions, and areas of the body covered by hair (e.g., back of neck, groin, buttock, and armpit). Most MRSA skin infections can be effectively treated by drainage of pus with or without antibiotics. More serious infections, such as pneumonia, bloodstream infections, or bone infections, are very rare in healthy people who get MRSA skin infections. Some settings have factors that make it easier for MRSA to be transmitted. These factors, referred to as the 5 Cs, are as follows: Crowding, frequent skin-to-skin Contact, Compromised skin (i.e., cuts or abrasions),

Contaminated items and surfaces, and lack of Cleanliness. The 5 Cs are commonly found in schools, dormitories, military barracks, households, correctional facilities, and daycare centers. The rates of MRSA infections in these settings continue to increase. Each year nearly one million hospital patients get infections while being treated for something else, although invasive MRSA infections decreased 28 percent from 2005 to 2008 in hospital settings. The best measure to prevent spreading infection in any setting is to practice proper hand hygiene.[73] View the CDC podcast on hand hygiene at www2a.cdc.gov/podcasts/browse.asp. When signs and symptoms of MRSA are experienced, the person should cover the area with a bandage and contact a health care professional, particularly if the signs and symptoms are accompanied by fever.

Streptococcal Disease

Group A streptococcus (GAS) is a bacterium found in the throat and on the skin. Most infections caused by GAS are relatively mild, such as "strep throat" or impetigo. Transmission is through direct contact with mucus or infected wounds or sores on the skin. Treatment with an antibiotic for 24 hours or longer will generally eliminate the spread of the bacteria in mild cases. In rare situations, the bacteria can get into the blood, muscle, or lungs and cause severe or life-threatening diseases such as necrotizing fasciitis or streptococcal toxic shock syndrome (STSS). STSS is not the same as toxic shock syndrome (from tampon use). Good hand washing is the best preventive measure against streptococcal disease, especially after coughing and sneezing and before food preparation and eating.[74]

Group B strep is the most common cause of life-threatening infection in newborns. One in five women carries group B streptococcal bacteria in her body, usually in the intestine, vagina, or rectum. While women who carry the bacteria are often asymptomatic, transmission through childbirth can cause sepsis, meningitis, or pneumonia in the newborn. CDC guidelines recommend that pregnant women be tested for group B strep at 35–37 weeks. If they test positive, they are given antibiotics at the time of delivery. This standardized protocol has dramatically reduced the number of cases in newborns, by more than 50 percent in some places.

In adults, group B strep can range from no symptoms to mild symptoms (e.g., urinary tract or bladder infections) to serious diseases (e.g., pneumonia, bloodstream disorders). The elderly are particularly vulnerable. Group B strep infections are diagnosed by culture tests and are treated with penicillin or other common antibiotics.[75]

Varicella (Chickenpox and Shingles)

Varicella is an acute, contagious disease caused by varicella zoster virus, a member of the herpes virus group. Primary infection manifests as chickenpox, after an incubation period of around 14–21 days. Symptoms include a rash of blister-like skin eruptions, fever, and fatigue. The virus is spread by coughing, sneezing, or contact with lesions. Prior to the introduction of a vaccine in 1995, nearly 4 million cases of chickenpox were reported every year, with 11,000–13,500 hospitalizations and 100–150 deaths. Since that time, three vaccines have been approved for vaccination against chicken pox. Varicella vaccine is 98 percent effective in preventing disease when two doses are administered. Immunity persists for more than 20 years. Vaccination is recommended for all children without an underlying condition or factor that increases the risk of complications. Nearly 89 percent of children are vaccinated and the annual death total is less than 10. The vaccination protects not only the young child but also the adult who has not been vaccinated nor had chickenpox as a child. The vaccination program has resulted in dramatic reductions in hospitalizations and deaths.[76]

Latent varicella infection, herpes zoster or shingles, occurs when the virus reactivates and causes a recurrent disease, usually in older adults. The risk of shingles is more common after age 50. A vaccine for shingles was *approved* in 2006. The vaccine is recommended for adults 60 years or older. Shingles can cause numbness, itching, or severe pain followed by clusters of blister-like lesions. Pain can persist for weeks, months, or years, and persons with shingles can be contagious to others who have not had chickenpox.[77]

Encephalitis

Arboviruses are a leading cause of viral encephalitis worldwide. In the United States, St. Louis encephalitis, Eastern and Western equine encephalitis, LaCrosse virus, and West Nile virus are transmitted by mosquitoes to humans. Symptoms can range from fever with headaches to temporary paralysis, seizures that occur despite treatment, coma, and death, depending on the strain.

West Nile virus is a seasonal epidemic in the United States that occurs in the summer through fall months. One in 150 infected persons will develop severe illness, including high fever, headache, neck stiffness, coma, tremors, convulsions, muscle weakness, loss of vision,

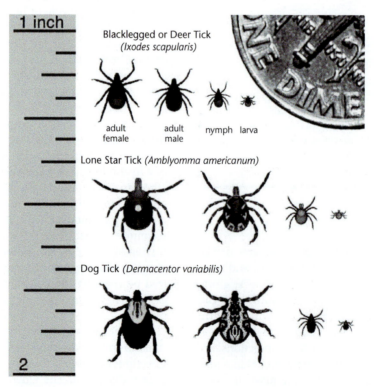

Comparison of ticks by appearance and relative size. Only deer ticks (*Ixodes scapularis*) are known to transmit Lyme disease.

SOURCE: www.cdc.gov/ncidod/dvbid/lyme/ld_transmission.htm (retrieved August 10, 2006).

or paralysis. Nearly 20 percent of infected persons will have some symptoms, but nearly 80 percent will show no symptoms at all.

Mosquito control is the primary method of preventing the spread of encephalitis and West Nile virus. This involves avoiding outside activities at dawn and dusk, using insect repellent and wearing long sleeves and pants, draining areas where pooled water allows mosquito larvae to incubate, and keeping windows closed or ensuring that screens are free from tears or holes. Persons over age 50 are at greater risk for severe illness, and those who spend a lot of time outdoors have a greater chance of contracting the virus.[78]

Lyme Disease

Lyme disease is caused by a bacterium transmitted by the bite of infected blacklegged (or deer) tick. Typical symptoms include fever, headache, and fatigue, and the first sign is usually a circular rash called erythema migrans at the site of the tick bite. The rash gradually expands over a period of several days, reaching up to 12 inches across. Untreated, the infection spreads to other body parts within a few days to weeks, producing a variety of symptoms. Later symptoms can include Bell's palsy (loss of muscle control in the face), shooting pains, heart palpitations, dizziness, and pain that moves from joint to joint. Many symptoms resolve, even without treatment, but for some people, chronic neurological complaints can persist. Early treatment is usually antibiotics, and most treatments are successful. In 2009, Lyme disease was the fifth most common nationally notifiable disease. Nearly 22,561 confirmed cases and 7,397 probable cases of Lyme disease were reported in 2010 in the United States, with the majority of cases on the East Coast and in the upper Midwest. In fact, 94 percent of cases were reported in 12 states in 2010: Connecticut, Delaware, Maine, Maryland, Massachusetts, Minnesota, New Jersey, New Hampshire, New York, Pennsylvania, Virginia, and Wisconsin. Prevention of Lyme disease includes using insect repellent, removing ticks promptly, and avoiding unnecessary exposure to areas that are infested with ticks during late spring and summer.[79]

Chapter Summary

- Nearly fifty STI-related organisms and syndromes are recognized today.
- The United States has one of the highest STI rates of the industrialized countries.
- Teenagers account for 25 percent of all STIs.
- Chlamydia is the most frequently reported infectious disease in the United States and must be reported to the CDC by all fifty states.
- Chlamydia is treated with antibiotics, either in a 7-day or single-dose regimen.
- The number of cases of gonorrhea has declined since the 1970s except in teenagers and some minority groups. A large discrepancy in cases exists between African American and white teenagers.
- Syphilis is caused by the spirochete *Treponema pallidum*.
- Syphilis has four phases: primary, secondary, latent, and tertiary. Congenital syphilis is transmitted to the infant during pregnancy.
- Genital herpes is incurable and difficult to control. Acyclovir has some effectiveness in preventing a herpes outbreak.
- Several types of human papilloma viruses (genital warts) are associated with cancer. HPV vaccine is recommended for girls ages 9–26.
- Hepatitis B is a viral infection causing inflammation of the liver. HBV is transmitted through exposure to infected blood and unprotected sexual intercourse. There is a vaccine to prevent HAV and HBV.
- Pelvic inflammatory disease causes chronic pelvic pain, infertility, and ectopic pregnancies.
- Most vaginitis is classified as trichomoniasis, bacterial vaginosis, or candidiasis.
- AIDS is the fifth leading cause of death in women between the ages of 25 and 44, the third leading cause of death in African American women between the ages of 15 and 44, and the fourth leading cause of death in Hispanic women ages 35–44.
- Invasive cervical cancer has been added to the list of AIDS-defining diseases. Invasive cervical cancer can be prevented with early detection.
- Epstein-Barr virus is a member of the herpes virus family. Ninety-five percent of healthy people carry the virus in their saliva.
- The peak flu season in the United States is late December through March. The flu shot and nasal-spray flu vaccine are available in the United States.
- Nearly 1 million hospital patients are infected with MRSA while being treated for something else. Hand hygiene is an important deterrent.
- Strep A and strep B are bacterial infections that can have serious complications.
- West Nile virus and encephalitis are transmitted by mosquitoes to humans.
- Lyme disease is transmitted by the blacklegged (or deer) tick.

Review Questions

1. Which STI has the highest incidence rate? What complications are associated with this STI?
2. Describe the four stages of syphilis.
3. What are the demographic characteristics that make a person more susceptible to STIs and/or HIV/AIDS?
4. Which individuals and groups are most susceptible to hepatitis B virus?
5. What complications can occur when pelvic inflammatory disease remains untreated?
6. What is the importance of the window period for determining the presence of HIV antibodies?
7. What are the known modes of transmission of HIV?
8. What measures can you take to prevent AIDS and other STIs?
9. Which STIs have vaccines available to prevent the disease?
10. Which STIs have antibiotics available to cure the disease?
11. Which infectious diseases have the most potential to lead to pandemics?
12. Which infectious diseases are most likely to impact college-age students?

Resources

Organizations and Hotlines

American Social Health Association
919-361-8400
www.ashastd.org/index.cfm

CDC National Prevention Information Network (NPIN)
800-458-5231
www.cdcnpin.org

CDC National AIDS Clearinghouse
1-800-458-5231
TTY: 1-800-243-1098
International: 1-404-679-3860
Monday–Friday, 9:00 A.M.–6:00 P.M. (Eastern)

National Herpes Hotline
919-361-8488
Monday–Friday, 9:00 A.M.–6:00 P.M. (Eastern)

National Institute of Allergy and Infectious Diseases
866-284-4107
www.niaid.nih.gov

National STD Hotline
1-800-232-4636
TTY: 1-888-232-6348

National Women's Health Resource Center
877-986-9472
www.healthywomen.org

Planned Parenthood Federation of America
800-230-PLAN
www.plannedparenthood.org

Sexuality Information and Education Council of the United States (SIECUS)
202-265-2405
www.siecus.org

Travelers' Health Information
1-800-232-4636
wwwnc.cdc.gov/travel

References

1. Centers for Disease Control and Prevention. Summary of notifiable diseases United States, 2009. *MMWR* 2009; 58 (No. 53): 3.
2. Centers for Disease Control and Prevention. 2006. *Elements of successful HIV/AIDS prevention programs.* http://www.cdcnpin.org/scripts/hiv/programs.asp
3. Centers for Disease Control and Prevention. 2010. *Sexually transmitted diseases treatment guidelines.* 59 (No. RR-12): 3.
4. Centers for Disease Control and Prevention. 2010. *Sexually transmitted diseases treatment guidelines.* 59 (No. RR-12): 44–9.
5. Ibid.
6. Ibid.
7. Ibid.
8. Ibid.
9. Ibid.
10. Centers for Disease Control and Prevention. 2000. *Tracking the hidden epidemic: Trends in STDS in the United States.* http://www.cdc.gov/nchstp/dstd/Stats_Trends/STD_Trends.pdf
11. Centers for Disease Control and Prevention. 2011. *Gonorrhea – CDC Fact Sheet.* http://www.cdc.gov/std/gonorrhea/stdfact-gonorrhea.htm

12. Centers for Disease Control and Prevention. 2010. *Sexually transmitted diseases treatment guidelines.* 59 (No. RR-12): 49–6.

13. Centers for Disease Control and Prevention. 2011. *Sexually transmitted disease surveillance 2010.* Atlanta: U.S. Department of Health and Human Services.

14. Centers for Disease Control and Prevention. 2010. *Sexually transmitted diseases treatment guidelines.* 59 (No. RR-12): 49–6.

15. Centers for Disease Control and Prevention. 2011. *Syphilis – CDC Fact Sheet.* http://www.cdc.gov/std/syphilis/STDFact-Syphilis.htm

16. Ibid.

17. Ibid.

18. Centers for Disease Control and Prevention. 2010. *Sexually transmitted diseases treatment guidelines.* 59 (No. RR-12): 26–0.

19. Ibid.

20. Ibid.

21. Centers for Disease Control and Prevention. 2011. *Sexually transmitted disease surveillance 2010.* Atlanta: U.S. Department of Health and Human Services.

22. Centers for Disease Control and Prevention. 2010. *Sexually transmitted diseases treatment guidelines.* 59 (No. RR-12): 19–20.

23. Centers for Disease Control and Prevention. 2012. *Genital herpes.* http://www.cdc.gov/std/Herpes/default.htm

24. Centers for Disease Control and Prevention. 2010. *Sexually transmitted diseases treatment guidelines.* 59 (No. RR-12): 20–5.

25. Centers for Disease Control and Prevention. 2012. *Genital herpes.* http://www.cdc.gov/std/Herpes/default.htm

26. Centers for Disease Control and Prevention. 2010. *Sexually transmitted diseases treatment guidelines,* 59 (No. RR-12): 69–74.

27. Centers for Disease Control and Prevention. 2011. *Sexually transmitted disease surveillance 2010.* Atlanta: U.S. Department of Health and Human Services.

28. Ibid.

29. Centers for Disease Control and Prevention. 2012. *Genital HPV infection – Fact sheet.* http://www.cdc.gov/std/HPV/STDFact-HPV.htm

30. Ibid

31. Centers for Disease Control and Prevention. 2010. *Sexually transmitted diseases treatment guidelines.* 59 (No. RR-12): 69–74.

32. Ibid.

33. National Cancer Institute. 2011. *Human papillomavirus (HPV) vaccines.* http://www.cancer.gov/cancertopics/factsheet/prevention/HPV-vaccine

34. Ibid.

35. Centers for Disease Control and Prevention. 2011. *Sexually transmitted disease surveillance 2010.* Atlanta: U.S. Department of Health and Human Services.

36. Centers for Disease Control and Prevention. 2010. *Bacterial vaginosis – CDC Fact sheet.* http://www.cdc.gov/std/bv/STDFact-Bacterial-Vaginosis.htm

37. Centers for Disease Control and Prevention. 2011. *Trichomoniasis – CDC Fact sheet.* http://www.cdc.gov/std/trichomonas/STDFact-Trichomoniasis.htm

38. Centers for Disease Control and Prevention. 2010. *Sexually transmitted diseases treatment guidelines.* 59 (No. RR-12): 58–61.

39. Centers for Disease Control and prevention. 2010. *Sexually transmitted diseases treatment guidelines.* 59 (No. RR-12): 61–3.

40. Centers for Disease Control and Prevention. 2011. *Pelvic inflammatory disease – CDC Fact sheet.* http://www.cdc.gov/std/PID/STDFact-PID.htm

41. Centers for Disease Control and prevention. 2010. *Sexually transmitted diseases treatment guidelines.* 59 (No. RR-12): 43–4.

42. Centers for Disease Control and Prevention. 2011. *HIV among women.* http://www.cdc.gov/hiv/topics/women/index.htm

43. World Health Organization. 2011. *Global HIV response: 2011 Progress report update.* http://www.who.int/hiv/pub/progress_report2011/summary_en.pdf

44. National Institutes of Health. 2011. *HIV infection.* http://www.nlm.nih.gov/medlineplus/ency/article/000602.htm

45. Food and Drug Administration. 2009. *Testing yourself for HIV-1 questions and answers.* http://www.fda.gov/BiologicsBloodVaccines/SafetyAvailability/HIVHomeTestKits/ucm126460.htm

46. Ibid.

47. National Institute of Allergy and Infectious Diseases. 2011. *Treatment of HIV infections.* http://www.niaid.nih.gov/topics/HIVAIDS/Understanding/Treatment/Pages/default.aspx

48. World Health Organization. 2011. *Global HIV response: 2011 Progress report update.* http://www.who.int/hiv/pub/progress_report2011/summary_en.pdf

49. National Institute of Allergy and Infectious Diseases. 2011. *Treatment of HIV infections.*

50. Bailey, J. V., et al. 2004. Sexually transmitted infections in women who have sex with women. *Sexually Transmitted Infections* 80: 244–6.

51. Adapted from American College Health Association. 2006. *Safer sex.*

52. Centers for Disease Control and Prevention. 2010. *Sexually transmitted diseases treatment guidelines.* 59 (No. RR-12): 5.

53. Ibid., p. 6.

54. Ibid., p. 45.

55. National Institute of Allergy and Infectious Diseases. 2009. *HIV/AIDS.* http://www.niaid.nih.gov/topics/HIVAIDS/Research/prevention/Pages/intervention.aspx

56. Centers for Disease Control and Prevention. *Epstein-Barr virus and infectious mononucleosis.* http://www.cdc.gov/ncidod/diseases/ebv.htm

57. WebMD. 2009. *Epstein-Barr virus Linked to MS.* http://www.webmd.com/multiple-sclerosis/news/20090504/epstein-barr-virus-linked-to-ms

58. Centers for Disease Control and Prevention. 2011. *Key Facts about influenza (flu) and flu vaccine.* http://www.cdc.gov/flu/keyfacts.htm

59. Ibid.

60. Centers for Disease Control and Prevention. *Hepatitis A vaccine.* http://www.cdc.gov/vaccines/pubs/vis/downloads/vis-hep-a.pdf

61. Ibid.

62. National Library of Medicine. 2010. *Hepatitis B.* http://www.ncbi.nlm.nih.gov/pubmedhealth/PMH0001324/

63. Centers for Disease Control and Prevention. 2010. *Hepatitis B: General information.* http://www.cdc.gov/hepatitis/HBV/PDFs/HepBGeneralFactSheet.pdf

64. National Library of Medicine. 2010. *Hepatitis B.* http://www.ncbi.nlm.nih.gov/pubmedhealth/PMH0001324/

65. Ibid.

66. Ibid.

67. Centers for Disease Control and Prevention. 2012. *Hepatitis B vaccination.* http://www.cdc.gov/hepatitis/HBV/HBVfaq.htm#-

68. Centers for Disease Control and Prevention. 2012. *Overview and statistics.* http://www.cdc.gov/hepatitis/HBV/HBVfaq.htm#a2

69. National Library of Medicine. 2010. *Hepatitis C.* http://www.ncbi.nlm.nih.gov/pubmedhealth/PMH0001329/

70. Centers for Disease Control and Prevention. 2012. *Overview and statistics.* http://www.cdc.gov/hepatitis/HCV/HCVfaq.htm#section1

71. Centers for Disease Control and Prevention. 2011. *Tuberculosis facts.* http://www.cdc.gov/tb/publications/factseries/prevention_eng.htm

72. Centers for Disease Control and Prevention. 2011. *Trends in tuberculosis, 2010.* http://www.cdc.gov/tb/publications/factsheets/statistics/TBTrends.htm

73. Centers for Disease Control and Prevention. 2011. *Methicillin-resistant Staphylococcus aureus (MRSA) infections.* http://www.cdc.gov/mrsa/index.html

74. Centers for Disease Control and Prevention. 2011. *Group A streptococcal (GAS) disease.* http://www.cdc.gov/ncidod/dbmd/diseaseinfo/groupastreptococcal_g.htm

75. Centers for Disease Control and Prevention. 2011. *Group B strep (GBS).* http://www.cdc.gov/groupbstrep/about/index.html

76. Centers for Disease Control and Prevention. 2011. *Chickenpox (varicella).* http://www.cdc.gov/chickenpox/index.html

77. Centers for Disease Control and Prevention. 2011. *Shingles (herpes zoster).* http://www.cdc.gov/shingles/

78. National Library of Medicine. 2010. *Encephalitis.* http://www.ncbi.nlm.nih.gov/pubmedhealth/PMH0002388/

79. Centers for Disease Control and Prevention. 2011. *Lyme disease.* http://www.cdc.gov/lyme/

Preventing and Controlling Chronic Health Conditions

CHAPTER OBJECTIVES

When you complete this chapter, you will be able to do the following:

◇ Describe how the cardiovascular system functions

◇ Differentiate among the types of heart disease

◇ Compare and contrast the various chronic conditions

◇ Determine risk factors for heart disease and other chronic conditions

◇ Describe ways to increase the protective factors that prevent heart disease and other chronic conditions

◇ Compare the early warning signals for heart disease and other chronic conditions

◇ Explain the current treatment protocols for heart disease and other chronic conditions

INACTION IS UNACCEPTABLE

Chronic diseases, including heart disease, cancer, type 2 diabetes, and stroke, are largely preventable. Nearly 80 percent of heart disease, stroke, and type 2 diabetes, and 40 percent of all cancers are related to lifestyle choices, impacting low- and middle-class families disproportionately. Obesity, sedentary lifestyles, and choosing to use tobacco are the major lifestyle risk factors identified as contributing to chronic diseases. The myth that chronic diseases occur in rich people in rich countries must be dispelled. The preponderance of chronic diseases occur in poor or middle-class people in all countries. Modifying or eliminating lifestyle risk factors requires governments to assume some responsibility for supporting healthy eating, increased physical activity, and non-smoking. Governments can do more to provide easy access and resources for purchasing fresh fruits and vegetables, can provide safe and accessible exercise areas, and can control or eliminate tobacco products.

Heart disease is the leading cause of all deaths worldwide. In the United States, chronic diseases account for 88 percent of all deaths, approximately 2.1 million people a year.[1] The National Center for Chronic Disease Prevention and Health Promotion leads the American effort in preventing and controlling chronic diseases. Check out the Centers for Disease Control and Prevention (CDC)'s chronic disease cost calculator that provides estimates of each state's Medicaid spending related to treating six chronic diseases: congestive heart failure, heart disease, stroke, hypertension, cancer, and diabetes.[2]

The next two chapters address the major chronic diseases, heart disease and cancer, and several familiar chronic diseases that women are particularly interested in knowing more about. The key to reducing the mortality and morbidity of chronic diseases is prevention, and this is made possible by governments and individuals taking action to save and improve the lives of the citizens. This chapter discusses strategies for preventing and managing chronic diseases, because inaction is unacceptable.

THE LEADING CAUSE OF DEATH IN WOMEN

Public awareness has come a long way since the days when men received nearly all the media, medical, and research attention concerning heart disease. The Framingham Heart Study, a landmark longitudinal study of heart disease that began in 1948, initially focused on premature heart disease and fatal heart attacks that occurred mainly in men. These researchers did not discover until decades later that, compared to men, women died in equal numbers from coronary heart disease (CHD); they just developed heart disease 10 or more years later than men! So, by age 65, the number of deaths from ischemic (restricted blood supply) heart disease is actually higher in women.

The first conference related to women's heart health, sponsored by the American Heart Association, was held in 1964. Its main focus was *how women could help protect their husbands' hearts.* It isn't surprising that the focus was on husbands because heart research often studied only male subjects, and when females were included, they were underrepresented. The findings and recommendations of heart research involving men were then projected to include women. Not recognizing the impact of heart disease in women was an unfortunate mistake. Women's warning signs and symptoms were taken less seriously than men's, treatment was less aggressive, and research on heart disease was limited in number or excluded women altogether. Clinical trials often excluded women because researchers worried about conducting tests on women of childbearing age. They thought that hormonal fluctuations in these women would influence drug trials, and if they unknowingly became pregnant, drug exposure might harm the fetus. Women over age 65 with heart disease and other health problems were often excluded in clinical trials because of researchers' concerns that their illnesses might produce inaccurate results. Today, U.S. women surpass men in the number of deaths related to heart disease.

Cardiovascular disease (CVD)—which includes CHD, high blood pressure (BP), heart failure, and stroke—accounts for one in three deaths or nearly one death every 39 seconds. CVD costs more than any other diagnostic group of diseases. The total direct and indirect costs of CVD in the United States are estimated at $297.7 billion in 2008 compared to cancer, with an estimated cost of $228 billion.[3] By 2020, the U.S. Public Health Service has set a goal to improve cardiovascular health of all Americans by 20 percent, while reducing deaths from cardiovascular diseases and stroke by 20 percent. This goal is challenging, given the increases in obesity and sedentary behavior over the past 30 years. For instance, the prevalence of obesity in children ages 6–11 increased from about 4 percent to 20 percent during this time frame. Today, 67.3 percent of adults age 20 and older are overweight or obese, with 33.7 percent classified as obese. Women's total energy consumption between 1971 and 2004 increased 22 percent, from 1542 to 1886 kcal/d. And the prevalence of metabolic syndrome, a cluster of major cardiovascular risk factors related to overweight/obesity and insulin resistance, has reached 32.6 percent among women.[4] The American Heart Association uses seven metrics for ideal cardiovascular health. Figure 15.1 shows how U.S. adults fared on the seven metrics as determined from NHANES data from 2007 to 2008.[5] How will U.S. adults fare between 2012 and 2020? What are you doing to reach the ideal status by achieving all seven metrics?

CARDIOVASCULAR DISEASES

Normal Cardiovascular Functioning

The **cardiovascular system** includes the heart and blood vessels. The heart is a four-chamber pump composed of cardiac muscle. This muscular pump sends blood throughout the body from early conception until death. The heart is located in the middle of the chest, behind the sternum, and is about the size of a clenched

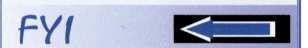

Coronary Arteries

The heart muscle has arteries to provide oxygen to itself. These arteries are the right coronary, the left anterior descending, and the left circumflex. The right coronary artery nourishes the back of the heart. The left anterior descending artery nourishes the front part of the heart. The left circumflex nourishes the side of the heart. Smaller coronary arteries called collateral arteries connect to larger arteries and help nourish the heart and may replace the function of larger arteries if they malfunction. Collateral vessels grow and enlarge in some individuals and act as alternative routes of blood flow when larger arteries are obstructed, causing myocardial ischemia (reduced blood flow to the muscular tissue of the heart). While women's hearts tend to be smaller than men's because of smaller body size, their coronary arteries may or may not be smaller than men's. The myth that coronary arteries are always smaller in women has resulted in some women not getting coronary bypass surgery when it was needed.

FIGURE 15.1 Age standardized prevalence estimates for poor, intermediate, and ideal cardiovascular health for each of the 7 metrics of cardiovascular health in the American Heart Association 2020 goals, among United States adults aged ≥ 20 years, National Health and Nutrition Examination Survey (NHANES) 2007-2008 (available data as of June 1, 2011).

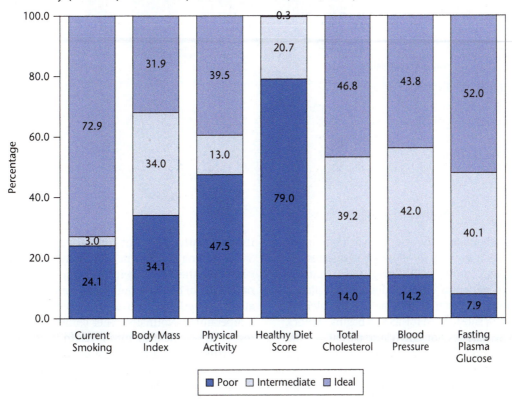

fist. In general, a woman's heart is smaller than a man's because the size of the heart is proportional to the size of the body. The two upper chambers, called atria, receive blood. The right atrium receives deoxygenated blood from all parts of the body, and the left atrium receives oxygenated blood from the lungs. The two lower chambers, called ventricles, send blood. The right ventricle pumps deoxygenated blood into the lungs, and the left ventricle pumps oxygenated blood to the entire body. The blood in the heart passes through valves that separate these chambers. The opening and closing of the valves (tricuspid, pulmonic, mitral, and aortic) cause the familiar pumping sound heard in a stethoscope. If these valves fail to function properly, blood may flow back into a chamber and cause a murmur.

The Vascular System The vascular system is composed of arteries, veins, capillaries, arterioles, and venules. The **arteries** carry blood away from the heart and are larger closest to the heart. (See *FYI:* "Coronary Arteries.") As the arteries move farther from the heart, they become the arterioles that feed the **capillaries**. The capillaries filter the blood, taking food and oxygen from the arterioles and sending waste products and carbon

dioxide to the venules. The venules carry blood into increasingly larger **veins** as blood flows to the heart.

Types of Heart Disease

The development of heart disease and the progression of atherosclerosis are influenced by a number of factors, including genetic predisposition, gender, race, advancing age, and lifestyle choices. CHD develops gradually as narrowing of the coronary vessels causes changes in the blood flow to the heart. The changes to the coronary vessels evolve into lesions that further obstruct blood flow. Initially, partial obstruction of a major vessel or its branches may occur. However, over time, a blood clot from somewhere above the obstruction may break free and lodge in the obstruction, thus causing a total blockage of the vessel.

Atherosclerosis **Atherosclerosis** is a gradual thickening and hardening of artery walls caused by a complicated process starting in childhood. The process begins with inner vessel wall (endothelium) injury and ends with a buildup of fatty deposits that harden over time. Although heredity is often implicated, the primary factor is excess cholesterol circulating in the bloodstream. When

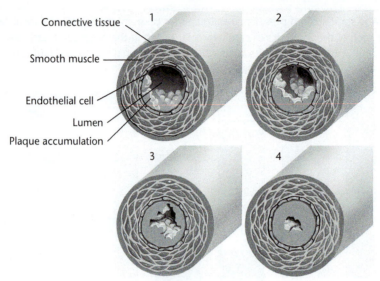

Connective tissue
Smooth muscle
Endothelial cell
Lumen
Plaque accumulation

Progression of atherosclerosis.

excess cholesterol bombards the arteries over a prolonged period, several reactions may develop: fat permeates the tissue macrophages, artery walls break down, muscle tissue is replaced with less elastic material, and plaque (accumulated fats, cholesterol, cellular debris, calcium, platelets, and other substances) forms and begins to block the artery.[6] These plaques not only cause partial or total obstructions to blood flow but they can rupture, causing a blood clot (thrombus) to break off and travel to other parts of the body. A traveling blood clot is known as an embolus and can cause a heart attack, stroke, pulmonary embolism, or gangrene, depending on where it lodges.

The primary risk factors for developing atherosclerosis are dietary intake of saturated fatty acids, elevation of systemic BP, cigarette smoking, and glucose intolerance. Other factors include diabetes, obesity, sedentary lifestyle, stress, hormone therapy, and heavy alcohol consumption. Women with sleep apnea have a higher risk of developing atherosclerosis. Sleep apnea is a disorder in which a woman stops breathing or has very shallow breathing. Untreated sleep apnea can increase the risk of having high BP, obesity, diabetes, heart attack, or stroke.[7] Tobacco smoke, whether mainstream or secondary, greatly worsens and speeds up the process of atherosclerosis in coronary and other arteries of the body.

Angina Pectoris

Chest pain is a common complaint heard by health care providers. **Angina**, from a Greek word that means "to strangle," describes a cluster of symptoms associated with oxygen deprivation. All attacks of angina begin as **ischemia** of the working heart muscle, forcing the heart to work in an anaerobic state (i.e., in the absence of oxygen). Chemical substances accumulate in the anaerobic state, and these substances are believed to initiate the pain associated with angina.

Older women in particular appear to have a higher incidence of angina than men, and for many, it may be the first warning sign of coronary artery disease (CAD). Stable angina (or chronic) is usually predictable and occurs when there is oxygen deprivation due to blockage or narrowing of one or more of the heart's arteries. It is initiated by physical exertion, strong emotions, or extreme temperatures. Normally, relief comes within minutes of rest or use of the drug nitroglycerin. Unstable angina results when the heart does not get enough oxygen, often because atherosclerosis blocks or constricts a portion of the artery. It usually occurs at rest, and the discomfort is usually more severe and prolonged. Prinzmetal's (variant) angina is a type of unstable angina caused by a coronary artery spasm near the atherosclerotic blockage. It usually occurs at rest and typically between midnight and 8 A.M.

Angina is *not* a heart attack, and once the pain passes (usually in less than a minute) blood returns to the heart muscle and the cells function normally. Angina manifests as a feeling of heaviness, squeezing, pressure, or burning in the chest, with pain radiating into the back, jaw, neck, and stomach and sometimes into the inner part of the left arm. Feelings of suffocation and impending death are quite common. Other symptoms include cold sweat, nausea, or light-headedness. Women who experience angina often exhibit signs dissimilar to typical angina symptoms. In fact, the signs are often more subtle in women than in men and can be very confusing. Women frequently experience inconsequential chest pains and fleeting rhythm disturbances when they are young. Therefore, they may be more likely to mistake angina for heartburn, gastric disorders, asthma, allergies, and bronchitis because they mimic the symptoms of angina. Some women describe a feeling of weakness and unusual fatigue. However angina manifests itself, women need to inform their health care provider when they experience chest pain.

A condition known as silent ischemia occurs when the heart is deprived of oxygen. A woman may not know she has this condition because she does not sense the typical symptoms of angina. Silent ischemia is most common in diabetics, particularly those who suffer from a sensory disturbance (not feeling body sensations). Silent ischemia that ends in tissue death is considered a silent myocardial infarction, or heart attack.

Angina is *not* a minor symptom and should be taken seriously by a woman and her health care provider. Although nearly 80 percent of angina pains will not develop into heart attacks, these pains may be a precursor to heart disease and may precede a full-blown heart attack. The factors that may reduce or control angina include quitting smoking; exercising regularly and managing weight; avoiding high altitudes and cold air; avoiding excessive alcohol, salt, or heavy meals; and decreasing emotional stress and physical exertion.[8]

Too often, women tend to ignore their chest pain and do not have it checked by the health care provider. The primary objectives for treatment of angina are to improve coronary blood flow and to reduce the amount of oxygen needed by the heart. Health care providers may prescribe nitroglycerin, beta blockers, calcium antagonists, or antiplatelet agents such as aspirin for ischemic heart disease.

Surgical procedures such as **coronary artery bypass grafting** (CABG) and percutaneous coronary intervention (PCI), formerly known as coronary angioplasty (PTCA), are designed to increase coronary blood flow. In PCI, a small tube (catheter) is used to access the heart and major blood vessels, usually through the femoral artery in the groin area. Under radiographic guidance, the catheter is threaded from the puncture site in the groin to the heart where the blocked coronary artery is opened using a balloon at the end of the catheter. Previously, many women sustained complications during angioplasty from tears to the arteries caused by the large balloons used to expand the collapsed artery. Today's smaller and finer balloons have improved the prognosis for women. Newer techniques include laser angioplasty, a procedure to vaporize the plaque, and atherectomy, a procedure to remove plaque from arteries by grinding it away. These procedures are typically followed by a stent procedure (use of a wire mesh tube, or stent, to prop open an artery) and can be done in conjunction with angioplasty. In CABG, the internal mammary artery or segments from the saphenous vein (leg) are used to bypass the obstructed coronary artery.[9] Transmyocardial revascularization has been used for those who had severe angina but who were not candidates for bypass surgery or PCI. This procedure involves exposing the heart through an incision on the left chest and using a laser to "drill" 20 to 40 holes from the outside of the heart into the ventricle.

Myocardial Infarction When **myocardial infarction (MI)** occurs, blood flow to the affected heart area ceases. This condition is commonly created when a moving blood clot (embolus) lodges in a coronary vessel and causes complete occlusion of the vessel. Occlusion occurs at a point where the vessel is too small for the clot to pass through. The heart tissue normally served by this vessel begins to experience almost immediate ischemia, and tissue death occurs unless collateral vessels provide the needed oxygen.

Angina pain occurs immediately and intensely in most MI cases. The difference between angina and MI is that the pain with MI cannot be alleviated by drugs because the tissue is depleted of blood flow. Some tissue

Health Tips

Warning Signs of a Heart Attack[10]

Women often experience more vague symptoms than men when it comes to heart attacks. Knowing the possible warning signs of a potential heart attack is important. Every minute counts. Remember: *Don't wait.* Women tend to delay seeking treatment, a dangerous choice.

Chest pain or discomfort
Uncomfortable pressure, fullness, squeezing in the center of the chest
Shortness of breath
Nausea or vomiting
Unusual fatigue
Spreading pain in the back, stomach, or abdomen
Neck or jaw pain
Cold sweats
Light-headedness (feelings of fainting)

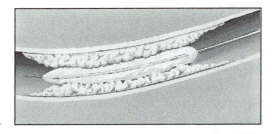

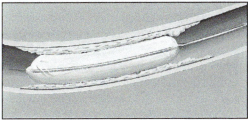

Angioplasty. (A) "balloon" is surgically inserted into the narrowed coronary artery. (B) The balloon is inflated, compressing plaque and fatty deposits against the artery walls.

death occurs with all MIs, but the extent of damage is dependent on the size and location of the artery supplying oxygen and the degree to which the tissue area remains deprived of oxygen. If collateral arteries are present, they can aid in supplying oxygen to tissue after an MI, thus reducing infarct size.

Regardless of age and treatment, MI is often more lethal for women than for men. Women are more likely to die within a year of the first heart attack or to have a second MI within 6 years. Studies continue to indicate that gender gaps still exist in the diagnosing and treatment of women with heart disease. Women who experience a more severe type of heart attack have been found to have persistently higher death rates than men with the same MI. Recent findings suggest that women's heart attacks get treated less aggressively with recommended medicines or procedures than men, or it takes them longer to receive them. Unfortunately, women themselves tend to wait longer than men in seeking medical assistance when having symptoms of a heart attack.[11] (See *Health Tip:* "Warning Signs of a Heart Attack.")

Congenital Heart Disease Congenital heart disease describes a structural problem in the heart that occurs during the development of the baby's heart before birth. A second type of heart disease, acquired, develops during childhood. Approximately thirty-five heart defects have been identified, including holes in the wall of the heart or blood vessels and problems with heart valves, the development of the heart, and the placement or development of the blood vessels near the heart. According to the American Heart Association (AHA), at least 8 of every 1000 infants born each year have a heart defect. In the United States, approximately 35,000 babies are born each year with cardiovascular defects, most of which can be helped by surgery even when the defect is severe.[12]

Advances in medical treatment have dramatically altered the outlook for children with congenital heart disease. Many who previously would have died as children can expect to live a full adult life. About 1 million Americans alive today have congenital heart defects.[13] In the United States, the number of women living with congenital heart disease is growing. These women need health care providers who understand the nuances of this disease. Many had surgery as children but did not recover completely. Thus, as adults, they face the possibility of long-term medical surveillance and further treatment.

It is important for adults with congenital heart disease to seek medical professionals who specialize in the treatment of their disease because congenital heart defects in adults are not common. Increasing numbers of specialty centers are being formed as the need for them increases. Adolescents face problems such as scars and chronic illness and have to deal with questions about types of exercise, sexual activity, type of contraception,

and so on. The levels of physical activity and exercise are individualized for people with heart defects. These levels are dependent on the type and severity of the heart defect and can be determined by a cardiologist with the aid of tests such as echocardiogram, Holter monitor, or exercise test. According to the AHA, most people with heart defects can work in virtually any occupation, but if a person's heart condition has a high risk for fainting or dizziness, safety may be a consideration when choosing an appropriate job.

Young women with congenital heart disease have further considerations. Menarche occurs slightly later in adolescents with congenital heart disease, especially in women who are cyanotic (blue) from insufficient oxygen. Women with cyanosis are also more likely to have irregular menstrual periods. If women with heart defects are considering whether to have children, they need adequate counseling for family planning. Although many women with heart defects can have successful pregnancies, they should still discuss this with their cardiologist before becoming pregnant. In some cases, pregnancy may not be recommended.

Pregnancy for women taking anticoagulants (drugs that prevent clotting) as a result of their heart disease will require special consideration from the health care provider. Adjustments in their medication will probably need to be made during the pregnancy. The changes in a woman's body, especially in the second and third trimesters, can make symptoms of congenital heart disease worse. Even in women who have not had prior symptoms, these body changes can cause problems to develop. The mother's heart condition, as well as medications commonly prescribed for heart disease, can also pose added risks to the fetus. The AHA indicates that the risk of heart disease in the fetus is higher if either parent has a congenital heart defect. Whether the affected parent is the mother or father, the frequency of heart defects increases from less than 1 percent in the general population to 2–20 percent when the parent is affected. Having close family members with congenital heart disease further increases the risk of having a child with a heart defect.

Advancements in science and genetics are improving our ability to predict the presence of heart disease in some people. Genetic counseling should be considered for women with heart defects who want to become pregnant. A slight increase in the incidence of birth defects, including heart defects, has also been shown for children with mothers who have diabetes. Information regarding noninherited risk factors for congenital heart disease is limited but some general guidelines are given to minimize potential prenatal exposure to risk factors for congenital heart defects. Mothers who want to become pregnant should discuss any medications (even over-the-counter) they are taking with their health care provider, take a daily multivitamin with folic acid, avoid contact with people who have influenza or other illnesses causing a fever, avoid exposure to organic solvents, be vaccinated for rubella, and have prenatal care to detect or manage diabetes and phenylketonuria. Nonconclusive trends included parental (paternal and maternal) cigarette smoking, use of illicit drugs, alcohol intake, paternal older age and maternal stress levels as potential risk factors for congenital heart disease.[14]

Women who have congenital heart disease should get regular medical care from their primary care provider and cardiologist. Regular dental care is also recommended to minimize the chance of oral infections that could affect the heart. In addition, antibiotics usually are recommended by the dentist prior to dental work for persons with congenital heart disease to prevent the occurrence of heart infection as a result of the dental care. A woman with heart disease needs to be cautious before taking any over-the-counter medications, vitamins, or herbal preparations and should discuss the potential for cardiac side effects or drug interactions with her health care provider or pharmacist.

Arrhythmia   Arrhythmia refers to disturbances in the normal sequence of cardiac electrical activity that causes irregular or abnormal heart rhythms. The normal electrical conduction for heart rhythm is generated in the sinoatrial or sinus node ("natural pacemaker") found in the right atrium. The electrical impulse then travels through the heart's conduction pathway to cause synchronized contractions of the atria and ventricles. Arrhythmias include a variety of abnormal electrical disturbances, and their effects range from insignificant "skipped" beats to more serious, pump-impairing irregularities that can be life-threatening. The prevalence of arrhythmias tends to increase with age. Women with certain congenital conditions or acquired heart disease are more prone to develop arrhythmias. In addition, conditions causing higher or lower concentrations of various minerals in the body such as potassium, magnesium, or calcium can lead to impaired electrical conduction in the heart. Arrhythmias can be brought on by the use of alcohol, caffeine, cigarettes, recreational drugs, hyperthyroidism, and some prescribed medications.[15] Tachycardia refers to a fast heart rate of more than 100 beats per minute. Bradycardia is a slow heart rate of fewer than 60 beats per minute. No treatment is needed for many arrhythmias. Once an arrhythmia has been documented, it is important to determine where it originates. Some arrhythmias (such as "skipping a beat") are quite normal in children and adolescents. Others require regulation with medications, an implanted pacemaker, cardioversion (medically controlled electrical shock to the heart), ablative techniques using a radiofrequency or electrocautery approach, or an automatic implantable defibrillator.

Atrial fibrillation is the most common serious heart rhythm abnormality, and an estimated 2.7 million Americans live with this arrhythmia.[16] Atrial fibrillation is a result of uncoordinated electrical signals originating in the atria that cause fast, irregular contractions from the upper heart chambers. Symptoms from atrial arrhythmias may include dizziness, light-headedness, fainting or near fainting, anxiety, weakness, palpitations (noticeable heart fluttering), shortness of breath, and chest pain. Heart disease can cause arrhythmias, but other causes include stress, caffeine, tobacco, alcohol, diet pills, electrolyte imbalance, and cough/cold medications. Atrial fibrillation may not be life-threatening, but it can lead to conditions that are, such as stroke. According to the AHA, a person with atrial fibrillation has a five times greater chance of having a stroke than someone without this condition. Fifty percent of those who do experience a stroke will die within one year.[17]

An artificial **pacemaker** is a medical device implanted under the skin of the chest under the collarbone with wires that are positioned in the heart. Pacemakers can sense when the heart rhythm is too fast or too slow and fire impulses to restore the proper (preset) rhythm and speed. (See *Her Story:* "Mandi: From Pacemaker to Mother.") Many misconceptions exist about artificial pacemakers because older models had more potential problems than do newer models. Women with pacemakers do *not* need

Her Story

Mandi: From Pacemaker to Mother

Mandi experienced heart palpitations and fatigue from a young age. It seemed that every time she got up from a chair or cleaned up after a meal, she would feel light-headed. She was always tired. But when she ran long distances on the track team, she didn't notice any symptoms. At age 16, she fainted while talking to friends in the school hallway. She went to her family health care provider, who recommended further tests. The tests showed bradycardia and the cardiologist recommended a pacemaker. The cardiologist was not accustomed to implanting a pacemaker in a young, thin woman. After the surgery, Mandi felt like a new person. She had more energy and the symptoms had disappeared.

Last year, at the age of 23, Mandi gave birth to a healthy baby girl. Mother and baby experienced no problems through the natural birth process. Do you know someone with a pacemaker? What symptoms did they have before getting the pacemaker? How do they feel today?

to be concerned about microwave ovens, most home appliances, or tools, but they do need to be cautious with cell phones, traveling through airports, some dental equipment, diagnostic radiation, and standing near electronic article surveillance or metal detectors including hand-held ones.[21] Women with pacemakers should always carry their pacemaker identification cards and know the pre-programmed lower and/or upper heart rate limits of her particular pacemaker. By learning how to take her pulse, a woman can monitor her heart rate as well as her heart rhythm. Any heart rate that is above or below the preset rate needs to be reported to her health care provider. Pacemakers use batteries to function and eventually need to be replaced in a minor surgical procedure. A woman's doctor uses special pacemaker analyzers to detect when the battery life is getting low, thus, it is important for her to keep her pacemaker check-up appointments.[18] (See *Health Tip:* "Devices Affecting Pacemakers.")

Congestive Heart Failure (CHF)   **Congestive heart failure** (or simply, heart failure or cardiac failure) is generally a chronic and progressive heart condition in which the heart becomes too weak to adequately pump blood to the body. The course of the disease varies from woman to woman and may include intermittent exacerbations within periods of stability. Although heart failure usually affects the left ventricle of the heart, it can involve any part of the heart. Left-sided heart failure is distinguished as being systolic or diastolic failure. Systolic failure occurs when the left ventricle loses its ability to contract normally, thus creating ineffective pumping force for circulating blood. Diastolic failure occurs if the left ventricle muscle stiffens and does not allow the chamber to fill properly with blood. Drug treatment varies depending upon the type of left-sided failure. Right-sided heart failure, usually a result of left-sided failure, causes blood to back up in the body's venous system as the right side of the heart loses its pumping strength. This right ventricular (RV) failure causes symptoms such as swelling in the legs and ankles.[20]

A woman's heart failure will be classified under two divisions by her doctor according to the severity of her symptoms. The *functional capacity class* has four categories, I through IV, with IV being the most limited physical activity. The *objective capacity class* ranges from A to D with the "D" category demonstrating the most objective evidence of severe cardiovascular disease.[21]

Overworked or damaged heart muscle results from a variety of possible factors: prior heart attacks, coronary artery disease, hypertension, heart valve disease, cardiomyopathy (a disease of heart muscle), congenital heart disease, severe lung disease, diabetes, severe anemia, hyperthyroidism, arrhythmia, or infection of the heart valves or muscle itself.[22] The best treatment is prevention of further damage. Gender differences in CHF are known to exist. While men tend to experience weakening of the heart muscle, women tend to experience stiffening and loss of elasticity of the heart muscle. Hormone deficiencies, such as occur with hypothyroidism, may accelerate the loss of elasticity. Women with hypothyroidism should seek medical attention and may need thyroid replacement therapy.[23]

Symptoms of CHF include shortness of breath, nausea, lack of appetite, weight gain, edema (swelling), especially of the lower extremities or abdomen, dry and hacking cough, heart palpitations and shortness of breath in lying position. Women with CHF tire easily and have difficulty exerting effort. Various medications can be prescribed to decrease the workload of a weakened heart. These include angiotensin-converting enzyme (ACE) inhibitors ((lowers the limit of angiotensin II), angiotensin II receptor blockers (blocks receptor sites from angiotensin II), anticoagulant or antiplatelet agents, beta blockers, diuretics (water pills), digitalis, and vasodilators (blood vessel dilators). In addition, a fluid-restricted or salt-restricted diet (less than 1500 mg) may be recommended. Coronary artery bypass or PCI

Health Tips

Devices Affecting Pacemakers[19]

Little or no risk

Home appliances such as microwave ovens, CB radios, electric drills
Dental equipment
Diagnostic radiation (radiographs)
Electroconvulsive therapy

More risk

Metal detectors and electronic article surveillance (including hand-held devices)
Cellular phones (excluding those of less than 3 watts)
Extracorporeal shock-wave lithotripsy (used to dissolve kidney stones)
Magnetic resonance imaging (MRI)
Medical equipment (carry a wallet ID with you)
Power-generating equipment (arc welding, powerful magnets in medical devices, etc.)
Radiofrequency ablation (radio waves used to manage arrhythmias)
Short-wave or microwave diathermy (high-frequency, high-intensity signals)
Therapeutic radiation (cancer therapy, etc.)
Transcutaneous electrical nerve stimulation (used to relieve pain)
MP3 player headphones (keep head phones at least 1.2 inches away from pacemaker)

may be needed to improve blood flow to the heart muscle itself, and in some severe cases a heart transplant may be considered.

Endocarditis

Endocarditis has also been called infective endocarditis and valve infection. It is an inflammation or infection of the inside lining of the heart chambers and heart valves that can damage or destroy the heart valves. Endocarditis occurs when certain organisms in the bloodstream lodge on preexisting abnormal heart valves or other damaged heart tissue, and it rarely occurs in people with normal hearts.

Bacterial infection is the most common source of endocarditis although other organisms such as fungi can be causative. Given that certain bacteria are "normal" inhabiters on parts of the body such as the mouth, upper respiratory system, skin, and intestinal and urinary tracts, some surgical and dental procedures cause a brief bacteremia (bacteria in the bloodstream). Bacteremia is common after many invasive procedures, but only certain bacteria can cause endocarditis. Procedures that create greater risk of endocarditis include professional teeth cleaning; tonsillectomy and adenoidectomy; rigid bronchoscopy (examination of respiratory airways with a scope); certain urinary and gastrointestinal tract procedures; injected drug use; prior valve, gallbladder, and prostate surgery, and the existence of central venous access lines.

Women with a known history of a heart condition, including congenital heart defects, a heart murmur, mitral valve prolapse, or other heart valve problems, should inform their health care provider and dentist of this condition. Preventive antibiotics are often prescribed prior to procedures that could predispose high-risk individuals to endocarditis. Women with existing heart conditions may consider carrying an endocarditis wallet card issued by the AHA that informs health care professionals of their particular condition. Good oral hygiene is important for all women but especially for those with heart conditions.

Symptoms of endocarditis may develop slowly or suddenly, and it is difficult to diagnose because multiple organ systems may become involved. A few symptoms include fever, chills, excessive sweating, reddish brown lines under the nails known as "splinter hemorrhages," Janeway lesions (red, painless skin spots on the palms and soles), Osler's nodes (red, painful nodes in the pads of the fingers and toes), joint pain, weakness, cardiac murmur, weight loss, and night sweats.[24] Hospitalization with intravenous antibiotic administration often is required. Antibiotic therapy generally is given for 4–6 weeks. Complications from endocarditis can include **dysrhythmia** (abnormality of an otherwise normal rhythmic pattern), CHF, brain abscess stroke, and other organ damage as a result of blood clots traveling from the infected valves.

Mitral Valve Prolapse

Mitral valve prolapse (MVP) is a condition in which one or both flaps of the mitral valve are enlarged and fail to close properly as they prolapse or "flop" back into the left atrium during contraction of the left ventricle. MVP may or may not be accompanied by mitral regurgitation in which blood flows back into the left atrium, causing an auditory "murmur." The cause is unknown although some studies suggest that MVP is an inherited disorder. The majority of individuals with MVP do not know they have the condition because they have no symptoms. Women who may have symptoms with MVP might experience palpitations, shortness of breath with exertion or lying flat, chest pain that comes and goes, dizziness, migraine headaches, or symptoms that mimic a panic attack.

All women with MVP should be under health care supervision because of the risk for bacterial endocarditis that may require her to take antibiotics prior to certain medical procedures, including dental work. The AHA no longer recommends routine antibiotics before dental procedures except for those with the highest level of risk for bacterial endocarditis.[25] Sometimes medications such as beta blockers may be required, and in more serious valve prolapse, surgery for valve replacement could be indicated. Women with MVP should have regular checkups with their cardiologist during pregnancy because the changes in and the stress of pregnancy place added strain on the heart. However, in most cases, the chances are good for an uncomplicated, successful pregnancy.

Risk Factors for Heart Disease

The AHA has identified several factors that increase the risk of heart disease and stroke. A woman's chance of having a heart attack or stroke increases when more risk factors are present. Research indicates that having just one risk factor doubles the chance of developing heart disease.[26] Some of the factors cannot be controlled, but most of them can be modified, treated, or controlled to reduce a woman's chances of developing heart disease or having a stroke. (See *FYI:* "Risk Factors for Cardiovascular Disease.")

Unchangeable risk factors for heart disease include increasing age, family health history, race, and gender. In addition, women with prior histories of heart attack or stroke are at higher risk for future CVD episodes. The risk factors that can be modified, treated, or controlled include tobacco smoke, high BP, high blood cholesterol, physical inactivity, obesity and overweight, and diabetes. Other contributing factors for women include menopause and estrogen loss, oral contraceptives, high triglyceride levels, excessive alcohol consumption, and stress.

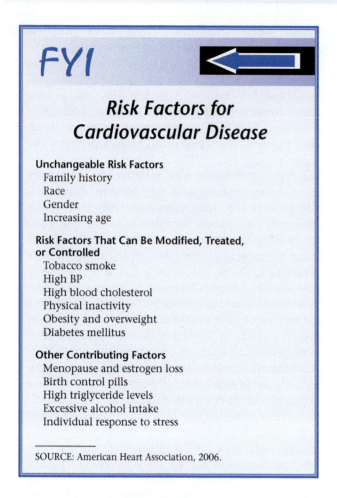

FYI

Risk Factors for Cardiovascular Disease

Unchangeable Risk Factors
Family history
Race
Gender
Increasing age

Risk Factors That Can Be Modified, Treated, or Controlled
Tobacco smoke
High BP
High blood cholesterol
Physical inactivity
Obesity and overweight
Diabetes mellitus

Other Contributing Factors
Menopause and estrogen loss
Birth control pills
High triglyceride levels
Excessive alcohol intake
Individual response to stress

SOURCE: American Heart Association, 2006.

Unchangeable Risk Factors

Increasing age As women age, their risk of heart disease and stroke begins to increase. At older ages, women who experience heart attacks are more likely than are men to die within a few weeks.

Family health history A woman's chances of developing heart disease or having a stroke are increased if her close blood relatives have had a heart attack or stroke.

Race African American women have a greater risk of heart disease and stroke than white women, which is largely attributed to their higher average BP levels. In comparison, African American women are also more likely to die of stroke than are white women. Mexican Americans, American Indians, native Hawaiians, and some Asian Americans also have higher risk, most likely due to higher rates of obesity and diabetes.

Gender Men have a greater risk of heart attack than women, and they have attacks earlier in life. Although more than half of the total stroke deaths occur in women, there is an overall equal incidence of stroke for men and women. Heart disease is the leading cause of death in both men and women.

Risk Factors That Can Be Modified, Treated, or Controlled

Tobacco smoke The nicotine and carbon monoxide in tobacco smoke reduce the amount of oxygen in the blood and damage blood vessel walls, causing plaque to build up. Tobacco smoke worsens atherosclerosis and speeds its buildup in arteries. In addition, tobacco smoke can trigger the formation of blood clots, cause arrhythmias in persons with chest pain or previous heart attacks, and promote heart disease by reducing HDL ("good" cholesterol). Smokers have a two to four times greater risk for developing CHD. In addition, smokers have much greater risks for developing peripheral artery disease (PAD), stroke, heart failure, sudden cardiac death, and abdominal aortic aneurysm.[27] Nearly 46,000 *nonsmokers* die each year from CHD resulting from exposure to environmental (secondhand or passive) tobacco smoke. Nearly 800 *infant deaths* also occur annually as a result of women smoking throughout the pregnancy. Use of oral contraceptives by women smokers is discouraged because of a higher risk for heart attack or stroke.

High blood pressure Hypertension, often called the silent killer, remains a major risk factor in heart attack, stroke, congestive heart failure, blindness, and kidney failure. Essential or primary hypertension, the most common type, has no known underlying cause. Although the causes of hypertension in 90 percent of the cases are not known, the contributing factors of uncontrolled hypertension are understood. Secondary hypertension, caused by an underlying disease and less common overall, is more common in women than in men.

Hypertension occurs when the heart is forced to exert more pressure to pump blood through the arteries to the body. This pressure not only overworks the heart but also contributes to atherosclerosis, hardening of the arteries. BP is, simply, the force of blood against artery walls. It is measured with a sphygmomanometer: A rubber cuff is wrapped around the arm, temporarily stopping blood flow to the brachial artery, and a stethoscope is used to listen for blood flow as it begins to flow through the brachial artery. **Systolic blood pressure** is the amount of pressure the blood exerts against the arteries while the heart is contracting. **Diastolic blood pressure** is the amount of pressure the blood exerts against the arteries while the heart is filling and resting between beats. When stating BP, systolic and then diastolic are given (e.g., 120/80). Normal BP is below 120 mm Hg systolic and below 80 mm Hg diastolic. Prehypertension is 120–139 mm Hg systolic *or* 80–89 mm Hg diastolic. Prehypertension means that there is a greater likelihood of developing hypertension later, but lifestyle changes may delay the onset. Over half of all Americans, 60 years of age and older, have high BP and women over 45 have an increased risk for high BP. Nearly 90 percent of persons over the age of 55 are likely to experience hypertension in their lifetime. Stage 1 hypertension in adults has been defined as BP between 140 and 159 mm Hg systolic *or* between 90 and 99 mm Hg diastolic. Stage 2 hypertension is a systolic reading equal to or greater than 160 mm Hg *or* a diastolic reading equal to or greater than 100 mm Hg.[28] Lifestyle changes are encouraged for persons with stage 1 and stage 2 hypertension, and drug therapy is usually prescribed. (See Table 15.1.)

Most American women will develop high BP during their lifetime. Even slight elevations in BP double the risk for the development of cardiovascular disease. Cardiovascular disease risk doubles for each increment of 20/10 mm Hg starting at BP of 115/75 mm Hg.[30] High BP is the most important risk factor for stroke. High BP tends to run in families, but it has no known cause and appears without symptoms. Other uncontrollable factors include age (BP tends to rise with age), race, and gender. High blood pressure occurs more often among African Americans than whites. Obesity, diabetes, smoking, sleep apnea, and regular alcohol use increase the likelihood of developing high BP. Some medications such as cold relief products and corticosteriods can raise a woman's blood pressure. Oral contraceptive use can occasionally contribute to hypertension, and it may be necessary for hypertensive women to use other birth control methods. In one study, women aged 40–59 with high BP were expected to encounter five times the normal rate of angina, heart attack, or sudden death. Losing weight, quitting smoking, avoiding second hand smoke,

reducing sodium intake, exercising regularly, and taking medication can act as protective factors. However, hypertension controlled by drug therapy remains a risk factor because it does not decrease the risk of CHD.

Complications from high BP during pregnancy are also possible. Gestational hypertension is high BP that develops during pregnancy and usually disappears within weeks after delivery. High BP can be detrimental for both the mother and the fetus, potentially causing harm to the mother's kidneys and other organs, and low birth weight and early delivery of the infant. Preeclampsia, a toxic condition that typically starts after the 20th week of pregnancy, is associated with an increase in BP and protein in the urine. Other symptoms associated with preeclampsia include persistent headaches, abdominal pain, blurred vision, and sensitivity to light. Preeclampsia has increased by nearly one-third in the past decade. When preeclampsia leads to eclampsia (preeclampsia with seizures), the condition becomes much more serious and is recognized as the second leading cause of maternal death in the United States.[31] (See Chapter 9.) A woman who has hypertension should discuss pregnancy beforehand with her health care provider.

High blood cholesterol High blood cholesterol is a major risk factor for heart disease, with the risk increasing as the blood level rises. Cholesterol is a normal fatty substance of the body that is used to form cell membranes and some hormones. Cholesterol enters the blood in two

TABLE 15.1 Classification and Management of Blood Pressure for Adults*[29]

BP CLASSIFICATION	SBP MMHG	DBP MMHG	LIFESTYLE MODIFICATION	INITIAL DRUG THERAPY WITHOUT COMPELLING INDICATIONS	INITIAL DRUG THERAPY WITH COMPELLING INDICATIONS
Normal	<120	and <80	Encourage		
Prehypertension	120–139	or 80–89	Yes	No antihypertensive drug indicated.	Drug(s) for compelling indications.‡
Stage 1 Hypertension	140–159	or 90–99	Yes	Thiazide-type diuretics for most. May consider ACEI, ARB, BB, CCB, or combination.	Drug(s) for the compelling indications.‡ Other antihypertensive drugs (diuretics, ACEI, ARB, BB, CCB) as needed.
Stage 2 Hypertension	≥160	or ≥100	Yes	Two-drug combination for most† (usually thiazide-type diuretic and ACEI or ARB or BB or CCB).	

*Treatment determined by highest BP category.

†Initial combined therapy should be used cautiously in those at risk for orthostatic hypotension.

‡Treat patients with chronic kidney disease or diabetes to BP goal of <130/80 mm Hg.

NOTE: DBP, diastolic blood pressure; SBP, systolic blood pressure. Drug abbreviations: ACEI, angiotensin-converting enzyme inhibitor; ARB, angiotensin receptor blocker; BB, beta blocker; CCB, calcium channel blocker.

ways: through absorption in the small intestine from animal products that are consumed and from its production in the body, mainly the liver. The body makes about 75 percent of its own cholesterol, so very little is needed from dietary sources. Since cholesterol and other fats cannot dissolve in the blood, cholesterol is transported through the blood on lipoproteins of varying densities. Low-density lipoprotein (LDL) has become known as the "bad" cholesterol because high levels of cholesterol in this lipoprotein increase a person's risk for coronary heart disease. Cholesterol carrying LDL can slowly build up in the inner walls of the arteries and, thus, narrow the lumen of the vessel. High levels of LDL are a better predictor of heart disease risk than total cholesterol levels. Lipoprotein(a) cholesterol is a genetic variation of plasma LDL and is an important risk factor for the development of premature atherosclerosis. Cholesterol in high-density lipoprotein (HDL) is commonly known as the "good" cholesterol because high levels of HDL *decrease* the risk of coronary heart disease. (See Table 15.2.) Medical experts

believe that HDL carries cholesterol away from the arteries back to the liver, where it is processed to pass out of the body. It is thought that HDL, thus, slows the progress of plaque build-up.

Young women appear to have higher HDL than men, particularly during childbearing years when estrogen levels are higher. However, by age 55, women tend to have higher *total* cholesterol as well, which decreases the protective advantage against coronary heart disease. The goals for reducing cholesterol in women are to lower total cholesterol and LDL levels and to raise HDL levels.

Total cholesterol and LDL cholesterol levels can be reduced by a diet low in saturated fat and cholesterol. Food products with monounsaturated and polyunsaturated fats should replace those with high saturated fats, trans fats, and triglycerides. High levels of trans-fatty acids in foods can raise a woman's cholesterol level. Food products containing hydrogenated oils are high in trans-fatty acids and should be avoided when trying to lower a cholesterol level. Reducing the amount of saturated fat and trans fats in the diet is more important in reducing blood cholesterol than is reducing the intake of cholesterol itself.

The average HDL cholesterol level for women is 50–60 mg/dL. Keeping HDL levels high (60 mg/dL or more) by quitting smoking, maintaining a healthy weight, and being physically active is important in fighting atherosclerosis. Smoking lowers HDL and increases the tendency for blood to clot. Women should be familiar with the absolute numbers of their total cholesterol and HDL because these levels are important in determining appropriate treatment by a health care provider.

While female sex hormones (estrogen) raise HDL cholesterol levels, male sex hormones (testosterone), progesterone, and certain steroids lower the HDL level. Hormone replacement therapy (HRT) is no longer recommended to prevent heart disease in postmenopausal women. Women whose blood cholesterol levels remain elevated despite dietary changes, regular physical activity, and weight loss may need to take cholesterol-lowering medications. Women should be aware that some cholesterol-lowering medications may interact with grapefruit, grapefruit juice, pomegranate, and pomegranate juice and should discuss these interactions with their doctor or pharmacist.[33] The most effective and widely tested cholesterol-lowering drugs for women are called statins. Statins not only lower LDL, they have modest effects on lowering triglycerides and raising HDL cholesterol. These medications, like most medications, have potential side effects and should not be a substitute for healthy lifestyle changes. Although most of statins' side effects are mild and disappear after the body has adjusted, muscle problems and liver abnormalities can occur. A woman on statins should have regular liver function tests as indicated by her health care provider. Women who are

TABLE 15.2 Healthy Levels of Cholesterol[32]

The following tables provide some general guidelines for optimal cholesterol and triglyceride levels. However, you should always discuss your own results with your doctor.

Total Cholesterol Level	Classification
Less than 200 mg/dL	Desirable
200–239 mg/dL	Borderline high
240 mg/dL and above	Very high

LDL Cholesterol Level	Classification*
Less than 100 mg/dL	Optimal
100–129 mg/dL	Near optimal/above optimal
130–159 mg/dL	Borderline high
160–189 mg/dL	High
190 mg/dL and above	Very high

HDL Cholesterol Level	Classification
Less than 40 mg/dL for men; less than 50 mg/dL for women	Major heart disease risk factor
60 mg/dL or higher	Gives some protection against heart disease

Triglyceride Level	Classification
Less than 150 mg/dL	Normal
150–199 mg/dL	Borderlin–high
200–499 mg/dL	High
500 mg/dL or higher	Very high

*Risk factors for heart disease include: family history of early heart problems (before age 55 for men, and before age 65 for women), smoking, high BP, diabetes, being male and over 45 or female and over 55, and having HDL levels below 40 mg/dL for men and 50 mg/dL for women.

Last update May 2008. © 2007 American Heart Association, Inc. All rights reserved. Unauthorized use prohibited.

pregnant or have active or chronic liver problems should not take statins. At times, cholesterol-lowering medications are used in combination with one another for more effectiveness. Other medications known as fibrates are used specifically to lower triglycerides. According to National Cholesterol Education Program (NCEP) guidelines, all adults 20 or older should have a fasting lipoprotein profile which includes a measurement of LDL, HDL, triglycerides, and total cholesterol. NCEP also recommends that this fasting (9–12 hours without food, liquids, or pills) test be done every 5 years.[34]

Physical inactivity   Women who are inactive have twice the risk of heart disease as women who exercise regularly. This risk is comparable to high blood cholesterol, high BP, or cigarette smoking. African American and Mexican American women report less leisure activity than Caucasian women. Exercise has many benefits, including decreasing levels of LDL and triglycerides and increasing levels of HDL, building a stronger immunity, boosting both physical and mental wellness, improving circulation, relieving tension and stress, countering anxiety and depression, and keeping weight under control. Most importantly, exercise can reduce CHD in women by 30–40 percent. National guidelines recommend that adults get 150 minutes (30 minutes on 5 days of the week) of moderate exercise or 75 minutes of vigorous physical activity per week.[35] The physical activity does not require one duration, but can occur in short spurts, that is, 10–15 minutes of activity several times a day.

Obesity and overweight   **Overweight** is defined as a body mass index (BMI) of 25 kg/m² or greater. **Obesity** is considered to be a BMI of 30 or greater, and **extreme obesity** is a BMI greater than 39. You can determine your BMI by accessing the Web site www.cdc.gov/bmi.

Estimates suggest that nearly 62 percent of American women (ages 20–74) are overweight, 34 percent are obese, and 6 percent are extremely obese. Obesity is the second leading preventable health problem in the United States, and among middle-aged women it has increased approximately 2 percent or more each year over a 40-year span. Obesity has a strong inverse relationship with socioeconomic status (that is, obesity increases as income level decreases) and women with college degrees are less likely to be obese compared with women with less education.[36]

Non-Hispanic black women have the highest prevalence of overweight and obesity, followed by Mexican American women. The risk of chronic disease such as heart disease increases with an increase in BMI. In fact, when BMI exceeds 30, the risk of death related to obesity increases by 50 percent. Women who have too much fat are at higher risk for multiple health problems, including premature death, type 2 diabetes, high BP, gallbladder disease, respiratory dysfunction, gout, insulin resistance,

osteoarthritis, and dyslipidemia (a lipid disorder that results in increases in cholesterol and/or triglyceride levels). Stroke and heart disease are health problems that are significantly related to women who carry their weight around the waist. Fat distribution around the central abdominal area (apple shape) is associated with greater health risk but research is ongoing regarding this risk. Further research is being done on fat tissue itself.

Two major types of adipose tissue are white adipose tissue, which stores energy (most body fat), and brown adipose tissue, which burns calories to maintain body heat. More evidence is demonstrating that these two body fats influence systemic energy metabolism and possibly influence obesity and type 2 diabetes.[37] (See *FYI:* "Countering the Myths of Some 'Protective Factors'.")

Diabetes   Women with diabetes are at higher risk for multisystem diseases, especially cardiovascular disease, than women without diabetes. Adults with diabetes have 2–4 times higher risk for heart disease and stroke. (See Diabetes Mellitus on page >>>). Women with diabetes have more than 2 times the risk of heart attack than nondiabetic women and double the risk of a second heart attack.[38]

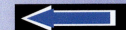

FYI

Countering the Myths of Some "Protective Factors"

Three previous factors that were believed to protect women from heart disease have now been found to show no benefit. First, HRT was believed to protect women from heart attacks. A study by the Women's Health Initiative found that HRT may *cause* heart attacks, stroke, or blood clots in *some* women. HRT is no longer recommended. Second, antioxidant supplements such as vitamin E and beta carotene were believed to reduce cardiovascular disease risk and have other health-promoting properties. Several clinical trials have shown no benefit, and in some studies, an increase in hemorrhagic strokes was found. Some antioxidant supplements may actually interfere with statin therapy. The role of antioxidants in stopping the progression of heart disease remains an area of study. Third, aspirin was believed to lower the risk of heart disease. However, potential benefits may be outweighed by risks such as stomach bleeding or ulcers in low-risk women. Aspirin therapy is recommended only for women at highest risk for heart attack (those who already have cardiovascular disease, diabetes, or chronic kidney disease), but regular use is contraindicated in this group if certain conditions exist.[39]

Other Contributing Factors

Menopause and estrogen loss Although the evidence is not clear, it is believed that estrogen acts as a protective factor against heart disease. Due to the natural loss of estrogen after menopause or the surgical removal of the ovaries, evidence suggests that an increased risk of heart disease occurs. At one time it was believed that HRT was beneficial in decreasing this risk in menopausal women. In 2002, clinical trials showed that HRT did *not* reduce the risk of cardiovascular disease and stroke in postmenopausal women. In fact, the Women's Health Initiative discontinued its HRT study because of the undue risk of blood clots and stroke for women participating in the study. In 2004, the National Institutes of Health discontinued the estrogen-only trial because of an apparent increased risk of stroke.

Oral contraceptives Women's risk of heart disease and stroke for those who take low-dose oral contraceptives has decreased over previous high-dose oral contraceptives. The risk still remains high for women who have high BP or choose to smoke while taking oral contraceptives. Using oral contraceptives is contraindicated for women who smoke and are 35 years of age and older, and women who develop high BP while taking oral contraceptives may be advised to stop taking them. Recent studies have shown that the risks of blood clots in legs and lungs are higher for women using Ortho Evra, the birth control patch, compared to women using birth control pills.

High triglyceride levels Triglycerides are a form of fat that comes from food and are also made in the body. Most fats eaten, including butter, margarines, and oils, are in triglyceride form, but excess calories from sugars and alcohol are converted into triglycerides and then stored in fat cells distributed throughout a woman's body. Triglycerides are fatty substances also known as lipids. Cholesterol is a lipid and a fat-like substance, not a fat. Women with high triglyceride levels may need to modify their lifestyle by controlling weight, choosing foods low in saturated fats and cholesterol, increasing physical activity, not smoking, and, in some cases, drinking less alcohol. Limiting the intake of carbohydrates to no more than 40–50 percent of total calories is sometimes encouraged. It is not clear whether high triglycerides alone are a risk factor for heart disease, but the AHA suggests that high triglyceride levels may increase the risk of heart disease more for women than for men. High triglyceride levels seem to be found along with high cholesterol levels, obesity and diabetes.[40]

Excessive alcohol intake Women who drink moderate amounts (an average of one drink daily) have a lowered risk of heart disease compared to nondrinkers. Despite this finding, it is not recommended that nondrinkers start using alcohol or that drinkers increase their use of alcohol. Excessive alcohol intake can lead to high triglyceride levels, high BP, heart failure, and stroke, and it can produce irregular heartbeats. Drinking too much alcohol also can contribute to obesity, alcoholism, unintended injuries, and suicide.

Stress Although research has not defined the role that stress plays in the development of heart disease, a woman's individual response to stress can be a contributing factor to heart disease. Negative responses such as overeating, smoking, or excessive alcohol intake are examples of how one's response to stress can contribute to the risk for heart disease.

Screening and Diagnosis

Women who suspect they have heart disease should be assertive in getting a proper diagnosis. Many of the traditional tests used for screening for heart disease were developed for men. For example, women often have been falsely diagnosed with heart disease from the traditional stress test, which is a treadmill test. The stress test is not specific or sensitive enough for women. Women can receive better results from a stress echocardiogram, which is a noninvasive technique that uses a treadmill test and ultrasound pictures of the heart. The ultrasound pictures allow the cardiologist to view the heart muscle contractions at peak exercise. Another test that uses radioactive tracers to assess blood flow during rest and exercise is equally accurate in women and men.

STROKE

Stroke is the fourth leading cause of death in women and the leading cause of adult disability, yet few women know the warning symptoms. (See *Health Tips:* "Warning Symptoms of Stroke.")

Although stroke is more common in men in most age groups, more women die from stroke at all ages. After a stroke, women tend to have more disability and find it difficult to return to their normal activities of daily living. Nearly 75 percent of all strokes occur in people over the age of 65, with the risk of stroke doubling each decade after the age of 55.

One-half of all African American women will die from stroke or heart disease. It is not clear why blacks are twice as likely to die from a stroke than whites, but some factors point to the higher percentage of blacks with high BP, diabetes, obesity, and sickle cell anemia. Black women have a lower 1-year survival rate following an ischemic stroke compared with white women.[42]

Stroke is a form of vascular disease with many causes and levels of severity. An artery carrying oxygen-rich blood to the brain may suddenly become clogged or burst, preventing blood flow to the brain. The two

Health Tips

Warning Symptoms of Stroke[41]

Common stroke symptoms in both women and men:

- Sudden weakness or numbness on one side of the body, usually the face, arm, or leg
- Sudden severe headaches with no known cause
- Sudden confusion, trouble speaking or understanding
- Sudden trouble seeing in one or both eyes
- Sudden trouble walking, dizziness, loss of balance or coordination

Unique stroke symptoms that women may report:

- Sudden face and limb pain
- Sudden hiccups
- Sudden nausea
- Sudden general weakness
- Sudden chest pain
- Sudden shortness of breath
- Sudden palpitations

primary types of stroke include **hemorrhagic** and **ischemic** stroke. Hemorrhagic strokes are further subdivided into subarachnoid stroke and intracerebral stroke, depending on the location in the brain of the burst blood vessel. Hemorrhagic strokes account for about 13 percent of all strokes. Ischemic stroke, which is about 87 percent of all strokes, occurs when a blood vessel is blocked and oxygen is prevented from flowing to the brain. Ischemic stroke results from an embolism, large artery thrombosis, or small penetrating artery thrombosis.[43]

Risk Factors for Stroke

The risk factors for stroke include those that cannot be changed, those that can be reduced with medical treatment, and those that can be reduced with lifestyle changes. The risk factors that cannot be altered include increasing age, race (African American and Hispanic women are at increased risk), heredity, gender, and the experience of a prior stroke or heart attack. Transient ischemic attacks (TIAs) are "mini" or small strokes that produce stroke-like symptoms but are only temporary. TIAs are strong predictors of stroke, since studies have shown that 40 percent of all people who have had a TIA will have an actual stroke in the future.

The risk factors that can be reduced with medical treatment include hypertension, heart disease, diabetes, high red blood cell count, atrial fibrillation, carotid or other artery disease, sickle-cell anemia, severe anemia, and high blood cholesterol.

Hypertension, or high BP, is the most important risk factor for stroke. As a woman's BP goes up, so does her risk of stroke. Treatment for high BP (higher than 140/90) is the key to reducing the chances of future strokes. The use of anticoagulants (blood thinners) or antiplatelet medicines such as aspirin can be helpful in the prevention of ischemic strokes. These agents would probably not be recommended for a woman who has had or is at risk of hemorrhagic stroke.

Another risk factor that can be altered with medical treatment is atrial fibrillation, a type of irregular heartbeat. Atrial fibrillation increases the risk of a blood clot breaking free and moving to the brain. Women with atrial fibrillation are five times more at risk for stroke. Research suggests that blood thinners can dramatically reduce the risk of stroke from atrial fibrillation by preventing clots from forming.

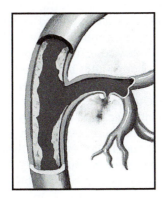

Hemorrhage
The sudden bursting of a blood vessel.

Coronary intervention

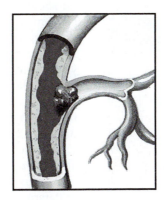

Embolus
A clot that moves through the circulatory system and becomes lodged at a narrowed point within a vessel.

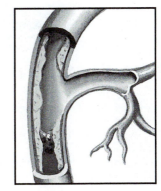

Thrombus
A clot that forms within a narrowed section of a blood vessel and remains at its place of origin.

Those risk factors that can be altered through lifestyle choices include tobacco use/smoking, excessive alcohol use, obesity, physical inactivity, and the use of some illegal drugs. Other risk factors that are unique to women include taking birth control pills, being pregnant, using HRT to relieve symptoms of menopause, having a history of migraines, and having a thick waist (larger than 35.2 inches) or high triglyceride levels (greater than 128) in postmenopausal women.[44]

Treatment

Stroke should be treated as an emergency. Two million brain cells die every minute during a stroke, which increases the risk of permanent brain damage, disability, or death. Hence, recognizing symptoms and acting F.A.S.T. can save a life and limit disability.[45] (See *FYI:* "F.A.S.T. Action Saves Lives.")

Knowing the warning signs is important because new drugs (e.g., tPA, or tissue plasminogen activator) can break up clots and limit damage to the brain if administered within 3 hours of the start of symptoms. Treatment approaches differ depending on the type of stroke a woman experiences. Health care providers find it far easier to predict survival than functional outcome. Level of consciousness is the best predictor of short-term survival, whereas recovery during the first 30–60 days predicts potential functional outcome.

A surgical procedure, carotid endarterectomy, has prevented thousands of strokes. This surgery removes fatty buildup (atherosclerosis) in the carotid arteries (blood vessels in the neck that supply oxygen to the brain). This procedure was shown to be less beneficial for women, the elderly, and those with disabilities.

Other surgical procedures include angioplasty and the placement of stents (meshlike tubes), which help keep a carotid artery open and prevent reblockage.

For hemorrhagic stroke, a procedure may be done to place a "coil" at the site of an aneurysm or arteriovenous malformation to prevent rupture of the vessel. In this procedure a catheter is inserted into a major artery of the leg or arm and guided to the weakened vessel site where the device is placed. Also, surgery can be performed to "clip off" or remove the aneurysm or malformed vessels.

Disability from Stroke

The devastation from stroke can include severe impairment of mental and bodily functions. The physical disability depends on the area of the brain affected such as sight, sound, motor skills, autonomic body systems (heart rate, respiration, body temperature), or language. Physical changes (permanent paralysis, impaired speech or thought processes, and memory loss) and emotional changes (loss of sexual desire, poor body image, depression) are common. The rehabilitation of a stroke patient begins as soon as possible, with health care staff and family members offering support and encouragement. The key to helping a woman recover from a stroke is access to rehabilitation. If she has private insurance to cover the cost of rehabilitation, her prognosis for recovery is better.

OSTEOPOROSIS

Osteoporosis (porous bone), a bone-weakening disease, results in bone mineral loss and increases the risk of skeletal frailty and fracturing. Bone is a living, growing tissue that consists primarily of a flexible protein (collagen) framework and the mineral calcium phosphate, which adds strength to the framework. Except for about 1 percent of calcium in the blood, the body's calcium is found in teeth and bone. During a woman's lifetime, old bone is continually removed (resorption) and replaced with new bone (formation). In her earlier years, a woman's body builds bone faster than it is removed, allowing for denser, growing bones. After peak bone mass is reached around the age of 30 years, bone resorption gradually begins to exceed bone formation. Although perceived as a disease of old age, osteoporosis starts in childhood. It has been described as a "pediatric disease with a geriatric outcome." Genetics, age, menopausal status, diet, and exercise play major roles in determining peak bone mass, an indicator of future bone density. Primary prevention focuses on increasing peak bone mass and reducing bone loss in later life. The greatest loss in bone density occurs in women during the first 5–10 years after menopause before leveling to approximately 1 percent a year. Osteoporosis

---

FYI

F.A.S.T. Action Saves Lives

Face Ask the person to smile. Does one side of the face droop?

Arms Ask the person to raise both arms. Does one arm drift downward?

Speech Ask the person to repeat a simple sentence. Are the words slurred? Can she repeat the sentence correctly?

Time If the person shows any of these symptoms, time is important. Call 911 or get the person to the hospital immediately.

SOURCE: National Stroke Association, 2010.

is often called the "silent disease" because bone loss occurs without symptoms. Without early diagnosis, the first symptom in many cases is a bone fracture.

Osteoporosis threatens the bone health of 44 million Americans (55 percent of all persons over age 50). An estimated ten million Americans have osteoporosis, and an estimated 34 million have low bone mass, which puts them at increased risk for osteoporosis and fractures. Eight million (80 percent) of those affected by osteoporosis are women, particularly postmenopausal women.[46] Twenty percent of non-Hispanic white and Asian women, 10 percent of Hispanic women, and 5 percent of African American women are estimated to have osteoporosis. Loss of height, spinal deformities such as kyphosis, and severe back pain, all resulting from collapsed vertebrae, are signs of advanced osteoporosis. Nearly half of all women over the age of 50 are predicted to have a bone fracture during their lifetime related to bone loss.

Bones of the spine, hips, ribs, and wrists are especially susceptible to osteoporosis-related fractures. Of special concern are fractures of the hip and spine because these fractures can lead to prolonged or permanent disability or even death. Nearly 24 percent of hip fracture patients age 50 and over die in the year following their fractures. Although the rate of hip fractures is two to three times higher in women than in men, men have twice the mortality rate in the first year following a hip fracture. Twenty percent of persons who were able to walk prior to a hip fracture will require long-term care, and only 15 percent of long-term care persons will be able to walk unassisted 6 months after the fracture.[47]

Heredity also influences the risk of osteoporosis. Common genetic differences have been found to account for 7 to 10 percent of the difference in bone density, particularly at the hip and spine.

Young women who are at increased risk for osteoporosis include highly trained female athletes with amenorrhea and those suffering from eating disorders. Complete *Assess Yourself:* "Determine Your Risk for Osteoporosis."

Female athletes who attempt to reduce body fat by extreme measures can suffer loss of bone mass from a set of factors called the female athlete triad. The triad of eating disorders, amenorrhea, and weak bones can lead to severe health complications other than osteoporosis. Athletes, knowing that exercise is strengthening their bones, should not fool themselves. Extreme exercise that causes exercise-induced amenorrhea can lead to irreversible bone loss within 6 months to 2 years.[48]

Exercise-induced amenorrhea is not a minor problem. Any female athlete who experiences more than 6 months of amenorrhea should be evaluated for loss of bone density and strongly encouraged to reduce training to a level at which menstruation resumes.

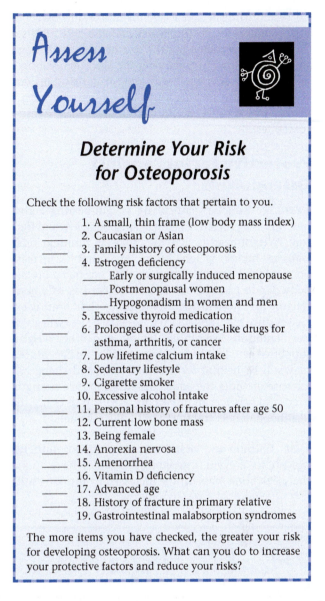

Assess Yourself

Determine Your Risk for Osteoporosis

Check the following risk factors that pertain to you.

_____ 1. A small, thin frame (low body mass index)
_____ 2. Caucasian or Asian
_____ 3. Family history of osteoporosis
_____ 4. Estrogen deficiency
     _____ Early or surgically induced menopause
     _____ Postmenopausal women
     _____ Hypogonadism in women and men
_____ 5. Excessive thyroid medication
_____ 6. Prolonged use of cortisone-like drugs for asthma, arthritis, or cancer
_____ 7. Low lifetime calcium intake
_____ 8. Sedentary lifestyle
_____ 9. Cigarette smoker
_____ 10. Excessive alcohol intake
_____ 11. Personal history of fractures after age 50
_____ 12. Current low bone mass
_____ 13. Being female
_____ 14. Anorexia nervosa
_____ 15. Amenorrhea
_____ 16. Vitamin D deficiency
_____ 17. Advanced age
_____ 18. History of fracture in primary relative
_____ 19. Gastrointestinal malabsorption syndromes

The more items you have checked, the greater your risk for developing osteoporosis. What can you do to increase your protective factors and reduce your risks?

Anorexia and bulimia nervosa can also contribute to rapid bone loss and fracture. Women who have these conditions may experience estrogen deficiency, malnutrition, and altered carbohydrate metabolism. Women who have exercise-induced amenorrhea or anorexia nervosa should be encouraged to gain weight to a level at which menstruation occurs naturally. Oral contraceptives can be prescribed for estrogen deficiency but are ineffective until weight gain and full endocrine function are restored.[49]

Smoking affects the processing of vitamin D and reduces the calcium absorption necessary for maintaining bone density. Thus, quitting smoking at any age may reduce bone loss. Results of studies related to excessive alcohol consumption, more than three drinks a day, and bone loss were mixed. Some studies suggested that excessive drinking interferes with calcium and vitamin D absorption, and others found no relationship between alcohol intake and osteoporosis. Some research implicates caffeine and high sodium intake as increasing the loss of calcium through the urine. Overall, women over the age of 65, younger postmenopausal women with one or more additional risk factors, and postmenopausal women who have a history of fractures should have a bone mass density (BMD) test.[50]

Protective Factors against Osteoporosis

Exercise Exercise, particularly weight-bearing activities, acts as a protective factor against bone loss and fracture. Weight-bearing activities such as running, brisk walking, hiking, weight lifting, and aerobics increase bone mineral density. A woman who has had a broken bone due to osteoporosis or is at higher risk of a bone fracture may need to do lower-impact weight bearing exercises since high-impact exercises may be less safe given her condition. Swimming, biking, and other weight-supported activities have less weight bearing benefits but may still be helpful for general health and strength.[51] Exercise provides the added benefit of muscle strength, tone, and balance, all important factors in reducing the likelihood of falls and fractures in older women.

Diet Calcium and vitamin D are two major nutrients needed to prevent osteoporosis. Studies have found that peak bone mass can be increased by drinking milk during childhood and adolescence and increasing calcium intake beyond the current Recommended Dietary Allowances. The most critical years for building bone mass are between preadolescence and age 30. (See *Health Tips:* "Recommended Calcium and Vitamin D Intakes.")

Calcium plays a variety of roles in body functioning besides increasing bone density. When blood levels of calcium drop, the heart, muscles, and nerves deplete the calcium from bones needed to function properly. Surveys have shown that American women and girls are taking in less than half the amount of calcium recommended for growth and maintenance of bone tissue. Approximately 1000–1300 milligrams of calcium per day are recommended. In addition to milk and other dairy products, good food sources of calcium include dark green, leafy vegetables such as broccoli, collard greens, bok choy, and spinach; sardines and salmon with bones; tofu; and almonds. Some foods like cereals, orange juice, and breads are fortified with calcium. Because the amount of calcium from food sources may not be adequate for some women, calcium supplements may be needed. It is important to recognize that a high calcium intake will not protect a woman against bone loss caused by estrogen deficiency, physical inactivity, smoking, alcohol abuse, and certain medical disorders and treatments. Getting too much calcium from supplements may increase a woman's chance of developing kidney stones and other health problems. Most experts indicate that 2000–2500 mg is the safe upper limit for total daily calcium intake from all sources.[53]

Health Tips

Recommended Calcium and Vitamin D Intakes*[52]

Children and Adolescents	Calcium (Daily)	Vitamin D (Daily)
1–3 years	500 mg	400 IU**
4–8 years	800 mg	400 IU**
9–18 years	1300 mg	400 IU**
Adult Women and Men	**Calcium (Daily)**	**Vitamin D (Daily)**
19–49 years	1000 mg	400–800 IU
50 years and over	1200 mg	800–1000 IU
Pregnant and Breastfeeding Women	**Calcium (Daily)**	**Vitamin D (Daily)**
18 years and under	1300 mg	400–800 IU
19 years and over	1000 mg	400–800 IU

*There are two types of vitamin D supplements: vitamin D-3 and vitamin D-2. Previous research suggested that vitamin D-3 was a better choice than vitamin D-2. However, more recent studies show that vitamin D-3 and vitamin D-2 are equally good for bone health. Vitamin D-3 is also called cholecalciferol. Vitamin D-2 is also called ergocalciferol.

**NOF does not have specific vitamin D recommendations for these age groups. These are the recommendations of the American Academy of Pediatrics.

Vitamin D, essential for building bone, must be present for calcium to be adequately absorbed through the small intestine. Vitamin D is synthesized by skin exposed to sunlight, and with aging, the skin seems to lose the ability to produce adequate amounts of vitamin D. Thus, milk and vitamin supplements are important sources of vitamin D in later years. Vitamin D also can be obtained from egg yolks, saltwater fish, and liver. The recommended intake is between 400 and 800 IU per day. Excessive amounts of vitamin D may be harmful; therefore, a woman should consult her health care provider before exceeding recommended doses of vitamin D.

Measuring Bone Density

A bone mineral density (BMD) test is the only way to diagnose osteoporosis and determine a woman's risk for future bone fracture. Early diagnosis is important because osteoporosis, a "silent disease," can go undetected for many years without symptoms. BMD testing not only determines bone health but also measures a woman's response to current osteoporosis treatment. There are many diseases, conditions, and disorders that may cause a woman to have bone loss. Bone loss may occur from autoimmune disorders or other conditions that require using steroid medicines, digestive and gastrointestinal disorders that impair the absorption of vitamins and minerals, hormonal or endocrine disorders that impact metabolism, blood disorders or cancers that cause bone loss or impact the function of the bone marrow, neurologic or nervous system disorders that impede activity of a woman, and a myriad of other conditions. Any of these health problems may necessitate closer monitoring of bone health through BMD tests.[54] The bone density of female athletes, women with eating disorders, postmenopausal women under age 65 with more than one risk factor for osteoporosis, any woman 65 years or older even without risk factors, women who have had significant loss of height, or perimenopausal women should be assessed.

Multiple types of BMD tests exist. These tests are painless and noninvasive. The most widely recognized and recommended BMD test is the DXA (dual-energy X-ray absorptiometry) which is similar to an X-ray but with much less exposure to radiation.[55]

DXA of the hip and spine are suggested over other areas such as the radius or heel. Peripheral BMD tests can be helpful in screening and predicting a woman's risk for fractures but central DXA is preferred for actual diagnosing of osteoporosis. BMD test results are based on a T-score, a standardized score. Women with low BMD (T-scores between –1.0 and –2.4) are diagnosed with osteopenia. A woman with osteopenia may have her bone density results further evaluated with the use of an online fracture risk assessment tool called FRAX.

FRAX estimates the changes of breaking a bone within the next 10 years and can help a woman make a decision about the need for treatment.[57]

Treatment

Osteoporosis has no cure, but it can be treated or prevented with different drug therapies. Antiresorptive drugs that are used to slow progressive thinning of bone include bisphosphonates such as Fosamax and Actonel, calcitonin, and estrogen analogs such as raloxifene. A bone-forming drug (anabolic drug) known as Forteo is the first Food and Drug Administration (FDA)-approved osteoporosis treatment that rebuilds bone. The injectable treatment is a form of parathyroid hormone approved for the treatment of osteoporosis in postmenopausal women and in women who are at high risk of breaking a bone due to long-term steroid medicine use. Forteo rebuilds bone and significantly increases bone mineral density, especially in the spine.[58]

Home safety and preventing falls should be concerns for women with osteoporosis, because falls can cause disabling fractures. Removing throw rugs or loose wires/cords in one's home is important. Walking paths should be cleared of clutter and stairways may need hand rails installed. Good lighting in rooms and hallways can prevent falls, especially at night, when drowsiness can increase a woman's risk for falls. Bathrooms may need various grab bars and nonskid tape installed in the tub or shower. Walking with proper safe footwear and using assist devices when warranted are also keys to prevention of falls. In brief, a woman's home and surrounding environment should be evaluated for safety. Drinking alcohol and taking medications that cause drowsiness or light-headedness can increase the risk of falls and therefore caution is advised with these activities.

DIABETES MELLITUS

Diabetes is a chronic disorder of carbohydrate metabolism with a deficiency in insulin production, insulin action, or both. Normally, insulin allows glucose (a form of sugar) to enter the cells so that energy can be produced. The disruption of normal carbohydrate metabolism causes high levels of glucose in the blood, which results in damage to many of the body's systems, especially blood vessels and nerves.

Diabetes is the seventh leading cause of death in the United States and can lead to complications resulting in permanent disability and premature debilitation. The risk for death among people with diabetes is about twice that of people of similar age but without diabetes.[59] Women with diabetes also have a two to four times increased risk for stroke, an increased risk for bladder and

Bone Density Test and FRAX Results and Treatment[56]

BONE DENSITY CATEGORY	WHEN TO CONSIDER TREATMENT WITH AN OSTEOPOROSIS MEDICINE—IN POSTMENOPAUSAL WOMEN AND MEN AGE 50 AND OLDER	T-SCORES	
		SCORES RANGE	POSSIBLE SCORE
Normal	Most people with T-scores of −1 or higher do not need to consider taking a medicine.	−1 and higher	+1.0 +0.5 0 −0.5 −1.0
Low Bone Density (Osteopenia)	People with T-scores between −1.0 and −2.5 should consider taking a medicine when there are certain risk factors suggesting an increased chance of breaking a bone in the next 10 years. FRAX score less than 3% at the hip or less than 20% at other sites may not need medicine FRAX score 3% or higher at the hip or 20% or higher at other sites may need to consider medicine.	−1.1 to −2.4	−1.1 −1.5 −2.0 −2.4
Osteoporosis	All people with osteoporosis should consider taking a medicine.	−2.5 and lower	−2.5 −3.0 −3.5 −4.0

http://www.nof.org/aboutosteoporosis/managingandtreating/medicinesneedtoknow

vaginal infections, and increased risk of complications during pregnancy.

Over 25 million Americans over 20 years of age have diabetes and the prevalence rises to over 26 percent among Americans 65 years or older. In addition, another 79 million people are estimated to have prediabetes.[60] The prevalence of type 2 diabetes is at least two to four times higher among black, Hispanic, American Indian, and Asian/Pacific Islander women than among white women.[61]

Complications associated with diabetes mellitus include diabetic retinopathy (a leading cause of blindness), kidney failure, heart disease, gum disease, diabetic neuropathy (sensory nerve damage to extremities), and diabetic foot disease, which can lead to amputation if left untreated. The three most common types of diabetes are type 1, type 2, and gestational diabetes. Cognitive decline and Alzheimer's disease have been found in some women with type 2 diabetes, particularly when blood-sugar levels are uncontrolled. Heredity, autoimmune factors, and environmental factors have been found to be possible causes of type 1 diabetes. Obesity is the leading contributor to the exponential increase in type 2 diabetes. 90–95 percent of all diagnosed diabetes

is type 2, but type 1 and gestational diabetes are also significant. Prediabetes is a condition that increases the risk for type 2 diabetes, heart disease, and stroke and is receiving more attention from the medical profession. Persons with prediabetes have impaired fasting glucose and/or impaired glucose tolerance. Prediabetics have higher than normal blood glucose or hemoglobin A1c levels but they are not high enough to be classified as diabetics. Hemoglobin A1c is a lab test that measures the average blood glucose control for the past 2–3 months. A1c is monitored two to three times a year but does not replace the daily testing of blood glucose that may be required for some diabetics. Losing weight and increasing physical activity can prevent or delay the onset of diabetes.[62]

Type 1 Diabetes

Type 1 diabetes was once called insulin-dependent or juvenile-onset diabetes. This form develops most frequently in young children and adolescents, but its rate is increasing among adults. It accounts for 5–10 percent of adults diagnosed with diabetes. In type 1 diabetes, the pancreas produces little or no insulin as a result of the body's immune system destroying its own pancreatic beta cells that make insulin. Daily insulin injections or the use of insulin pumps is required to maintain normal blood-sugar levels, thus providing the body's cells with energy. Physical activity and healthy eating are also important in managing this disease.[63] Ongoing research of islet cell transplantation and pancreas transplantation is being undertaken to find treatments so type 1 diabetics can live without daily injections of insulin.[64]

Type 2 Diabetes

Type 2 diabetes was once known as non–insulin-dependent or adult-onset diabetes. In this form of diabetes, the pancreas produces insulin but for some reason the body is resistant to the insulin and is unable to use it properly. As the insulin level rises, the pancreas loses more of its ability to produce insulin. Type 2 diabetes is the most common form of diabetes and appears more frequently in adults over the age of 45, but it is increasingly being found in adolescents and children. This type of diabetes is linked to obesity and physical inactivity and can be controlled by a healthy diet, physical activity, and weight control, and by insulin injections and/or oral medications. In addition, some studies have found that women who smoke have a higher risk of developing type 2 diabetes than women who never smoked or who quit smoking. (See *Health Tips:* "Warning Signs of Diabetes.")

Gestational Diabetes

Gestational diabetes affects 18 percent of pregnancies. A screening test that measures blood glucose level is usually done between the 24th and 28th weeks of pregnancy. Pregnant women with high blood glucose levels during pregnancy who had no previous signs of diabetes are said to have gestational diabetes. Women who become pregnant after age 25 are more likely to develop diabetes.[65]

Gestational diabetes usually appears around the 24th week of pregnancy. Although the cause is unknown, it may be related to the large quantities of hormones that the placenta starts producing at that time. These hormones may block or cause an insulin resistance in the mother's body that lasts until the pregnancy is over.

Many women who experience gestational diabetes will experience a return to normal blood-sugar levels after the pregnancy. However, studies show that these women remain more susceptible to gestational diabetes in future pregnancies, and more than half of them will develop type 2 diabetes later in life. Approximately 35–60 percent of women who had gestational diabetes develop diabetes within 10–20 years.[66]

Although babies born to mothers with gestational diabetes do not have any greater risk for birth defects than those delivered from nongestational diabetic mothers, they are more at risk for other problems. These include macrosomia (large or fat bodies), hypoglycemia (low blood glucose) after delivery, jaundice, and respiratory distress syndrome (RDS). Macrosomic babies may need to be delivered by cesarean section if they are too large for vaginal delivery. Large babies can cause difficult deliveries for both the mother and baby, with the baby being at risk for arm and shoulder injuries or even oxygen deprivation for a period of time. If an ultrasound shows that a woman is carrying a macrosomic baby, an amniocentesis test may be recommended to determine the baby's risk for RDS, because macrosomic babies are also at increased risk for premature birth.

Women with gestational diabetes are at higher risk for preeclampsia, urinary tract infections, and ketonuria. Preeclampsia is a potentially life-threatening condition in which a woman experiences pregnancy-induced high BP usually accompanied by edema (swelling) of the lower legs and hands. Ketonuria is the presence of ketones in the urine. Ketones are acidic byproducts of fat breakdown that build up in the blood and are excreted in the urine when a woman's body utilizes fat for energy when no other source is available. Gestational diabetic mothers should be monitored closely during pregnancy and should be encouraged to maintain a healthy diet and to exercise regularly.

Pregnancy for Women with Diabetes

Pregnancy in women with diabetes is risky, but with prompt preconception care and careful monitoring of blood sugar, these women will have healthy pregnancies and healthy babies. Women considering birth control methods should be aware that oral contraceptives

Health Tips

Warning Signs of Diabetes

Type 1 (usually occurs suddenly)	Type 2 (usually occurs gradually)
Frequent urination	Any of the insulin-dependent symptoms
Excessive thirst	Recurring or hard-to-heal skin, gum, or bladder infections
Extreme hunger	
Dramatic weight loss	Drowsiness
Irritability	Blurred vision
Weakness and fatigue	Tingling or numbness in hands or feet
Nausea and vomiting	Itching
	Very dry skin

can affect glucose levels and diabetes management and that IUD use can lead to infection. IUDs are typically contraindicated for women with diabetes because they already have a higher risk for infection.[67]

ASTHMA

Asthma is a chronic, incurable disease of the lungs, characterized by inflammation and temporary narrowing of the air passageways leading from the mouth and nose into the lungs. Asthmatics have inflamed airways that tend to react strongly to some inhaled substances causing surrounding muscles to tighten, thus leading to narrow passages and less air into the lungs. Women and children with asthma suffer periodic episodes, or attacks, with mild to severe symptoms that may include shortness of breath, wheezing, coughing (often occurring at night or early morning), chest pain or tightness, or any combination. In severe cases, an asthma attack can lead to the death of the individual. It is important to treat early symptoms during flareups to prevent the symptoms from worsening.

Asthma is one of the most common and costly diseases in the United States and affects nearly 20 million Americans. The rates of asthma have progressively increased during the past three decades. Although asthma is more common in male children, adult women outnumber adult men as asthma sufferers since women over age 20 are more likely to develop the condition. Each year, more women than men die of asthma-related complications, and women account for 65 percent of deaths due to the condition. African American women have the highest mortality rate and are at least 2.5 times more likely to die from asthma than non-Hispanic white women.[68]

While the root causes of asthma remain unknown, heredity is believed to play a role. A child with one parent having asthma has a one in three chance of developing asthma, while a child with two parents with asthma has a seven in ten chance of developing the condition.[69] While persons of any ethnic or socioeconomic group may develop asthma, living in poverty or with little access to health care or in urban areas where air quality is poor or working in occupations in which exposure to lung irritants is more likely, appears to account for more disparity in the disease than simply gender or ethnic differences.[70]

Types of Asthma

Asthma is divided into two types: allergic and nonallergic. *Allergic asthma* is most common, with nearly 50 percent of sufferers having this type. As its name implies, allergic asthma is triggered in susceptible individuals by exposure to common airborne pollutants and allergens, including mold spores, pollen, dust mites or roaches, animal dander, feather bedding, perfume, foods, tobacco smoke, or other environmental contaminants. *Nonallergic,* or *intrinsic,* asthma may be triggered by allergens but is often triggered by other factors including stress, anxiety, extreme weather changes, exercise, cold air, dry air, hyperventilation, viruses, and bronchial illnesses including colds and flu, and lung infections. Other triggers for asthma symptoms include sulfites in foods and drinks, medicines such as aspirin or other nonsteroidal anti-inflammatory drugs, and nonselective beta blockers (including eye drops). For women, monthly hormonal cycles or the hormonal changes that occur during pregnancy may trigger the onset of adult asthma. Menopausal women may also experience adult-onset asthma for the first time. For some patients, however, asthma symptoms may disappear or lessen in adulthood, as asthma is most often diagnosed during childhood.

Managing Your Asthma

If you have asthma, controlling the condition and your symptoms is important for your continuing health and quality of life. First, educate yourself about your asthma by staying current with new information and research. Checking your lungs for air flow on a daily basis with a device called a peak flow meter can help you detect potential changes in your condition that should be brought to the attention of your health care provider. If your asthma is triggered by food allergens, know which foods or food ingredients you are sensitive to and avoid them. Avoid exposure to fabrics or chemicals that are known irritants, and keep your living or work spaces as free of irritants and allergens as possible. Evidence suggests that exposure to cockroach allergens might be the most important risk factor for asthma in inner-city households; therefore, effective cockroach extermination can reduce allergen concentrations.[71] During warm weather, when ozone or air particulates are at high levels, you may wish to stay away from outdoor activities, as poor air quality may also trigger attacks. Uncontrolled asthma, which often flares up at night, can be managed with prescribed medications.

There are two groups of asthma medications: those that provide quick relief for immediate symptoms of an asthma attack and others that are used for long-term management of asthma. A woman should understand how and when to use them, whether the medicines are inhalers or pills.

There are many effective medications that help control symptoms, including some that are available over the counter. It is important to take all your medications as prescribed. Any changes to your current drug regimen or additions of over-the-counter medications should not be attempted without first consulting your health care provider, as this could cause potentially harmful drug interactions. Let your health care provider know if, over time, your condition does not improve or your symptoms worsen.

Asthma and Pregnancy

When an asthmatic woman becomes pregnant, controlling her symptoms is vital for both her health and the health of her unborn baby. A developing fetus depends on its mother's blood for its oxygen needs, and frequent asthma attacks may lead to a lessening of the oxygen supply available to a fetus. Having a sufficient level of oxygen in the fetal blood is essential for its healthy development, and inadequate oxygen at key times throughout this development could result in impaired growth or even in fetal death. As many as 4–8 percent of pregnant women may have asthma, making it one of the most common serious medical conditions affecting pregnancy.[72]

Uncontrolled asthma has been associated with a greater risk for a pregnant woman's developing hypertensive problems, including preeclampsia, a potentially serious or even life-threatening condition that affects some women. It may also cause other problems, including premature birth or having a low-birth-weight baby.[73] Because the risks of uncontrolled asthma on a pregnancy outweigh those of most asthma medications, a woman who is already on a prescribed drug regimen for this condition should not stop or change this regimen unless directed to do so by her physician or health care provider.

While some prenatal or postpartum problems are seen more frequently in women with uncontrolled asthma, medical experts are still uncertain as to the exact role asthma may play in causing these conditions. Until more is learned in this regard, keeping adequate medical control over her asthma is the best way for a woman to ensure both a healthy pregnancy and a healthy baby.

The National Institutes of Health provides the following summary of control measures for environmental factors that can make asthma worse during pregnancy. First, exposure to allergens that the pregnant woman may be sensitive to, including animal dander, house-dust mites, cockroaches, pollens, and indoor mold, should be reduced or eliminated. Indoor humidity should be reduced to less than 50 percent if possible. Tobacco smoke should be eliminated from the house and other areas, such as day care and workplace environments. Exposure to indoor and outdoor pollutants and irritants such as wood-burning stoves and fireplaces, unvented stoves or heaters, perfumes, cleaning agents, etc. also should be reduced or eliminated.[74]

Asthma and Tobacco Smoke

Tobacco smoke may contain up to 4000 trace chemicals, many of which are known toxins, including arsenic, formaldehyde, and cyanide. Secondhand smoke, the smoke that is emitted as a result of a lit cigarette, pipe, or cigar, has been rated as a Group A carcinogen by the U.S. Environmental Protection Agency, with Group A carcinogens ranked as the most serious.[75] As more is learned about the dangers from exposure to secondhand smoke (SHS), research indicates that children who are routinely exposed to SHS have a greater likelihood of developing asthma, allergies, and other serious lung conditions. The chance of a child dying from sudden infant death syndrome (SIDS) greatly increases if one or both parents are smokers.[76]

Because children's lungs are still maturing, they are more sensitive to the effects of tobacco smoke and the chemicals burned off in the process of smoking. Children exposed to these chemicals may experience impaired lung function, may have more infections of the respiratory tract, and may suffer from more allergies than children who are not exposed to tobacco smoke. Infants and children exposed to environmental tobacco smoke (ETS) are more likely to develop middle ear infections, many times necessitating the insertion of surgical ear tubes. Infants up to 18 months old who are exposed to secondhand smoke may be at greater risk for lung infections and infections of the lower respiratory tract, which incur high medical costs if the infant needs hospitalization.

If an adult must smoke, smoking should be done outside of a home and outside of areas such as cars, buildings, or play areas in which children are likely to spend time. In the long-term, ceasing the smoking habit, while difficult, remains the best strategy for adults to ensure not only their own lung and respiratory health, but that of their children as well.

EPILEPSY

Epilepsy, a chronic brain disorder characterized by recurrent seizures, is a general term for more than twenty different types of seizure disorders. It occurs when abnormal electrical activity in the brain causes an involuntary change in body movement or function, sensation, awareness, or behavior lasting from a few seconds to a few minutes. Any disturbance of the normal pattern of neuron (nerve cell) activity can lead to seizures. Epilepsy can result from abnormal electrical neuron activity, an imbalance of neurotransmitters, or a combination of these factors. Experts divide the different types of seizures into groups including generalized seizures, partial seizures, gelastic and dacrystic seizures, nonepileptic seizures and status epilepticus.[70] Symptoms during a seizure will depend on the site of the electrical activity in the brain. A person experiencing a grand mal seizure (a generalized tonic-clonic seizure) may lose consciousness, fall to the ground, and have rigidity and muscle jerks. During a complex partial seizure, a woman may seem confused or dazed and won't be able to answer questions or follow directions. Absence (petit mal) seizures can go undetected as the person may experience only a short period of rapid blinking or staring into space.

Gelastic ("laughing") and dacrystic ("crying") seizures are most commonly found in people with hypothalmic hamartomas. Gelastic seizures create forced laughter-like sounds in conjunction with a facial contraction resembling a smile or smirk. Dacrystic seizures create sounds with a crying quality and facial contraction causing a grimace expression.[77]

Approximately 3 million Americans have some form of epilepsy. Although epileptic seizures may be caused by lack of oxygen, head trauma, stroke, brain tumor, poisoning, infection/fever, inherited conditions, or fetal development complications, there is no known cause for the majority of them. Seizure-preventing drugs known as antiepileptic drugs are the most common form of treatment. Surgery, vagal nerve stimulation, and a special ketogenic diet are sometimes tried when drug therapies do not work. Various anticonvulsants can be used depending on the type of seizure experienced. If a woman has more than one type of seizure, it is possible that several medications will be prescribed. Surgery for epilepsy may be considered, although there is no guarantee that the seizures will be reduced or eliminated. Vagal nerve stimulation is a form of electrical stimulation of the brain through the vagus nerve in the neck. With this procedure, a small battery is placed in the chest wall and programmed to deliver short bursts of electrical energy to the brain. The ketogenic diet is a strict high-fat, low-carbohydrate diet that is reemerging as a possible treatment for epilepsy, especially for children whose seizures are not controlled by other means. This diet is a serious treatment with potential side effects including vitamin deficiencies. Further research is needed to evaluate this method of treatment for children and adults. Women on this diet may experience menstrual irregularities, pancreatitis, vitamin deficiencies, dehydration, constipation, decreased bone density, eye problems, and kidney stones or gallstones.[78] Additional research is being conducted with stem cell transplants, neuron stimulation, and on the development of a device to more readily predict seizures several minutes before they occur.

Photosensitivity epilepsy occurs in 3 percent of people with epilepsy, particularly in children and adolescents. With this condition, exposure to flashing lights of certain intensities or wavelengths can trigger seizures. Photosensitive epileptic seizures may be triggered by

Health Tips

First Aid for Seizures

What to Do

- Look for medical identification.
- Loosen collars and ties.
- Protect the head from injury.
- Protect the person from nearby hazards.
- Turn person on side to keep airway clear.
- Call for aid.

What Not to Do

- Do not place anything in the mouth. (The tongue cannot be swallowed.)
- Do not provide any liquids during or immediately after the seizure.
- Do not give artificial respiration, unless the person does not start breathing again after the seizure.
- Do not restrain the person.

television, video games, computer monitors, fire alarms, strobe lights, or even natural sunlight when there is a flickering or rapid flashing effect from the light.[79] (See *Health Tips:* "First Aid for Seizures.")

Initially, controlling the seizures is the primary concern of health care providers and the person with epilepsy. However, it doesn't take long to realize that the social stigma connected with epilepsy is often more difficult to overcome.

Psychosocial and Economic Considerations

The person with epilepsy and her caregiver (if dealing with a child) may know a lot about the illness, including what seizures are, what to do when one occurs, what medications do, how they should be taken, and their potential side effects. But what about the psychosocial, legal, and economic aspects of epilepsy? How are these addressed? Many questions arise: Should I tell my instructors? Is it safe to drive a car? Can I drink alcohol? What will my friends think, how will they act, if I tell them I have epilepsy? Is it safe to get pregnant? Educating the person with epilepsy and her caregiver is important, but so is educating the public. Education is the only way to reduce or eliminate the stigma associated with epilepsy. Employers, family, and friends of persons with epilepsy need to educate themselves about the disorder. Remember: Epilepsy is what a woman has, not what she is. She is a woman with epilepsy; not an epileptic woman.

Birth Control, Conception, and Pregnancy

Over 1 million girls and women in the United States live with a seizure disorder. Birth control, conception, and pregnancy create special circumstances and concerns for these women. Despite the special concerns, more than 90 percent of women with epilepsy who become pregnant give birth to normal, healthy infants.

Some antiepileptic medicines can lower estrogen concentrations by 40–50 percent, complicating the use of hormonal birth control methods. Women need to keep their health care provider informed when using these two medications concurrently because adjustments may need to be made if midcycle bleeding occurs, indicating poor birth control regulation. In addition, there is a 25–30 percent lower fertility rate for women with epilepsy. The reasons for the lower fertility rate are unknown but appear to range from genetic predisposition, seizure type and frequency, and side effects from antiepileptic medications to social pressures to refrain from having children.

Women with epilepsy should plan their pregnancies with a health care provider because medications will need to be monitored closely and adjusted before and throughout the pregnancy. The effects of medication on a developing fetus occur primarily in the first few weeks after conception. Not only do the antiepileptic medications pose special concerns, but seizure activity itself during the pregnancy can be hazardous for both the mother and the fetus. Breast-feeding is considered safe for most women with epilepsy but should be discussed with the health care provider. Safety for infants and children should also be discussed because the mother with epilepsy could have unexpected seizures.[80]

Research has brought advances in diagnosis and treatment of epilepsy effectiveness of medications, and knowledge of pregnancy issues. Women with epilepsy can help control their own seizures by taking medications as prescribed, avoiding unusual stress, maintaining regular sleep cycles, and complying with the health care provider's treatment protocol.[81]

ARTHRITIS

Arthritis is an inflammatory condition of the joints, characterized by swelling, pain, and/or difficulty moving that persists for more than 2 weeks. (See *Health Tips:* "SERIOUS: The Warning Signs of Arthritis.")

Over 100 types of arthritis and related diseases (known as rheumatic diseases) have been classified, with consequences ranging from mild to debilitating. The variety of arthritis and related diseases that women

Health Tips

SERIOUS: The Warning Signs of Arthritis

Swelling in one or more joints
Early morning stiffness
Recurring pain or tenderness in any joint
Inability to move a joint normally
Obvious redness and warmth in a joint
Unexplained weight loss, fever, or weakness combined with joint pain
Symptoms like these persisting for more than 2 weeks

often encounter include osteoarthritis, rheumatoid arthritis, systemic lupus erythematosus, fibromyalgia, carpal tunnel syndrome, gout, Marfan syndrome, and scleroderma. If you experience arthritis, you need to know which type because treatment protocols vary. Arthritis affects 50 million Americans and is the leading cause of disability. In addition, people who are obese, overweight, or physically inactive or who have less education are more likely to be affected by arthritis. Although the prevalence of arthritis is less for non-Hispanic blacks and Hispanics compared to whites, both groups report a higher incidence of arthritis-attributed activity limitation.[82] Women are more likely than men to have arthritis, and the prevalence of arthritis increases with age.

Treatment can include rest, relaxation, weight control, physical activity, the use of heat or cold, medications for pain and inflammation, surgery, and use of assistive devices. Two general rules to follow regarding physical activity with arthritis are that any physical activity is better than none and the benefits of physical activity outweigh the risks. Women with arthritis should start out at "lower" and "slower" levels of activity and build gradually to higher levels while using low-impact aerobic activities, muscle strengthening exercises and balancing exercises. Women may need to modify activity when arthritis symptoms worsen by lessening the frequency, duration or intensity of the activity. Physical activity should be "joint friendly" with low risk for injury or "pounding" on the joints and should take place in safe, unobstructed environments. Many traditional or alternative therapies exist that can be beneficial to a person suffering from arthritis, but as a consumer you need to be informed and watch carefully for quackery. Self-management programs that increase a person's ability to manage the chronic condition have also proven to be effective.

Osteoarthritis

Osteoarthritis (OA), or degenerative joint disease, occurs when cartilage that provides a smooth, gliding surface and cushion between the bones breaks down, resulting in pain, swelling, and altered joint function. It is the most common kind of arthritis and affects the weight-bearing joints, particularly the knees, hips, and ankles, but it can also affect the hands, lower spine, and neck. Osteoarthritis pain is often worse after overuse of the joint or periods of inactivity. Osteoarthritis is more common in women and people over age 45. The causes of OA are unknown, but factors such as heredity, aging, obesity, prior joint injury, muscle weakness, nerve injury, and overuse have been implicated in increased risk for the disease. Treatment focuses on minimizing the pain and improving joint movement. Management of the disease includes patient education, medications for inflammation and pain, weight control, heat/cold therapy, joint protection, physical activity to keep the joints flexible, and light weight lifting to improve muscle strength. Research indicates that in a person who is overweight even a modest weight loss (15 pounds) can improve symptoms of OA by almost 50 percent. Surgery is considered when other measures have proven ineffective against pain control and maintaining joint function.[83]

Rheumatoid Arthritis

Rheumatoid arthritis (RA) is a systemic, autoimmune, and chronic inflammatory disease of unknown cause that involves inflammation in the lining of the joints (synovium) and/or other internal organs. RA occurs two to three times more frequently in women than in men and is most prevalent in postmenopausal women. Symptoms often begin in women between the ages of 30 and 60. Research is being conducted to find the cause of RA so that better treatments might be found. Genetic and environmental factors, as well as endocrine, nerve, and immune system factors, are being studied. Research also is focused on the potential role of infectious agents as triggers of RA. The joints become swollen, red, and inflamed, and this condition lasts for an extended period of time. A pattern of flare-ups and remissions begins, and eventually the cartilage between the joints disappears and bone-to-bone irritation and pain ensue. RA can lead to long-term joint damage resulting in chronic pain, loss of function, and disability. Inflammation of RA most often affects joints in the hands and feet and is symmetrical (occurs equally on both sides of the body). This helps distinguish it from other forms of rheumatic (inflammatory) diseases.

Early diagnosis and treatment of RA are critical in preventing joint injury, thus limiting joint damage and

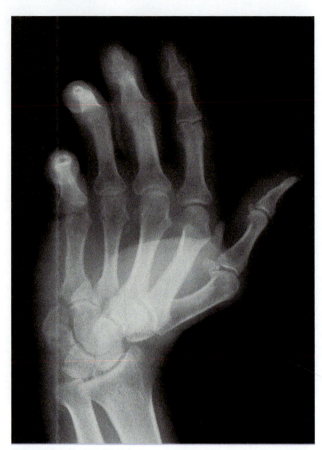

X-Ray of Arthritic Hands.

loss of movement. Treatment of RA is individualized according to the severity of a woman's arthritis and other medical conditions that she may have. Treatment focuses on pain relief, inflammation reduction, stopping or slowing joint damage or improving function. Three classes of drugs are commonly used in the treatment of RA: nonsteroidal anti-inflammatory agents (NSAIDs), corticosteroids, and disease-modifying antirheumatic drugs (DMARDs). DMARDs are being used more aggressively in the first 2 years to slow cartilage damage and bony erosions. A group of drugs known as biologic response modifiers are being used in conjunction with DMARDs to create a more effective treatment outcome. These biologic response modifiers inhibit proteins called cytoxines that contribute to inflammation.[84] In addition to drug therapy, physical activity, joint protection, and self-management techniques are used to improve the quality of life. A blood-filtering process, protein-A immunoadsorption therapy, which removes antibodies and immune complexes that promote inflammation, can be used in women with RA.[85] Various surgical procedures may also be used to reduce inflammation and pain or to enhance joint function. Pregnancy creates a difficult situation because most of the medications used are not recommended during

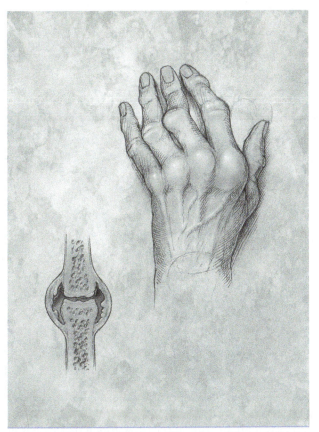

Rheumatoid arthritis can cause distortion of finger joints.

pregnancy and may need to be discontinued throughout the pregnancy.

Systemic Lupus Erythematosus (SLE)

Systemic lupus erythematosus (SLE) is the most common of three types of **lupus** and is recognized by the red, butterfly-shaped rash found across the bridge of the nose and cheeks. SLE is a chronic, autoimmune, rheumatic disease of connective tissue that causes inflammation affecting joints, muscles, and vital organs, especially the skin, kidneys, heart, lungs, and brain.

Lupus is an unpredictable disease of flare-ups and remissions that develops between the ages of 15 and 44, mostly in women of childbearing age. The symptoms of lupus can range from mild to life-threatening. Lupus affects women nearly 10 times more frequently than men but most women (80–90 percent) can live a normal life span with non–organ-threatening symptoms. Lupus is two to three times more common in women of color.[86]

The cause of lupus is unknown; however, a combination of genetic, environmental, and hormonal factors have been implicated as "triggers" for the illness or to bring on a flare. Some of these triggers include UV light from the sun, tanning beds, or florescent lights, certain drugs that make a woman more sensitive to the sun (e.g., sulfa drugs), penicillin and other antibiotics, viral or bacterial infections, physical and emotional stresses, and vaccinations containing live virus.[87]

Signs and Symptoms The most commonly reported symptoms of SLE are found in *FYI:* "The Most Common Symptoms of Lupus."[88] The pattern of remission and flare-ups is common and can be fatal if left untreated. Flare-ups are often precipitated by exposure to sunlight, an infection, or a drug reaction. For some women, the use of estrogen may induce or trigger a lupus flare-up. The risk of blood clots is a real concern for women who are taking estrogen, and estrogen is contraindicated in women whose blood tests show a presence of antiphospholipid antibodies.[89] Women with lupus are much more likely than other women to suffer fractures due to osteoporosis. The bone loss associated with lupus is due to the use of certain medications, stress, and less physical activity.

Diagnosis and Treatment The immunofluorescent antinuclear antibody (ANA) test is a screening test for the presence of autoantibodies and is used to diagnose SLE. Determining whether a woman has SLE depends on the results of the ANA test and a minimum of four supporting symptoms. Diagnosis of SLE can be difficult, and it may take some time to associate various symptoms of the past with newer symptoms in the present. There is no cure for SLE, but early treatment of

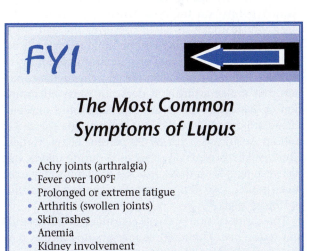

FYI

The Most Common Symptoms of Lupus

- Achy joints (arthralgia)
- Fever over 100°F
- Prolonged or extreme fatigue
- Arthritis (swollen joints)
- Skin rashes
- Anemia
- Kidney involvement
- Pain in the chest on deep breathing (pleurisy)
- Butterfly-shaped rash across the cheeks and nose
- Sun or light sensitivity (photosensitivity)
- Unusual loss of hair
- Pale or purple fingers from cold or stress (Raynaud's phenomenon)
- Mouth or nose ulcers
- Seizures
- Abnormal blood clotting problems

symptoms is important for long-term management of this highly individualized disease. Treatment can range from the use of NSAIDs and antimalarial drugs for less dangerous symptoms to the use of immune suppressants and high-dose corticosteroids for more threatening symptoms.

Prevention of Flare-ups Preventive measures are equally important, including avoidance of excessive sun exposure, use of sunscreens, regular exercise, stress management, no smoking, limited or no alcohol consumption, proper use of prescribed medications, prompt treatment of infections, and maintaining proper nutrition. Support from family and friends can help alleviate the effects of stress, especially when dealing with the unpredictable aspects of the disease.

Pregnancy and Lupus Health care providers suggest that women considering pregnancy try to time the pregnancy for a period when the disease is least active. For some women, the first symptoms of lupus may appear during pregnancy, and for others, they may occur immediately after childbirth. Careful monitoring is necessary to minimize harmful effects on the expectant mother or her fetus.

Fibromyalgia

Fibromyalgia is a common and chronic musculoskeletal syndrome characterized by fatigue; widespread pain in the muscles, ligaments, and tendons; and multiple "tender points" on the body where there is increased sensitivity to touch or slight pressure. The soft tissue pain of fibromyalgia, ranging from mild to severe, is described as deep-aching, radiating, gnawing, shooting, or burning. Fibromyalgia is considered a rheumatic condition, but unlike arthritis, it does not cause inflammation or damage to the joints. The American College of Rheumatology (ACR) states that fibromyalgia affects 3–6 million Americans, with 80–90 percent being women. Fibromyalgia is generally diagnosed during middle age (between ages 30 and 50), but the symptoms may exist much earlier. (See *FYI:* "Common Signs and Symptoms of Fibromyalgia.")

The cause of fibromyalgia continues to be debated and researched. The multiple precipitating factors may include traumatic physical or emotional events, repetitive injuries, illnesses such as HIV infection, Lyme disease, or flu-like viral infection. Hereditary and environmental causes are being studied. Women with certain rheumatic diseases such as RA, SLE, and ankylosing spondylitis (spinal arthritis) have a greater likelihood of developing fibromyalgia.[91]

Fibromyalgia is difficult to diagnose because the main symptoms of pain and fatigue overlap with numerous

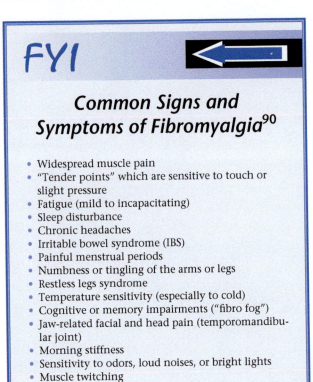

FYI

Common Signs and Symptoms of Fibromyalgia[90]

- Widespread muscle pain
- "Tender points" which are sensitive to touch or slight pressure
- Fatigue (mild to incapacitating)
- Sleep disturbance
- Chronic headaches
- Irritable bowel syndrome (IBS)
- Painful menstrual periods
- Numbness or tingling of the arms or legs
- Restless legs syndrome
- Temperature sensitivity (especially to cold)
- Cognitive or memory impairments ("fibro fog")
- Jaw-related facial and head pain (temporomandibular joint)
- Morning stiffness
- Sensitivity to odors, loud noises, or bright lights
- Muscle twitching
- Irritable bladder

other conditions. Diagnostic laboratory tests are unavailable for diagnosing the condition, so other potential causes must be ruled out prior to making a diagnosis of fibromyalgia. The ACR has set specific criteria for establishing a diagnosis, including eleven of eighteen designated "tender points" located on the body. (See Figure 15.2.)

Symptom-specific medications such as sleep medications, muscle relaxants, headache remedies, pain medications, and anti-inflammatory drugs may be used to treat the symptoms of fibromyalgia based on the woman's presenting complaints. The FDA has approved three medications for the treatment of fibromyalgia. Savella and Cymbalta were originally developed to treat depression, whereas Lyrica was developed to treat neuropathic pain. Antidepressants that increase brain chemicals including serotonin and norepinephrine are the most useful in treating symptoms by modulating sleep, pain, and immune system function.[92]

Women with fibromyalgia may also benefit by reducing stressors in their lives and getting deep-level (stage 4) sleep at night. Practical suggestions for enhancing quality of sleep can be found in numerous publications. Women can learn to balance daily activities with rest periods; eat more healthy foods; avoid or limit alcohol and caffeine intake; exercise to improve muscular strength, flexibility, and aerobic endurance; and seek external support to deal with depression, anxiety, and stress. Changes in weather, cold or drafty environments, as well as infections and allergies, can contribute to symptom flare-ups,

FIGURE 15.2 The location of the eighteen tender points that comprise the criteria for fibromyalgia.

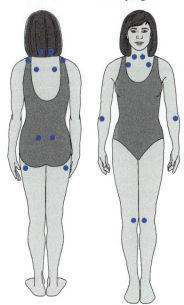

SOURCE: National Institute of Arthritis and Musculoskeletal and Skin Diseases, National Institutes of Health, Department of Health and Human Services. www.niams.nih.gov/hi/topics/fibromyalgia/fibrofs.htm (retrieved July 30, 2012).

so care should be taken to avoid them. Women with fibromyalgia need to know that it is not a progressive or life-threatening condition. It does not damage the joints, muscles, or internal organs, and with time, many women experience improvements in their condition.

MULTIPLE SCLEROSIS

Multiple sclerosis (MS) is a chronic, debilitating disease that affects the central nervous system (CNS) including the brain, spinal cord, and optic nerves. MS is thought to be an autoimmune disease that causes damage to and loss of myelin, the fatty white tissue that surrounds and protects the nerve fibers of the CNS and aids in the smooth conduction of electrical impulses. This injury and loss, called demyelination, results in areas known as plaques and scar tissue (sclerosis) that disrupt the normal conduction of electrical impulses causing the various symptoms of MS. The exact cause of this disease is still unknown, but it is believed that there is an abnormal response of the body's immune system that causes it to attack its own myelin. The autoimmune response in MS is believed to be triggered by multiple factors including genetics, gender, and environment. Some possible environmental triggers being studied are trauma, viruses, and heavy metals (toxins). Although there is no evidence that MS is inherited, genetic factors may make certain

people more susceptible to MS. The prevalence of MS is higher among persons who live in certain geographic regions farther from the equator that have cold, damp climates, particularly areas that are 40 degrees north in latitude. This prevalence has led researchers to investigate possible links of sunlight exposure and vitamin D as protective factors.

The onset or diagnosis of MS is usually between the ages of 20 and 50 years and is two to three times higher in women than in men. MS is a leading cause of neurologic disability in early adulthood and is found more commonly in non-Hispanic whites and people of northern European ancestry. The National Multiple Sclerosis Society estimates that approximately 400,000 Americans have MS and 200 more people are being diagnosed weekly.[93] Studies have demonstrated high rates among identical twins. If one identical twin develops MS, the other twin has a one in four chance of developing the disease.[94]

Signs and Symptoms

Precipitating events such as infection, trauma, or pregnancy can bring on or exacerbate the symptoms of MS. Symptoms of MS are unpredictable and depend on the site(s) of demyelination in the CNS. Symptoms vary from person to person and can even vary within the same person. (See *Health Tips:* "Possible Symptoms of Multiple Sclerosis.")

Health Tips

Possible Symptoms of Multiple Sclerosis[96]

- Gait (walking) disturbances
- Muscle weakness
- Spasticity and muscle rigidity
- Impairment of pain, temperature, and touch senses
- Pain (moderate to severe)
- Tremor
- Speech and swallowing disorders
- Vision disturbances (blurred or double vision, blindness in one eye, or green-red color distortion)
- Vertigo and dizziness
- Bladder, bowel, or sexual dysfunction
- Depression or emotional problems
- Cognitive abnormalities
- Headaches
- Fatigue
- Hearing loss
- Itching
- Numbness
- Seizures

The symptoms can be mild to severe, long or short in duration, and may appear in various combinations. Symptoms can worsen when women with MS are exposed to higher temperatures whether inside or outside the body. Environments or activities that raise a woman's core body temperature by one-quarter to one-half degree can cause temporary aggravation of MS symptoms.[95] The initial symptom of MS is often a visual disturbance that, inexplicably, has a tendency to clear up in the later stages of MS. Most people with MS experience muscle weakness of the extremities with impaired coordination and balance at some time during their lives. Nearly 50 percent of women with MS will have cognitive impairments of which they will not be aware. Cognitive disturbances may include problems with attention, concentration, memory, and good judgment. Cognitive impairments usually are mild and sometimes remain unnoticed. Although depression is a common symptom, other emotional changes can be experienced that cause a person with MS to have inappropriate emotional reactions or facial expressions such as the "laughing/weeping syndrome."

There are four major clinical courses that multiple sclerosis may follow.[97] Each form may vary from mild to moderate to severe. The relapsing-remitting form of MS is the most common (85 percent) and consists of clearly defined flare-ups of symptoms followed by partial or complete recovery periods. The primary-progressive form is a slow but nearly continuous worsening of the disease from the onset with no distinct relapses or remissions. A woman may experience varying rates of progression and temporary improvements. The secondary-progressive form includes an initial period of relapsing-remitting disease followed by a steady decline with or without flare-ups. Most persons with relapsing-remitting MS experience this form within 10 years of the initial diagnosis, but new drug therapies have slowed this tendency.

Diagnosis and Treatment

Overall, diagnosing MS by the presenting symptoms is difficult because of the unpredictable and varying nature of the disease. Many women endure years of tests before an accurate diagnosis is made. A diagnosis is made by reviewing a woman's history of symptoms, performing multiple tests and procedures, and evaluating the functioning of her present nervous system (e.g. reflexes and coordination). Diagnostic tests include magnetic resonance imaging (MRI), evoked potential tests, and a spinal tap. A physician must have three criteria in order to make a diagnosis of MS: evidence of damage in at least two separate areas of the CNS; evidence that the damage occurred at least 1 month apart; and all possible diagnoses must be ruled out.[98]

There is no cure for MS, but fortunately many women with the disease do not need any treatment. The aim of treatment is to enhance quality of life by addressing the symptoms and improving functionality. Exercise has numerous benefits including better cardiovascular endurance, increased muscular strength and endurance, an enhanced mental outlook and participation in social activities, and better bladder and bowel control. Cortico-steroids, which have anti-inflammatory properties, can be used to reduce the duration and intensity of a flare-up, particularly in women with motor or movement symptoms. However, steroids have a multitude of side effects, so they usually are not recommended for long-term use. Various MS disease-modifying agents are available that can reduce disease activity and progression. Cost and side effects are major issues with these agents; thus, careful consideration by each woman and her neurologist is necessary.[99]

Pregnancy and MS

A woman's ability to become pregnant is not affected by MS, and the course of pregnancy, labor, and delivery is not adversely affected by MS. The symptoms of MS often remit or stabilize during pregnancy. This is thought to be related to normal changes in a pregnant woman's immune system that allow her to carry a fetus that is in essence partially foreign tissue to her since the fetus carries genes from the father. The downside to this temporary reprieve is that 20–40 percent of women with MS have a relapse within 3 months following delivery. A woman with MS who is considering becoming pregnant should also consider the potential side effects of MS drugs on the fetus and the physical limitations that may make it difficult to carry a fetus to term.

Support System

Multiple sclerosis can affect the entire family or immediate support network of a woman with MS. The financial, physical, and emotional stresses of MS may require support groups and possible counseling to assist a woman and her support network in coping with the disease.

THYROID DISEASE

The butterfly or shield-shaped thyroid gland has two lobes on each side of the neck connected by a tissue bridge, the isthmus, and is located just in front of the trachea and below the larynx. The smaller parathyroid glands are found near or embedded in the posterior areas of the thyroid lobes. The thyroid gland cells are arranged into millions of saclike follicles that synthesize and contain the glycoprotein thyroglobulin. After various processes, the thyroglobulin attaches to iodide to create the two main thyroid hormones of T_3 (triiodothyronine) and T_4 (thyroxine). Another hormone, thyrocalcitonin, is also found in the thyroid and acts primarily to regulate the body's blood calcium and phosphate levels by directing the inhibition of bone-resorbing osteoclasts or promoting bone formation of the osteoblasts. In brief, the thyroid hormones are responsible for the rates of metabolism throughout the body so that the body's intake of oxygen and heat production keep pace with the body's needs and activities. Thus, the thyroid hormones regulate the rate of fat, protein, and glucose metabolism, are necessary for normal growth and development, and are needed for resistance to infection.

The malfunctioning of the thyroid or any of the other glands/organs (e.g., hypothalamus or pituitary gland) that the thyroid communicates with can result in abnormalities. The three basic types of abnormalities are: goiter, an enlargement of the thyroid; hyperthyroidism; and hypothyroidism. A goiter, which may also appear as a symptom of hyperthyroidism, can be caused by a lack of iodine intake, inflammation (thyroiditis), or benign or malignant tumors.

Hyperthyroidism is a result of overactivity or hyperfunctioning of the thyroid that leads to increased body metabolism and heat production. Hypothyroidism is a result of hyposecretion or underactivity of the thyroid causing a decreased body metabolism and heat production. The symptoms and treatment of hypothyroidism and hyperthyroidism are generally opposite of one another.

The most severe, rare form of hypothyroidism, myxedema coma, is a medical emergency in which metabolism slows to near death. Thyroid crisis or storm is the emergency extreme of hyperthyroidism and can lead to high fever, delirium, coma, or death.

Hypothyroidism[100]
Symptoms (varying from mild to severe):

- Weight gain
- Lethargic, sluggish, easily fatigues, complacent or disinterested, or depressed
- Sparse, coarse hair which tends to break
- Anorexia
- Coarse, flaky, and dry skin
- Thick, brittle fingernails
- Puffiness around eyes, upper eyelid droop
- Usually no goiter
- No cardiac changes initially but may develop slow heart rate or cardiac enlargement with low blood pressure if untreated
- Low temperature
- Constipation
- Menorrhagia (excessive menstrual bleeding)
- Lethargic but good muscular strength
- Intolerance to cooler environments

Hypothyroidism
Symptoms (varying from mild to severe):

- Decreased libido or infertility
- Somnolent
- Forgetful, slowing of intellectual activity
- Puffy face, hands and feet
- Decreased sweating
- Muscle cramps

Treatment:

- Gradual thyroid hormone replacement (eg., levothyroxine)

Hyperthyroidism[101]
Symptoms (varying from mild to severe):

- Weight loss
- Energetic, nervous, easily irritated, mood swings, emotional outbursts
- Fine hair, hair loss, failure to hold permanent wave
- Increased appetite
- Warm, flushed, fine skin with hyperpigmentation at pressure points
- Thin, easily broken fingernails
- Double vision, exophthalmos (bulging or protruding eyeballs), eyelid retraction
- Goiter
- Tachycardia, palpitations or dysrhythmia, hypertension
- High temperature
- Increased frequency of bowel movements, diarrhea
- Increasing muscle weakness and atrophy
- Amenorrhea or scant flow

Hyperthyroidism
Symptoms (varying from mild to severe):

- Intolerance to warmer environments
- Decreased libido or infertility
- Insomnia
- Difficulty concentrating
- Increased sweating
- Tremors

Treatment:

- Drug therapy (antithyroid)
- Radioactive iodine-131 therapy
- Surgery
- Beta blockers to control tachycardia, sweating, or anxiety

The two forms of hypothyroidism are cretinism and myxedema. Cretinism is caused by a thyroid hormone deficiency during fetal development or soon after birth and results in defective physical development and mental retardation. Severe iodine deficiency in the diet of an expectant mother can lead to cretinism.

Myxedema, adult hypothyroidism, is a disease of older persons and of women with risk factors including age over 50 years, being female, obesity, thyroid surgery, or exposure of the neck to X-ray or radiation treatment.

The most common cause of hypothyroidism is Hashimoto's thyroiditis, a long-term inflammatory autoimmune condition in which the body attacks its own thyroid gland.

Hyperthyroidism (thyrotoxicosis), like most other thyroid conditions, is more prominent in women than in men. Graves' disease, another autoimmune disorder, is the primary cause of hyperthyroidism. The principle hallmarks of Graves' disease are the bulging eyes (exophthalmos) and goiter in addition to hyperthyroidism. Other causes of hyperthyroidism include cancer of the thyroid, infections of the gland, and ingestion of too much thyroid hormone or iodine. Women with hyperthyroidism are at increased risk for osteoporosis.[102]

During and after pregnancy, women on thyroid medications for hyperthyroidism or hypothyroidism should be followed closely by their health care provider to ensure the best outcomes for them and their child.

IRRITABLE BOWEL SYNDROME (IBS)

Irritable bowel syndrome (IBS), a chronic gastrointestinal disorder that interferes with the colon's normal function, is characterized by abdominal pain, bloating, cramping, constipation, and diarrhea. The symptoms can vary from one woman to the next, but most women can control their symptoms through diet adjustments, stress management, and prescribed medications. One in six Americans have symptoms of IBS and it occurs nearly twice as often in women.[103] IBS usually begins before the age of 35 and, though it can be distressing at times, it does not seem to permanently harm the intestines or lead to serious diseases such as cancer. IBS is not related to inflammatory bowel disorders such as Crohn's or ulcerative colitis.

Symptoms of IBS seem to be caused when the normal contractions of the intestinal wall muscles become stronger and last longer than usual. This abnormal action propels food through the intestines, causing gas, pain, bloating, and diarrhea. However, in some women, food may pass slower causing constipation with the passing of hard, dry stools. The abnormal functioning of the intestines and altered sensations in IBS lead to its common symptoms. In addition to the symptoms mentioned, a woman may have mucous in her stool and may have alternating bouts of diarrhea and constipation. Worsening of IBS symptoms has been associated with triggers such as eating large meals; taking certain medications; drinking alcohol; drinking caffeine-containing products such as coffee, tea, or colas; ingesting wheat, rye or barley products, chocolate or milk products; and experiencing stressful or emotional upsets. Some women experience more IBS symptoms during their menstrual periods, suggesting a possible link between IBS and reproductive hormones. Women should know that symptoms of fever, weight loss, bleeding, persistent severe pain, or recurrent vomiting are not associated with IBS and should be reported to a health care provider.[104]

The cause of IBS cannot be linked to any specific factor. Theories about the cause of IBS range from bacterial infection, gluten product intolerance similar to celiac disease, and to diminished serotonin receptor activity along the GI tract. The immune system is also being researched for possible links to IBS.[105]

IBS is diagnosed by its signs and symptoms after other diseases have been ruled out, since other conditions have similar effects. Treatment of IBS includes: medications to regulate constipation or diarrhea, antispasmodics to control muscle spasms and reduce abdominal pain, antidepressants, fiber supplements, and Lotronex. Lotronex is an IBS-specific drug that is only approved for women with severe IBS who have not responded to other treatments and whose primary symptom is diarrhea. Lotronex is prescribed with great caution because of the serious potential side effects of severe constipation and decreased blood flow to the colon. Amitiza, a recently approved FDA drug, is used to treat women with IBS who experience constipation.[106]

A woman can help manage her IBS by altering her diet habits. In general, eating smaller meals more often or eating smaller portion sizes may help. It would benefit a woman to keep a food journal to find out what foods or beverages irritate her IBS since each woman will react differently to some of the same products. For instance, high fiber diet or diet supplements may help some women but only exacerbate symptoms in others. If dairy products are a problem, a woman may need to find other tolerable sources of calcium. Carbonated beverages, chewing ice or gum, or drinking through a straw may cause a woman to swallow air leading to gas, bloating, and discomfort, and should be avoided when possible. Avoiding caffeine-containing products or alcohol might limit IBS symptoms. Foods that cause gas such as cabbage, broccoli, or cauliflower may need to be eliminated from the diet.

Since women with IBS have colons that are more sensitive and reactive to triggers that might not affect others, a woman should stop smoking and may need to find ways to reduce stress. In addition, counseling for stress or depression, getting regular exercise, deep breathing, yoga, massage, and meditation may be helpful in preventing or alleviating IBS symptoms.

ALZHEIMER'S DISEASE

The normal brain contains approximately 100 billion nerve cells (neurons). These neurons communicate or send electrical messages to one another through connections known as synapses. Transmission of electrical charges from one neuron to the next involves chemicals known as neurotransmitters, that carry signals across the synaptic connections of the nerve cells. **Alzheimer's disease (AD)** is a disruption of the normal flow of electrical activity, both within the neurons themselves and from outside the neurons at the synapses. These changes cause a reduction in the number of synapses and lead to death of neurons.

Alzheimer's disease (AD), the most common form of dementia, causes a gradual, progressive loss of brain cells that eventually leads to death if death does not occur from another cause first (often from bronchiopneumonia). It is characterized by confusion, progressive memory loss, behavioral disturbances, loss of language skills, and decline in the ability to perform routine tasks. AD affects the brain cells that control memory and cognitive thinking skills first and then progresses to other regions of the brain. AD advances at different rates and may last 3–20 years. The average life span is 4–8 years after diagnosis.

The exact cause of AD is unknown. Scientists know that AD involves the malfunction or death of nerve cells and believe the triggers begin damaging the brain years before symptoms appear.

Along with brain tissue inflammation, two abnormal structures are found in the brain tissue of a person diagnosed with Alzheimer's disease. Plaques and tangles are being investigated as markers of the disease to determine the actual cause of death of neurons. Plaques, deposits of excess beta-amyloid protein fragments, are found clumped between neurons and cause blockage of the transfer of electrical information at the synapses. Tangles are twisted strands of a protein called tau that are found inside the dying neurons. Tau normally keeps the transportation tracks parallel within the cells so nutrients and essential supplies can move easily through the cells. When these protein tracks fail to function normally, the cell eventually dies. Although plaques and tangles can be found in most aging brains, they tend to form in a predictable pattern beginning in areas of important learning and memory and spreading to other regions.

Increasing age is the leading risk factor for developing AD, as most people with the disease are 65 years or older. The risk of developing AD doubles about every 5 years after age 65. Approximately half of all people 85 and older will have AD, but AD is not considered a normal part of aging. Women are more likely to have AD or dementia because women, on average, tend to live longer than men. Having a parent, sibling, or child with AD is another risk factor that increases a woman's risk of developing the disease; more familial AD means a higher risk for other family members. When AD tends to run in a family, genetic or environmental factors, or both, may contribute to increased risk. A protein called apolipoprotein (apoE) is being investigated for its relationship to AD. ApoE is a normal component in the body that helps carry cholesterol in the blood. The apoE gene has three forms, one of which (apoE4), seems to increase the likelihood of a person developing AD. Scientists are looking at other Alzheimer's risk genes that may increase a familial tendency for AD. Researchers have strong evidence that high cholesterol, high BP, and vascular disease elevate the risk of AD. The heart–head connection is important to recognize when looking at risks that might be controlled by diet, exercise, and maintaining good health behaviors. Increased risk of Alzheimer's disease is also associated with prior moderate and severe head trauma, head injury, and traumatic brain injury.[107] AD is a costly disease affecting nearly 5.4 million Americans and impacts the lives of nearly 15 million unpaid caregivers. It is the sixth leading cause of death in the United States and kills nearly 82,000 people annually.[108]

Signs and Symptoms

A key component of AD is memory loss, exhibited by forgetfulness. Actions such as missed appointments, unreturned telephone calls, trouble finding the right word, and difficulty understanding conversation may be signs to watch. Failing to recognize people, getting lost while alone, relinquishing important responsibilities (such as paying the bills), or reducing social circles may also be signs. The Alzheimer's Disease Association provides a list of ten warning signs to recognize AD.[109] (See *Health Tips:* "Ten Warning Signs to Recognize AD.")

Stages of Alzheimer's Disease

There are documented common patterns of symptom progression in AD that are categorized in seven stages. Stage 1 is considered the *unimpaired* or normal functioning brain with no memory problems identified. The *very mild cognitive decline* of stage 2 may be normal

Health Tips

Ten Warning Signs to Recognize AD

- Memory loss that disrupts daily life
- Challenges in planning or solving problems
- Difficulty completing familiar tasks at home or work
- Confusion with time or place
- Trouble understanding visual images and spatial relationships
- New problems with words in speaking or writing
- Misplacing things and losing the ability to trace steps
- Decreased or poor judgment
- Withdrawal from work or social activities
- Changes in mood and personality

may occur. Recollection of personal history and the names of significant family members or caregivers is difficult. The individual may still recall their own name and can generally distinguish between familiar and unfamiliar persons. Assistance with dressing and toileting is usually necessary and increased episodes of wandering and urinary/bowel incontinence may occur. Personality and behavioral changes that might be seen include: suspiciousness, delusions, hallucinations, and compulsive repetitive movements such as hand-wringing and tissue shredding. Stage 7 is the final stage of *very severe cognitive decline*. The individual loses her ability to respond to the environment, to speak, and to control movement. Recognizable speech is usually lost and the ability to walk, sit, smile or even hold her head up disappears. She will progress to being totally bed bound as the reflexes become abnormal and the muscles grow rigid. Since swallowing also becomes impaired, decisions about feeding alternatives arise for family and caregivers.

Diagnosis

An early diagnosis is important for the person with AD and her family so that they can plan for the future and initiate early treatment of symptoms. Although a definitive diagnosis cannot be made until an autopsy of the brain tissue reveals the plaques and tangles, a diagnosis of "probable" or "possible" AD can be made with about 90 percent accuracy. A complete medical history is required to review past and present medical conditions as well as testing to determine current mental and physical functioning. A diagnosis is made after ruling out other potential causes through mental status evaluation, physical examination, neurological exams, laboratory tests, psychiatric and psychological evaluation, and various brain scans.

Normal age-related memory changes may be distinguished from Alzheimer's disease symptoms by the following:[110]

Someone with Alzheimer's disease symptoms

- Poor judgment and decision making
- Inability to manage a budget
- Losing track of the date or the season
- Difficulty having a conversation
- Misplacing things and being unable to retrace steps to find them

Someone with typical age-related changes

- Making a bad decision once in awhile
- Missing a monthly payment
- Forgetting which day it is and remembering later
- Sometimes forgetting which word to use
- Losing items from time to time

age-related changes or the first sign of memory lapses associated with AD. The subtle forgetting of familiar words or names, or the location of everyday objects such as keys or eyeglasses may not be apparent to persons living or working with someone exhibiting AD. In stage 3, the *mild cognitive decline* is noticed by family, friends, and coworkers. Problems with word or name finding; inability to remember names of newly introduced individuals; decreasing performance at work or social settings; limited recall of material read; misplacing valuable objects; and inability to plan or organize become recognizable. The *moderate cognitive decline* of stage 4 demonstrates clear-cut deficiencies in specific areas such as decreased memory of recent events or occasions; impaired ability to perform complex tasks such as managing finances or planning social events; forgetting one's own personal history; and withdrawal from socially challenging situations. Major gaps in memory and deficits in cognitive function occur during stage 5 and require that the individual have some assistance with day-to-day activities. With the *moderately severe cognitive decline* an affected individual will become confused about where they are, the date, or the season. They also may not be able to recall their current address, telephone number, choose proper clothing for the season or occasion, or perform less challenging arithmetic. At this stage there is usually no need for assistance with eating or use of the bathroom. As AD progresses into *the severe cognitive decline* of stage 6 memory worsens and significant personality changes may emerge, requiring that the individual have extensive assistance with daily activities. During this stage significant loss of awareness regarding recent experiences, events, and surroundings

Treatment

No treatments can stop the progressive loss of brain cells in AD, but current drug treatments can help minimize or stabilize the symptoms for a period of time. Three medications known as cholinesterase inhibitors are commonly prescribed for the early treatment of AD (Donepezil, Rivastigmine, and Razadyne). They are designed to inhibit the breakdown of acetylcholine in the brain. Acetylcholine is a chemical messenger that is important for memory and other cognitive skills. Cholinesterase inhibitors keep the levels of acetylcholine high, helping to maintain cognitive functioning or improve cognitive symptoms. Memantine, a receptor antagonist, is now prescribed for moderate to severe AD. It appears to regulate the activity of glutamate, a chemical messenger that helps with learning and memory. Other medications may be necessary to help control behavioral symptoms such as agitation, wandering, depression, sleeplessness, and anxiety. Other substances, such as vitamin E, antidepressants, antianxiety medications, and antipsychotics, are being studied to determine their efficacy in slowing the progression of AD or to treat behavioral and psychiatric symptoms. Any supplement or medication used by an individual with AD should be discussed with a health care provider. For instance, vitamin E may not be recommended for persons taking "blood thinners." As AD progresses, the ability of the affected person to communicate experiences will require the caregiver to monitor for medication side effects or even symptoms of common illnesses that may go undetected.[111]

Nondrug therapies include providing the AD patient with a stable and familiar environment. During the mild to moderate stages of AD, the family should encourage the person with AD to function independently, and the daily routine should become familiar. A consistent schedule for daily activities reduces agitation, and safety can be enhanced by placing locks on doors. Collecting and sharing personal items helps to stimulate the memory of persons with AD. Nursing homes that accept persons with AD often provide alarms and codes to secure doors, visual pictures for communicating and stimulating memory, and measures to prevent wandering.[112]

Role of Caregiver

AD seriously impacts caregivers as well as persons with AD. Caregivers suffer from anxiety, depression, and anger. They can receive needed assistance by joining a support group. These support groups offer emotional support and current information about additional home health services, the behavior of persons with AD, and help in nursing home placement. Recent studies suggest that a person with AD can remain at home nearly a year longer if caregivers have a support system that offers emotional and informational support. Most urban areas provide support groups for care-givers, and the national office of the Alzheimer's Association provides information regarding the location of your local chapter.

Now complete *Journal Activity:* "Your Family Tree and Chronic Disease."

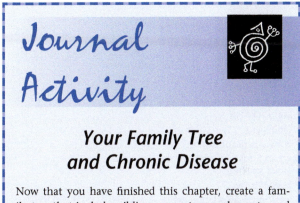

Journal Activity

Your Family Tree and Chronic Disease

Now that you have finished this chapter, create a family tree that includes siblings, parents, grandparents, and great-grandparents. Under each name, include the diseases or conditions that each person has or had. Select one disease or condition and write all the protective factors that you can practice to reduce your risk of contracting this disease.

Chapter Summary

- More women die from cardiovascular disease than any other disease.
- African American women are at greater risk than white women for coronary artery disease.
- Atherosclerosis is a gradual process of artery breakdown that causes plaque to accumulate and form occlusions.
- Heart attacks are more lethal for women than men.

- High BP is defined as a systolic pressure of 140 mm Hg and/or diastolic pressure of 90 mm Hg and/or taking antihypertensive medication.
- Stroke is the third leading cause of death and the leading cause of disability in women.
- Osteoporosis is a bone-weakening disorder causing bone mineral loss that can result in skeletal frailty and fractures.

- African American women compared to white women are 50 percent more likely to develop type 2 diabetes.
- The best way to overcome the stigma of epilepsy is by educating the public.
- Arthritis, an inflammatory condition of the joints, is the leading cause of work-related disability.
- Systemic lupus erythematosus affects primarily women of childbearing age.

- Multiple sclerosis affects primarily young white women, often between the ages of 30 and 40.
- Hyperthyroidism leads to increased body metabolism and heat production. Hypothyroidism results from underactivity of the thyroid gland.
- Alzheimer's disease is the most common dementia, and a key component is memory loss.

Review Questions

1. What is the leading cause of death in women?
2. What is atherosclerosis?
3. What are the signs and symptoms of angina?
4. What is the difference between a heart attack and congestive heart failure?
5. What are the primary risk and protective factors for heart disease?
6. How can hypertension be controlled?
7. What are the warning signs of stroke? type 2 diabetes? arthritis?
8. What are the risk and protective factors for osteoporosis?
9. What causes lupus? multiple sclerosis? Alzheimer's disease? thyroid disease?
10. What can you do to protect yourself against chronic conditions?

Resources

Organizations and Hotlines

Alzheimer's Association (National Office)
    800-272-3900
    www.alz.org

American Diabetes Association
    800-DIABETES
    (800-342-2383)
    www.diabetes.org

American Heart Association
    800-AHA-USA
    (800-242-8721)
    www.americanheart.org

American Stroke Association
    888-4-STROKE
    (888-478-7653)
    www.strokeassociation.org

Epilepsy Foundation
    800-332-1000
    www.efa.org

The Lupus Foundation of America, Inc.
    202-349-1155
    www.lupus.org

Multiple Sclerosis Foundation
    800-225-6495
    www.msfacts.org

National Heart, Lung, and Blood Institute
    301-592-8573
    www.nhlbi.nih.gov

National Multiple Sclerosis Society
    1-800-344-4867
    www.nationalmssociety.org

National Osteoporosis Foundation
    www.nof.org
    1-800-231-4222

National Stroke Association
    800-STROKES
    (800-787-6537)
    www.stroke.org

Related Diseases Association, Inc.
    (information on women and autoimmune diseases)
    1-800-598-4668
    www.aarda.org/women.html

Web Sites

American Lung Association
    www.lungusa.org

Centers for Disease Control and Prevention (CDC)
    www.cdc.gov

Diabetes Public Health Resource (CDC)
    www.cdc.gov/diabetes

Fibromyalgia Network
    www.fmnetnews.com

March of Dimes
    www.marchofdimes.com

National Fibromyalgia Association
    www.fmaware.org

National Institute of Arthritis and Musculoskeletal and Skin Diseases (NIAMS)
    www.niams.nih.gov

National Institutes of Health
    Osteoporosis and Related Bone Diseases
    National Resource Center
    www.niams.nih.gov/Health_Info/Bono/
    WISEWOMAN (a CDC initiative)

(Well-Integrated Screening and Evaluation for **Women** Across the Nation)
    www.cdc.gov/wisewoman

References

1. World Health Organization. *The impact of chronic disease in the United States.* http://www.who.int/chp/chronic_disease_report/usa.pdf

2. *Chronic disease cost calculator.* http://www.cdc.gov/chronic disease/resources/calculator/index.htm

3. Veronique, L. R., et al. Heart disease and stroke statistics – 2012 update: A report from the American Heart Association. *Circulation* 2011. http://circ.ahajournals.org/content/early/2011/12/15/CIR.0b013e31823ac046.full.pdf

4. Ibid.

5. Ibid.

6. National Library of Medicine. 2004. *Developmental process of atherosclerosis.* www.nlm.nih.gov/medlineplus/ency/image pages/18020.htm (retrieved December 12, 2008).

7. *What is sleep apnea?* http://www.nhlbi.nih.gov/health/health-topics/topics/sleepapnea/

8. *What is angina?* http://www.nhlbi.nih.gov/health/health-topics/topics/angina/

9. *What is coronary artery bypass grafting?* http://www.nhlbi.nih.gov/health/health-topics/topics/cabg/during.html

10. *Signs of a heart attack.* http://www.womenshealth.gov/heart-health-stroke/signs-of-a-heart-attack/

11. American Heart Association. 2008. Women are more likely than men to die in hospital from severe heart attack. *Circulation*

12. *What are congenital heart defects?* http://www.nhlbi.nih.gov/health/health-topics/topics/chd/

13. Ibid.

14. *Noninherited risk factors and congenital cardiovascular defects: current knowledge.* A scientific statement from the American Heart Association Council on Cardiovascular Disease in the Young. http://circ.ahajournals.org/content/115/23/2995.full.pdf

15. *Understand your risk for arrhythmia.* http://www.heart.org/HEARTORG/Conditions/Arrhythmia/UnderstandYourRiskforArrhythmia/Understand-Your-Risk-for-Arrhythmia_UCM_002024_Article.jsp

16. *What is atrial fibrillation (AFib or AF)?* http://www.heart.org/HEARTORG/Conditions/Arrhythmia/AboutArrhythmia/What-is-Atrial-Fibrillation-AFib-or-AF_UCM_423748_Article.jsp

17. Ibid.

18. *Devices that may interfere with pacemakers.* http://www.heart.org/HEARTORG/Conditions/Arrhythmia/PreventionTreatmentofArrhythmia/Devices-that-may-Interfere-with-Pacemakers_UCM_302013_Article.jsp

19. *Living with your pacemaker.* http://www.heart.org/HEARTORG/Conditions/Arrhythmia/PreventionTreatmentofArrhythmia/Living-With-Your-Pacemaker_UCM_305290_Article.jsp

20. *Types of heart failure.* http://www.heart.org/HEARTORG/Conditions/HeartFailure/AboutHeartFailure/Types-of-Heart-Failure_UCM_306323_Article.jsp

21. *Classes of heart failure.* http://www.heart.org/HEARTORG/Conditions/HeartFailure/AboutHeartFailure/Classes-of-Heart-Failure_UCM_306328_Article.jsp

22. *Understand your risk for heart failure.* http://www.heart.org/HEARTORG/Conditions/HeartFailure/UnderstandYourRiskforHeartFailure/Understand-Your-Risk-for-Heart-Failure_UCM_002046_Article.jsp

23. Legato, M. J. 2002. *Eve's rib: The groundbreaking guide to women's health.* New York: Three Rivers Press, Random House.

24. *Endocarditis.* http://www.ncbi.nlm.nih.gov/pubmedhealth/PMH0002088/

25. *Mitral valve and mitral valve prolapse.* http://www.heart.org/HEARTORG/Conditions/HeartAttack/PreventionTreatmentofHeartAttack/Mitral-Valve-and-Mitral-Valve-Prolapse_UCM_434087_Article.jsp

26. *What is heart disease?* http://www.nhlbi.nih.gov/educational/hearttruth/lower-risk/index.htm

27. *Highlights: Smoking among adults in the United States: Coronary heart disease and stroke.* http://www.cdc.gov/tobacco/data_statistics/sgr/2004/highlights/heart_disease/

28. *What is high blood pressure?* http://www.nhlbi.nih.gov/health/health-topics/topics/hbp/

29. Adapted from: *The Seventh Report of the Joint National Committee on Prevention, Detection, Evaluation, and Treatment of High Blood Pressure.* http://www.nhlbi.nih.gov/guidelines/hypertension/jnc7full.pdf

30. Ibid.

31. *What is preeclampsia?* http://www.nhlbi.nih.gov/hbp/issues/preg/preclamp.htm

32. Adapted from American Heart Association: *What your cholesterol levels mean.* http://www.heart.org/HEARTORG/Conditions/Cholesterol/AboutCholesterol/What-Your-Cholesterol-Levels-Mean_UCM_305562_Article.jsp

33. *Drug therapy for cholesterol.* http://www.heart.org/HEARTORG/Conditions/Cholesterol/PreventionTreatmentofHighCholesterol/Drug-Therapy-for-Cholesterol_UCM_305632_Article.jsp

34. *Third Report of the National Cholesterol Education Program (NCEP) Expert Panel on Detection, Evaluation and Treatment of High Blood Cholesterol in Adults (Adult Treatment Panel III),* NIH Pub. No. 02-5215, September 2002. http://www.nhlbi.nih.gov/guidelines/cholesterol/atp3full.pdf

35. *Physical activity improves quality of life.* http://www.heart.org/HEARTORG/GettingHealthy/PhysicalActivity/StartWalking/Physical-activity-improves-quality-of-life_UCM_307977_Article.jsp

36. *Adult obesity.* http://www.cdc.gov/obesity/data/adult.html

37. *Obesity.* http://www2.niddk.nih.gov/NR/rdonlyres/FD9F7372-519E-48C6-B9FD-7A1A8BB33507/0/DSP2011_7_Obesity_508.pdf

38. *Women and heart disease facts.* http://www.womensheart.org/content/HeartDisease/heart_disease_facts.asp

39. ????? keep ?????

40. *What are high blood cholesterol and triglycerides?* http://www.heart.org/idc/groups/heart-public/@wcm/@hcm/documents/downloadable/ucm_300308.pdf

41. Ibid.

42. *African Americans and stroke.* http://www.stroke.org/site/PageServer?pagename=AAMER

43. National Stroke Association. *Types of stroke.* http://www.stroke.org/site/PageServer?pagename=type

44. National Stroke Association *Women's stroke risk.* http://www.stroke.org/site/PageServer?pagename=womrisk

45. National Stroke Association. *Stroke 101.* http://www.stroke.org/site/DocServer/STROKE_101_Fact_Sheet.pdf?docID=4541

46. National Osteoporosis Foundation. *Fast facts.* http://www.nof.org/node/40

47. Ibid.

48. Sports Medicine Newsletter. *Exercise and osteoporosis.* sports medicine.about.com/od/women/a/osteoporosis.htm (retrieved October 4, 2008).

49. Warren, M. P. and A. I. Chua. 2008. Exercise-induced amenorrhea and bone health in the adolescent athlete. *Annals of the New York Academy of Sciences* 1135: 244–52.

50. About Osteoporosis. *Having a bone density test.* http://www .nof.org/aboutosteoporosis/detectingosteoporosis/bmdtest

51. About Osteoporosis. *Exercise for healthy bones.* http://www .nof.org/aboutosteoporosis/prevention/exercise

52. About Osteoporosis. *Calcium: What you should know.* http:// www.nof.org/aboutosteoporosis/prevention/calcium

53. Ibid.

54. About Osteoporosis. *Diseases and conditions that may cause bone loss.* http://www.nof.org/aboutosteoporosis/ detectingosteoporosis/diseaseboneloss

55. About Osteoporosis. *Detecting osteoporosis.* http://www.nof .org/aboutosteoporosis/detectingosteoporosis/diagnosing

56. *Bone density test and FRAX results and treatment.* http:// www.nof.org/aboutosteoporosis/managingandtreating/ medicinesneedtoknow

57. About Osteoporosis. *Detecting osteoporosis.* http://www.nof .org/aboutosteoporosis/detectingosteoporosis/diagnosing

58. About Osteoporosis. *Osteoporosis medicines: What you need to know.* http://www.nof.org/aboutosteoporosis/ managingandtreating/medicinesneedtoknow

59. CDC. 2011. *National diabetes fact sheet.* http://www.cdc.gov/ diabetes/pubs/pdf/ndfs_2011.pdf

60. Ibid.

61. CDC. *Diabetes & women's health across the life stages: A public health perspective.* http://www.cdc.gov/diabetes/pubs/pdf/ womenshort.pdf

62. CDC. 2011. *National diabetes fact sheet.*

63. *Type 1 diabetes.* http://www.ncbi.nlm.nih.gov/pubmedhealth/ PMH0001350/

64. American Diabetes Association. *Living with diabetes.* http:// www.diabetes.org/living-with-diabetes/treatment-and-care/ transplantation/

65. *Gestational diabetes.* http://www.ncbi.nlm.nih.gov/ pubmedhealth/PMH0001898/

66. CDC. 2011. *National diabetes fact sheet,* 2011 http://www.cdc .gov/diabetes/pubs/pdf/ndfs_2011.pdf

67. American Diabetes Association. *Diabetes basics.* http://www .diabetes.org/diabetes-basics/tips/tips-search-results.html?tip_ category=womens-health#is-there-any-birth-control.html

68. *Asthma facts and figures.* http://www.aafa.org/display .cfm?id=8&sub=42#fast

69. Ibid.

70. *Ethnic disparities in the burden and treatment of asthma.* https:// www.aafa.org/pdfs/Disparities.PDF

71. National Institute of Environmental Health Sciences. *Asthma and its environmental triggers.* http://www.niehs.nih.gov/ health/assets/docs_a_e/asthma_and_its_environmental_ triggers_.pdf

72. National Heart, Lung, and Blood Institute. 2004. *Managing asthma during pregnancy: Recommendations for pharmacologic treatment update.* http://www.nhlbi.nih.gov/health/prof/lung/ asthma/astpreg.htm

73. Asthma and Allergy Foundation of America. *Pregnancy and asthma.* http://www.aafa.org/display.cfm?id=8&sub= 16&cont=65

74. National Heart, Lung, and Blood Institute. 2004. *Managing asthma during pregnancy: Recommendations for pharmacologic treatment: Update.* http://www.nhlbi.nih.gov/health/prof/ lung/asthma/astpreg.htm

75. United States Environmental Agency. *Setting the record straight: secondhand smoke is a preventable health risk.* http:// www.epa.gov/smokefree/pubs/strsfs.html

76. CDC. *Health effects of secondhand smoke.* http://www.cdc .gov/tobacco/data_statistics/fact_sheets/secondhand_smoke/ health_effects/#sids

77. *Types of seizures.* http://www.epilepsyfoundation.org/about epilepsy/seizures/index.cfm

78. *Ketogenic diet.* http://www.epilepsyfoundation.org/aboutepi lepsy/treatment/ketogenicdiet/index.cfm

79. *Photosensitivity and seizures.* http://www.epilepsyfoundation .org/aboutepilepsy/seizures/photosensitivity/index.cfm

80. *Parenting concerns for the mother with epilepsy.* http://www .epilepsyfoundation.org/livingwithepilepsy/gendertopics/wo menshealthtopics/parentingconcerns.cfm

81. Health issues after your baby is born. http://www.epi lepsyfoundation.org/livingwithepilepsy/gendertopics/ womenshealthtopics/pregnancyandepilepsymedications/ health-issues-after-your-baby-is-born.cfm

82. *Differences in the prevalence and impact of arthritis among racial/ ethnic groups in the United States.* http://www.cdc.gov/arthritis/ data_statistics/race.htm

83. *How is osteoarthritis treated?* http://www.rheumatology.org/ practice/clinical/patients/diseases_and_conditions/osteoar thritis.asp

84. American College of Rheumatology. *Biologic treatments for rheumatoid arthritis.* http://www.rheumatology.org/practice/ clinical/patients/medications/biologics.asp

85. Hailey, D., and L. A. Topfer. 2002. Extracorporeal immunoadsorption treatment for rheumatoid arthritis. *Issues Emerg Health Technol* 28: 1–4. http://www.ncbi.nlm.nih.gov/ pubmed/11968222

86. *What is lupus?* http://www.lupus.org/webmodules/webarticle- snet/templates/new_learnunderstanding.aspx?articleid=2232 &zoneid=523

87. *Causes of lupus.* http://www.lupus.org/webmodules/webarticle snet/templates/new_learnmen.aspx?articleid=109&zone id=529

88. *What are the symptoms of lupus?* http://www.lupus.org/web modules/webarticlesnet/templates/new_learnunderstanding .aspx?articleid=2235&zoneid=523

89. *Living with lupus.* http://www.rheumatology.org/practice/ clinical/patients/diseases_and_conditions/lupus.asp

90. National Institute of Arthritis and Musculoskeletal and Skin Diseases, National Institutes of Health. *Fibromyalgia.* http:// www.niams.nih.gov/Health_Info/Fibromyalgia/

91. *Who gets fibromyalgia?* http://www.niams.nih.gov/Health_ Info/Fibromyalgia/default.asp#b

92. *How is fibromyalgia treated?* http://www.niams.nih.gov/ Health_Info/Fibromyalgia/default.asp#e

93. National Multiple Sclerosis Society. 2005. *Who gets MS?* www .nationalmssociety.org/about-multiple-selerosis/whogetsms/ indes.aspx

94. Ibid.

95. *Heat and temperature sensitivity.* http://www.nationalmssociety .org/about-multiple-sclerosis/what-we-know-about-ms/treat- ments/exacerbations/heattemperature-sensitivity/index .aspx

96. *Symptoms*. http://www.nationalmssociety.org/about-multiple-sclerosis/what-we-know-about-ms/symptoms/index.aspx

97. *What is multiple sclerosis?* http://www.nationalmssociety.org/about-multiple-sclerosis/what-we-know-about-ms/what-is-ms/index.aspx

98. *Diagnosing MS*. http://www.nationalmssociety.org/about-multiple-sclerosis/what-we-know-about-ms/diagnosing-ms/index.aspx

99. *Treatments*. http://www.nationalmssociety.org/about-multiple-sclerosis/what-we-know-about-ms/treatments/index.aspx

100. *Diseases and conditions*. http://www.mayoclinic.com/health/DiseasesIndex/DiseasesIndex

101. Ibid.

102. *Hyperthyroidism (overactive thyroid)*. http://www.mayoclinic.com/health/hyperthyroidism/DS00344/DSECTION=lifestyle-and-home-remedies

103. *Irritable bowel syndrome*. http://www.ncbi.nlm.nih.gov/pubmedhealth/PMH0001292/

104. http://www.digestive.niddk.nih.gov/ddiseases/pubs/ibs/

105. Ibid.

106. Ibid.

107. Ibid.

108. *Alzheimer's disease facts and figures*. 2011. http://www.alz.org/downloads/Facts_Figures_2011.pdf

109. Alzheimer's Foundation. 2005. *Ten warning signs of Alzheimer's disease*. www.alz.org/AboutAD/Warning.asp

110. *10 Signs of Alzheimer's*. http://www.alz.org/alzheimers_disease_10_signs_of_alzheimers.asp?type=alzFooter#typical

111. *Treatments for Alzheimer's disease*. http://www.alz.org/alzheimers_disease_treatments.asp

112. *Living with Alzheimer's*. http://www.alz.org/living_with_alzheimers_4521.asp

Chapter Sixteen

Reducing Your Risk of Cancer

CHAPTER OBJECTIVES

When you complete this chapter, you will be able to do the following:

◇ Distinguish differences between benign and malignant tumors

◇ Summarize the leading cancer sites by incidence and death

◇ Identify the seven warning signs of cancer

◇ Classify the common types of malignancies

◇ Explain possible lifestyle and genetic causes of various cancers

◇ Analyze various types of new research related to cancer treatments

◇ Describe the primary types of cancers related to women and the treatment and prevention for each

◇ Identify protective factors that help combat the development of cancer

◇ Compare and contrast medical and complementary treatment options

◇ Explain the importance of social support in recovery from cancer

THE BIG "C"

One in three women today can expect to have cancer in her lifetime, and nearly 50 percent of these cases involve the female reproductive system. Many women will someday hear the words, "Your Pap smear was positive; we need to do further tests," or "You have a lump in your breast; we need to schedule a biopsy." Despite reassurance from the health care provider that there is no cause for concern at this time, a woman would probably experience myriad feelings because the word "cancer" is stigmatized and usually evokes strong emotions.

This chapter provides information on the nature and sites of the most common cancers found in women, offers guidelines for early detection, suggests strategies for prevention and early intervention, and discusses various medical and complementary treatment protocols. The information can help you to develop a realistic plan for cancer prevention and management.

DEFINING CANCER

Women may have the perception that all tumors are cancerous, that all cancers are the same, and that cancer diagnosis is synonymous with death. However, most tumors are **benign** and are rarely life-threatening. Benign tumors are made up of cells that are encapsulated; they do not spread to other parts of the body and do not invade surrounding tissues. These tumors can usually be surgically removed and do not grow back. **Malignant tumors** are cancer and refer to numerous diseases characterized by abnormal cells that divide uncontrollably and have the ability to infiltrate and destroy normal cells. Cancer cells are not encapsulated, and they can break away from the primary tumor and **metastasize** (or travel) to other parts of the body through the bloodstream or the lymphatic system. Metastasized cancer cells can form new tumors and invade tissue and organs in the new area of the body.

Health Tips

Seven Warning Signs of Cancer

The American Cancer Society has identified seven major warning signs of cancer:

- A change in bowel or bladder habits
- A sore that does not heal
- Unusual bleeding or discharge from any place
- A lump in the breast or other parts of the body
- Chronic indigestion or difficulty in swallowing
- Obvious changes in a wart or mole
- Persistent coughing or hoarseness

There are more warning signs for other kinds of cancer that are not as common as those listed above. To learn more about the warning signs of cancer, contact your local chapter of the American Cancer Society or the National Cancer Institute at 1-800-4-CANCER. Visit their Web sites at www.cancer.org and www.cancer. gov.

TABLE 16.1 Leading Sites of New Cancer Cases and Death in Women, 2012 Estimates[1]

ESTIMATED NEW CASES	ESTIMATED DEATHS
Breast	Lung and bronchus
226,870	72,590
Lung and bronchus	Breast
109,690	39,510
Colon and rectum	Colon and rectum
70,040	25,220
Uterine corpus	Pancreas
47,130	18,540
Non-Hodgkin's lymphoma	Ovary
31,970	15,500
Melanoma of skin	Leukemia
32,000	10,040
Thyroid	Non-Hodgkin's lymphoma
43,210	8,620
Ovary	Uterine corpus
22,280	8,010
Pancreas	Liver
21,830	6,570
All sites	Brain and other nervous system
790,740	5,980
	All sites
	275,370

NOTE: Excludes basal and squamous cell skin cancer and in situ carcinoma except urinary bladder. Percentages may not total 100 percent due to rounding.

The prognosis for a woman with cancer depends on a variety of factors, including the nature of the tumor, its location, and its stage. The key to survival of cancer is early detection. The earlier cancer is diagnosed, the better the prognosis. The American Cancer Society (ACS) has identified seven warning signs of cancer. (See *Health Tips:* "Seven Warning Signs of Cancer.") If any of these signs are present, you should see your health care provider immediately. In 2012 the ACS estimated that 790,740 women would be diagnosed with cancer and 275,370 would die from it eventually.[2] (See Table 16.1.) The highest incidence and mortality rates for reported cancer cases in women are for cancers of the lungs, breast, and colon and rectum. (See *FYI:* "Cancer Incidence by Race and Ethnicity.")

CLASSIFICATIONS OF COMMON MALIGNANCIES

Each cancer is distinguished by the nature, site, or clinical course of the tumor. Generally, cancers are classified according to the part of the body in which they originate or by the type of cell as seen under the microscope. The World Health Organization has identified forty-six body sites, with numerous types of cancer at many sites, totaling well over a hundred different cancers.

The four most common categories of cancer are carcinoma, sarcoma, lymphoma, and leukemia. (See Table 16.2.) Carcinomas are the most common type of cancer in the United States, representing 80–90 percent of all reported cancers. Carcinomas originate in the glandular or epithelial cells, which line the organs of the body. Sarcomas are cancers that begin in the connective tissues of the body, either the bone, muscles, or cartilage and are relatively rare in the United States, accounting for less than 2 percent of all new cancers each year. Lymphomas are cancers of the lymphatic system and can be broadly subdivided into Hodgkin's disease and non-Hodgkin's lymphomas (a number of diseases). Leukemia is a cancer of the blood-forming tissues and can be one of many types. Early symptoms mimic those of other diseases, including mononucleosis, tonsillitis, mumps, and others. Blood tests and examination of the cells in the bone marrow are necessary for diagnosing leukemia.

In addition to the most common categories, it is important to understand the difference between in situ and invasive cancer. "In situ" refers to cancerous tumors that are usually early stage and localized. The survival rates are usually higher for in situ cancer than for *invasive* cancer, which has spread to other tissues. A variety of systems are used to determine the stage of cancer according to the major factors influencing prognosis. The most common system for determining the stage of cancer is

TABLE 16.2 Common Classifications of Cancer

Carcinoma
A malignant epithelial neoplasm that tends to invade surrounding tissue and to metastasize to distant regions of the body. Carcinomas develop most frequently in the skin, large intestine, lung, stomach, prostate gland, cervix, and breast. The tumor is firm, irregular, nodular, with a well-defined border.

Sarcoma
A malignant neoplasm of the soft tissues arising in fibrous, fatty, muscular, synovial, vascular, or neural tissue, usually first presenting as a painless swelling. About 40 percent of sarcomas occur in the lower extremities, 20 percent in the upper extremities, 20 percent in the trunk, and the rest in the head or neck. The tumor, composed of closely packed cells in a fibrillar or homogeneous matrix, tends to be vascular and is usually highly invasive.

Lymphoma
A neoplasm of lymphoid tissue that is usually malignant. Characteristically, the appearance of a painless, enlarged lymph node or nodes is followed by weakness, fever, weight loss, and anemia.

Leukemia
A malignant neoplasm of blood-forming tissues characterized by diffuse replacement of bone marrow with proliferating leukocyte precursors, abnormal numbers and forms of immature white cells in circulation, and infiltration of lymph nodes, the spleen, and the liver. Acute leukemia usually has a sudden onset and rapidly progresses from early signs, such as fatigue, pallor, weight loss, and easy bruising, to fever, hemorrhages, extreme weakness, bone or joint pain, and repeated infections. Chronic leukemia develops slowly, and signs similar to those of the acute forms of the disease may not appear.

TABLE 16.3 TNM Staging: Determining the Extent and Location of Cancers

T = tumor size
    TX means the tumor is immeasurable
    T0 means there is no evidence of primary tumor
    Tis means the cancer is in situ
    T1, T2, T3, T4: Less invasive to more invasive;
                    higher number is more invasive

N = nodal involvement
    NX means the nearby lymph nodes cannot be evaluated
    N0 means nearby lymph nodes do not contain cancer
    N1, N2, N3 describe the size, location, and/or the number of nodal involvement; the higher the N number, the more lymph nodes are involved

M = metastases to other locations in the body
    MX means metastasis cannot be evaluated
    M0 means that no distant metastases were found
    M1 means that distant metastases are present and have spread to other parts of the body

the **TNM** staging system, developed by the American Joint Committee on Cancer and the International Union Against Cancer. In the TNM system, T represents the tumor size and level of invasion ranging from 1 to 4. N represents the nodal involvement, the size and number of the nodes, and degree of spread to lymph nodes ranging from 1 to 4. And M represents the absence or presence of distant metastases, denoted as X, 0, or 1. For example, stage 0 for breast cancer refers to noninvasive or in situ cancers, whereas stage 4 means the carcinoma extends beyond the breast to another part of the body such as bone, liver, or lung. Each cancer site has a different staging, unique to the site.[3] (See Table 16.3). Gynecologic cancers are frequently classified according to the guidelines of the International Federation for Gynecologic Oncology. This system divides the disease into five stages from stage 0, a carcinoma in situ, to stage IV, the metastasis to other sites. The stages were further subdivided into three grades with grade 1 being well-differentiated with the best prognosis and grade 3 being least-differentiated with the poorest prognosis.[4] For example, stage I for endometrial cancer refers to carcinoma in situ, whereas stage IV means the carcinoma extends beyond the pelvis and involves the bladder or rectum.

CAUSES OF CANCER

Scientists remain uncertain about the exact causes of cancer, although external (chemicals, radiation, and viruses) and internal (hormones, immune conditions, and inherited mutations) factors are recognized. Lifestyle and environmental factors account for most cancer risk, and a number of known **carcinogens** have been identified. Cigarette smoking, diet, exposure to carcinogenic chemicals, ionizing radiation, and ultraviolet rays account for the vast majority of cancers. Researchers also study the patterns of cancer to determine the risk factors and protective conditions that increase or decrease the likelihood of getting cancer. Cancer is *not* caused by injuries, bruises, or bumps and is *not* contagious. Cancer develops over time. Still, most women who get cancer have no known risk factors. And many women who have risk factors do not get cancer. This section discusses lifestyle and environmental factors contributing to cancer, and the biological changes that develop to increase the risk of developing cancer.

Lifestyle Factors Implicated in Cancer

Cigarette Smoking　Cigarette smoking is associated with cancers of the lung, larynx, pharynx, oral cavity, esophagus, pancreas, bladder, kidney, uterus, and cervix. Cigarette smoking accounts for 87 percent of lung cancer deaths and 30 percent of all cancer deaths. Passive (or secondhand) smoke causes disease, including lung cancer, in healthy nonsmokers. An estimated 45 million Americans are current smokers, which includes one in five U.S. women.[5] However, the per capita consumption of cigarettes continues to decline. Smoking cigarettes remains the most significant factor in premature death of women, particularly in the areas of cancer and heart disease.

Diet and Physical Activity　Approximately one-third of cancer deaths in the United States are due to diet and lack of physical activity, according to research studies. Other than use of tobacco, dietary choices and physical activity are the most important changeable behaviors that determine risk of developing cancer. The types of food consumed, the amount of fat rather than the specific type of fat consumed, food preparation methods, and overall caloric balance are risk factors for some cancers in women, particularly cancers of the breast, colon, and rectum.

Consuming a healthy diet, high in fruits and vegetables (especially green vegetables) and low in animal fat, meat, and highly caloric foods can reduce the risk of developing the most common cancers.[6] The 5-A-Day program, a partnership between grocers, produce suppliers, and federal and state agencies, is a nationwide campaign to encourage people to eat five or more servings of fruits and vegetables each day as a part of a low-fat, high-fiber diet. By adopting a physically active lifestyle, women can achieve a healthy weight and gain the multiple benefits of engaging in an exercise program. Physical activity helps move food through the intestine, thus reducing the time the intestinal tract is exposed to food carcinogens; activity also decreases the exposure of breast tissues to circulating estrogen. Reducing circulating concentrations of insulin and increasing metabolism, as a result of physical activity, can reduce the risks of developing breast, colon, and other types of cancers. In addition to reducing potential for cancer development, regular physical activity also reduces the risk of hypertension, heart diseases, diabetes, osteoporosis, stress, and depression.

Growing Older　Perhaps the most important risk factor for cancer is aging. Most cancer occurs in people over the age of 65. However, people of all ages, even children, can develop cancer. The death rates for most other age-related cancers have leveled off, and for people younger than 55 the cancer death rate has declined. Over 50 percent of all cancers occur in persons over the age of 65, and the age-related death rate for people aged 55 and older is still rising.

Viruses　A number of viruses have been linked to an increased risk of cancer, including hepatitis B, human T-lymphotropic virus (HTLV-1), herpes simplex virus-2 (HSV-2), Epstein-Barr, and some types of human papillomavirus (HPV). Hepatitis B has been linked to liver cancer, whereas HSV-2 and HPV have been associated with an increase in cervical cancer.[7]

Alcohol Consumption　Heavy alcohol consumption, particularly in conjunction with cigarette use or chewing tobacco, contributes to an increased risk of cancer. These cancers include mouth, esophagus, liver, larynx, pharynx, breast, and stomach. Moderate alcohol use is associated with a slightly increased risk of breast cancer among women, but the reason is unknown. Some studies suggest that drinking alcohol is related to changes in hormonal levels, particularly an increase in estrogen levels in women.[8]

Close Relatives with Certain Types of Cancer　Some cancers (including melanoma and cancers of the breast, ovary, prostate, and colon) tend to occur more frequently in some families. It is unclear whether these cancers are related to heredity, factors in a family's environment, lifestyle patterns, or pure chance.

Hormone Replacement Therapy (HRT)　Studies have shown that high cumulative exposure to estrogen increases the risk of endometrial cancer. Estrogen alone (ERT) may be prescribed for women who have had a hysterectomy because they are not at risk for uterine cancer. A more solid link between breast cancer and combined HRT has been strengthened due a recent study published in the *Journal of the American Medical Association*. The study had a longer patient follow-up period than previous studies and revealed that estrogen and progestin should be used very conservatively to treats symptoms of menopause. It was also found that death rates from breast cancer were higher among women receiving the hormones, compared with women using a placebo.[9]

views in regard to whether screening can detect lung cancer early with the goal of decreasing deaths from lung cancer. New results have been reported that people who had low-dose helical computed tomography (CT) scans did have a lower chance of dying from lung cancer than people who had chest radiography.[14] Research continues that will provide important information about the effectiveness of more modern screening tests. Because advanced-stage lung cancer causes such high mortality and screening has little effect on mortality rates, the best hope is prevention and better techniques for detection and treatment. More effective imaging methods and increased emphasis on smoking cessation are necessary for reducing lung cancer mortality. The presence of lung cancer is determined by examining tissue from the lung. A **biopsy,** the removal of small sample tissue, is done by bronchoscopy, needle aspiration, thoracentesis, or thoracotomy. If lung cancer is detected, it is then staged to determine the treatment plan.

Treatment Treatment depends on a number of factors, including the type of cancer, the size, the location, and the extent of the tumor. By the time a woman knows she has lung cancer, the cancer has likely metastasized to other areas of the body or to a greater portion of the lung. Lung cancer is classified as small cell (14 percent) or non–small cell (85 percent) carcinomas.[15] The prognosis for survival from lung cancer is poor, with only 15 percent of women diagnosed with lung cancer managing to survive 5 years or more. Surgery is the most common treatment for non–small cell lung cancer. Small cell lung cancer spreads rapidly, and chemotherapy and radiation are the first treatments of choice. Photodynamic therapy (PDT), a type of laser therapy, may be used when the cancer cannot be removed through surgery. Additional types of treatment include oral medications that target growth of cancer cells and blood supply to tumors.[16]

Breast Cancer

In the United States, breast cancer is the second leading cancer killer of all women and the leading cause of cancer death in African American women. Even though white women have the highest incidence rate of breast cancer, African American women have the highest death rate. Some researchers speculate that the higher death rate is probably due to diagnosis at a later stage of the disease. These women wait longer, are less likely to have clinical breast examinations, and have fewer mammograms. The incidence of breast cancer has declined since 2000 and accounts for 29 percent of all cancers in women. The American Cancer Society estimates that 226,870 women will get breast cancer and 39,510 women will die from it in 2008.[17]

Risk and Protective Factors What do you think your risk for breast cancer is (high, medium, low)? Would you think it was low if your mother or grandmother didn't have breast cancer? Many women conclude that if their family history is free of breast cancer, they are free from risk. Not true! Although family history is a recognized risk factor, 85–95 percent of all women who develop breast cancer have no family history of the disease. In fact, the majority of all breast cancers occur in women with no known risk factors. All women are at risk because the two main risk factors are (1) being a woman and (2) getting older.

Age is a leading risk factor for breast cancer; the accumulative risk of developing breast cancer increases with age. After age 40, non-Hispanic white women are more likely to be diagnosed with breast cancer than African American women, but African American women are more likely to die.[18] The median age of diagnosis for women is 61.[19] Women aged 75–79 have the highest incidence of breast cancer.

Identifiable risk factors include family history, previous breast biopsy (with abnormal cell growth), previous breast exposure to radiation (from childhood cancer treatment), HRT (5 years or more after menopause), alcohol (two to five drinks daily), obesity and high-fat diets, personal history of breast cancer (mother, grandmother, or aunt), genetic alterations (*BRCA1, BRCA2,* and others), menarche at an early age (before age 12), late menopause (after age 50), never having children, use of DES during pregnancy, late childbearing (first child after age 30), dense breast tissue (more likely to occur in breasts with more lobular and ductal tissue). Identifiable protective factors include breast feeding and having children. One research study of 100,000 women found that for every 12 months of breast feeding a woman reduces her risk of breast cancer by 4.3 percent.[20] For every birth, she reduces her risk by 7 percent. Recent studies have also explored the relationship between physical activity and breast cancer. There is continual evidence that exercise reduces the risk of developing breast cancer. The big unknown is how much exercise produces the best results. One study out of the Women's Health Initiative found that 1.25–2.5 hours per week of brisk walking reduced a woman's risk by 18 percent. However, walking 10 hours a week reduced the risk of developing breast cancer slightly more.[21]

For postmenopausal (not premenopausal) women, obesity increases the risk of developing breast cancer. One study found that women who gained 55 pounds or more after age 18 had a 1.5 times the risk of breast cancer than of women who maintained their weight. A gain of 22 pounds or more post-menopause increased the risk of breast cancer by 18 percent, whereas women who lost 11 pounds or more after menopause had a 20 percent lower breast cancer risk.[22] Having more fat tissue increases estrogen levels in the body and increases the likelihood of developing breast cancer. The epidemic of obesity and weight gain in women in the United States is of grave concern due to the increased potential for developing many chronic diseases, including breast cancer.

The best protection for a woman is early detection, that is, regular screening mammograms (see *FYI:* "Guidelines for Breast Cancer Detection"), breast exams by a health care provider, and monthly breast self-exams. A second protective factor is immediate treatment if breast cancer is diagnosed.

What to Look For The two most common warning signs are lumps or thickening in the breast. Most lumps are benign, particularly lumps that are soft, round, smooth, or movable. Generally, an irregular, hard lump that feels attached to breast tissue is more likely to be malignant. Most breast cancers (70–80 percent) begin in the cells of the ducts, usually of the upper outer portion of the breast. In situ breast cancers are confined within the ducts or lobules; they have not spread beyond the

area where they began. Lobular carcinoma in situ is sometimes believed to be a marker of increased risk for developing invasive cancer rather than a cancer itself. The seriousness of cancerous tumors that are invasive is determined by the staging at first diagnosis: local stage (confined to the breast), regional stage (spread to the lymph nodes), and distant stage (metastasized to other sites).

Additional warning signs include a change in the size or shape of the breast, discharge from the nipple, or a change in the color or texture of the skin of the breast or around the areola. Any discharge from the nipple should be brought to the attention of your health care provider!

Mammography **Mammography** allows health care providers to detect breast cancer up to 2 years before a lump can be felt. Early detection increases the likelihood that the cancer has not metastasized. High-quality mammography, an X-ray technique to visualize the internal structure of the breast, helps health care providers identify very small lumps, areas of calcification, or other tissue changes. Mammography is the best method for detecting breast cancer, but it is not perfect. Dense breast tissue, common in younger women, reduces the mammographic image and makes early diagnosis of breast cancer more difficult. Young women in particular may experience more false positives, that is, suspicious lesions found through mammography that when biopsied are shown to be benign. One of the reasons for the controversy regarding mammography for young women is the additional monetary cost and emotional turmoil of false positives. False-negative results are rare, particularly with better imaging techniques. However, because they can occur, breast self-examination and clinical breast examination are important. Women with high lifetime risk may need annual magnet resonance imaging (MRI)in addition to a mammogram.

Women with breast implants should know that mammographic images have limited effectiveness. They should inform the technician before the mammogram is taken. The facility needs to use special techniques designed for women with implants, and technicians need to be familiar with doing mammograms for women with breast implants.

Biopsies What happens if a lump is detected on a manmogram? A second mammogram may be required if a positive result occurs. However, mammography cannot distinguish benign from malignant lesions with absolute certainty. A biopsy is the only method to determine if cancer cells are present. The health care provider may proceed with fine-needle aspiration, a procedure involving a very thin needle and a syringe. Fine-needle aspirations are most common in women who have large,

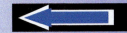

FYI

Guidelines for Breast Cancer Detection

The American Cancer Society, the National Cancer Institute, and other medical groups recommend routine mammograms for all women over the age of 40. There is still some discrepancy for women in their 40's. The American Cancer Society recommends mammograms *every year* for all women over the age of 40, and the National Cancer Institute recommends mammograms *every year or two* for all women over the age of 40. Both groups agree that mammograms should be conducted annually for women over age 50. Mammograms today can detect cancer in very early stages, well before physical symptoms can be detected by the woman or her health care provider. Studies show that women in their forties who had regular mammograms compared to those who did not have periodic mammograms were less likely to die of breast cancer and had more treatment options.

The American Cancer Society still recommends monthly breast self-examination (BSE) for women aged 20 and over. (See Chapter 7 for BSE instructions.) Clinical breast examinations are recommended every 3 years for women 20 and over and every year for women 40 and over.

palpable lesions. A needle is placed into the lump to determine if the lesion is solid or a fluid-filled **cyst.** If it is fluid-filled, the health care provider drains the fluid and the cyst collapses. If the cyst reappears, it can be drained again. No further treatment is necessary if the cyst does not reappear.

If the lesion is solid, the health care provider may attempt to draw out some cells for microscopic analysis. Fine-needle aspiration of a solid lesion requires great skill by the health care provider. If the lesion is malignant, it is important that cancerous cells be prevented from leaking out of the lesion into the body cavity.

Needle biopsy requires local anesthesia and uses a larger needle with a special cutting edge. A small core of tissue is removed, which may cause some bruising but rarely leaves a scar. Oftentimes, needle biopsies will be verified by surgical biopsies before further treatment is recommended.

A biopsy is the only method to determine if cancer cells are present. Whether surgical breast biopsy or needle aspiration is chosen by the health care provider depends on the nature and location of the lump. Surgical breast biopsy increases the tissue damage, is more costly, and is currently the only available method for women with non-palpable or small lesions (less than an inch in diameter). An *excisional* biopsy removes *all* of the lump or suspicious tissue mass. This procedure is performed under a local anesthetic and typically on an outpatient basis; the woman goes home the same day. An *incisional* biopsy removes a portion or cross-section of the lump. This procedure is performed under a local anesthetic as well and is recommended for lumps larger than an inch in diameter. Fully 80 percent of women in the United States who undergo surgical breast biopsies do *not* have cancer.

Treatment Research has led to better treatment, a lower risk of death, and an improved quality of life for women who have breast cancer. The treatment prescribed by the **oncologist** should be based on the most current research. Treatment will be based on the stage of cancer and the woman's surgical preference.

An oncologist is a physician who has special training to study, diagnose, and treat all types of cancer.

Special lab tests help the oncologist learn more about the cancer. Hormone receptor tests can determine whether hormones help the cancer grow. Other tests help determine whether the cancer is likely to spread or to return after treatment. Additional tests of the bones, liver, or lungs may be ordered to determine if distant sites have been impacted.

In some instances, a second opinion may be required or wanted. A brief delay (3 to 4 weeks) does not reduce the effectiveness of treatment. Finding a doctor for a second opinion can be achieved in a variety of ways:

through a referral from her primary physician, by calling 1-800-4-CANCER, through the local medical society directory or nearby medical school, or through the American Board of Medical Specialties directory found in the local library or online at www.certifieddoctor.org.

Breast cancer can be treated with local and/or systemic therapy. Local therapy (surgery or radiation therapy) is used to remove or destroy breast cancer at the site. Systemic treatments (chemotherapy, hormonal therapy, and biological therapy) are used to destroy or control cancer throughout the body. Surgery is the most common treatment for breast cancer. Breast-conserving surgery, an operation to remove the cancer but not the breast, includes **lumpectomy** (see Figure 16.1) and segmental mastectomy (partial mastectomy). At the time of surgery, some of the axillary (underarm) lymph nodes are often removed and examined under a microscope to see if the breast cancer has spread to the lymph nodes. After surgery, most women will receive **radiotherapy** (radiation treatment).

Mastectomy is surgery that removes the breast. In **total mastectomy** (see Figure 16.2), the whole breast is removed and some lymph nodes under the arm may also be removed. In **modified radical mastectomy** (see Figure 16.3), the whole breast, most of the lymph nodes under the arm, and often, the lining over the chest muscles, are removed. In radical mastectomy, the breast, both chest muscles, all of the lymph nodes under the arm, and some additional fat and skin are removed. Radical mastectomy is rarely used today although it was the standard procedure for many years; more effective, less invasive surgeries reduce potential risks of major surgeries. Mastectomy can be complemented by radiation therapy, chemotherapy, and hormonal therapy in combination or alone. See *Viewpoint:* "Should Women Opt for Preventative Mastectomies?"

Researchers are studying other facets of cancer treatment. They are testing new anticancer drugs, doses, and treatment schedules. They are seeking ways to reduce the side effects of treatment, such as lymphedema (swelling under the arm caused by fluid buildup due to faulty lymphatic drainage) and the reduced ability of bone marrow to make blood cells. Procedures such as neoadjuvant chemotherapy (using chemo before surgery), sentinel lymph node biopsy, colony-stimulating factors, autologous bone marrow transplants, and peripheral stem cell transplants are being explored. Now see *Viewpoint:* "Lumpectomy or Mastectomy?" and *Her Story:* "Arlette: Surviving Breast Cancer."

Drug therapy is proving to be beneficial in reducing the risk of breast cancer reccurring. *Tamoxifen* is an antiestrogen drug, taken on a daily basis in pill form, that reduces the chances of the cancer coming back by about 50 percent for women with early breast cancer for cancers that had estrogen or progesterone receptors.

FIGURE 16.1 In lumpectomy, the surgeon removes the breast cancer and some normal tissue around it. (Sometimes an excisional biopsy serves as a lumpectomy.) Often, some of the lymph nodes under the arm are removed.

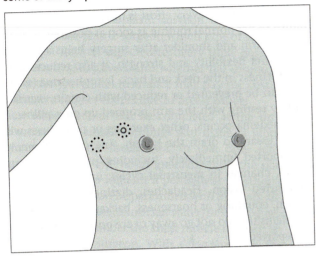

FIGURE 16.3 In modified radical mastectomy, the surgeon removes the whole breast, most of the lymph nodes under the arm, and often the lining over the chest muscles. The smaller of the two chest muscles also may be taken out to help in removing the lymph nodes.

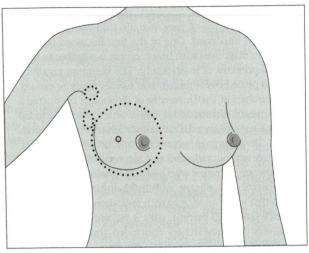

FIGURE 16.2 In total mastectomy, the surgeon removes the whole breast. Some lymph nodes under the arm may also be removed.

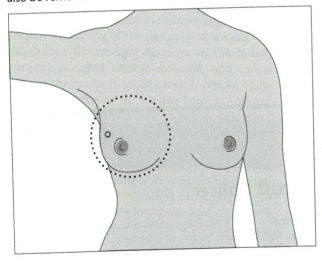

Aromatase inhibitors (AIs), such as letrozole (Femara), anastrozole (Arimidex), and exemestane (Aromasin), work by blocking an enzyme responsible for producing small amounts of estrogen in postmenopausal women. Clinical trials have been performed both comparing one of the AIs to tamoxifen for a total of 5 years and adding treatment with an AI following 2–6 years of tamoxifen. These studies have shown there is a clear advantage to using either an AI instead of tamoxifen for a total of 5 years, or switching to an AI after several years of

Viewpoint

Should Women Opt for Preventive Mastectomies?

Should women elect to have a mastectomy in order to prevent potential breast cancer? Research reveals that women who have harmful mutations in the *BRCA1* and *BRCA2* genes have an 80 percent chance of developing breast cancer at some point during their lifetime. (See section on gene mutation research.) A recent study published in the April 1, 2009, issue of *Cancer* found that women who learned that they have *BRCA* genes are likely to consider a preventive mastectomy as the best way to reduce the risk and the fear of developing breast cancer.[18] However, there are numerous other options that safeguard against this cancer. These include frequent mammograms, breast magnetic resonance imaging (MRI), clinical breast exams, tamoxifen therapy, and risk reduction surgery, such as prophylactic mastectomy. What are your thoughts on this type of preventive surgery? What would you do if you found that you had *BRCA* genes? Are the costs and the medical personnel needed to perform this surgery justified?

tamoxifen, rather than keeping postmenopausal women on tamoxifen alone for 5 years. However, AIs have been found to have fewer side effects than tamoxifen because

ACTIONS TO TAKE WHEN CANCER IS DIAGNOSED

When the diagnosis of cancer occurs, a common reaction is to feel like life is out of control. A woman can take a number of steps toward regaining control over her life. First, get more information about the particular cancer. As stated earlier, there are over 100 different cancers, and each primary site could be one of several different kinds of cancers. Once a woman knows the type of cancer, she can call the National Cancer Institute (1-800-4-CANCER) or the American Cancer Society for more information. Reliable websites provide guidance and valuable information. See websites in Resources at the end of the chapter.

Second, get a second opinion before deciding on a particular treatment protocol. Seeking confirmation is reasonable and common. The second oncologist should be informed about the initial diagnosis. She or he will likely be more direct and straightforward with recommendations, particularly because an expert opinion is being solicited rather than a request for involvement in the patient's progress.

Third, a woman should feel certain about her options. Any questions and responses that are not fully understood should be addressed. If a National Cancer Institute–designated comprehensive or clinical cancer center is nearby, choose it. The specialists at these centers are most familiar with current treatment protocols and any recent research developments. The primary health care provider and surgeon should be board certified in cancer care, such as an oncologist or an oncology surgeon.

SOCIAL SUPPORT

Social support is a critical factor in recovery from a stressful event such as cancer. Support from family and friends plays a major role in the speed and level of recovery. Unfortunately, women with cancer seem to lose the level of support they enjoyed before the diagnosis of cancer. The fear of cancer causes some people to avoid contact with anyone or anything that reminds them of it. Cancer, compared to other chronic diseases, is a stigmatized condition. In fact, many people still believe that the diagnosis of cancer is a death sentence, and some may even believe cancer is contagious. Cancer support groups provide a confidential environment where patients and their families can discuss all aspects of the disease, such as managing side effects, sharing their feelings, and work-related concerns.[44]

Women who have undergone a modified radical mastectomy may be concerned about the inability to engage in vigorous physical activity, the fear that the cancer will return, and resentment or worry regarding the quality of care received. Women with chronic diseases such as heart disease feel some control over their destiny, such as when they can modify their diet and increase their physical activity level. This control provides them with a sense of doing something to improve their chance of survival. However, women living with cancer do not have the same opportunity to exhibit control.

Cancer survivors who reported energy losses due to treatment also indicated a reduction in discretionary activities and social network size. These reductions may lead to lower levels of emotional and physical support at a time when support is most needed. The American Cancer Society has recognized the need for support and provides numerous services for women and their families, including the following: online communities and support where one can explore *What Next* (cancer support network); *Circle of Sharing*™ (personalized cancer information); *Cancer Survivors Network* (an online community where persons with cancer can connect with others with cancer). Other support services include *Reach to Recovery* (for breast cancer support), *I Can Cope* (cancer education classes), *Road to Recovery* (a program that provides transportation to and from treatment for patients), *Patient Navigator Program* (connects patient with a patient navigator at a cancer treatment center), and, *Look Good . . . Feel Better* (help with appearance-related side effects of treatment). All of these resources can be found on the ACS web site.[45]

COMPLEMENTARY AND ALTERNATIVE TREATMENT IN CANCER MANAGEMENT

This chapter would not be complete without mention of the complementary and alternative medicine (CAM) used to treat or cope with cancer. *Complementary treatments* are medical products and practices that are not considered standard medical care, but are used along with usual medical treatment. *Alternative medicine* is treatments used instead of usual medical treatments.[46] Usual or standard medical treatments are based on research studies and usually follow a recognized and approved protocol. The American Cancer Society and other respected organizations continually review current practices, attempting to determine the benefit in the treatment of cancer. The National Cancer Institute provides insight into various types of CAM approaches.[46]

Mind-Body

Mind-body treatments are used to improve the psychological and emotional capability to improve bodily functions in a way that assist in healing and coping with cancer. These treatments include use of *aromatherapy* with essential oils to improve the quality of life for cancer patients by reducing stress and anxiety as chemical messages are sent to the area of the brain that affects mood and emotion. *Hypnosis or self-hypnosis* has been found to reduce pain and anxiety during procedures such as breast biopsy.[47] Cancer patients often feel supported by *spirituality* or beliefs and practices of religion. While spirituality practices differ with culture and traditions, patients may find relief of anxiety or fear and help determining major life decisions through prayer, religious support groups, and/or the medical team beliefs. Another mind-body practice is *yoga,* which tends to relieve stress and anxiety through physical postures, breathing and relaxation. Yoga also promotes fitness and therefore may enhance the immune system to help find cancer in the body. *Meditation, biofeedback,* and *imagery* can also be beneficial to coping with the disease of cancer.

A variety of relaxation techniques have been touted as beneficial for women with cancer, not so much as cures but rather as *adjuvant* therapy, meaning practices that enhance the body's ability to heal. Creative visualization (imagining scenes, pictures or experiences to visual the healing of the body), affirmations, biofeedback, humor, art and music therapy, and meditation are all helpful practices in coping with cancer and improving quality of life. Each of these is discussed in greater detail in Chapter 5.

Nutritional Treatments

Vegetarian diets have been tried by women with cancer in an effort to slow the progression of the disease. Vegetarians do not eat meat, fish, or poultry but some will eat products with animal by-products. Vegans consume only foods with plant origin, whereas lacto-vegetarians consume foods with plant origins and dairy products. The Zen macrobiotic diet emphasizes eating cereals, such as rice. It is a low-fat complex carbohydrate diet with no animal products, no refined sugar, and limited fluids. Low-fat diets with fruits and vegetables are shown to be health enhancing and helpful to preventing cancer.

Herbal and vitamin therapy. An array of complementary treatments have been touted to help either prevent, cure, or limit cancer spread. These include megavitamin therapy, enzyme therapy, shiitake mushrooms, shark cartilage, Essiac herbs, wheatgrass, coffee enemas, milk thistle, mistletoe extracts, and others. Hoxsey therapy, a special herbal tonic, evolved when a farmer decided to collect herbs that had healed his cancerous horse. This therapy was banned by the Food and Drug Administration in 1960 but is still available in Mexico. Shark cartilage therapy evolved because sharks are believed to seldom get cancer. Thus, proponents suggest that shark cartilage should be tested for its cancer-inhibiting ability. There are numerous other suggested remedies that are outside the realm of standard medicine. Cancer patients should always consult their oncologist when considering the use of any of these CAM treatments.

Magnetic and Energy Treatments

Magnetic and electronic devices use gamma rays, X rays, light waves, or radio waves are types of treatment meant to cure or slow the progression of cancer. These are intended to balance life forces, the energy of the body. Some standard therapies may also use a variety of electronic devices; however, these procedures have been accepted by the medical community (i.e., radiation therapy, MRI, diagnostic, and other therapies.)

Tai Chi , which has slow, gentle movement focusing on breath and concentration, *Reiki,* which claims to balance energy by placing hands on or near the person, or *Therapeutic Touch,* involving the movement of hands over energy fields of the body, are all examples of *energy medicine,* intended to used for healing and improved health.[48]

CHOOSING A TREATMENT PLAN

A woman diagnosed with cancer or a recurrence of cancer faces myriad decisions, including the choice of medical and complementary treatments. Complementary methods have been touted by too many individuals to be dismissed, yet grasping at straws does not provide a sense of control. Knowledge and accurate evaluation of the effectiveness of conventional therapy and alternative treatment protocols are the best methods to begin recapturing control. The first step for any woman is to focus on those things most within her control, including becoming more familiar with the treatment options available to her. Deciding whether to follow conventional therapy alone, or a combination of conventional and complementary/alternative therapies, depends on an accurate diagnosis by an oncologist and a clear picture of the prognosis for that particular type of cancer. A woman needs to be involved in the process of decision making throughout the treatment and recovery phase. Remember: Early detection is important to your well-being!

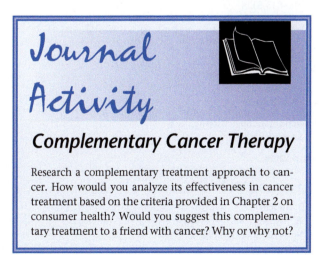

Journal Activity

Complementary Cancer Therapy

Research a complementary treatment approach to cancer. How would you analyze its effectiveness in cancer treatment based on the criteria provided in Chapter 2 on consumer health? Would you suggest this complementary treatment to a friend with cancer? Why or why not?

Chapter Summary

- Half of all cancers affecting women are cancers of the reproductive system.
- There are significant differences in benign and malignant tumors.
- The World Health Organization has identified forty-six body sites and numerous cancers at each site, over a hundred different cancers.
- The American Cancer Society has identified seven major warning signs of cancer.
- Lifestyle and environmental factors account for most cancer risks.
- The amount of fat a person consumes is a risk factor for some cancers.
- Cigarette smoking accounts for 85 percent of all lung cancer deaths and 30 percent of all cancer deaths.
- Lung cancer is the leading cause of cancer deaths in women.
- Breast cancer is the most prevalent type of cancer in women.
- If a woman has a diagnosis of cancer, she should get information about the cancer, get a second opinion from another physician, learn about all the treatment options for her type of cancer, and seek a support group to help her through the treatment and recovery.
- Screening mammography complemented by monthly breast self-examinations and clinical breast examinations are the best methods for early detection of breast cancer.
- Cervical and endometrial cancers are extremely curable if detected early.
- Skin cancer is the most prevalent and most curable type of cancer found in women.
- Melanoma can be detected by attention to asymmetry, border irregularity, color change, and diameter greater than 6mm.
- Tanning beds emit UVA rays that contribute to skin wrinkling, irregular pigmentation, and immunosuppression.
- Social support is a critical factor in recovering from cancer.
- Many women explore complementary therapies as an adjunct to conventional health care.

Review Questions

1. What are the seven warning signs of cancer?
2. What are the definitions for the following terms: benign, malignant, metastasis, in situ, and invasive?
3. What are the four most common categories of cancer?
4. What are some of the lifestyle and environmental causes of cancer?
5. What are the leading cancer sites in women based on race and ethnicity?
6. What are the early signs and symptoms for each of the following cancers: lung, breast, uterine, and ovarian?
7. What are the five best preventive measures a woman can practice to reduce the risk of cancer? What criteria did you use to determine these choices?
8. Explain all treatment options for a woman who has been diagnosed with cancer.
9. What are the newer medications that are used for treatment of cancer?
10. What are some of the complementary therapies a woman might select to supplement conventional therapy?

Resources

Web Sites

American Cancer Society
  800-ACS-2345
  www.cancer.org/index

American Institute for Cancer Research
  800-843-8114
  www.aicr.org

Center for Complementary and Alternative Medicine
  www.nccam.nih.gov

Corporate Angel Network, Inc.
  866-328-1313
  www.corpangelnetwork.org

Intercultural Cancer Council
  iccnetwork.org/

Mayo Clinic
  800-446-2279
  www.mayoclinic.com

M.D. Anderson
  877-MDA-6789
  www.mdanderson.org

Memorial Sloan-Kettering Cancer Center
  800-525-2225
  www.mskcc.org

National Breast Cancer Coalition (NBCC)
  www.stopbreastcancer.org
  800-622-2838

National Cancer Institute
  www.cancer.gov
  800-4-cancer

NOAH: New York Online Access to Health
  www.noah-health.org

Ovarian Cancer National Alliance (OCNA)
  www.ovariancancer.org
  866-399-6262

The Susan G. Komen Breast Cancer Foundation
  ww5.komen.org/
  877-465-6636

Y-ME National Breast Cancer Organization, Inc.
  www.y-me.org
  800-221-2141

References

1. American Cancer Society: 2012. *Cancer facts and figures.* Atlanta, GA: ACS, p. 10.
2. Ibid.
3. National Cancer Institute. 2010. *Staging cancer.* http://www .cancer.gov/cancertopics/factsheet/detection/staging, (retrieved April 8, 2012).
4. Ibid.
5. U.S. Department of Health and Human Services. 2004. *Women, tobacco, and cancer: An agenda for the 21st century.* Rockville, MD: U.S. Department of Health and Human Services, National Institutes of Health, National Cancer Institute, p. 5.
6. Centers for Disease Control and Prevention. 2008. *Five-a Day-Program.* Atlanta, GA: CDC.
7. Liao, J. B. 2007. Viruses and human cancer. *Yale Journal of Biology and Medicine.* 79(3-4): 115–22.
8. American Cancer Society: 2012. *Cancer facts and figures.* Atlanta, GA: ACS, p. 49.
9. Chlebowshi, R. T. 2010. Estrogen plus progestin and breast cancer Incidence and mortality in postmenopausal women. *JAMA* 304(15).
10. American Cancer Society: 2012. *Cancer Facts and Figures.* Atlanta, GA: ACS, p.21.
11. U.S. Department of Commerce, National Oceanic & Atmospheric Administration. 2010. *WMO/UNEP scientific assessment of ozone depletion.* http://www.esrl.noaa.gov/csd/ assessments/ozone/ (retrieved April 8, 2012).
12. American Cancer Society. 2011. *Stem cell transplant (peripheral blood, marrow, and cord blood transplants: Problems in the post-transplant period.* http://www.cancer.org/Treatment/ TreatmentsandSideEffects/TreatmentTypes/BoneMarrowand PeripheralBloodStemCellTransplant/stem-cell-transplant-problems-shortly-after-transplant (retrieved April 10, 2012).
13. American Cancer Society. 2012. *Cancer Facts and figures.* Atlanta, GA: ACS, p. 10.
14. National Lung Screening Trial Research Team. 2011. Reduced lung cancer mortality with low-dose computed tomographic screening. *New England Journal of Medicine* 365(5): 395–409.
15. American Cancer Society. 2012. *Cancer facts and figures.* Atlanta, GA: ACS, p. 16.
16. MD Anderson Cancer Center. 2012. *Lung cancer treatment.* http://www.mdanderson.org/patient-and-cancer-information/ cancer-information/cancer-types/lung-cancer/treatment/ index.html (retrieved April 10, 2012).
17. American Cancer Society. 2012. *Cancer facts and figures.* Atlanta, GA: ACS, p. 9.
18. Ibid, p. 43–4.
19. Howlader, N., Noone, A. M., Krapcho, M., et al. (Eds.). *SEER Cancer Statistics Review, 1975–2008: Fast Stats.* Bethesda, MD: National Cancer Institute. http://seer.cancer.gov/ csr/1975_2008/, 2011.
20. Collaborative Group on Hormonal Factors in Breast Cancer. 2002. Breast cancer and breast feeding: Collaborative re-analyses of individual data from 47 epidemiological studies in 30 countries, including 50,302 women with breast cancer and 93,973 women without the disease. *Lancet* 360: 187–95.
21. American Cancer Society. 2006. *Breast cancer.* http:// documents.cancer.org/acs/groups/cid/documents/ webcontent/003090-pdf.pdf p. 17. (Retrieved April 30, 2012)
22. Eliassen, A. H., Colditz, G. A., Rosner, B., et al. 2006. Adult weight change and risk of postmenopausal breast cancer. *JAMA* 296(2): 193–201.
23. American Cancer Society. 2012. *Cancer facts and figures: 2012.* Atlanta, GA: ACS. p. 10.
24. Susan G. Komen Foundation. 2012. *Breast reconstruction.* http://ww5.komen.org/BreastCancer/BreastReconstruction .html (retrieved April 30, 2012).
25. American Cancer Society. 2012. *Cancer Facts and Figures: 2012.* Atlanta, GA: ACS. 10.
26. Ibid, p. 23.
27. Ibid, p. 17.
28. Johns Hopkins Ovarian Cancer Center of Excellence. *Genetic testing and risk assessment.* http://www.hopkinsmedicine.org/ kimmel_cancer_center/types_cancer/ovarian_cancer.html (retrieved on April 30, 2012).
29. M.D. Anderson Cancer Center. 2012. *Ovarian cancer diagnosis.* http://www.mdanderson.org/patient-and-cancer-information/ cancer-information/cancer-types/ovarian-cancer/diagnosis/ index.html (retrieved April 30, 2012).
30. Johns Hopkins Ovarian Cancer Center of Excellence. *Genetic testing and risk assessment.* http://www.hopkinsmedicine.org/ kimmel_cancer_center/types_cancer/ovarian_cancer.html (retrieved on April 30, 2012).
31. American Cancer Society. 2012. *Cancer facts and figures: 2012.* Atlanta, GA: ACS. p. 21.
32. Ibid.
33. Ibid.
34. Skin Cancer Foundation. 2012. *Skin cancer information.* http:// www.skincancer.org/skin-cancer-information (retrieved May 7, 2012).
35. American Cancer Society. 2012. *Cancer facts and figures: 2012.* Atlanta, GA: ACS. p. 21.
36. Abramson Cancer Center of the University of Pennsylvania: OncoLink. 2012. *Melanoma: The Basics.* http://www.oncolink .org/types/article.cfm?c=18&s=63&ss=497&id=8600&CFID=4 5571738&CFTOKEN=42566272 (retrieved May 7, 2012)
37. American Cancer Society. 2012. *Cancer facts and figures: 2012.* Atlanta, GA: ACS. p. 10.
38. Ibid, p. 12.
39. National Cancer Institute. 2012. *Colorectal cancer screening.* http://www.cancer.gov/cancertopics/factsheet/detection/ colorectal-screening (retrieved on May 7, 2012).
40. American Cancer Society. 2012. *Colorectal cancer early detection.* http://www.cancer.org/Cancer/ColonandRectumCancer/ MoreInformation/ColonandRectumCancerEarlyDetection/ colorectal-cancer-early-detection-screening-tests-used. (retrieved May 7, 2012).
41. American Cancer Society. 2012. *Cancer facts and figures: 2012.* Atlanta, GA: ACS. p. 12–3.
42. Ibid, p. 13.
43. Ibid.
44. National Cancer Institute. 2002. *Cancer support groups: Questions and answers.* www.cancer.gov/cancertopics/ factsheet/support/support-groups (retrieved May 9, 2012)
45. American Cancer Society. 2012. *Find support and treatment.* http://www.cancer.org/Treatment/SupportProgramsServices/ index (retrieved on May 9, 2012)

goals, target dates for completion, rewards, intervention strategies, and witnesses to the agreement.

behavioral counseling—A style of psychotherapy designed to teach clients new skills by providing instructions, modeling new behaviors, promoting behavioral rehearsal, and providing feedback on performance.

benign—Not cancerous; harmless.

binge drinking—Consuming four or more drinks in a row for women (five or more for men).

binge eating disorder—Involves binge eating but not purging (vomiting and laxative abuse) afterward.

bioavailability—Rate and extent to which the active ingredient is absorbed from a drug product and becomes available at the site of action.

biofeedback—The use of electronic equipment to monitor the physiological state of the body while the individual learns techniques to voluntarily regulate the body's systems and reduce unwanted symptoms.

bipolar disorder—Mixture of major depressive episodes and manic episodes.

birth control—Umbrella term for all the strategies used to prevent childbirth, including contraception.

blastocyst—A cluster of embryonic cells; the stage of development between the zygote and embryo.

body composition—The amount of lean and fat tissue in the body.

body dysmorphic disorder (BDD)—The classification of body-image disturbance reserved for the non–eating disorder population.

body mass index (BMI)—Numerical expression of body weight based on height (expressed in meters) to weight (expressed in kilograms) to help determine healthy body weight.

brand name—Patented name given to a drug by the manufacturer that developed the drug.

Braxton Hicks—Contractions or irregular tightening of the uterus during pregnancy, sometimes called false labor.

breast augmentation—Surgical method to increase the size of the breast by implanting synthetic materials into the chest wall behind the breast tissue.

breast reduction surgery—Surgery performed to reduce the size of the breasts.

bulimia nervosa—Eating and then vomiting soon afterward or using a laxative in order to avoid weight gain.

C

caffeinism—Chronic consumption of high levels of caffeine.

calipers—A device that measures the thickness of skin-folds taken at different sites on the body; the data are used to determine an individual's percent body fat.

capillaries—Blood vessels with thin membranes that allow for the exchange of carbon dioxide and waste by-products for oxygen and food.

carcinogenic—The ability to cause the development of cancer.

carcinogens—Substances that can cause the growth of cancer.

cardiorespiratory endurance—The ability to perform physical activities for long periods of time while oxygen is supplied to various tissues of the body.

cardiovascular system—Body system that includes the heart and blood vessels.

caveat emptor—Let the buyer beware; opposite of *caveat vendor,* or let the seller beware.

cervical cap—Small rubber cup fitted over the narrow lower end of the uterus to prevent sperm from entering the cervical canal.

cervicitis—Acute or chronic inflammation of the uterine cervix.

cervix—Part of the uterus that protrudes into the vaginal opening.

chemical name—The name that describes the molecular structure of a drug.

chemotherapy—Use of drugs to treat disease, most often cancer.

childhood abuse—Physical or mental injury, sexual abuse or exploitation, negligent treatment, or maltreatment of a child before age 18, by a person who is responsible for the child's welfare.

chlamydia—The most common sexually transmitted infection found in U.S. women; caused by microorganisms that live as parasites within cells.

choice theory and reality therapy—A style of psychotherapy that emphasizes client choice and responsibility for choosing behaviors that meet client's needs.

cilia—Small, hairlike structures that produce motion to help clear the lungs.

clitoris—Pea-shaped projection made up of nerves, blood vessels, and erectile tissue.

closed adoption—Confidential and no contact between birth and adoptive parents.

codependency—A preoccupation with a particular individual and her problems to the point of self-neglect. This results from prolonged association with an addict who has an oppressive set of rules that prevent the open expression of feelings, concerns, and problems.

cognitive appraisal—The process of categorizing an encounter with respect to its significance for well-being.

cognitive-behavioral therapy—A style of psychotherapy that focuses an identifying and challenging irrational client beliefs that contribute to maladaptive feelings and behaviors.

cohabitation—Two people living together in a committed relationship without marriage.

coitus interruptus—An unreliable birth control method in which the penis is withdrawn from the vagina prior to ejaculation.

colostrum—The initial breast milk produced by the mother.

complementary medicine—A practice used in conjunction with conventional medicine.

complicated grief—Delayed or incomplete adaptation to loss.

comprehensive fitness program—A fitness program encompassing all components essential to overall fitness: cardiorespiratory endurance, muscle strength and endurance, flexibility, and body composition.

compulsive exercise—A compelling emotional drive to exercise excessively to achieve an ideal but unrealistic image rather than for health improvement.

computerized tomography (CT) scan—A beam that rotates around the body and provides a series of X-rays of a particular area of the body from various angles.

condom—A latex sheath designed to cover the erect penis and hold semen upon ejaculation.

congestive heart failure (CHF)—Circulatory congestion caused by heart damage that inhibits adequate blood flow to the body.

continuous abstinence—Not having sex with a partner.

contraception—A variety of methods used to prevent fertilization of the ovum.

coronary artery bypass grafting (CABG)—Any one of many types of surgery that allows blood to travel past or around a blockage.

corticoids—Hormones generated by the adrenal glands that influence the body's control of glucose, protein, and fat metabolism.

cosmetic surgeon—A physician who specializes in beauty-enhancing surgery such as face-lifts or breast augmentation.

counseling model—A style of psychotherapy from which a counselor typically conceptualizes and counsels a client.

cross-fiber friction massage—Massaging an area where injury or surgery has occurred to break up possible adhesions and scar tissue.

cyberstalking—The use of the Internet, e-mail, or other electronic communications devices to stalk another person. Stalking generally involves harassing or threatening behavior that an individual engages in repeatedly, such as following a person, appearing at a person's home or place of business, making harassing phone calls, leaving written messages or objects, or vandalizing a person's property.

cycle-based method—Natural family planning method that relies on abstinence during the time of ovulation.

cyclothymic disorder—A chronic fluctuating mood disturbance involving numerous periods of mania and depression.

cyst—A closed sac in or under the skin containing liquid or semisolid material.

D

date rape—Sexual assault of a woman by a man she has agreed to see socially.

delirium tremens (DTs)—A condition resulting from withdrawal from chronic alcohol abuse and causing uncontrollable tremors, confusion, and vivid hallucinations.

democratic parenting style—A parenting style that seeks to raise a responsible child by setting limits for the child and giving the child choices within those limits.

Depo-Provera—Trademark name for a contraceptive method utilizing progestin injection into the gluteal or deltoid muscle once every 3 months.

depression—An emotional state of persistent dejection ranging from mild discouragement and gloominess to feelings of extreme despondency and despair.

detoxification—A period of time when an addict does not drink to rid the body of alcohol and its toxic chemicals.

diabetes mellitus—Group of metabolic diseases identified by high blood sugar levels.

diaphragm—Oval, dome-shaped device that covers the lower end of the uterus to prevent sperm from entering the cervical canal.

diaphragmmatic breathing—Slow, relaxed, deep breathing to calm emotions and fully oxygenate the body.

diastolic blood pressure—Amount of pressure the blood exerts against the arterties while the heart is relaxing.

Dietary Reference Intakes (DRIs)—Generic term that includes three types of reference values in the diets of particular age and gender groups.

dilation and currettage (D&C)—Medical procedure that dilates the cervix and scrapes the uterine lining to remove contents.

dilation and evacuation (D&E)—Medical procedure that dilates the cervix and aspirates the contents of the uterus.

disaccharide—A compound made up of two monosaccharides, or simple sugars; examples include sucrose, maltose, and lactose.

discouraged child—A child who feels she has no place of significance in the family.

distress—Stress that diminishes the quality of life, commonly associated with disease, illness, and maladaptation.

divorce—A legal dissolution to a marriage.

domestic abuse—Abuse committed in the home by an intimate associate, usually the spouse.

doula—A person who is trained to provide guidance and support to a woman during pregnancy and childbirth.

dysmenorrhea—Painful menstrual periods characterized by severe cramps, headaches, lower-back and/or leg pain; occasionally incapacitating pain.

dynamic stretching—A form of stretching using momentum to steadily increase speed and reach and move into an extended range of motion; this type of stretching moves you carefully to the limits of your range of motion.

dysrhythmia—Disturbances in the normal sequence of cardiac electric activity; sometimes referred to as arrythmia.

dysthymic disorder—Involves the presence of two of the following symptoms for most of the day for at least 2 years (1 year for adolescents and children): poor appetite or overeating, insomnia, low energy or fatigue, low self-esteem, poor concentration or difficulty making decisions, or feelings of hopelessness.

E

eclampsia—Acute toxemia of pregnancy characterized by convulsions and coma.

ectopic pregnancy—Implantation of the embryo in the fallopian tube, ovary, abdominal cavity, or cervix.

EDNOS (Eating Disorder Not Otherwise Specified)—Missing a diagnosis of anorexia or bulimia by only one criterion; afflicts 2 to 6 percent of the population.

effective communication—Components are appropriate body language, encouraging responses, paraphrasing, clarification, and summarization.

effective listening—Components are appropriate body language, encouraging responses, paraphrasing, clarification, and summarization.

elder abuse—Elder abuse is doing something or failing to do something that results in harm to an elderly person or puts a helpless older person at risk of harm. This includes

- Physical, sexual and emotional abuse
- Neglecting or deserting an older person you are responsible for
- Taking or misusing an elderly person's money or property

ELISA test—Abbreviation for enzyme-linked immunosorbent assay, a screening test for the HIV antibody.

embryo—The developing egg from the time of implantation (about 2 weeks after conception) in the uterus until the 5th week of pregnancy.

emotional intelligence—The ability to recognize your emotions and those of the people around you and have the competence to work with those emotions to resolve problems, especially in the workplace.

emotional intimacy—A feeling of knowing and being known.

emphysema—Chronic shortness of breath caused by tissue deterioration characterized by increased air retention and reduced exchange of gases.

endocarditis—Inflammation or infection of the inside lining of the heart chambers and/or valves.

endocrine system—Bodily system that consists of endocrine glands in order to maintain and regulate body activities. It is activated by the anterior section of the hypothalamus.

endogenous factors—Events that occur within you.

endometriosis—Chronic growth of endometrial tissue outside the uterus; can be painful and debilitating.

endometrium—Mucous membrane lining the uterus.

epidemiology—The study of relationships of the various factors determining the frequency and distribution of diseases in a human community.

epilepsy—A group of nervous system disorders caused by uncontrolled electrical discharge from nerve cells of the surface of the brain marked by recurrent seizures.

epinephrine and norepinephrine—Powerful adrenal hormones whose presence in the bloodstream prepares the body for maximal energy production and skeletal muscle response.

episiotomy—Surgical procedure to widen the vaginal opening during childbirth.

erotic love—A relationship built on passion and sexual desire.

ethyl alcohol—A clear, somewhat tasteless liquid found in various types of beverages that produce intoxication; ethanol.

eustress—Stress that adds a positive, enhancing dimension to the quality of life.

exercise adherence—Consistent involvement in an exercise program to gain long-term health benefits.

existential counseling—A style of psychotherapy that assists a client to live a more authentic and fulfilling life by resolving feelings of anxiety and guilt.

exogenous factors—External events that influence you.

extreme obesity—A body mass index (BMI) greater than 39.

F

fall and winter SAD—A category of Seasonal Affective Disorder (SAD) that occurs in fall and winter. Symptoms, may include depression, hopelessness, anxiety, loss of energy, social withdrawal, oversleeping, loss of interest in activities, appetite changes and difficulty concentrating.

female condom—Thin, polyurethane pouch with two flexible rings; one covers the cervix and the other partially covers the vagina.

femininity—Possessing a high number of attributes defined as feminine and a low number of attributes defined as masculine.

feminist—A person who advocates for equal rights for all persons with a special focus on women's concerns.

feminist therapy—Also referred to as gender equity therapy; empowers women through an egalitarian (equity-based) relationship with the therapist.

fermentation—Process by which sugars are converted into grain alcohol through the action of yeast.

fetal alcohol effects (FAE)—A limited number of the characteristic birth defects associated with fetal alcohol syndrome such as below normal IQ, learning disabilities, hyperactivity, short attention span, and often similar physical malformations as with FAS; completely preventable.

fetal alcohol syndrome (FAS)—A cluster of birth defects including irreversible mental and physical disabilities that develop as a result of expectant mothers consuming excessive amounts of alcohol.

fibrocystic breast condition—Catchall phrase for any signs or symptoms not related to breast cancer.

fibromyalgia—A common and chronic musculoskeletal syndrome characterized by fatigue, widespread pain in the muscles, ligaments, and tendons, and multiple "tender points" on the body where there is increased sensitivity to touch or slight pressure.

fight-or-flight response—The body's innate response to stress by either confrontation or avoidance.

five stages of grief—A grief process model that includes the stages of denial, anger, sorrow/despair/depression, bargaining, and acceptance.

flexibility—The range of motion of a particular joint.

follicular phase—First stage of a woman's menstruation and ovarian cycle.

Food and Drug Administration (FDA)—The federal agency charged with approval and control of drug-related products in the United States.

free radicals—Toxic chemicals in the body that cause damage to body cells and can lead to serious illnesses such as cancer.

Freudian psychoanalytic theory—An original psychological theory developed by Sigmund Freud, that provides the basis for psychoanalytic counseling which assist a client to gain conscious awareness of unconscious patterns of thinking to work through anxiety.

G

gamete intrafallopian transfer (GIFT)—Use of a laparoscope to guide the transfer of unfertilized eggs and sperm into the woman's fallopian tubes through an incision in the abdomen.

gender-relations theory—Originally self-in-relation theory; a response to traditional Western psychology that emphasizes separation and individuation, but neglects the intricacies of human interconnection.

gender-role socialization—The tendency to interact with a child or to limit the experiences of a child in ways that seem more suitable to traditional roles relative to the child's gender.

general adaptation syndrome (GAS)—A pattern of responses in reaction to life demands or threats.

generic name—Common name for a drug.

gestalt counseling—A style of psychotherapy designed to assist a client to identify, explore and resolve unfinished business of a client which interferes with living life more fully and freely.

glamorization—Basing the desirability of a woman on her body shape, mainly thinness in the arms, legs, face, and waist, and largeness of the breasts and hips (the hourglass figure). Thought to have begun in the 1830s when the camera was invented.

glycemic index—Measures the speed by which foods raise the blood glucose level.

gonorrhea—A sexually transmitted infection caused by the bacterium *Neisseria gonorrhoea*.

grief—The emotional experience of loss.

grief process—Different methods of examining the ways in which people deal with the loss of loved ones, usually defined as having different stages or processes.

gynecology—The study and treatment of medical concerns specific to women.

H

health care maintenance—The continuation of what one is doing to maintain one's current health status.

health education—Involves research and study in the causes, prevention, and treatment of disorders. Also involves the publication and distribution of this information to the public.

health intervention—The act or fact of interfering so as to modify.

health maintenance organization (HMO)—A type of health insurance that provides a full-range of health care services using specific physicians and specialists for a prepaid amount of money.

health promotion—(a) Dissemination through literature and workshops of information regarding healthy lifestyles, enhancement of life quality, and illness prevention; (b) includes the idea that health is something to be nurtured and by doing so we prevent the onset of illness and disease.

health-related components of fitness—Cardiorespiratory endurance, muscular strength and endurance, flexibility, and body composition.

heme iron—Iron found in animal tissue in the form of hemoglobin and myoglobin.

hemodialyis—A medical procedure that removes impurities or wastes from the blood.

hemoglobin—The iron-bearing molecules found in red blood cells that carry oxygen to and carbon dioxide away from body cells.

hemorrhagic stroke—Results when a blood vessel bursts inside the brain.

hepatitis A virus (HAV)—A disease of the liver caused by the hepatitis A virus.

hepatitis B virus (HBV)—A viral infection causing inflammation of the liver; may be severe and result in prolonged illness or death.

hepatitis C virus (HCV)—A disease of the liver caused by the hepatitis C virus.

herpes simplex virus (HSV)—A viral infection that attacks the skin and nervous system, usually producing short-lasting, fluid-filled blisters on the skin and mucous membranes.

heterosexism—A belief or attitude that results in bias or discrimination toward anyone who is not heterosexual.

HIPAA—Policy that requires health care providers to develop procedures that protect the privacy of patients' health care information and records.

homeostasis—Relative balance in the internal environment of the body; naturally maintained by adaptive responses that promote healthy survival.

homophobia—The fear or dislike of someone who is homosexual.

hot flashes—Short periods of extreme warmth experienced by some women around the time of menopause; also called hot flushes.

human immunodeficiency virus (HIV)—The organism that causes AIDS.

human papilloma virus (HPV)—A group of more than one hundred viruses including genital warts; some types increase the risk of cancer.

hymen—Fold of mucous membrane, skin, and fibrous tissue covering the vaginal opening.

hypertension—Common disorder marked by high blood pressure; divided into stage 1 and stage 2.

hypothalamus—Activates the endocrine system and the autonomic nervous system.

hysterectomy—An operation to remove a woman's uterus and, sometimes, the fallopian tubes, ovaries, and cervix.

I

infant mortality—Statistical rate of infant death during the first year of birth expressed as the number per 1,000 live births.

intracytoplasmic sperm injection (ICSI)—A type of in vitro fertilization (IVF) in which a single sperm is injected into the center of an egg; can be used with sperm that are less mobile or weaker.

intrauterine device—Contraceptive method made of plastic or other material that is inserted into the uterus to prevent pregnancy.

intrauterine growth retardation—Abnormal process in which the development and maturation of the fetus is impeded or delayed by a number of factors, including genetics, drugs, and malnutrition.

in vitro fertilization (IVF)—Surgical retrieval of eggs, fertilization in the laboratory, and transfer of the embryo into the uterus.

ischemia—Lack or absence of oxygen.

ischemic stroke—Results when an inadequate supply of blood and oxygen gets to the brain, often due to a blood clot or fatty deposit.

isokinetic—Exercise in which muscular force is exerted at a constant speed against an equal force that is exerted by a strength-training machine.

isometric—Exercise that increases muscle tension by applying pressure against stable resistance; accomplished by opposing different muscles.

isotonic—Muscle contraction in which force is generated while the muscle changes in length.

J

jaundice—Yellowing of the skin, mucous membranes, and eyes caused by too much bilirubin in the blood.

K

Kegel exercises—Exercises in the genital area that help strengthen the muscles of the pelvic floor.

ketones—Chemical by-products resulting from the incomplete breakdown of fats.

L

labia majora—Two folds of skin, one on each side of the vaginal opening.

labia minora—Two folds of skin between the labia majora, from the clitoris to the vaginal opening.

liberal feminism—A philosophy that sees the oppression of women as a denial of equal rights, representation, and access to opportunities.

lightening—The descent of the uterus and fetus into the pelvic cavity, which occurs 2 to 3 weeks before the onset of labor.

love addict—An unhealthy pattern of becoming involved with a partner to mask fear of abandonment.

ludic love—A relationship built on game playing and maintaining distance.

lumpectomy—Surgical removal of breast cancer and some normal tissue surrounding it.

lupus—Systemic lupus erythematosus is a chronic, autoimmune disease of connective tissue that causes inflammation and affects vital organs.

luteal phase—Part of the menstrual cycle that includes the development of the corpus luteum.

M

macrominerals—Nutrients required in the body in amounts exceeding 100 mg/day.

macrophage—Any large cell that can surround and digest foreign substances in the body.

magnetic resonance imaging (MRI)—Magnetic fields that absorb radio waves to produce images of organs and processes inside the body.

mainstream smoke—Smoke drawn through the cigarette and inhaled and exhaled by the smoker.

major depressive disorder—Typically the recurrence of a major depressive episode.

major depressive episode—The presence of at least five of the following symptoms for most of the day for at least a 2-week period: feelings of sadness or emptiness, diminished interest or pleasure, weight loss, insomnia, feelings of worthlessness or inappropriate guilt, diminished ability to think or concentrate, recurrent thoughts of death or suicide.

malignant tumors—Cancerous tumors; characterized by abnormal cells that divide uncontrollably and have the ability to infiltrate and destroy normal cells.

mammography—Imaging of the breast produced by low-dose X ray.

manic love—A consuming or obsessive relationship built on a strong need for love and affection.

marital rape—Sexual assault of a woman by her husband.

masculinity—Possessing a high number of attributes defined as masculine and a low number of attributes defined as feminine.

massage—Systematically stroking, kneading, and pressing the soft tissues of the body to induce a state of total relaxation.

maternal mortality—Death of a woman while pregnant or within 42 days of termination of the pregnancy.

meditation—A technique to calm the mind and body through a conscious mental process that induces a relaxation response.

melanoma—Any of a group of skin cancers made up of melanocytes.

menarche—The first menstrual cycle for a female.

menopause—The end of ovulation and menstruation.

menstruation—The sloughing off of the endometrium.

metabolic rate—Rate or intensity at which the body produces energy.

metastasis—The process by which cancer is spread to distant parts of the body.

methylxanthines—A family of chemical compounds that function as mild central nervous system (CNS) stimulants, includes caffeine.

midwife—A person who is trained to assist a woman during pregnancy and childbirth delivery.

misogyny—An attitude or behavior of hatred toward women.

mitral valve prolapse (MVP)—Condition in which one or both flaps of the mitral valve are enlarged and fail to close properly.

modified radical mastectomy—Surgical removal of the whole breast, most of the lymph nodes under the arm, and often, the lining of the chest muscles.

monoclonal antibodies—A group of identical antibodies made from a single antibody.

monosaccharides—Simple sugar molecules; examples include glucose, fructose, and galactose.

mons pubis—The triangular, mounding area of fatty tissue that covers the pubic bone.

mourning—The actual expression of loss, or the behaviors that take place as a result of the grief experience.

multiple sclerosis (MS)—Chronic, debilitating disease that affects the central nervous system and causes damage to or loss of myelin.

muscular endurance—The ability for a muscle to generate force over a period of time or for a number of repetitions.

muscular strength—Ability of a muscle to generate force against some type of resistance.

myocardial infarction (MI)—A heart attack.

N

negative reinforcer—Removal of something uncomfortable to increase the likelihood that a behavior will be repeated.

neoadjuvant therapy—The use of drugs to shrink a cancer before surgical removal.

neurotherapy—Training the brain waves to enhance cognitive performance or recover from emotional or physical trauma or drug addiction.

nicotine—Physically and psychologically addictive stimulant substance found in tobacco.

nonheme iron—Iron found in plant sources and tissues in animals other than heme iron tissues.

nonoxynol-9 (N-9)—A lubricant that is no longer recommended for the prevention of HIV or other STIs.

nutrient density—The ratio of nutrients to energy in a food product; high-density means the food has more nutrients than calories. Soda pop has low nutrient density.

O

obesity—A body mass index greater than 30.

omnivorous—Consuming both plant and animal food sources.

oncogenes—Genes that may cause a cell to be changed to cancer.

oncologist—A physician who specializes in cancer care.

ongoing mindfulness—The process of exploring the impact that sociocultural influences have on you and your life development.

open adoption—Contact between birth and adoptive parents occurs as the child is being raised; contact can be occasional to regular depending on the agreement.

oral contraceptives—Pills that contain estrogen and/or progestin and inhibit ovulation through suppressing follicle stimulating and lutenizing hormones.

osteoarthritis (OA)—A degenerative joint disease.

osteoporosis—A bone-weakening disorder in which normal bone density is lost; marked by thinning of bone tissue and growth of small holes in bone.

outercourse—Dry sex or sexual interaction without penile penetration.

ovaries—Reproductive organs found on each side of the lower abdomen beside the uterus.

overweight—A body mass index (BMI) of 25 or greater.

ovulation—The release of the mature egg from the ovary.

ovulatory phase—Part of the menstrual cycle that includes the release of the mature egg from the ovary.

oxidation—Any process in which the oxygen content of a compound is increased.

P

pacemaker—A medical device implanted to treat slow heart rate (bradycardia).

patellofemoral knee pain—An injury to the knee that is characterized by nonspecific pain under the kneecap.

patent medicines—Those medicines available to the general public without a prescription; information pertaining to the drug is usually available on the label.

peer marriage—Egalitarian partnership between two people.

pelvic inflammatory disease (PID)—Any inflammation of the female reproductive tract, especially one caused by bacteria.

perimenopause—A decline in monthly hormonal cycles before menopause.

perineum—Part of muscle and tissue located between the vaginal opening and the anal canal.

periodic abstinence—No sexual intercourse for a period of time, often used in fertility awareness methods.

person-centered counseling—A nondirective style of psychotherapy designed to assist a client to feel fully accepted by the therapist so the client can feel safe to discuss and resolve personal fears and anxieties.

physical dependency—Body cells dependent upon a chemical substance to maintain homeostasis.

phytochemicals—Nonnutrient substances found in plant foods that have a positive effect on the body's physiology phytonutrients.

pituitary gland—A gland of the brain that releases adrenocorticotropic hormone as part of the stress response.

placenta—The structure inside the uterus that provides the communication between the mother and the fetus.

plastic surgeon—A physician who specializes in reconstructive surgery and also performs beauty-enhancing procedures.

PNF—Contraction and relaxation of a muscle prior to stretching it; allows for longer stretches and faster development of joint flexibility.

polycystic ovarian syndrome (PCOS)—Occurs when the ovaries produce excessive amounts of male hormones (androgens) and multiple small cysts develop.

polysaccharides—Compounds composed of numerous saccharide units; complex carbohydrates.

positive reinforcer—Presentation of a reward to increase the likelihood that a behavior will be repeated.

positive therapeutic relationship—A relationship between a client and a therapist based on trust and a sense of safety that enables a client to benefit from psychotherapy.

postmenopause—Begins when menstruation has ceased for 1 year.

posttraumatic stress disorder (PTSD)—A variety of symptoms (for example, irritability, insomnia, anxiety) that result from viewing or being involved in a traumatic event.

pragmatic love—A relationship built on practical needs between partners.

preeclampsia—A disorder encountered early in the pregnancy characterized by hypertension or swelling.

preferred provider organization (PPO)—Physicians who agree to provide their services for a reduced rate to insurance companies.

premenstrual dysphoric disorder (PMDD)—Bouts of marked premenstrual depressed mood, anxiety, sadness, or anger that occur a few days before menstruation; the most severe type of menstruation related mood distress.

premenstrual syndrome (PMS)—Nervous tension, irritability, and so forth that occur a few days before menstruation.

preventive health action—Measures serving to avert the occurrence of illness or disease.

primary infertility—Inability to conceive after a year of unprotected sexual intercourse.

primary prevention—An extension of health education.

proactive care—Designing and living a lifestyle that reduces the risk of illness and also improves one's current health status.

problem solving—Step-by-step approach of planning and negotiating and involves all parties to be affected.

progressive relaxation—A technique that involves alternately tensing and releasing the muscles of the body and resulting in greater relaxation.

proof—Measurement of ethyl alcohol content found in beverages; stated in terms of percentages.

psychological abuse—Use of children, intimidation, threats, and economic domination to control, manipulate, and cause anxiety in one's partner.

psychological dependence—Dependence on the feeling produced by the presence of the drug in the body; an emotional or psychological desire to continue using the drug; habituation.

psychosomatic disorders—Physical illnesses generated by the effects of stress.

punishment—Presentation of something uncomfortable to reduce behavior.

Q

quackery—The promotion of a medical remedy that does not work or has not been proven to work.

quickening—A mother's first perception of fetal movement.

R

radiotherapy—High-energy radiation therapy using X rays or gamma rays to treat cancer; also called radiation therapy.

reactive care—The treatment of any illness, disorder, or disease that may develop.

Recommended Dietary Allowances (RDAs)—Recommended nutrient intakes that meet the needs of healthy people of similar age and sex based on current knowledge.

reflexology—The use of compression massage on designated areas on the hands and feet.

relaxation response—A brief technique to quiet the body and the mind that involves slow, deep breathing combined with muscle relaxation.

resiliency—The ability to recover, overcome adversity, and bounce back following difficult situations.

reverse SAD—A category of Seasonal Affective Disorder (SAD) that involves a set of symptoms that occur only during a particular time of the year. Symptoms may include persistently elevated mood, increased social activity, hyperactivity, and disproportionate enthusiam. Symptoms may be described as the opposite of fall and winter SAD symptoms.

rheumatoid arthritis (RA)—An autoimmune, chronic inflammatory disease of unknown cause that involves the joints and/or internal organs.

RICE—Rest, ice, compress, elevate; temporary care of a minor injury that does not need a physician's attention.

ring—Clear, flexible, thin polymer ring that provides a continuous low dose of etonogesterel (progestin) and ethinyl estradiol (estrogen) to prevent pregnancy.

RU-486—Trademark name for a drug therapy used to induce abortion.

S

saline implant—A pouch filled with salt water used to reconstruct or increase the size of the breast.

sandwich generation—Women in middle adulthood.

Seasonal Affective Disorder (SAD)—A set of symptoms that come and go at the same time every year. See types: Full and winter SAD, reverse SAD, and spring and summer SAD.

secondary infertility—Difficulty conceiving after already having conceived and carried a normal pregnancy.

secondary prevention—Identifies persons who are in the early stages of "unhealth," which may lead to the development of disorders or illnesses.

secondary reinforcer—A less obvious reinforcer that may be contributing to resistance to change.

self-caring—Taking care of one's own personal physical, emotional, and spiritual needs.

self-efficacy—The conviction that one can successfully execute the behavior or behaviors required to produce desired outcomes.

self-esteem—How good one feels about oneself, measured by the distance between the perceived self and the ideal or preferred self.

sexism—An attitude or act of bias or discrimination against a person because of the person's gender.

sexual assault—Sexual improprieties or sexual violence directed toward another person, including rape.

sexual discrimination—Discrimination (usually in employment) that excludes one sex (usually women) to the benefit of the other sex.

Sexual function—The ability to experience desire, arousal, orgasm, and satisfaction.

sexual harassment—Unwanted sexual advances, requests for sexual favors, and other verbal or physical conduct of a sexual nature that negatively affects the work environment.

shin splints—Strains of the muscles that move the foot and ankle at their attachment point to the shin; can result in a stress fracture to the long bone in the leg.

side effects—Undesirable, uncomfortable, or unsafe reactions when using any type of drug in which the effects are unexpected.

side-stream smoke—Smoke from the lit end of the cigarette; contains more tar, nicotine, and carbon monoxide than mainstream smoke.

silicone gel–filled implant—A pouch filled with silicone gel used to reconstruct or increase the size of the breast.

smoking cessation program—A program to quit smoking that includes behavioral modification techniques, group support, program meetings, and occasionally includes nicotine substitutes.

sociocultural influences (SCIs)—Include (but not limited to) family members, family history, family values, religious doctrine, media, school activities and personnel, community events, national events, world events, historical events, friends, famous persons, and significant others.

solution focused therapy—A style of psychotherapy that involves helping clients shift from talking about problems to focusing on finding solutions.

spermicide—A chemical substance that kills or immobilizes sperm.

spina bifida—Congenital birth defect in which the spine fails to enclose the spinal cord; usually occurs within the first month of pregnancy.

spring and summer SAD—a category of seasonal Affective Disorder (SAD) that occurs in spring and summer. Symptoms may include anxiety, insomnia, irritability, agitation, weight loss, poor appetite, and increased sex drive.

static stretching—Stretching muscles in a slow and gentle manner and holding that position for 10–30 seconds.

storgic love—A relationship built on security and friendship.

stress—A physiological and psychological state of arousal caused by the perceived presence of a challenging or threatening event.

stress amenorrhea—Cessation of the mentrual flow caused by stress.

stressors—Factors or events, real or imagined, that elicit a state of stress.

stroke—A vascular disease caused when a blood vessel bursts or becomes clogged in the brain; a brain attack.

sudden infant death syndrome (SIDS)—Sudden and unexpected death of an apparently normal and healthy infant that occurs during sleep, and with no physical or autopsy evidence of disease.

support network—Resources consisting of three systems that focus on clarifying how you define meaning from life through your beliefs and values, how you access support from those around you, and how you draw upon your own personal strengths and abilities.

surrogacy—A woman, other than the partner, who agrees to become pregnant and carry the fetus to full term.

symptothermal method—Natural family planning method that combines basal body temperature and the cycle-based method.

syphilis—A sexually transmitted infection caused by the bacterium (spirochete) *Treponema pallidum.*

systolic blood pressure—Amount of pressure the blood exerts against the arteries while the heart is contracting.

T

tar—Sticky black particulate matter in tobacco.

tertiary prevention—The application of an intervention to treat an existing disorder or illness.

tetrahydrocannabinol (THC)—The active ingredient in the hemp plant *Cannabis sativa;* found in marijuana, hashish, and ganja.

thought stopping—An important technique for altering negative self-suggestions.

TNM—A staging system for determining the stage of cancer.

total mastectomy—Surgical removal of the whole breast and possibly some lymph nodes under the arm.

toxemia—Presence of bacterial toxins in the blood; also called blood poisoning.

transdermal patch—A contraceptive patch that releases progestin and estrogen through the skin into the bloodstream.

trans fat—The fatty acids formed when hydrogen is pumped into liquid vegetable oils to make them more firm.

transient ischemic attacks (TIAs)—Small strokes that produce strokelike symptoms that are temporary.

treatment interventions—Actions that are taken to halt the progress of a discomfort, disorder, or disease and, if possible, move the individual away from the discomfort and toward increased health.

trichomoniasis—An STI that commonly infects the vagina.

trigger-point massage—Placing pressure on a muscle where the ligaments or tendon is attached.

tubal ligation—Sterilization process in women in which the fallopian tubes are blocked to prevent pregnancy.

type 1 diabetes—A disease in which the pancreas produces little or no insulin; once called insulin-dependent or juvenile diabetes.

type 2 diabetes—A disease in which the pancreas produces insulin but the body is resistant or cannot utilize it.

U

United States Pharmacopeia (USP)—Describes the properties of medicines and ensures the purity of the drug.

uterus—Pear-shaped female organ of reproduction in which the ovum implants and develops.

V

vacuum aspiration—Suction method by which the fetus and placenta are removed up to the 14th week.

vagina—Part of female genitals that form a canal from the vaginal opening to the cervix.

vaginitis—An inflammation of the vaginal area; often characterized by discharge or itching.

vasectomy—Sterilization process in men in which the vas deferens are blocked to prevent pregnancy.

vasoconstrictors—Substances that constrict the blood vessels of the body causing an elevation in blood pressure and heart rate.

vasovasostomy—Microsurgical procedure used to reverse a vasectomy.

veins—Blood vessels that carry deoxygenated blood and waste by-products to the heart and lungs.

vulva—The pudendum; the outer genitals of a female.

W

Western blot test—Laboratory test used to detect the presence of HIV antibodies; regarded as more accurate than the ELISA.

withdrawal symptoms—Unpleasant symptoms such as tremors, insomnia, and seizures when drug use is discontinued.

Y

Yasmin—A low-dose oral contraceptive.

yoga—Body postures and poses to improve health.

Z

zygote—The developing egg from the time it is fertilized until implantation in the uterus.

zygote intrafallopian transfer (ZIFT)—Fertilization of the eggs in the laboratory and use of the laparoscope to transfer the fertilized eggs (zygote) into the woman's fallopian tube.

Credits

Photos

Chapter 1
p. 7: Courtesy of Cynthia K. Chandler; **p. 23:** Courtesy of Cynthia K. Chandler.

Chapter 2
p. 32: © Jose Luis Pelaez Inc./Blend Images LLC; **p. 42:** Keith Brofsky/ Getty Images.

Chapter 4
p. 93: Courtesy of Cynthia K. Chandler.

Chapter 5
p. 120: Eric Audras/Photoalto/PictureQuest; **p. 130:** PhotoDisc/Getty Images; **p. 143:** Duncan Smith/Getty Images; **p. 148:** Courtesy of Cynthia K. Chandler; **p. 148:** Courtesy of Cynthia K. Chandler.

Chapter 7
p. 193: Keith Brofsky/Getty Images.

Chapter 9
p. 233 (Fig 9.2): The McGraw-Hill Companies, Inc./Christopher Kerrigan, photographer; **p. 233 (Fig. 9.3);** Getty Images/Brand X; **p. 234 (Fig. 9.4)** © McGraw-Hill Companies, Inc./Jill Braaten, photographer; **p. 234 (Fig. 9.5):** The McGraw-Hill Companies, Inc./Christopher Kerrigan, photographer; **p. 235 (Fig. 9.7a):** The McGraw-Hill companies, Inc./Christopher Kerrigan, photographer; **p. 240 (Fig. 9.9):** McGraw-Hill Companies, Inc.

Chapter 10
p. 271: © PhotoDisc/Getty Images; **p. 289:** © PhotoDisc/Getty Images.

Chapter 11
p. 305 (Figs. 11.1, 11.2, 11.3): Courtesy of Danny Ramsey Ballard; **p. 306 (Fig. 11.4):** Courtesy of Danny Ramsey Ballard.

Chapter 13
p. 343: Ingram Publishing; **p. 349:** Monkey Business Images Ltd./ Photolibrary.

Chapter 14
p. 378: Reprinted by permission of The National Association of People with AIDS, www.napwa.org.

Chapter 15
p. 416: Scott Bodell/Getty Images; **p. 417:** Jim Wehtje/Getty Images.

Text

Chapter 2
p. 49 (FYI): Barrett, et al., Consumer Health: *A Guide to Intelligent Decisions, Eighth Edition.* New York, New York. The McGraw-Hill Companies,Inc. © 2007.

Chapter 6
p. 157 (Assess Yourself): From Payne, W., Hahn, D., and Lucas, E., *Understanding Your Health*, 9th ed., New York: McGraw-Hill, 2007.

Reprinted by permission of the McGraw-Hill Companies; **p. 163 (FYI) and (Health Tips):** From *Verbally Abusive Relationship,* 2nd Edition, Copyright © 1992, 1996, Patricia Evans. Published by Adams Media, an F+W Media, Inc. Co. All rights reserved.

Chapter 7
p. 190 (Health Tips): From Payne, W., Hahn, D., and Lucas, E., *Understanding Your Health*, 9th ed., New York: McGraw-Hill, 2007. Reprinted by permission of the McGraw-Hill Companies; **p. 200 (Poem):** © 1993 Portia Nelson, from *There's a Hole in My Sidewalk*, Hillsboro, OR: Beyond Words Publishing, Inc. Reprinted by permission.

Chapter 15
p. 400 (FYI) p. 402 and (Table 15.2): Reprinted with Permission www.heart.org ©2012 American Heart Association, Inc.

Line Art

Chapter 3
p. 70 (Fig. 3.1): Reprinted from *Journal of Counseling and Development,* 71 (2): 171 © 1992 ACA. Reprinted with permission. No further reproduction without written permission of the American Counseling Association; **p. 76 (Fig. 3.2):** Adapted from Maslow, Abraham H., Frager, Robert D., and Fadiman, James, *Motivation and Personality*, 3rd ed., 1997, Pearson Education, Inc., Upper Saddle River, NJ. Reprinted with permission.

Chapter 5
p.117 (Fig. 5.2): From Payne, W., Hahn, D., and Lucas, E. 2007. *Understanding YourHealth.* 9th ed. New York: McGraw-Hill. Reprinted by permissionof the McGraw-Hill Companies; p. 131 (Assess Yourself): Copyright © 1997 AMS Press Inc. All rights reserved.

Chapter 8
p. 222 (Fig. 8.5): Reprinted from Payne, W., Hahn, D., and Lucas, E., 2007. *Understanding Your Health.* 9th ed. New York: McGraw-Hill. Reprinted by permission of the McGraw-Hill Companies; **p. 223 (Fig. 8.6)** Basson, R. 2001. Using a different model for female sexual response to address women's problematic low sexual desire. *Journal of Sexual and Marital Therapy,* 27:395–403. Reprinted by permission of the publisher (Taylor & Francis Ltd., http://www.tandf.co.uk/journals).

Chapter 9
pp. 231, 233, 235, 235, 249 (Figs. 9.1, 9.2 bottom, 9.6, 9.7 bottom, 9.12): Reprinted from Payne, W., Hahn, D., and Lucas, E., 2007. *Understanding Your Health.* 9th ed. New York: McGraw-Hill. Reprinted by permission of the McGraw-Hill Companies; **p. 252 (FYI):** © World Health Organization. Reprinted by permission; **pp. 257, 259 (Figs. 9.14, 9.15):** Source: Guttmacher Institute, Facts on induced abortion in the United States, In Brief, New York: Guttmacher Institute, 2008, <www .guttmacher.org/pubs/fb_induced_abortion.html> (retrieved July 2008).

Chapter 10
p. 273, (Fig. 10.1) USDA Center for Nutrition Policy and Promotion.

Chapter 11
p. 310 (Fig. 11.5): Reprinted from Payne, W. A., and Hahn, D. B., *Understanding Your Health*, New York: McGraw-Hill, 1998, artwork by Jeanne Robertson. Reprinted by permission of the McGraw-Hill Companies.